EFFECTS OF DRUGS ON THE CELL NUCLEUS

BRISTOL-MYERS CANCER SYMPOSIA

Series Editors
MAXWELL GORDON / STANLEY T. CROOKE
Bristol Laboratories
Syracuse, New York

1. Harris Busch, Stanley T. Crooke, and Yerach Daskal (Editors). *Effects of Drugs on the Cell Nucleus, 1979.*

EFFECTS OF DRUGS ON THE CELL NUCLEUS

Edited by

HARRIS BUSCH
Department of Pharmacology
Baylor College of Medicine
Texas Medical Center
Houston, Texas

STANLEY T. CROOKE
Bristol Laboratories
Syracuse, New York
Department of Pharmacology
Baylor College of Medicine
Texas Medical Center
Houston, Texas

YERACH DASKAL
Department of Pharmacology
Baylor College of Medicine
Texas Medical Center
Houston, Texas

ACADEMIC PRESS 1979
A Subsidiary of Harcourt Brace Jovanovich, Publishers
New York London Toronto Sydney San Francisco

ACADEMIC PRESS, INC.
111 Fifth Avenue, New York, New York 10003

United Kingdom Edition published by
ACADEMIC PRESS, INC. (LONDON) LTD.
24/28 Oval Road, London NW1 7DX

Library of Congress Cataloging in Publication Data

Main entry under title:

Effects of drugs on the cell nucleus.

Papers presented at a symposium entitled "Drug effects
on the cell nucleus, " held at the Baylor College of
Medicine in Nov. 1978.
  Includes bibliographies.
  1. Cancer cells--Drug effects--Congresses.
2. Cell nuclei--Drug effects--Congresses. 3. Cells--
Drug effects--Congresses. 4. Antineoplastic agents--
Physiological effect--Congresses. I. Busch, Harris.
II. Crooke, Stanley T. III. Daskal, Yerach.
IV. Baylor University, Waco, Tex. College of Medicine,
Houston. [DNLM: 1. Cell nucleus--Drug effects--
Congresses. 2. Antineoplastic agents--
Pharmacodynamics--Congresses. QV595 E27]
RC271.C5E33   616.9'94'061   79-51690
ISBN 0-12-147654-5

PRINTED IN THE UNITED STATES OF AMERICA

79 80 81 82   9 8 7 6 5 4 3 2 1

Dedication

This volume is affectionately dedicated to the memory of Wilhelm Bernhard, M.D., whose untimely death in October, 1978, was a great loss to the scientific world and, specifically, to the students of the cell nucleus.

Bernhard received his M.D. at the University of Berne in 1946. He joined Professor Oberling in Villejuif in 1948, where he became the head of the Electron Microscopy Laboratory. He led a distinguished group of colleagues in research on ultrastructure and, subsequently, received numerous prizes and awards. His splendid achievements served as an inspiration to workers around the world.

Bernhard was a man of great enthusiasm and keen insight concerning the problems of cell and nuclear structure and function. In addition, he was keenly appreciative of life and its many beautiful aspects. We will all miss him.

Harris Busch

Contents

1

Localization of Nuclear Functions at the Cellular and Molecular Level
MICHEL BOUTEILLE and ANNE MARIE DUPUY-COIN

2

The Molecular Biology of Cancer: The Cancer Cell and Its Functions
HARRIS BUSCH

3

Studies on Silver-Stained Nucleolar Components
KAREL SMETANA and HARRIS BUSCH

12 Drug Effects on tRNA
K. RANDERATH

13 Potentiation by 2′-Deoxycoformycin of the Inhibitory Effects of Cordycepin and Xylosyladenine on Nuclear RNA Synthesis in L1210 Cells
ROBERT I. GLAZER

14 Effects of Chemical Mutagens on Chromosomes
T.C. HSU and WILLIAM AU

15 The Influence of Nitrosoureas on Chromatin Nucleosomal Structure and Function
MARK E. SMULSON, S. SUDHAKAR, K.D. TEW, T.R. BUTT, and D.B. JUMP

16 Gene Regulation in Steroid-Responsive Cells

GEORGE E. SWANECK, MING-JER TSAI, and BERT W. O'MALLEY

17 Biochemical and Morphological Changes Stimulated by the Nuclear Binding of the Estrogen Receptor

JAMES H. CLARK, SHIRLEY A. McCORMACK, HELEN A. PADYKULA,
BARRY MARKAVERICH, and JAMES W. HARDIN

18 Testosterone Effects on the Prostatic Nucleus

KHALIL AHMED, MICHAEL J. WILSON,
SAID A. GOUELI, and MARY E. NORVITCH

19 Drug Effects on the Cell Cycle
SAM C. BARRANCO

20 G_2 Arrest Induced by Anticancer Drugs
POTU N. RAO

21 Perspectives on the Research of New Anticancer Agents
A. DI MARCO

22 Isoproterenol-Stimulated Induction of Lactate Dehydrogenase and Modulation of Nuclear Protein Kinase Activity in C_6 Rat Glioma Cells
RICHARD A. JUNGMANN, MARY L. CHRISTENSEN, and DENNIS F. DERDA

23

Action of Nitrous Oxide and Griseofulvin
on Microtubules and Chromosome Movement
in Dividing Cells

S.M. COX, P.N. RAO, and B.R. BRINKLEY

List of Contributors

Numbers in parentheses indicate the pages on which the authors' contributions begin.

KHALIL AHMED (419), Toxicology Research Laboratory, Department of Laboratory Medicine and Pathology, Veterans Administration Center, University of Minnesota, Minneapolis, Minnesota 55417

WILLIAM AU (315), Section of Cell Biology, The University of Texas System Cancer Center, M. D. Anderson Hospital and Tumor Institute, Houston, Texas 77030

SAM C. BARRANCO (455), Department of Human Biological Chemistry and Genetics, University of Texas Medical Branch, Galveston, Texas 77550

MICHEL BOUTEILLE (1), Laboratory of Cell Pathology, Institut Biomédical des Cordeliers, Université Pierre et Marie Curie, 75270 Paris, France

B.R. BRINKLEY (521), Department of Cell Biology, Baylor College of Medicine, Houston, Texas 77030

HARRIS BUSCH (35, 89), Department of Pharmacology, Baylor College of Medicine, Houston, Texas 77025

T.R. BUTT (333), Department of Biochemistry. and The Vincent T. Lombardi Cancer Research Center, Georgetown University School of Medicine and Dentistry, Washington, D. C. 20007

MARY L. CHRISTENSEN (507), Department of Biochemistry, Northwestern University Medical School, Chicago, Illinois 60611

JAMES H. CLARK (381), Department of Cell Biology, Baylor College of Medicine, Houston, Texas 77030

S.M. COX (521), Department of Cell Biology, Baylor College of Medicine, Houston, Texas 77030

STANLEY T. CROOKE (127), Research and Development, Bristol Laboratories, Syracuse, New York 13201, and Department of Pharmacology, Baylor College of Medicine, Houston, Texas 77025

Y. DASKAL (107), Electron Microscopy Unit, Department of Pharmacology, Baylor College of Medicine, Houston, Texas 77030

DENNIS F. DERDA (507), Department of Biochemistry, Northwestern University Medical School, Chicago, Illinois 60611

A. DI MARCO (491), Division of Experimental Oncology B, Instituto Nazionale per lo Studio a la Cura dei Tumori, 20133 Milano, Italy

ANNE MARIE DUPUY-COIN (1), Laboratory of Cell Pathology, Institut Biomédical des Cordeliers, Université Pierre et Marie Curie, 75270 Paris, France

ROBERT I. GLAZER (301), Applied Pharmacology Section, Laboratory of Medicinal Chemistry and Biology, National Cancer Institute, National Institutes of Health, Bethesda, Maryland 20014

SAID A. GOUELI (419), Toxicology Research Laboratory, Department of Laboratory Medicine and Pathology, Veterans Administration Center, University of Minnesota, Minneapolis, Minnesota 55417

JAMES W. HARDIN (381), Department of Cell Biology, Baylor College of Medicine, Houston, Texas 77030

SUSAN B. HORWITZ (181), Department of Molecular Pharmacology, Albert Einstein College of Medicine of Yeshiva University, Bronx, New York 10461

T.C. HSU (315), Section of Cell Biology, The University of Texas System Cancer Center, M. D. Anderson Hospital and Tumor Institute, Houston, Texas 77030

D. B. JUMP (333), The Vincent T. Lombardi Cancer Research Center, Georgetown University School of Medicine and Dentistry, Washington, D. C. 20007

RICHARD A. JUNGMANN (507), Department of Biochemistry, Northwestern University Medical School, Chicago, Illinois 60611

KURT W. KOHN (207), Laboratory of Molecular Pharmacology, Division of Cancer Treatment, National Cancer Institute, National Institutes of Health, Bethesda, Maryland 20014

SHIRLEY A. McCORMACK (381), Department of Cell Biology, Baylor College of Medicine, Houston, Texas 77030

BARRY MARKAVERICH (381), Department of Cell Biology, Baylor College of Medicine, Houston, Texas 77030

WERNER E.G. MÜLLER (161), Physiologisch-Chemisches Institut, Abteilung Angewandte Molekularbiologie, Universitat Duesbergweg, 6500 Mainz, West Germany

MARY E. NORVITCH (419), Veterans Administration Medical Center, Minneapolis, Minnesota 55417

BERT W. O'MALLEY (359), Department of Cell Biology, Baylor College of Medicine, Texas Medical Center, Houston, Texas 77030

HELEN A. PADYKULA (381), Laboratory of Electron Microscopy, Wellesley College, Wellesley, Massachusetts 02181

SETH D. PINSKY (241), Vincent T. Lombardi Cancer Research Center, Georgetown University Medical Center, Washington, D. C. 20007

K. RANDERATH (275), Department of Pharmacology, Baylor College of Medicine, Houston, Texas 77030

POTU N. RAO (475, 521), Department of Developmental Therapeutics, The University of Texas System Cancer Center, M. D. Anderson Hospital and Tumor Institute, Houston, Texas 77030

EDWARD A. SAUSVILLE (181), Department of Molecular Pharmacology, Albert Einstein College of Medicine of Yeshiva University, Bronx, New York 10461

PRAVINKUMAR B. SEHGAL (251), The Rockefeller University, New York, New York 10021

KAREL SMETANA (89), Institute of Experimental Medicine, Czechoslovak Academy of Sciences, Prague 2, Albertov 4, Czechoslovakia

MARK E. SMULSON (333), Department of Biochemistry, and The Vincent T. Lombardi Cancer Research Center, Georgetown University School of Medicine and Dentistry, Washington, D. C. 20007

HENRY M. SOBELL (145), Department of Chemistry, The University of Rochester, Rochester, New York 14627

S. SUDHAKAR (333), Department of Biochemistry, and The Vincent T. Lombardi Cancer Research Center, Georgetown University School of Medicine and Dentistry, Washington, D. C. 20007

GEORGE E. SWANECK (359), Department of Cell Biology, Baylor College of Medicine, Houston, Texas 77030

IGOR TAMM (251), The Rockefeller University, New York, New York 10021

K.D. TEW (333), Department of Biochemistry, and The Vincent T. Lombardi Cancer Research Center, Georgetown University School of Medicine and Dentistry, Washington, D. C. 20007

MING-JER TSAI (359), Department of Cell Biology, Baylor College of Medicine, Houston, Texas 77030

MICHAEL J. WILSON (419), Toxicology Research Laboratory, Department of Laboratory Medicine and Pathology, University of Minnesota, Veterans Administration Center, Minneapolis, Minnesota 55417

PAUL V. WOOLEY, III (241), Georgetown University Hospital, Washington, D. C. 20007

Editors' Foreword

The editors are pleased to be associated with the Bristol-Myers Cancer Symposia series. Inasmuch as each symposium is organized by a different institution with its own program chairmen, we thought it would be useful to have series editors who could provide continuity in format and presentation.

The first Bristol-Myers Cancer Symposia was organized by Baylor College of Medicine. For the second symposium, the Yale University School of Medicine will serve as the host. Succeeding symposia are tentatively scheduled at the Pritzker School of Medicine of the University of Chicago, at the Johns Hopkins University Medical School, and at the Stanford University Medical School.

We hope that these symposia will contribute to a better understanding of oncologic disease and will point the way toward more rational design of chemotherapeutic agents and other diagnostic and treatment modalities.

Among the topics on cancer research presented and discussed at this symposium were morphological and biochemical aspects of the cell nucleus, drug effects on nuclear morphology and biochemistry, drug interactions with nuclear DNA, effects of microbial products on nuclear DNA-synthesizing systems, drug effects on nuclear proteins and RNA, and hormonal effects on the nucleus and on nuclear regulatory mechanisms.

M. Gordon
S. T. Crooke
Series editors

Foreword

The history of medicine is filled with examples of discovery that came despite imperfect knowledge. One hundred years before a virus was identified, Jenner introduced smallpox vaccine. Twenty-two years before the rationale of liver therapy was understood, the cure for pernicious anemia was available. In 1932, investigators discovered that Prontosil red dye was active in strep infections. It took several years to determine the active moiety—sulfanilamide—and more than a decade to reveal its mode of action.

The progress reported in this volume represents the substance of the first Bristol-Myers Symposia on Cancer Research, covering the vital subject of the effects of drugs on the cell nucleus. The host institution for this symposium was Baylor College of Medicine, and the program was developed under the cochairmanship of Drs. Harris Busch, Stanley T. Crooke, and Yerach Daskal. It is especially fitting that the first Bristol-Myers symposium was held at Baylor Medical School because of the unique relationship between Bristol-Myers and Baylor, serving we believe as a model for constructive interactions between pharmaceutical companies and academe. This symposium makes contributions in a time-honored way both to understanding cell biology and to the empirical development of cancer chemotherapeutic agents. The findings of the participants of this symposium, and at succeeding ones, may prove important in cancer treatment—especially in developing new chemotherapeutic agents.

As a scientist, that would excite me. As a citizen it would please me. But whether that happens or not, the contributions of the participants in this symposium are scientifically important and thus endorse the worth of our company's commitment to cancer research. Bristol-Myers Company is proud to be a meaningful part of the important work of this symposium's participants.

Herman Sokol
President
Bristol-Myers Company

Preface

When the Bristol-Myers Company made the decision to develop its prize and special grants program, it also decided to support special symposia at each of the five major institutions that were the recipients of the grants.

The first such symposium was developed at Baylor College of Medicine in November, 1978. The symposium was entitled "Drug Effects on the Cell Nucleus" and was divided into three major parts: (1) a general review of the morphology and biochemistry of the cell nucleus and the morphological and biochemical end results of drug treatment, (2) the biochemical effects of a variety of anticancer agents on the cell nucleus, and (3) interactions of hormones directly and indirectly with structures and functions of the cell nucleus.

The speakers selected for the symposium were chosen on the basis of the special features of their work and the timeliness of the topics in their general area. It was clear from the outset that, at a symposium such as this, only a few of the many topics could be presented. The organizing committee regrets that both time and resources did not permit presentation of a larger series of speakers or topics. Despite this limitation, however, it was felt by all that we had been treated to an outstanding series of presentations.

Harris Busch
Stanley T. Crooke
Yerach Daskal

1

Localization of Nuclear Functions at the Cellular and Molecular Level

MICHEL BOUTEILLE AND ANNE MARIE DUPUY-COIN

I. What Is New?

The present chapter is intended to describe recent progress in studies where the electron microscope has been used essentially to relate nuclear

EFFECTS OF DRUGS ON THE CELL NUCLEUS

1

structure to nuclear function as defined by means of biochemistry and molecular biology. As a matter of fact, electron microscope examination by itself would have provided little information in past years if it had not been combined with the powerful tools available to investigators: ultrastructural autoradiography and cytochemistry. The methods of ultrastructural cytochemistry used in the 1960s to obtain some idea of the chemical nature of nuclear structures have been much less employed in the last 10 years. In the latter period, emphasis was put on the localization of functions, and in this work electron microscope autoradiography has proved much more powerful. However, it is now clear that immunocytochemistry whose development was so successful in its recent applications, will certainly become a major method of investigation for nuclear function and structure.

Most data are now less controversial than they were a few years ago (Bouteille *et al.,* 1974). However, in most cases, the generality of the information cannot be established. For instance, fibrillar centers are now believed to represent the nucleolar organizing region (NOR), but this structure is only conspicuous in some cell lines, especially *in vitro,* and is hardly visible in other cells such as hepatocytes. In this respect, the present observations should be considered as defining a working direction, rather than representing a complete description of the correlation between structure and function in eukaryotic cells.

The methodology is assumed to be familiar to the reader. As far as electron microscope autoradiography is concerned, to the extensive reviews by Jacob (1971) and by Bouteille *et al.* (1975) are now added reviews and reports on the use of this technique for the localization of nuclear functions (Angelier *et al.,* 1976a; Bouteille, 1976; Bouteille *et al.,* 1976; Fakan, 1976, 1978). The usefulness of quantitative analyses and especially statistical approaches in the analysis of autoradiographs should be stressed. Several methods have been described (Blackett and Parry, 1973; Salpeter *et al.,* 1969; Williams, 1969), and their use in the localization of nuclear functions at the cellular level has been reported (e.g., Dupuy-Coin and Bouteille, 1975; Moyne, 1977; Moyne *et al.,* 1978). This is especially true when autoradiography of isolated molecules—fiber autoradiography (see, e.g., Cairns, 1962; Hand, 1975; Petes and Williamson, 1975; Van't Hof, 1975)—is used at the ultrastructural level for biomolecular complexes spread on grids and shadowed. The methodology and results have been extensively described in investigations where such statistical approaches have been used for DNA molecules (Delain and Bouteille, 1979; Leibovitch *et al.,* 1975) and transcription units (Angelier *et al.,* 1976b, 1979).

As for the description of the nuclear structure (Fig. 1), the steps in the increase in knowledge of this topic can be followed in a number of consec-

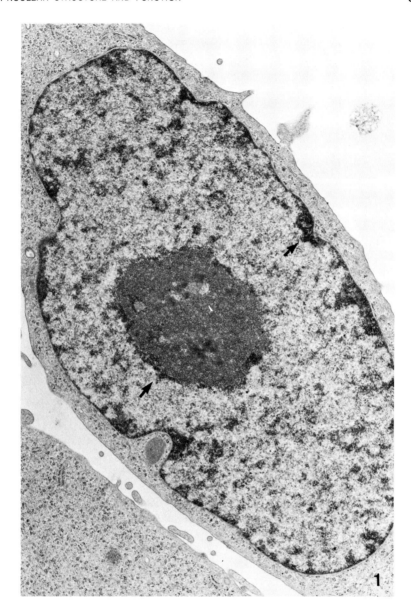

Fig. 1 General aspect of a typical interphase nucleus in a cell from an established cell line in culture (TG cells). The chromatin is observed in condensed form on the periphery of the nucleus and around the nucleolus (arrows). The remaining nucleoplasm contains dispersed chromatin. ×16,000. Micrograph of C. A. Bourgeois.

utive reviews (Bernhard and Granboulan, 1968; Bouteille, 1972; Bouteille *et al.*, 1974; Busch and Smetana, 1970; Fakan, 1978; Franke and Scheer, 1974; Frenster, 1974; Monneron and Bernhard, 1969; Simard *et al.*, 1974; Smetana and Busch, 1974). Therefore there is no need in this chapter to present lengthly descriptions, and most of this information is only summarized, specific points on recent progress being stressed. Likewise, biochemical and molecular aspects are left out, since specific chapters are devoted to this topic elsewhere in this volume. The effects of drugs on nuclear morphology have also been excluded for the same reason.

The most conspicuous change in our current view of the correlation between structure and function in the cell nucleus has clearly been the transition from the cellular to the molecular level. The discovery of the possibility of visualizing transcription units (Miller and Bakken, 1972; Miller and Beatty, 1969a,b), as well as new insights into the intimate structure of chromatin—nucleosomes (Callan and Klug, 1978)—have resulted in an entirely new level of investigation that we can call supramolecular. While most knowledge up to now was obtained at the cellular level by using morphological, cytochemical, and autoradiographic data for the nucleus within the entire cell either *in vivo* or *in vitro* on cellular fractions—isolated nuclei and isolated nucleoli—it is now possible to analyze electron microscopically such processes as replication and transcription directly on molecular spreadings. This has presented an exciting new goal, namely, to bridge our knowledge at the cellular level with these pieces of information obtained at the molecular level. The present chapter is based on both points of view.

II. Structure and Localization of Chromatin

An entirely new aspect of this question is associated with the discovery of the intimate structure of chromatin in the form of repeating units called nucleosomes, whose definition is now both biochemical and morphological. On the contrary, little information has been gained on the localization of chromatin. As stressed below, our efforts will be directed in the next years to description of the three-dimensional distribution of the chromatin both dispersed and condensed within the nuclear volume.

A. Intimate Structure of Chromatin

It is clear that the DNA of an eukaryotic chromosome, in which it is likely to be represented by a single molecule, must be highly folded under its condensed aspect as visible in interphase chromatin. Independently of its segmentation into genetic units of different functional significance, the physical distribution of DNA within the volume of chromatin is at the present time one of the most investigated topics. This structure has been known for a long time to be associated with the linking of DNA with basic proteins—histones, nonhistone proteins including polymerases, various enzymes, probably other regulatory proteins, and RNA.

The idea of a regular structure behind the filamentous arrangement conspicuous in any electron micrograph arose from X-ray diffraction of nucleohistones, suggesting the presence of repeating units (Luzzati and Nicolaieff, 1959; Wilkins *et al.*, 1959). However, it was not before 1973 that DNA could be cut into multiples of unit size by the use of an endogenous nuclease in rat liver cells (Hewish and Burgoyne, 1973).

From observations that H3 and H4 histones could be observed in solution as a specific tetramer (Kornberg and Thomas, 1974) a definite model has been provided for the basic unit of chromatin consisting of beads approximately 10 nm in diameter, with about 200 base pairs of DNA located externally around a protein core containing 8 histones molecules—a $(H3)_2(H4)_2$ tetramer and two each of H2a and H2b. The external location of the DNA was suggested by neutron-scattering experiments (Hjelm *et al.*, 1977; Pardon *et al.*, 1975), the radius of gyration of DNA being larger than the proteins.

It is interesting to note the critical role played by electron microscopy in this story (Fig. 2): The particulate nature of chromatin was actually demonstrated on electron micrographs (Olins and Olins, 1974; Woodcock, 1973). Chromatin was shown to be made out of beads called nu bodies, separated from each other by segments of DNA, the length of which was compatible with the presence of 40–80 base pairs. Besides the experiments where correlation was demonstrated between the discrete peaks of nuclease-digested chromatin after sedimentation in a sucrose gradient with the number of beads observed in electron microscopy (Finch *et al.*, 1975; Noll, 1974), and immunochemical experiments tending to show the identity of the histone content from one nucleosome to the other (Bustin *et al.*, 1976), the correspondence of the biochemically defined units to electron microscopically visible nucleosomes was demonstrated by electron microscope visualization of complexes resulting from mixing *in vitro* histones and adenovirus (Oudet *et al.*, 1975) or SV40 (Germond *et al.*, 1975) DNA. Further evidence for the exact histone content of nucleosomes and its identity in all nucleosomes was provided by reconstitution experiments *in vitro* of viral DNA with the various histones and their correlation with electron microscopically visible particles (Oudet *et al.*, 1975).

At the present time the exact relationship of the "core particle" (Shaw *et al.*, 1976), of rather distinct molecular constitution, to more complete

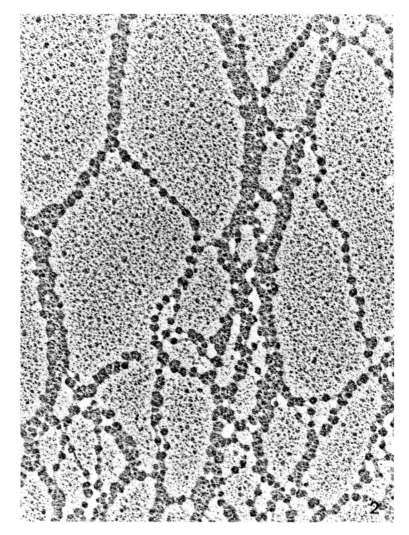

Fig. 2 Chromatin isolated from a KB cell during interphase. Spreading and platinum shadowing. The DNP fibers are easily identified by their repeating structure: nucleosomes (18 nm). × 110,000. Micrograph of D. Bouvier and J. Hubert.

and less well-defined nucleosomes is still under investigation. So is the exact number of DNA base pairs associated with the nucleosomes— probably 244 at the present time. The number of base pairs included in the linker DNA, the localization of histone H1, and the attachment of nonhistones proteins, will soon be defined by further experiments. Of extreme importance is the exact role of histone H1—or H5 in avian erythrocytes—if histones have anything to do with the degree of compaction of chromatin. A lot of information is currently drawn from the application of biophysical methods and crystallographic analysis of chromatin, from which the exact dimensions of nucleosomes are expected to be soon determined. The same can be said about the exact morphology of DNA folding around nucleosomes, especially the possible presence of sharp bends or kinks (Crick and Klug, 1975; Sobell *et al.*, 1976).

B. Superstructure

As the nucleosomal structure of chromatin is not sufficient to explain, even if highly folded, the usual appearance of chromatin in electron micrographs of intact nuclei, a higher level of organization has been postulated. In electron micrographs, 100-Å-thick fibrils have been reported to be the basic structure of chromatin, both in interphase nuclei (Hay and Revel, 1963) and in mitotic or meiotic chromosomes (for review, see Zirkin and Wolfe, 1972). Thicker fibrils, 100–150 Å in diameter, were described in erythrocyte heterochromatin (Davies, 1968), in frog spermiogenesis (Zirkin, 1971), and in lily pachytene chromosomes (Ris and Kubai, 1970). On the whole these figures were observed by studies on whole-mount chromosome specimens and isolated fibrils (Ris and Kubai, 1970). In fact different classes of diameters ranging from 80 to 118 and from 161 to 177 were statistically determined in sections of various cell types (Zirkin and Wolfe, 1972), suggesting significant variations from one type of cell to the other.

More recently, electron microscope studies of micrococcal digested nuclei—presumably native chromatin—in the presence of chelating agents or Mg^{2+} ions, after H1 depletion or not, suggested the nucleofilaments to be coiled into a superhelix, the turns of which were closely packed together in the form of a solenoid (Finch and Klug, 1976). The exact role played by H1 and nonhistone proteins in this superstructure will be of considerable importance, since the mechanism of the condensation of the chromatin has not yet been determined. The exact number of nucleosomes per turn of the solenoid is of course still to be established, and this would give an exact idea of the compaction ratio for the DNA in chromatin.

Another important question is whether nucleosomes are a specific structure for inactive chromatin, or whether such repeating units can be found in transcription units as suggested but not evidenced by electron microscopy.

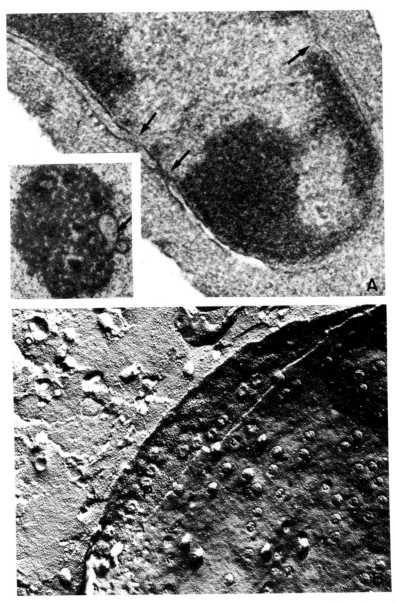

Fig. 3 Nucleocytoplasmic exchanges are assumed to take place through nuclear pores (arrows) shown here in a section (A) and in a replica of freeze-fractured preparations (B). However, they may also occur through other structures such as nucleolar channels (inset). (A) Reactivated chick erythrocyte nucleus in a reconstituted cell obtained by cell fusion from a chick nucleus and rat fibroblast enucleated cytoplasm.

C. Localization of Chromatin in Intact Nuclei

Chromatin, originally defined as nuclear material taking basic stains (Flemming, 1882), is electron microscopically recognized after uranyl and lead salt staining as divided into two main parts: condensed and dispersed chromatin. Condensed chromatin is found in two contiguous locations, the peripheral chromatin, observed as dense clumps of irregular shape, apparently attached to the inner leaflet of the nuclear envelope and perinucleolar chromatin. At the point of attachment, chromatin displays a specific arrangement of granule like appearance with periodic distribution. This is particularly visible when the dense lamina is conspicuous (Fawcett, 1966; Kalifat *et al.*, 1967; Schatten and Thoman, 1978; Stelly *et al.*, 1970). This gave morphological support to the attachment of chromosomes to the nuclear membrane during mitosis or even interphase (Comings, 1968; DuPraw, 1965). Condensed chromatin is also found in close connection with the nucleolus but is still contiguous with the rest of the condensed chromatin. Whether this nucleolus-associated chromatin has also a nucleolar function is still to be determined.

Dispersed chromatin is assumed to occupy the rest of the volume of the nucleus, i.e., the so-called interchromatin region of the nucleus, which is believed to be the part of chromatin that is active in terms of replication and/or transcription (see below). Most of the evidence for this comes from electron microscope autoradiography (see below; for reviews, see Bouteille *et al.*, 1974; Fakan, 1976, 1978) and from studies where perichromatin fibrils have been associated with transcription either by means of electron microscopy and cytochemistry (Fakan, 1976, 1978) or by a combination of biochemical analysis and electron microscope study (Stevenin *et al.*, 1976). However, it is interesting to point out that so far no cytochemical method has ever demonstrated the presence of chromatin in a dispersed state in this region. The usual uranyl and lead salts do not stain much material in this region, and the Feulgen-like electron-dense stains are not able to detect this dispersed chromatin (Cogliati and Gautier, 1973; Moyne, 1973).

×95,000. (From A. M. Dupuy-Coin *et al.*, 1976, reproduced by permission of Academic Press.) (B) Mouse hepatocyte. Freeze-fracture. Nuclear pores are numerous on the E face; the P face has more particles. ×40,000. Micrograph of C. Masson. Inset: TG cell. Nucleolar channel cross section (arrow). Such channels can be observed in a variety of cell types as a common attachment mode of the nucleolus to the nuclear envelope. ×15,000. (From C. A. Bourgeois *et al.*, 1979.)

The boundary between condensed and dispersed chromatin being rather ill-defined, one is left with the idea that there is a gradient of density of chromatin from the most condensed state in the periphery of the nucleus to the most dispersed state in the interchromatin region. In between, a gradient of material which has been called perichromatin fibrils, following the EDTA regressive technique of Bernhard (1969), is likely to be the active form of chromatin in interphase intact nuclei.

D. Three-Dimensional Arrangement of Chromatin

It is amazing that after so many years of morphological investigation of the cell nucleus almost nothing is known about the three-dimensional arrangement of the clumps of condensed chromatin within the nuclear volume. In ultrathin sections, these clumps seem to be distributed in a rather random fashion. Considering the high degree of complexity of chromatin arrangement at the molecular and subcellular levels, as described above, this is certainly not the case. There are reasons to believe that chromosomes at the end of telophase join a definite region of the nucleus. In order to clarify this point, it seems necessary to obtain, on the one hand, points of reference in the nucleus and, on the other, genetic or molecular probes which could be used for localization of genes in the interphase nucleus. In somatic mammalian cells at least, this has not yet been possible. One of the only points of reference available is the presence of the nucleolus with its highly condensed associated chromatin; this is probably due to the fact that ribosomal (rDNA) is highly repetitive so that nucleolar genes are visible in the form of a definite nuclear organelle, contrary to the others genes.

Another interesting point is the difficulty in figuring out how condensed chromatin becomes dispersed, and vice versa; while it is conceivable that transcriptionally active genes are made accessible to RNA polymerases at the boundary between condensed and dispersed chromatin, since only a little part of the genome is supposed to be in the active phase, it is much more difficult to understand the replication process known to involve all the genome during a given cell cycle. This would mean that the entire chromatin material goes from the condensed to the dispersed state within a cell cycle, so that any instant electron micrograph can be considered as picturing a single moment of a complex and dynamic process.

Finally, little is known about the position of the nucleus and its nuclear organelles relative to the cytoplasmic organelles. There are reasons to believe that, at least in highly polarized cells, the nuclear position with respect to the cytoplasm is not random (Bouteille, 1977). On the other hand, microcinematography has shown very complex movements of the nucleus within its cytoplasmic location (Baud, 1959). A lot of information is expected from studies where the respective positions of nuclear versus cytoplasmic organelles can be statistically described, especially as far as the complexity of nucleocytoplasmic exchanges of RNAs and proteins is concerned (Fig. 3).

III. Sites of Replication

A. Replication in Intact Nuclei

Current concepts of the location of DNA replication in the interphase nucleus are now fairly well established (for reviews, see Bouteille *et al.*, 1974; Fakan, 1978). Contrary to earlier experiments, electron microscope autoradiography following tritiated thymidine incorporation showed that the active part of chromatin in terms of replication was the dispersed chromatin region—the interchromatin region—and was not especially associated with the nuclear envelope as suggested in bacteria. This is known from early experiments by Ockey (1972) where the toxic effect of the synchronizing drugs was taken into account and the conclusion was drawn that diffused chromatin was the normal site of replication, at least in early S-phase, and the peripheral labeling was considered as resulting from a concentration of DNA breakdown products. Further evidence for this point was given by Fakan *et al.* (1972) using short pulses of thymidine in untreated mouse cells, where the normal site of replication was found to be the diffused chromatin and the activity was not found to be preferentially associated with purified nuclear envelope fractions.

Very much is still to be investigated, however, concerning the possible effect of the cell cycle on the location of replication; as pointed out above, it must be assumed that all the genome has to be replicated during a given cell cycle, and this process is not yet clearly understood.

The same can be said about the variation in incorporation of thymidine during the course of cell differentiation. Early observations by Milner (1969a,b) and others showed that the amount of thymidine incorporation was readily correlated with chromatin dispersion in phytohemagglutinin-stimulated lymphocytes. A thorough study of the correlation between thymidine incorporation and chromatin dispersion was carried out in stimulated lymphocytes of antiperoxidase immunized animals, where the various stages of differentiation toward antibody production could be traced by immunocytochemistry (Kuhlmann *et al.*, 1975). It was clear that replication was restricted to intermediate stages of differentiation where chromatin was in a highly dispersed state, while in undifferentiated lymphocytes or fully differentiated plasma cells chromatin was condensed and thymidine incorporation was very low (Fig. 4).

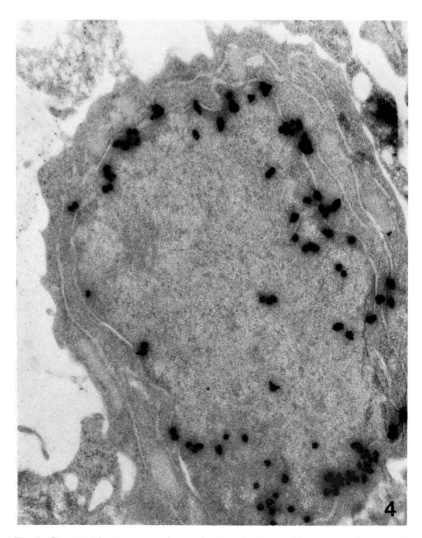

Fig. 4 Blast cell from a mouse immunized against peroxidase; secondary reaction. In contrast with the high degree of condensation of lymphocytes, this blast cell exhibits fully dispersed chromatin. The autoradiographic labeling after [³H]thymidine incorporation for 2 hours is, however, restricted to the periphery of the nucleus. Shorter pulses would have resulted in labeling in the dispersed chromatin. × 175,000. (From Kuhlmann et al., 1975, reproduced by permission of Academic Press.)

The conclusion of all these studies is that most if not all DNA replication takes place at the boundary between condensed and dispersed chromatin, but the three-dimensional and the dynamic aspects of this process are not well understood.

Finally, as far as the nucleolus is concerned, it remains possible that rDNA replication does not take place simultaneously with the replication of other genes (Blondel, 1968; Charret, 1969; Erlandson and de Harven, 1971).

B. Replication at the Molecular Level

While replication is now a fairly well-known molecular process, especially in prokaryotes, we still have little information on the way this process takes place in the chromatin of eukaryotes. As pointed out above, we still do not know whether nucleosomes are structures specific for inactive chromatin or whether transcription units contain nucleosomes defined both biochemically and electron microscopically.

Nucleosome-like beads have been shown both in transcription units of amphibian oocytes nucleoli and in somatic mammalian cells (Angelier and Lacroix, 1975; Angelier et al., 1979; Puvion-Dutilleul et al., 1977a,b, 1978). However, in essence these pictures cannot be controlled biochemically, so that the existence of core particles with their normal set of histones has not yet been proved in such situations. We therefore still do not know whether nucleosomes are at all compatible with replication. Efforts have been recently put forward to determine whether the constitution of nucleosomes as octamers makes it possible for them to open up into two symmetric substructures. Such models, where the nucleosome structure can be separated into two halves, have been proposed (Richards et al., 1977; Weintraub et al., 1976). Electron microscopy has confirmed this possibility (Oudet et al., 1978).

Even less is known about the exact way DNA can replicate when higher levels of organization—solenoid—are taken into consideration. Furthermore, we still have no information, as pointed out above, on the three-dimensional distribution of replication sites in chromatin.

Recent progress in the association of electron microscope autoradiography with molecular spreading and shadowing has made it possible to obtain significant labeling of naked DNA molecules on grids (Delain and Bouteille, 1979; Leibovitch et al., 1975). A quantitative evaluation of the results according to a widely used method (Salpeter et al., 1969) illustrated the possibility of individualizing labeled segments of the molecules as compared to cold segments. The use of highly labeled probes could therefore be expected to provide us with information on the localization of replication within the nuclear volume by means of electron microscope autoradiography. On a long-term basis, it should be possible, considering the progress of genetic engineering, to map the interphase nucleus.

IV. Pre-rRNA and Nucleolar Transcription

Most of the work carried out on the localization of transcription in interphase nuclei has involved nucleolar transcription. This is partly because the nucleolar genes are the only ones that are actually visible during interphase in the form of a well-defined nucleolus; the other genes cannot be separated morphologically. The conspicuous character of nucleolar genes is certainly related to their high degree of repetitivity. Furthermore, they display a quite specific intimate ultrastructure in which fibrillar centers can be described as surrounded by the RNA fibrillar part which is itself surrounded by the granular part; these three nucleolar portions, which are clearly visible in most if not all nucleoli in eukaryotic cells, are often described as forming the nucleolar body which is itself surrounded by nucleolus-associated chromatin (Fig. 1). A considerable amount of work has been performed in order to parallel these morphological parts of the nucleolus with the biochemically well-known rRNA processing. With the use of different pulses of tritiated uridine, electron microscope autoradiography experiments have succeeded in developing the idea of morphological RNA processing in nucleoli. This is summarized in the next section. In recent years, however, most of the interest was devoted to the nucleolar counterpart of the dispersed chromatin known in the nucleoplasm. The rationale consisted of looking at interphase nucleoli for the equivalent of the well-known NOR as defined in chromosomes during mitosis. At the present time the NOR region is associated with the fibrillar centers of interphase nucleoli as described below. Finally the spectacular progress of electron microscope visualization of transcription units following the initial work in amphibian nucleoli (Miller and Beatty, 1969a), and the recent combination of such techniques with electron microscope autoradiography on molecular spreadings (Angelier et al., 1976b, 1979), enables us to propose a comprehensive view of rRNA transcription at the supramolecular level.

A. Morphological Processing of rRNA

There is now a full line of electron microscope autoradiographic evidence that labeling takes place in a given part of the nucleolus and that, with the use of pulses of increasing duration, the labeled product can be followed from one nucleolar compartment to another (Fig. 5). Earlier studies (Bernhard and Granboulan, 1968; Fakan and Bernhard, 1971; von Gaudecker, 1967; Granboulan and Granboulan, 1965; Karasaki, 1965; La Cour and Crawley, 1965; Simard and Bernhard, 1967; Unuma *et al.,* 1968) gave abundant support to this concept of morphological processing. This process was best illustrated by electron microscope autoradiography combined with segregation of the various nucleolar components as obtained with actinomycin D (Geuskens and Bernhard, 1966). From these studies, it is clear that the first place where the labeling appears after short pulses is the fibrillar part of the nucleolus (Fig. 6). Only some time afterward does the labeling appear in the granular component. An interesting study by Royal and Simard (1975) supplied evidence that a parallel could be shown between this morphological processing and biochemical rRNA processing by means of an interesting correlation between the autoradiographic kinetics and the biochemical kinetics at the scintillation counter. From this study it appears that the first stages of molecular processing take place in the fibrillar part of the nucleolus, while later stages occur in the granular part.

B. Identification of the Nucleolar Organizing Region (NOR) during Interphase

In recent years considerable effort has been made to obtain a better understanding of the exact localization of the DNA that acts as a template for rRNA transcription. This rDNA has obviously been postulated to be contained within the nucleolus, but up to recently this localization was controversial, since the exact location and even the existence of dispersed chromatin within the nucleolar volume were not determined (Bouteille *et al.,* 1974).

The main progress in the last 10 years or so has been to reconcile the various definitions of the nucleolus as given by different types of investigations. From an ultrastructural point of view (Bernhard and Granboulan, 1968) the nucleolus is described as consisting of a fibrillar portion, a granular part, nucleolus-associated condensed chromatin, and the more recently demonstrated fibrillar centers (Goessens, 1976b; Goessens and Lepoint, 1974; Recher *et al.,* 1969). The functional counterpart of this ultrastructural definition has been provided by means of electron microscope autoradiography as described above. This picture represents the fully developed nucleolus, but numerous morphological variations have been observed according to the cell cycle, the physiology of the cell, and the cell species (for review, see Smetana and Busch, 1974). Likewise, the biochemical concept involving the various steps of rRNA processing has been fairly well correlated with the morphological parts of the nucleolus

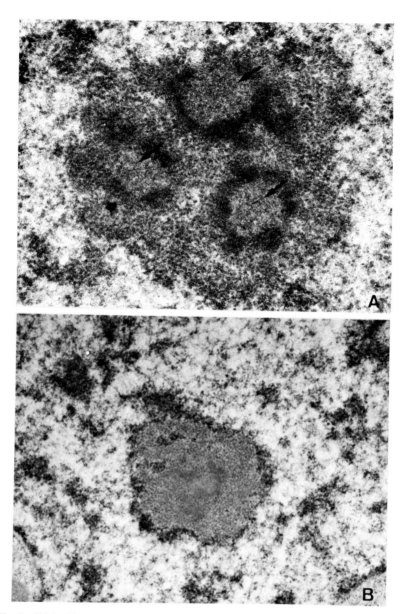

Fig. 5 (A) Architecture of normal nucleoli granulosa cell of *Lacerta vivipara*. Three fibrillar centers (arrows) are visible, surrounded by the RNA fibrils and RNA granules. × 40,000. Micrograph of J. Hubert. (B) Same cell type stained with thallium according to Moyne (1973). The fibrillar centers, RNA fibrils, and granules retain little contrast, while peri- and intranucleolar chromatin is conspicuous.× 35,000. Micrograph of J. Hubert.

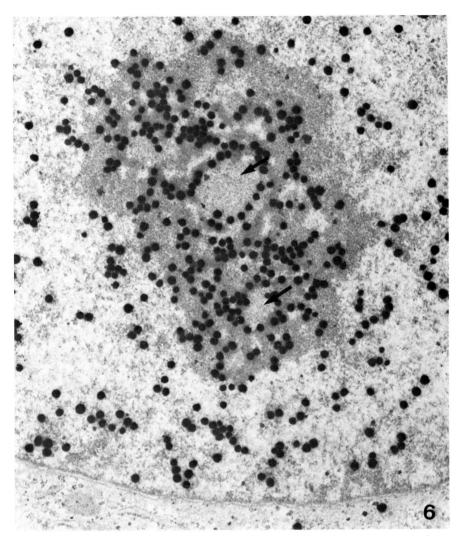

Fig. 6 Incorporation of [³H]uridine in a nucleolus of a TG cell in culture. The autoradiographic labeling is essentially restricted to the fibrillar component around the fibrillar centers (arrows). × 13,000. Micrograph of D. Hernandez.

as pointed out above. However, there is another way of considering the nucleolus, which points to the rDNA as its most essential component, since it carries the transcription units as visualized electron microscopically as the very first step of rRNA processing (Miller and Beatty, 1969a). This is the cytogenetic point of view. Cytogeneticists long ago identified rRNA genes at definite chromosomal sites called NORs. These NORs are readily visible in some chromosomes as secondary constrictions (Birnsteil *et al.*, 1966; Henderson *et al.*, 1972, 1974a,b, 1976a,b, 1977; Hsu *et al.*, 1975; Ritossa and Spiegelman, 1965; Scheuermann and Knalmann, 1975). These secondary constrictions are also identified in electron microscopy as well-defined electron-lucid regions (Goessens and Lepoint, 1974; Hsu *et al.*, 1967; Lafontaine, 1968; Lafontaine and Lord, 1974).

An important contribution to the problem of localizing the NOR during interphase was made by the demonstration in plant cells (Chouinard, 1971a, 1975) and animal cells (Goessens and Lepoint, 1974) that the NOR as identified electron microscopically was precisely the part of the nucleus around which nucleoli were observed to develop at the end of telophase. Strong support for this idea was provided by following nucleologenesis under conditions where it was possible to observe the appearance of a newly formed nucleolus from nuclei which did not contain a nucleolus nor were involved in RNA transcription, namely, in chick erythrocyte nuclei reactivated by cell fusion (Dupuy-Coin *et al.*, 1976; Hernandez-Verdun and Bouteille, 1979 (Fig. 7) and colchicine-induced micronuclei (Hernandez-Verdun *et al.*, 1979).

The current concept concerning the localization of the NOR during interphase itself is that it can be somehow identified with the fibrillar centers of the nucleolus first described by Recher *et al.* (1969). This is based upon similarity in ultrastructural appearance (Chouinard, 1971b; Goessens, 1973, 1974, 1976a,b; Jordan and Luck, 1976; Mirre and Stahl, 1976, 1978). Further support was provided by the use of *in situ* hybridization in the quail oocyte (Knibiehler *et al.*, 1977). However, these experiments were only carried out light microscopically, so that exact localization of the ribosomal cistrons was not possible. Therefore, although it is reasonable for the time being to consider the fibrillar centers the interphasic counterpart of the NOR as visible in chromosomes, the precise localization of the transcription units, as visualized using the technique of Miller, is still opened to question. This is discussed in the next section.

C. rRNA Transcription at the Molecular Level

Progress of considerable importance was made by Miller and Beatty (1969a) who demonstrated that electron microscopy was able to visualize the activity of nucleolar genes that code for precursor molecules of rRNA (Fig. 8). The first data were obtained for amphibian oocyte nucleoli. The nuclear content is dispersed manually in distilled water under definite conditions and centrifuged onto a grid for electron microscopy. The prin-

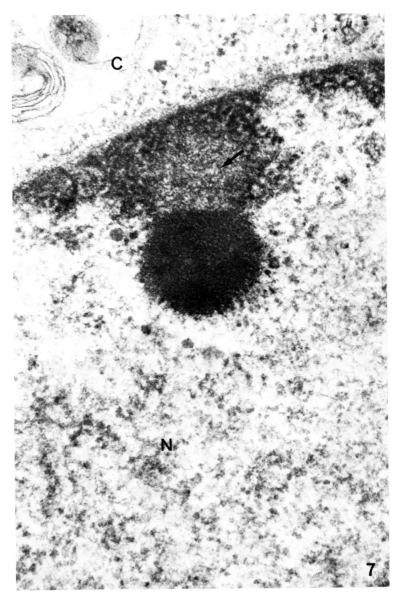

Fig. 7 Newly formed nucleolus in a reactivated chick erythrocyte nucleus, injected into a TG cell by cell fusion—heterokaryons. This nucleolus is observed at an early stage of nucleologenesis and consists only of a fibrillar center (arrow), i.e., the NOR, surrounded by condensed chromatin and a fibrillogranular portion which is a sign of resumed RNA synthesis. N, Nucleus; C, cytoplasm. ×80,000. Micrograph of D. Hernandez.

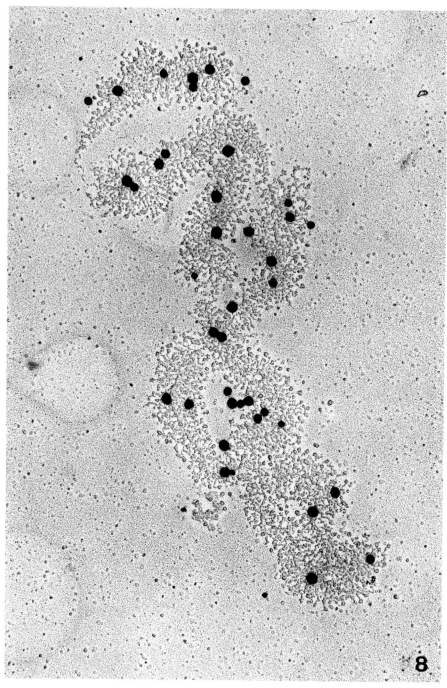

Fig. 8 Transcription unit of *Pleurodeles waltii* oocyte nucleoli. Spreading according to Miller and EM autoradiography following [³H]uridine incorporation. × 30,000. Micrograph of N. Angelier.

ciple of this technique is therefore to disorganize the nuclear structures and then to spread them out on a grid. The nucleolar spreadings can either be stained by phosphotungstic acid or contrasted by platinum rotative shadowing.

The activity of nucleolar genes has then been observed in a variety of systems (Hennig *et al.*, 1973; McKnight and Miller, 1976; Miller and Beatty, 1969a,b; Miller *et al.*, 1970; Spring *et al.*, 1974; Trendelenburg, 1974), and it is now clear that the typical organization exhibits a high degree of similarity in various species. The only intra- and inter-specific variations noticed by investigators concerned the size of the transcription units. The cellular systems investigated so far are various animal and plant cells (Scheer *et al.*, 1976b; Spring *et al.*, 1974), prokaryotes (*Escherichia coli*; Miller and Bakken, 1972; Miller *et al.*, 1970), embryonic cells, rat hepatocytes (Foe *et al.*, 1976; Hamkalo *et al.*, 1973; McKnight and Miller, 1976; Puvion-Dutilleul *et al.*, 1977a,b), insects (Trendelenburg, 1974; Trendelenburg *et al.*, 1973, 1974), and spermatocytes (Glatzer, 1975; Meyer and Hennig, 1974).

The typical morphological aspect is a DNA fiber which is the template axis along which fibrillar sequences of similar length, polarized in the same direction, are disposed. These RNA fibrils increase in size from the beginning to the end of the transcription unit. Between the sequences, the spacer is apparently devoid of transcription.

While the general character of the morphology of rRNA transcription in a variety of species has been evidenced, some specific points remain to be elucidated: the heterogeneity of the transcription units, especially in terms of the size of the units themselves and of the spacers (Scheer *et al.*, 1973, 1977; Spring *et al.*, 1974, 1976; Trendelenburg *et al.*, 1976) in *Xenopus*, *Acetabularia*, and *Dytiscus*; and the possibility of some degree of transcription in the spacers (Franke *et al.*, 1976). The question is whether the striking similarity in shape if not in size of the transcription units reflects a high degree of homogeneity in the mechanism of transcription in the various ribosomal genes involved. In terms of size, a high degree of heterogeneity has been reported from one DNP axial fiber to another (Wellauer *et al.*, 1976a,b) and even in the same DNP axial fiber (Scheer *et al.*, 1973, 1977). Even the polarity of the transcription units has been reported to be variable (Spring *et al.*, 1974, 1976).

With respect to variability and heterogeneity, recent information has been obtained using electron microscope autoradiography on molecular spreadings of transcription units in nucleoli of amphibian oocytes (Angelier *et al.*, 1976b, 1979). The conclusion was that in fact a high degree of heterogeneity could be observed in the labeling of the transcription units as compared to each other, suggesting that the mechanism of transcription and probably the rate of transcription were not exactly the same in all the transcription units of a same nucleolus and from one nucleolus to another. The same type of investigation has been used in an attempt to elucidate the mechanism of release of RNA transcripts from the DNA axial fiber. The data have been found to be compatible with the possibility that RNA processing begins before the transcript has been released from the DNA template, as suggested by Franke *et al.* (1976), or that the transcripts, once achieved, are stored along the DNA fiber (Angelier *et al.*, 1979).

V. Pre-mRNA and Nucleoplasmic Transcription

A. Cellular Level

This process is certainly much less well known than nucleolar transcription. This is partly due to the lack of information now available on the precise morphological substrates for the various steps of pre-mRNA formation. While specific techniques for revealing DNA in the nucleus — Feulgen-like methods — are now widely employed, we have no specific technique available for detecting RNA. The only cytochemical tool available is the EDTA staining technique of Bernhard (1969). Unfortunately this is a regressive method and the time at which the regression has to be stopped is decided by the investigator. This varies to a large extent from one tissue to another, and therefore this technique must be regarded as a useful tool rather than a specific method. After using such a technique the interchromatin granules and the perichromatin granules are visible. These two types of granules are actually observed also after usual uranyl and lead salt staining. A third structure appears after EDTA staining — perichromatin fibrils. A complete description of our present knowledge of these various nuclear structures can be found in reviews by Bouteille *et al.* (1974) and by Fakan (1978). These data are only briefly summarized here.

1. *Interchromatin Granules*

First described by Swift (1959) these granules have long been considered to contain RNA, although no definite evidence has been provided for this fact except that they remain stained after the EDTA technique. Although they are widely distributed in all eukaryotic cells so far investigated, we have at present not the slightest idea as to their possible role in nuclear function.

2. *Perichromatin Granules (Fig. 9)*

These granules have been more amply documented. They are at the present time the best candidates for pre-mRNA carriers. Their location

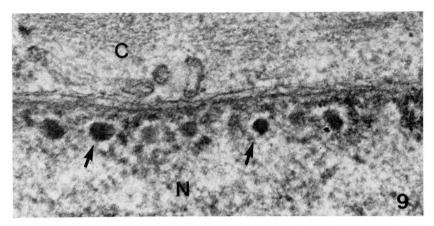

Fig. 9 Perichromatin granules (arrows) in a glial cell infected with herpes simplex hominis type 2 (HSV₂). The granules are found in an unusual amount but still exhibit their typical structure and relationship with peripheral chromatin. N, Nucleus; C, cytoplasm. × 72,000. Micrograph of A. M. Dupuy-Coin.

around the clumps or chromatin pictures, suggesting that they may be found in interchromatin channels, in nuclear pores, and even in the perikaryotic cytoplasm, and their response to experimental situations where pre-mRNA is biochemically known to be altered, are strong arguments for this conclusion. However, no definite answer to this question will be provided before such granules are isolated and proved to contain pre-mRNA (See Daskal, Chap. 4, this book). Recent arguments have been provided by examining nuclei of cells infected with herpesvirus, where such perichromatin granules are suggested to represent viral RNA, supporting their function as pre-mRNA carriers (Dupuy-Coin *et al.*, 1979).

3. Perichromatin Fibrils

These fibrils are observed on the periphery of the chromatin clumps after the EDTA staining technique has been applied. They were earlier suggested to be related to extranucleolar RNA synthesis because of their location in the perichromatin region (Monneron and Bernhard, 1969) and their similarity to Balbiani granules (Vasquez-Nin and Bernhard, 1971). Subsequent experiments suggested changes in their amount in experimental situations where pre-mRNA was modified. Interesting studies on this problem were carried out by Stevenin *et al.* (1976), where the morphological appearance of fibrils from nuclear extracts containing biochemically pre-mRNA was correlated with the aspect of perichromatin fibrils *in situ*, and by Puvion-Dutilleul *et al.* (1977a), who investigated the presence of these fibrils around clumps of isolated chromatin. Together with the well-known fact that the main site of extranucleolar transcription in the nucleus is precisely this perichromatin region (for reviews, see Bouteille *et al.*, 1974; Fakan, 1978), these data point to this fibrillar region as being the active region in pre-mRNA transcription. However, it remains to outline precisely this region which depends strongly on the degree of dispersion of chromatin. While this region is very easy to define in cells where chromatin is condensed—that is, in cells that are inactive in transcription, it is impossible to give a precise definition when cells are highly active in replication and/or transcription, such as blast cells.

As pointed out above, the exact relationship between condensed and dispersed chromatin is still to be described. Another important point is that, as already mentioned, the number of so-called perichromatin fibrils depends strictly on the time during which regression with the EDTA solution is carried out. This makes it rather difficult to make comparisons between different time points, between different experimental situations, and between experimental nuclei and control nuclei. In particular, the correlation between these data and the observations at the molecular level as described in the next section is still an open question.

B. Supramolecular Level

If this considerable amount of data definitely shows that the morphological mechanism of rRNA is fairly well understood, the picture is quite different as far as pre-mRNA is concerned. The bulk of the data has so far been obtained in three different situations: lampbrush chromosomes, as observed in meiotic prophase and especially during the diplotene period in oocytes and spermatocytes. (Angelier and Lacroix, 1975; Miller *et al.*, 1970; Scheer *et al.*, 1976a), chromosomes of dipters (for reviews, see Case and Daneholt, 1977, 1978), and in mammalian cells—isolated hepatocytes (Puvion-Dutilleul *et al.*, 1977a,b, 1978) and cultured cells (Villard and Fakan, 1978).

In the two first situations, the general morphology of the transcription units is fairly comparable to that of pre-rRNA units, except for the size which is larger.

In lampbrush chromosomes (Fig. 10), the RNA transcripts can be as long as 5 μm. As in nucleolar units, the size of these transcripts increases from the origin to the end of the transcription unit. However, the morphological heterogeneity of the units is striking. Some loops seem to be entirely transcribed, while others display only one fibrillar sequence and others show several transcription units. The polarity of the sequences can be either similar or opposed, while some complexes do not show any apparent polarity. The same variability is observed in the spacers whose size can be observed to vary to a large extent. The picture is made even

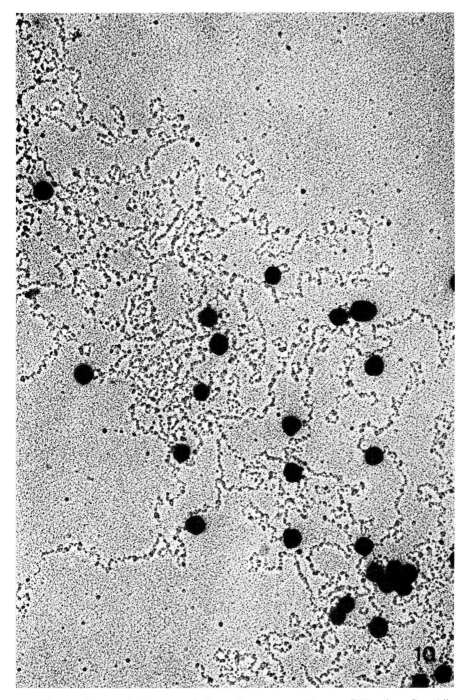

Fig. 10 Extranucleolar transcription units—presumably pre-mRNA—from *P. waltii* oocytes. Spreading according to Miller and platinum shadowing. Autoradiographic labeling after [³H]uridine incorporation. × 21,000. Courtesy of N. Angelier (Ivry-France).

more complicated by the fact that the RNA transcripts tend to display a superstructure—to coil and to tangle as a network.

Another situation in which a clear correlation can be made between the molecular and the cellular level is the salivary gland of dipters which is known to contain giant-sized polytene chromosomes which have been widely used in mapping the chromosomal location of defined genes. Among the dipters usually employed, *Drosophila* has been for several decades the best system for genetic investigation. For electron microscope studies, *Chironomus* has even been more widely studied because of the existence of chromosomal puffs—Balbiani rings—now considered to be loci of genetic activity (Beermann, 1952). In fact the similarity in shape and presumably in function of Balbiani granules and perichromatin granules observed in mammalian cells (Vasquez-Nin and Bernhard, 1971) explains in large part the interest which devoted to this system in recent years (Stevens and Swift, 1966). Balbiani ring 2 is the most important puff in the salivary glands of *Chironomus tentans*. Experiments using autoradiography (Pelling, 1964), biochemistry (Edström and Beermann, 1962), and hybridization with radioactive BR2 RNA (Lambert, 1972; Lambert *et al.*, 1972) showed that this ring was a type of RNA synthesis. Its ultrastructure was shown to exhibit a lampbrushlike appearance (Beermann and Bahr, 1954) and linked Balbiani granules. The connection of these granules to the deoxyribonucleoprotein axis has been evidenced, suggesting the packing up of the transcripts before its release from the ribonucleoprotein fiber (for review, see Case and Daneholt, 1977). Because of the exceptional size of this 75 S RNA, the use of the Miller and Beatty technique permitted visualization of long transcription units up to 8 μm in length and carrying about 125 transcripts. In this case it is even possible to recognize the "Christmas tree" in ultrathin sections, which is an ill-defined axis of the loops, carrying stalked granules and uncoiled fibrillar structures (Case and Daneholt, 1978). These observations are to be compared with similar investigations on *Drosophila melanogaster* (Laird and Chooi, 1976; Laird *et al.*, 1976; McKnight and Miller, 1976) and *Oncopeltus fasciatus* (Foe *et al.*, 1976; Laird *et al.*, 1976).

Interestingly enough, the species where transcriptional complexes other than rRNA have allowed a thorough study of their ultrastructure in molecular spreadings are not vertebrates, but green algae (Scheer *et al.*, 1976a), embryos, and spermatocytes of insects (Amabis and Nair, 1976; Foe *et al.*, 1976; Glatzer, 1975; Laird and Chooi, 1976; Laird *et al.*, 1976; McKnight and Miller, 1976). Nevertheless these data, added to those obtained for lampbrush chromosomes and dipter salivary gland giant chromosomes, provide a clear picture of what is probably the generality of the structure of presumably pre-mRNA transcription at the molecular level.

In contrast, little information is now available on premessenger transcription in the chromatin of mammalian cells (Fig. 11). With the exception of a few morphological data obtained in somatic or germinal cells (Kierszenbaum and Tres, 1975; Miller and Bakken, 1972; Oda and Omura, 1975) the most complete investigations were reported by Puvion-Dutilleul *et al.* (1977a,b, 1978) in isolated rat liver cells, and by Villard and Fakan (1978) in cultured mouse cells (Fig. 12). In both cases, the transcription fibrils

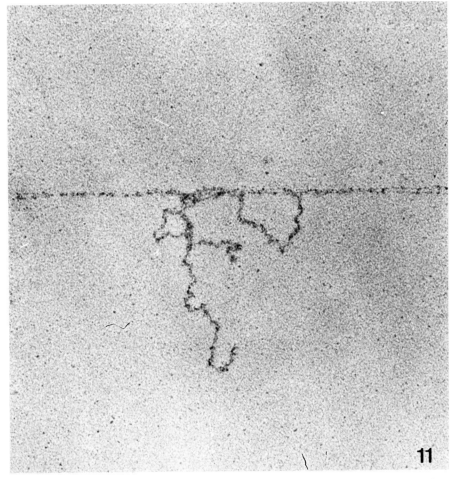

Fig. 11 Chromatin isolated from a KB cell during interphase. Spreading and positive staining with PTA. The DNP fiber supports RNP fibrils—presumably pre-mRNA with a higher degree of superstructure. × 80,000. Micrograph of D. Bouvier and J. Hubert.

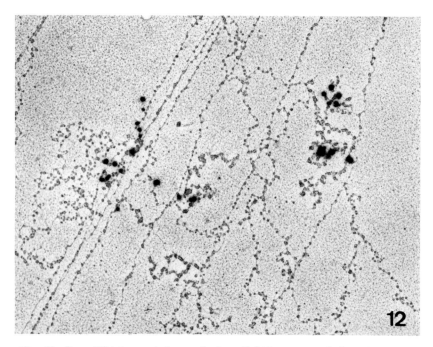

Fig. 12 Pre-mRNA transcription units from P 815 mouse cells in culture labeled with tritiated uridine for 5 minutes. Spreading as described elsewhere (Villard and Fakan, 1978). Elon ascorbic development. The labeling enables one to distinguish between RNA and DNA fibrils. ×50,000. Courtesy of Dr. S. Fakan (Lausanne, Switzerland).

are of irregular length, and their position on the DNP fibril seems at first glance random. On rare occasions a regular gradient of growth of the same type as that observed in ribosomal transcription units was found. In all cases one of the difficulties is to identify the transcript from the deoxyribonucleoprotein fiber, although the transcript is usually of nodular appearance and exhibits a high degree of superstructure. In this respect the use of electron microscope autoradiography was found to be helpful (Villard and Fakan, 1978). As for the existence of true "Christmas trees," a quantitative evaluation of the length of the fibrils and the examination of its regression line support this hypothesis (Puvion-Dutilleul *et al.*, 1978).

If the irregularity in the length of the fibrils and generally speaking in the morphological shape of the transcription units, if any, is present in somatic vertebrate cells, this could provide a partial explanation for the difficulties encountered in correlating these molecular data with the still complex picture of the nonribosomal transcription process in the nucleus at the cellular level. There is no doubt, however, that by augmenting the present number of data, and especially the systems in which they accumulate, such a correlation will soon be as easy as in the case of ribosomal transcription.

VI. Conclusions

In this chapter an attempt has been made to put together the data that both at the molecular and at the cellular level may help our interpretation of the localization of the main functions of the interphase nucleus. As compared to a few years ago (Bouteille *et al.*, 1974), we now understand fairly well the basic mechanisms of replication and transcription as visualized by electron microscopy on molecular spreadings. In comparison little progress has been made at the cellular level, and this is certainly due to the fact that we now have a rather complete picture of the ultrastructure of the interphase nucleus. It is clear therefore that most of our effort in the next years will be devoted to bridging these two levels of investigation. For the ultimate goal, however, i.e., the construction of a map of the interphase nucleus, it will obviously be necessary to wait for specific probes that can be inserted in the genome and localized by tracing methods such as electron microscope autoradiography and immunocytochemistry.

References

Amabis, J. M., and Nair, K. K. (1976). *Z. Naturforsch., Teil C* **31**, 186.

Angelier, N., and Lacroix, J. C. (1975). *Chromosoma* **51**, 323.

Angelier, N., Bouteille, M., Charret, R., Curgy, J. J., Delain, E., Fakan, S., Geuskens, M., Guelin, M., Lacroix, J. C., Laval, M., Steinert, G., and Van Assel, S. (1976a). *J. Microsc. Biol. Cell.* **27**, 215.

Angelier, N., Hémon, D., and Bouteille, M. (1976b). *Exp. Cell Res.* **100**, 389.

Angelier, N., Hémon, D., and Bouteille, M. (1979). *J. Cell Biol.* **80**, 277.

Baud, C. A. (1959). *In* "Problèmes d'ultrastructures et de fonctions nucleaires" (J. A. Thomas, ed.), Vol. 1, p. 29. Masson, Paris.

Beermann, W. (1952). *Chromosoma* **5**, 139.

Beermann, W., and Bahr, G. F. (1954). *Exp. Cell Res.* **6**, 195.

Bernhard, W. (1969). *J. Ultrastruct. Res.* **27**, 250.

Bernhard, W., and Granboulan, N. (1968). *In* "Ultrastructure in Biological Systems" (A. J. Dalton and F. Hagueneau, eds.), pp. 81–149. Academic Press, New York.

Birnsteil, M. R., Wallace, H., Sirlin, J. L., and Fishberg, M. (1966). *Natl. Cancer Inst., Monogr.* **23**, 431.

Blackett, N. M., and Parry, D. M. (1973). *J. Cell Biol.* **57**, 9.

Blondel, B. (1968). *Exp. Cell Res.* **53**, 348.

Bourgeois, C. A., Hemon, D., and Bouteille, M. (1979). *J. Ultrastruct. Res.* (In press.)

Bouteille, M. (1972). *Acta Endocrinol. (Copenhagen), Suppl.* No. 168, 11.

Bouteille, M. (1976). *J. Microsc. Biol. Cell.* **27**, 121.

Bouteille, M. (1977). *Life-Sci. Res. Space, Symp., Cologne/Porz* Eur. Space Ag. Publ. SP-130, p. 311.

Bouteille, M., Laval, M., and Dupuy-Coin, A. M. (1974). *In* "The Cell Nucleus" (H. Busch, ed.), Vol. 1, pp. 3–71. Academic Press, New York.

Bouteille, M., Dupuy-Coin, A. M., and Moyne, G. (1975). *In* "Hormone Action, Part E, Nuclear Structure and Function" Methods in Enzymology, Vol. 40, (B. W. O'Malley and J. G. Hardman, eds.), pp. 3–41. Academic Press, New York.

Bouteille, M., Fakan, S., and Burglen, M. J. (1976). *J. Microsc. Biol. Cell.* **27**, 171.

Busch, H., and Smetana, K. (1970). "The Nucleolus." Academic Press, New York.

Bustin, M., Goldblatt, D., and Sperling, R. (1976). *Cell* **7**, 297.

Cairns, J. (1962). *Cold Spring Harbor Symp. Quant. Biol.* **27**, 311.

Callan, H. G., and Klug, A. (1978). *Philos. Trans. R. Soc. London, Ser. B* **283**, 231.

Case, S. T., and Daneholt, B. (1977). *Int. Rev. Biochem.* **15**, 45.

Case, S. T., and Daneholt, B. (1978). *J. Mol. Biol.* **124**, 223.

Charret, R. (1969). *Exp. Cell Res.* **54**, 353.

Chouinard, L. A. (1971a). *Adv. Cytopharmacol.* **1**, 69.

Chouinard, L. A. (1971b). *J. Cell Sci.* **9**, 637.

Chouinard, L. A. (1975). *J. Cell Sci.* **19**, 85.

Cogliati, R., and Gautier, A. (1973). *C. R. Acad. Sci., Ser. D* **276**, 3041.

Comings, D. E. (1968). *Am. J. Hum. Genet.* **20**, 440.

Crick, F. H., and Klug, A. (1975). *Nature (London)* **255**, 530.

Davies, H. G. (1968). *J. Cell Sci.* **3**, 129.

Delain, E., and Bouteille, M. (1979). To be published.

DuPraw, E. J. (1965). *Proc. Natl. Acad. Sci. U.S.A.* **53**, 161.

Dupuy-Coin, A. M., and Bouteille, M. (1975). *Exp. Cell Res.* **90**, 111.

Dupuy-Coin, A. M., Ege, T., Bouteille, M., and Ringertz, N. R. (1976). *Exp. Cell Res.* **101**, 355.

Dupuy-Coin, A. M., Arnoult, J., and Bouteille, M. (1978). *J. Ultrastruct. Res.* **65**, 60.

Edström, J. E., and Beermann, W. (1962). *J. Cell Biol.* **14**, 371.

Erlandson, R. A., and de Harven, E. (1971). *J. Cell Sci.* **8**, 353.

Fakan, S. (1976). *J. Microsc. (Paris)* **106**, 159.

Fakan, S. (1978). *In* "The Cell Nucleus" (H. Busch, ed.), Vol. 5, pp. 3–52. Academic Press, New York.

Fakan, S., and Bernhard, W. (1971). *Exp. Cell Res.* **67**, 129.

Fakan, S., Turner, G. N., Pagano, J. S., and Hancock, R. (1972). *Proc. Natl. Acad. Sci. U.S.A.* **69**, 2300.

Fawcett, D. W. (1966). *Am. J. Anat.* **119**, 129.

Finch, J. T., and Klug, A. (1976). *Proc. Natl. Acad. Sci. U.S.A.* **73**, 1897.

Finch, J. T., Noll, M., and Kornberg, R. D. (1975). *Proc. Natl. Acad. Sci. U.S.A.* **72**, 3320.

Flemming, W. (1882). "Zell substanz, Kern und Zelltheilung." Vogel, Leipzig.

Foe, V. E., Wilkinson, L. E., and Laird, C. D. (1976). *Cell* **9**, 131.

Franke, W. W., and Scheer, U. (1974). *In* "The Cell Nucleus" (H. Busch, ed.), Vol. 1, p. 219. Academic Press, New York.

Franke, W. W., Scheer, U., Spring, H., Trendelenburg, M. F., and Khrone, G. (1976). *Exp. Cell Res.* **100**, 233.

Frenster, J. H. (1974). *In* "The Cell Nucleus" (H. Busch, ed.), Vol. 1, p. 565. Academic Press, New York.

Germond, J. E., Hirt, B., Oudet, P., Gross-Bellard, M., and Chambon, P. (1975). *Proc. Natl. Acad. Sci. U.S.A.* **72**, 1843.

Geuskens, M., and Bernhard, W. (1966). *Exp. Cell Res.* **44**, 579.

Glatzer, K. H. (1975). *Chromosoma* **53**, 371.

Goessens, G. (1973). *C. R. Acad. Sci., Ser. D* **277**, 325.
Goessens, G. (1974). *C. R. Acad. Sci., Ser. D* **279**, 991.
Goessens, G. (1976a). *Exp. Cell Res.* **100**, 88.
Goessens, G. (1976b). *Cell Tissue Res.* **173**, 315.
Goessens, G., and Lepoint, A. (1974). *Exp. Cell Res.* **87**, 63.
Granboulan, N., and Granboulan, P. (1965). *Exp. Cell Res.* **38**, 604.
Hamkalo, B. A., Miller, O. L., and Bakken, A. H. (1973). *Cold Spring Harbor Symp. Quant. Biol.* **38**, 915.
Hand, R. (1975). *J. Histochem. Cytochem.* **23**, 475.
Hay, E. D., and Revel, J. P. (1963). *J. Cell Biol.* **16**, 29.
Henderson, A. S., Warburton, D., and Atwood, K. C. (1972). *Proc. Natl. Acad. Sci. U.S.A.* **69**, 3394.
Henderson, A. S., Eicher, E. M., Yu, M. T., and Atwood, K. C. (1974a). *Chromosoma* **49**, 155.
Henderson, A. S., Warburton, D., and Atwood, K. C. (1974b). *Chromosoma* **44**, 367.
Henderson, A. S., Atwood, K. C., and Warburton, D. (1976a). *Chromosoma* **59**, 147.
Henderson, A. S., Eicher, E. M., Yu, M. T., and Atwood, K. C. (1976b). *Cytogenet. Cell Genet.* **17**, 307.
Henderson, A. S., Warburton, D., Megraw-Ripley, S., and Atwood, K. C. (1977). *Cytogenet. Cell Genet.* **19**, 281.
Hennig, W., Meyer, G. F., Hennig, I., and Leoncini, O. (1973). *Cold Spring Harbor Symp. Quant. Biol.* **38**, 673.
Hernandez-Verdun, D., and Bouteille, M. (1979). *J. Ultrastruct. Res.* (In press.)
Hernandez-Verdun, D., Bouteille, M., Ege, T., and Ringertz, N. R. (1979). *Exp. Cell Res.* (in press).
Hewish, D. R., and Burgoyne, L. A. (1973). *Biochem. Biophys. Res. Commun.* **52**, 504.
Hjelm, R. P., Kneale, G. G., Suau, P., Baldwin, J. P., and Bradbury, E. M. (1977). *Cell* **10**, 139.
Hsu, T. C., Brinkley, B. R., and Arrighi, F. E. (1967). *Chromosoma* **23**, 137.
Hsu, T. C., Spirito, S. E., and Pardue, M. L. (1975). *Chromosoma* **53**, 25.
Jacob, J. (1971). *Int. Rev. Cytol.* **30**, 91.
Jordan, E. G., and Luck, B. T. (1976). *J. Cell Sci.* **22**, 75.
Kalifat, S. R., Bouteille, M., and Delarue, J. (1967). *J. Microsc. (Paris)* **6**, 1019.
Karasaki, S. (1965). *J. Cell Biol.* **26**, 937.
Kierszenbaum, A. L., and Tres, L. L. (1975). *J. Cell Biol.* **65**, 258.
Knibiehler, B., Navarro, A., Mirre, C., and Stahl, A. (1977). *Exp. Cell Res.* **110**, 153.
Kornberg, R. D., and Thomas, J. O. (1974). *Science* **184**, 865.
Kuhlmann, W. D., Bouteille, M., and Avrameas, S. (1975). *Exp. Cell Res.* **96**, 335.
La Cour, L. F., and Crawley, J. W. C. (1965). *Chromosoma* **16**, 124.
Lafontaine, J. G. (1968). *In* "The Nucleus" (A. J. Dalton and F. Hagueneau, eds), pp. 151–196. Academic Press, New York.
Lafontaine, J. G., and Lord, A. (1974). *J. Cell Sci.* **16**, 63.
Laird, C. D., and Chooi, W. Y. (1976). *Chromosoma* **58**, 193.
Laird, C. D., Wilkinson, L. E., Foe, V. E., and Chooi, W. Y. (1976). *Chromosoma* **58**, 169.
Lambert, B. (1972). *J. Mol. Biol.* **72**, 65.
Lambert, B., Wieslander, L., Daneholt, B., Egyhazi, E., and Ringborg, U. (1972). *J. Cell Biol.* **53**, 407.
Leibovitch, S., Delain, E., and Bouteille, M. (1975). *J. Microsc. Biol. Cell.* **23**, 23a.
Luzzati, V., and Nicolaieff, A. (1959). *J. Mol. Biol.* **1**, 127.
McKnight, S., and Miller, O. L. (1976). *Cell* **8**, 305.
Meyer, G. F., and Hennig, W. (1974). *Chromosoma* **46**, 121.

Miller, O. L., and Bakken, A. H. (1972). *Acta Endocrinol. (Copenhagen)*, *Suppl.* No. 168, 155.

Miller, O. L., and Beatty, B. R. (1969a). *J. Cell. Physiol.* **74**, 225.

Miller, O. L., and Beatty, B. R. (1969b). *Science* **164**, 955.

Miller, O. L., Beatty, B. R., Hamkalo, B. A., and Thomas, C. A. (1970). *Cold Spring Harbor Symp. Quant. Biol.* **35**, 505.

Milner, G. R. (1969a). *Nature (London)* **221**, 71.

Milner, G. R. (1969b). *J. Cell Sci.* **4**, 569.

Mirre, C., and Stahl, A. (1976). *J. Ultrastruct. Res.* **56**, 186.

Mirre, C., and Stahl, A. (1978). *J. Cell Sci.* **31**, 79.

Monneron, A., and Bernhard, W. (1969). *J. Ultrastruct. Res.* **27**, 266.

Moyne, G. (1973). *J. Ultrastruct. Res.* **45**, 102.

Moyne, G. (1977). *Cytobiologie* **15**, 126.

Moyne, G., Pichard, E., and Bernhard, W. (1978). *J. Gen. Virol.* **40**, 77.

Noll, M. (1974). *Nature (London)* **251**, 249.

Ockey, C. H. (1972). *Exp. Cell Res.* **70**, 203.

Oda, T., and Omura, S. (1975). *Acta Histochem. Cytochem.* **8**, 303.

Olins, A. L., and Olins, D. E. (1974). *Science* **183**, 330.

Oudet, P., Gross-Bellard, M., and Chambon, P. (1975). *Cell* **4**, 281.

Oudet, P., Germond, J. E., Bellard, M., Spadafora, C., and Chambon, P. (1978). *Philos. Trans. R. Soc. London Ser. B* **283**, 241.

Pardon, J. F., Worcester, D. L., Wooley, J. C., Tatchell, K., Van Holde, K. E., and Richards, B. M. (1975). *Nucleic Acids Res.* **2**, 2163.

Pelling, C. (1964). *Chromosoma* **15**, 71.

Petes, T. D., and Williamson, D. H. (1975). *Exp. Cell Res.* **95**, 103.

Puvion-Dutilleul, F., Bachellerie, J. P., Zalta, J. P., and Bernhard, W. (1977a). *Biol. Cell.* **30**, 183.

Puvion-Dutilleul, F., Bernadac, A., Puvion, E., and Bernhard, W. (1977b). *J. Ultrastruct. Res.* **58**, 107.

Puvion-Dutilleul, F., Puvion, E., and Bernhard, W. (1978). *J. Ultrastruct. Res.* **63**, 118.

Recher, L., Whitescarver, J., and Briggs, L. (1969). *J. Ultrastruct. Res.* **29**, 1.

Richards, B., Pardon, J., Lilley, D., Cotter, R., and Wooley, J. (1977). *Cell Biol. Int. Rep.* **1**, 107.

Ris, H., and Kubai, D. F. (1970). *Annu. Rev. Genet.* **4**, 263.

Ritossa, F. M., and Spiegelman, S. (1965). *Proc. Natl. Acad. Sci. U.S.A.* **53**, 737.

Royal, A., and Simard, R. (1975). *J. Cell Biol.* **66**, 577.

Salpeter, M. M., Bachmann, L., and Salpeter, E. E. (1969). *J. Cell. Biol.* **41**, 1.

Schatten, G., and Thoman, M. (1978). *J. Cell Biol.* **77**, 517.

Scheer, U., Trendelenburg, M. F., and Franke, W. W. (1973). *Exp. Cell Res.* **80**, 175.

Scheer, U., Franke, W. W., Trendelenburg, M. F., and Spring, H. (1976a). *J. Cell Sci.* **22**, 503.

Scheer, U., Trendelenburg, M. F., and Franke, W. W. (1976b). *J. Cell Biol.* **69**, 465.

Scheer, U., Trendelenburg, M. F., Krohne, G., and Franke, W. W. (1977). *Chromosoma* **60**, 147.

Scheuermann, W., and Knalmann, M. (1975). *Exp. Cell Res.* **90**, 463.

Shaw, B., Herman, T., Kovacic, R., Beaudreau, G., and Van Holde, K. E. (1976). *Proc. Natl. Acad. Sci. U.S.A.* **73**, 505.

Simard, R., and Bernhard, W. (1967). *J. Cell Biol.* **34**, 61.

Simard, R., Langelier, Y., Mandeville, R., Maestracci, N., and Royal, A. (1974). *In* ''The Cell Nucleus'' (H. Busch, ed.), Vol. 3, p. 447. Academic Press, New York.

Smetana, K., and Busch, H. (1974). *In* "The Cell Nucleus" (H. Busch, ed.), Vol. 1, p. 75. Academic Press, New York.

Sobell, H., Tsai, C., Gilbert, S., Jain, S., and Sakore, T. (1976). *Proc. Natl. Acad. Sci. U.S.A.* **73,** 3068.

Spring, H., Trendelenburg, M. F., Scheer, U., Franke, W. W., and Herth, W. (1974). *Cytobiologie* **10,** 1.

Spring, H., Krohne, G., Franke, W. W., Scheer, U., and Trendelenburg, M. (1976). *J. Microsc. Biol. Cell.* **25,** 107.

Stelly, N., Stevens, B. J., and André, J. (1970). *J. Microsc. (Paris)* **9,** 1015.

Stevenin, J., Devilliers, G., and Jacob, M. (1976). *Mol. Biol. Rep.* **2,** 385.

Stevens, B. J., and Swift, H. (1966). *J. Cell Biol.* **31,** 55.

Swift, H. (1959). *Symp. Mol. Biol., Univ. Chicago* pp. 266–303.

Trendelenburg, M. F. (1974). *Chromosoma* **48,** 119.

Trendelenburg, M., Scheer, U., and Franke, W. W. (1973). *Nature (London), New Biol.* **245,** 167.

Trendelenburg, M. F., Spring, H., Scheer, U., and Franke, W. W. (1974). *Proc. Natl. Acad. Sci. U.S.A.* **71,** 3626.

Trendelenburg, M. F., Scheer, U., Zentgraf, H., and Franke, W. W. (1976). *J. Mol. Biol.* **108,** 453.

Unuma, T., Arendell, J. P., and Busch, H. (1968). *Exp. Cell Res.* **52,** 429.

Van't Hof, J. (1975). *Exp. Cell Res.* **93,** 95.

Vasquez-Nin, G., and Bernhard, W. (1971). *J. Ultrastruct. Res.* **36,** 842.

Villard, D., and Fakan, S. (1978). *C. R. Acad. Sci., Ser. D* **286,** 777.

von Gaudecker, B. (1967). *Z. Zellforsch. Mikrosk. Anat.* **82,** 536.

Weintraub, H., Worcel, A., and Alberts, B. (1976). *Cell* **9,** 409.

Wellauer, P. K., Dawid, I. B., Brown, D. D., and Reeder, R. H. (1976a). *J. Mol. Biol.* **105,** 461.

Wellauer, P. K., Reeder, P. H., Dawid, I. B., and Brown, D. D. (1976b). *J. Mol. Biol.* **105,** 487.

Wilkins, M. H. F., Zubay, G., and Wilson, H. R. (1959). *J. Mol. Biol.* **1,** 179.

Williams, M. A. (1969). *Adv. Opt. Electron Microsc.* **3,** 219.

Woodcock, C. L. F. (1973). *J. Cell Biol.* **59,** 368a.

Zirkin, B. R. (1971). *J. Ultrastruct. Res.* **34,** 159.

Zirkin, B. R., and Wolfe, S. L. (1972). *J. Ultrastruct. Res.* **39,** 496.

2

The Molecular Biology of Cancer: The Cancer Cell and Its Functions

HARRIS BUSCH

I. Introduction

Virtually every cell type in the human body represents a highly specialized structure whose phenotype contributes in one way or another to the elegant functioning of the physiology and adaptability of the individual. The phenotype of cancer cells (Busch, 1976a) differs in several important respects from that of any nontumor tissue (Figs. 1–3). Cancer cells have a dysplastic phenotype, represented by (1) uncontrolled cell growth and division, (2) invasiveness, and (3) metastasis, which is transmitted genetically or epigenetically to the daughter cells (Busch, 1974). The evidence is clear that a single cancer cell is sufficient to produce cancer in susceptible hosts and that cancer represents a disordered state of biochemical genetics (Furth and Kahn, 1937; Hosokawa, 1950; Ishibashi, 1950).

Clinically, cancer (like diseases such as syphilis) appears to be "many disease states," depending on the phenotype of the tissue of origin (Busch, 1974). In studies on neoplastic disease, it is clearly important to distinguish between the manifestations of the disease and the fundamental pathological events. For example, patients with severe hypoglycemic states as a result of insulinomas may not exhibit any late effects of cancer at all. In this case, the organ-specific phenotypic changes related to the neoplastic process dominate the clinical picture. However, the underlying cancerous disease state is the same as in other human neoplasms.

Moreover, in neoplasms of any given tissue, there is a broad range of

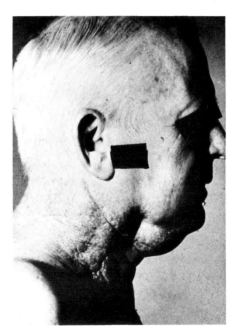

Fig. 1   Patient with epidermoid carcinoma of the neck, showing a line of partial healing after resection.

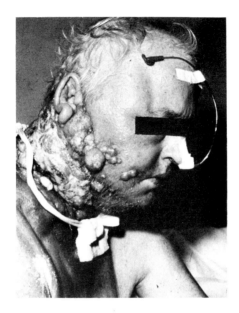

Fig. 2 Same patient as in Fig. 1, 3 hours premortem. The ulceration of the surface and presence of fibrin are apparent, as well as local metastatic lesions. The patient also suffered from mediastinal penetration of the tumor.

quantitative variants. Insulinomas are a good example of variation from high levels of insulin production and secretion to very low levels or none at all. Accordingly, the investigator has the problem of defining events that are critical to the disease process and directly related to it, and differentiating those that either are results of indirect events of the process or are totally unrelated.

The Relationship of Cytoplasmic Processes to the Cancer Phenotype

All the common lethal characteristics of cancer cells (Figs. 1 and 2) are related to cytoplasmic functions, particularly invasiveness (Figs. 3 and 4) and metastasis (Fidler, 1979). Of course, many biosynthetic activities involved in growth are carried out by cytoplasmic systems. For the most part, none of the mechanisms involved in these biosynthetic reactions appear to differ from those of nontumor systems. Accordingly, a key question is, Where is the locus of the cancer lesion in the neoplastic cells, or in what way is there a differentiation of the neoplastic cells so that they exhibit their special common features?

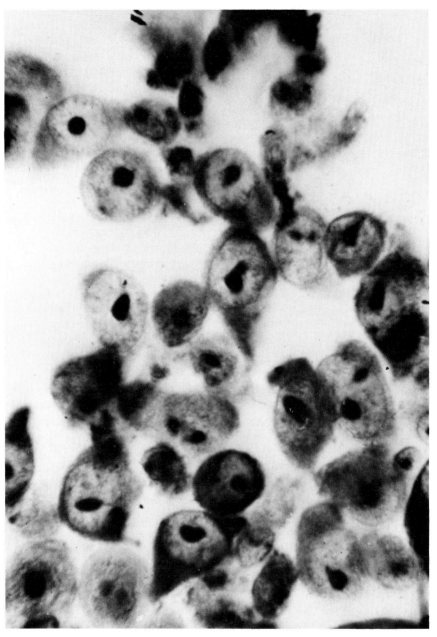

Fig. 3A Light microscope view of cancer cells stained with azure C. The pleomorphism of the nucleoli is apparent.

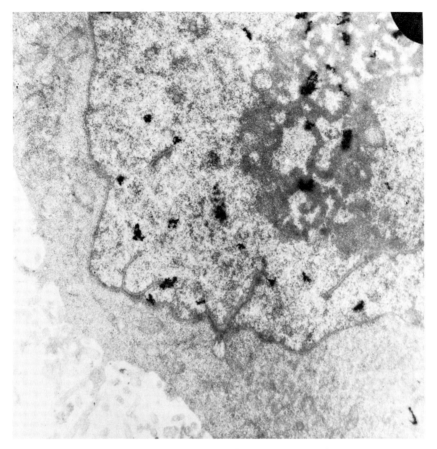

Fig. 3B Electron micrograph of a Novikoff hepatoma showing the enlarged nucleolus and the enlarged nucleus with a large ratio of nucleus to cytoplasm. Note the microvilli on the cell surface. Labeling with tritiated uridine for short times shows partial localization to the nucleolus.

All major properties of cancer cells are exhibited by nontumor cells at some point in ontogeny (Busch, 1976a). For example, growth is a property of all cells, invasiveness is a property of several types of white cells, and metastasis is a common embryonic phenomenon (Figs. 4–8). Although the production of abnormal chromosomes is an uncommon and pathological event in nontumor cells and generally leads to destruction of the affected cell, alterations in chromosome number such as polyploidy commonly occur in liver cells with maturation and aging (Sandberg and Sakurai, 1974).

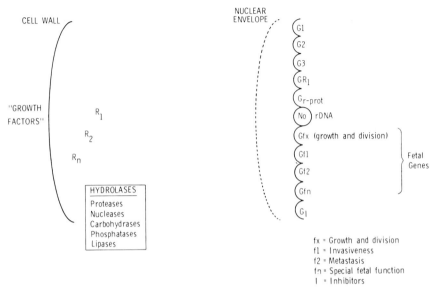

Fig. 4 Elements of cellular response to external stimuli in the resting or ground state. It is envisioned that growth factors and other stimuli are almost continuously present in the cellular periphery in equilibrium with intracellular elements. R_1–R_n, Cytoplasmic receptor proteins; G1–GR_1, structural genes including genes for receptor proteins (GR_1); G_{r-prot}, Genes for ribosomal proteins; No, rDNA genes; Gf1–Gfn, fetal genes with functions indicated; and G_I inhibitor genes.

As recently pointed out in studies from many laboratories (Fishman and Sells, 1976; Fishman and Busch, 1979), the "tumor antigens" of human cells and nonviral animal tumors frequently represent fetal gene readouts (Fig. 6) ranging from late fetal stages to early elements of sperm and ovum. Simply expressed, along with neoplastic transformation, there frequently is fetal gene activation which is apparently quite random in terms of the "biological clock." Of course, it is by no means proven that such fetal gene readouts have any more to do with meaningful neoplastic processes than the activation of genes for production of the many isozymes reported to exist in various tumors (Sato and Sugimura, 1974; Weinhouse, 1972).

The concept that fetal genes are active in the process of neoplasia is an attractive one (Busch, 1976a). If one considers the genome a large mass of potential gene readouts (Fig. 4) subject to the influence of factors and various stimuli that may act through receptor intermediates or directly on the genome, it may be considered that in each cell (Fig. 5) a limited population of genes is operative. Their products, which are mRNA species of various types, interact with ribosomes originating in the nucleolus to form

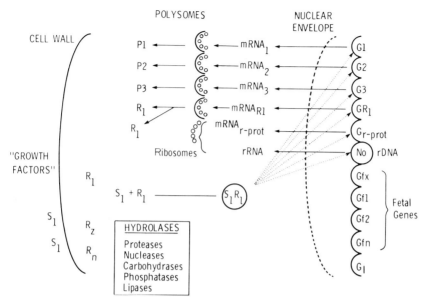

Fig. 5 Response of cells to a stimulus (S_1) with the formation of a stimulus–receptor complex (S_1R_1) which impinges upon a group of genes (G1–GR_1, G_{r-prot}, and No-rDNA) to produce a series of mRNAs, ribosomes, and polysomes that in turn synthesize specific products including R_1. The "battery" of fetal genes is not involved in these normal responses. P1–P3, Protein readouts. R_z, other receptor protein. See Fig. 4 for other symbols.

the polysomes that are the units of protein synthesis in the cytoplasm. These are involved in the production of specific proteins (P1–P3, R1, and so on) that define the phenotype of the specific cell. The key point is that the fetal genes are "silent" in these mature cells of normal individuals.

In fetal cells (Fig. 6) there is a complex series of events in progress, related largely to the time point on the biological clock. As Fig. 6 indicates, the fetal cells operate with their own set of signals, which are coupled with special readouts that produce the incredible number of events that not only involve growth, specialization, and migration of cells but also specify organization with an incredible degree of accuracy. As many have noted, special events occur in ontogenesis that do not recur during normal life. For example, the processes involved in limb bud formation, including initiation, elongation, and termination of growth, can be interfered with by thalidomide, resulting in the arrested states characteristic of phocomelia. Even if the drug is removed, there is no repetition of the phenomenon; i.e., the limb buds do not continue to grow. Accordingly, there is only a defined "time window" during which limb bud growth and development occur.

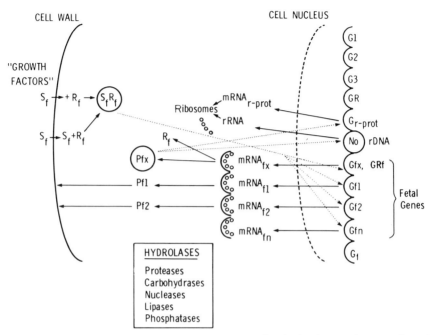

Fig. 6 A pattern similar to that in Fig. 5 is shown for the fetal state when a variety of fetal genes are activated by stimulus S_f (fetal stimulus factors) and receptor R_f to form S_fR_f, which acts in the same way as the factors controlling structural genes of the adult. See Fig. 4 for other symbols.

Needless to say, these special time points in the biological clock must be under the control of special "start" and "stop" signals which are probably active only during specific phases of ontogenesis. There is a rigid timing of these events in embryogenesis; either a series of feedback loops or specific inhibitors must exist that "turn off" specific fetal functions. Among the types of shutoff mechanisms that could exist are (1) loss of S_f or (2) inhibition by fetal factors of the function of S_f (Fig. 6). If in cancer cells special fetal genes are activated (Figs. 7 and 8), suppression of function may not occur in the adult because associated factors have long been inoperative. It is thus conceivable that a variety of functions of neoplastic cells could be controlled if specific fetal control elements were available (Illmensee and Mintz, 1976).

Figure 7 indicates that, at the time of exposure to carcinogens, three or possibly more major effects may occur in which a carcinogen interacts with (1) receptors, (2) activators, or (3) cellular or chromatin enzymes or other proteins or directly or indirectly with the genome. The carcinogen may exert a direct effect on the genome (Fig. 7). The primordial cell that

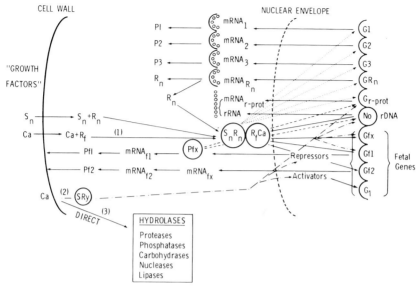

Fig. 7 Effects of carcinogenic agents on cellular responses. It is envisioned that carcinogens permit structural genes to function in the production of normal products but that, through several mechanisms, fetal genes are activated to produce a variety of fetal products, including Pf1 and Pf2, which are important to invasiveness and metastasis. The carcinogen may act with a fetal receptor to interact directly with the genome or may cause a new stimulus within the cell to interact with a receptor that will interact with the genome. Alternatively, the carcinogen may interfere with degradative reactions involved in normal growth controls. Ca, carcinogen; see Fig. 4 for other symbols.

becomes a cancer cell is thrown into genomic disarray leading to the dysplasia referred to by Sugimura (1976). Carcinogens may destroy most affected cells. Others undergo a wide variety of phenotypic alterations ranging from total loss of phenotypic function to excessive production of specialized products. At some crucial time, the genome becomes "set" for its altered functional activity in which both fetal and specialized genes are expressed (Fig. 8). In recent studies from this laboratory, it appears that in cancer cells the genome set occurs even before telophase has been completed (Busch *et al.*, 1979).

The cancer cells that emerge from the oncogenic event have a fundamental fixed mechanism that includes the operation of fetal genes. In these cells, many normal receptors are deleted (Fig. 8). Other receptors may be produced (R_n or R_z). However, the key genes, Pfx, Pf1, and Pf2, that are derepressed represent the fetal gene elements that are the key to the biology of cancer, including cell growth and division, invasiveness,

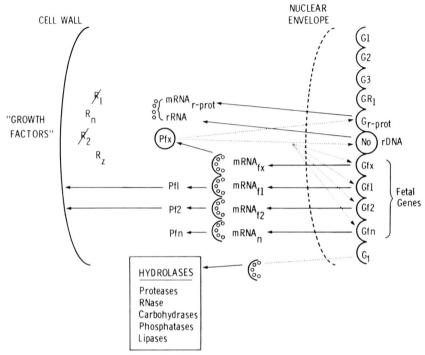

Fig. 8 This diagram indicates the expression of cancer as a continuous production of gene products involved in growth, invasiveness, and metastasis. Such cells no longer produce R_1, R_2 (blocked, $\mathcal{R}_1$, $\mathcal{R}_2$), or other products that may have phenotypic specificity. It is envisioned that these gene products and their derepressors are produced or maintained in high concentration throughout mitosis and keep these genes activated during new cell formation. Moreover, the lack of fetal extracellular regulatory mechanisms does not permit these genes to be inactivated as they would be during fetal growth and development. See Fig. 4 for other symbols.

and metastasis. The cellular mechanisms involved and their control are the primary interests of the following elements of our program (Busch, 1976a).

II. The Cell Nucleus

Much new information has accumulated on the structures (Figs. 9 and 10) and products of the cell nucleus (Tables I and II) (Busch, 1974; Elgin and Weintraub, 1975; Stein and Kleinsmith, 1975; Busch, 1978a,b,c).

For the purpose of the present chapter, the topic is segregated into four general divisions: (1) the structure and content of the cell nucleus, (2)

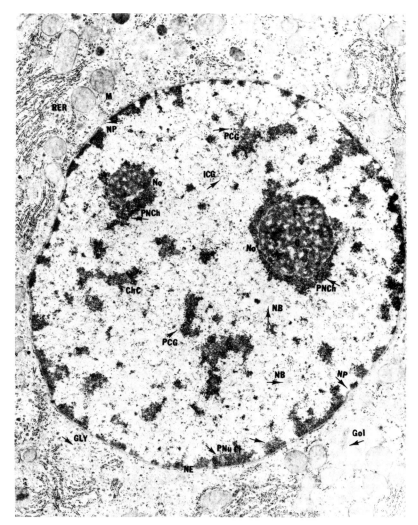

Fig. 9 Electron micrograph of a rat liver cell nucleus. Within the nucleus, nucleoli (No) are surrounded by perinucleolar chromatin (PNCh). The nucleoli consist of granular (G) and fibrillar (F) elements. Chromocenters (ChC) are distributed randomly within the nucleoplasm. Frequently, perichromatin granules (PCG) are associated with these chromocenters. Within the nucleus nuclear bodies (NB) and interchromatin granules (ICG) are occasionally seen that are apparently cross sections of the nuclear RNP network. The inner layer of the nuclear envelope (NE) surrounds a conspicuous layer of dense chromatin (PNuCh). The clear areas within this heterochromatin layer usually mark the location of the nuclear pores (NP). In the cytoplasm, glycogen elements (GLY) are present. Mitochondria (M) and rough endoplasmic reticulum (RER) are distributed throughout the cytoplasm. Occasionally Golgi (Gol) complexes are seen around the nuclear periphery. Lead citrate–uranyl acetate staining. × 18,000. Courtesy of T. Unuma and Y. Daskal.

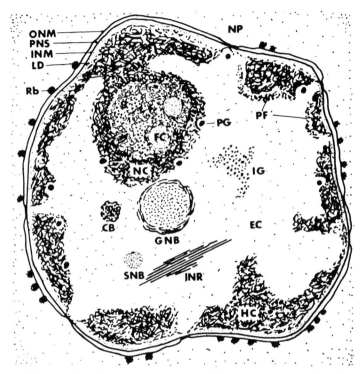

Fig. 10 Ideal section of a nucleus, showing all the main components. The nucleus is surrounded by the outer (ONM) and inner nuclear (INM) membranes that enclose the perinuclear space (PNS) which is a part of the rough endoplasmic reticulum and has ribosomes (Rb) attached. Between the chromatin and the inner membrane lies the lamina densa (LD) which is thinner in front of the nuclear pores (NP). The chromatin is found as heterochromatin (HC), nucleolus-associated chromatin (NC), and euchromatin (EC). The nucleolus shows the granular (g) components and fibrillar centers (FC). In the borderline of the chromatin, many perichromatin granules (PG) and a layer of perichromatin fibrils (PF) (of which only a portion has been drawn) are found. Finally, in the interchromatin space, a cluster of interchromatin granules (IG), a granular nuclear body (GNB), a simple nuclear body (SNB), a coiled body (CB), and an intranuclear rodlet (INR) are seen. (From Bouteille *et al.*, 1974.)

chromatin, its constituents, and the synthesis of mRNA, (3) the nucleolus and synthesis of rRNA, and (4) special features of the nucleolus of cancer cells.

In any consideration of the nucleus, it should be recalled that, whether it represents a small structure in a large cell or a giant structure in a relatively small cell, there is always a layer of cytoplasm, no matter how small, between it and the cell's plasma membrane. This structure plays an important role in the feedback interactions of the nucleus with the whole

TABLE I

Nuclear Structures[a]

Nuclear envelope
  Outer layer—continuation of the endoplasmic reticulum
  Inner layer
  Nuclear pores
  Juxtaenvelope chromatin
Chromatin—chromosomes
  Interphase chromatin
    Euchromatin—dispersed chromatin
    Heterochromatin—condensed chromatin
  Meiotic chromatin
    Chromatin in various states of condensation
    Defined metaphase chromosomes
The nucleolus
  Nucleoli in various stages of cell function
  Nucleolar chromosomes
  rDNA and its controls
  Pre-rRNA
  Interlocks of rRNA and ribosomal protein synthesis
  The nucleolar channel system
Nuclear RNP network
Nuclear particles
  Perichromatin granules
  Interchromatin granules
  Nuclear bodies
  Nuclear rodlets
  Nuclear inclusions
  mRNP precursor particles (informosomes)

[a] From Busch et al (1975).

array of stimuli to which the cell is exposed (Figs. 3B, 4, and 9). In this sense, the nucleus is part of an integrated system by which cells of various organs respond to extracellular and intracellular stimuli (Fig. 5). These stimuli interact with the nuclear informational system to produce specific products (Table II) that permit response of the cytoplasm to the environment and its functional demands. The charm of the cell nucleus rests in the remarkable variety of its potential products which alter cellular function so remarkably from tissue to tissue and organ to organ (Busch, 1974).

A. The Role of the Cell Nucleus

The nucleus contains the major repository of genetic information, chromatin, which comprises DNA and its associated proteins. Very small amounts of DNA are in the mitochondria and, if there is a significant amount of DNA in the cell membrane or the endoplasmic reticulum, it is

TABLE II

Nuclear Products[a]

DNA
  Complete DNA replication during cell division
  Gene amplification or repetition
RNA
  mRNA
    mRNA sequences
    poly(A) 3'-termini
    The 5'-cap (? nucleus)
  rRNA
    28 S rRNA
    18 S rRNA
    5.8 S rRNA
    5 S rRNA
  tRNA
    tRNA nucleotide sequence
    Many modified tRNA nucleotides
  LMWN RNA
    Uridine-rich nuclear RNA U1, U2, U3
    Other species including 4.5 S RNA_{I-III}, 5 S RNA_{III}, 8 S RNA
  Precursor-processing reactions for each RNA species
RNP particles
  mRNP particles
  Informosomes
  Polysomes
  rRNA particles
  Granular nucleolar elements
  Completed ribosomes

---

[a] From Busch *et al* (1975).

at such a low level that thus far reports of its presence have not been uniformly reproducible. The genetic information of the cell nucleus becomes operational in the form of polysomes which contain mRNA (template RNA), ribosomes, and associated biosynthetic elements (Table II).

A major question in cell and molecular biology concerns the nature of the control systems that regulate the genome. Since the DNA is the same in virtually all cells of an individual (red blood cells and haploid cells excepted), it remains totipotent throughout the life of the cell (Gurdon, 1974). The substances that govern the gene readouts must be derived from the cytoplasm or external cellular milieu directly or by interaction with appropriate receptor or carrier molecules that interact with gene loci. The mechanisms of transport and function of these substances are discussed later.

Many beautiful light microscope studies have been made on nuclei and nucleoli (Busch and Smetana, 1970; Montgomery, 1898). Recent elegant advances in scanning and electron microscopy have provided improved two- and three-dimensional analyses of the nuclear structures as well as their spatial interrelationships (Table I). The fundamental structure of the cell nucleus is rather simple. As seen in Figs. 9 and 10, isolated nuclei essentially consist of a highly permeable double-layered envelope which circumscribes a semihomogeneous structure. The basic nuclear framework is the nuclear ribonucleoprotein (RNP) network (nuclear matrix), the hub of which is the nucleolus (Fig. 9). The nuclear envelope and the nuclear matrix provide both the basic elements of nuclear structure and the sites of attachment of critical nuclear elements (Figs. 9 and 10). In general, the nucleus may be considered a unit structure containing an internal matrix surrounded by a double-layered envelope of high porosity (Franke and Scheer, 1974).

Although at one time the nucleus was thought to be an amorphous structure, with the exception of the nucleoli, improved methods have shown that it contains a series of particulate structures (Bouteille *et al.*, 1974) that play special and important roles in its function (Figs. 9 and 10).

B. The Double-Layered Nuclear Envelope

The nuclear envelope (Fig. 5) consists of two portions, the outer layer, which is frequently covered by ribosomes and is in intimate contact with the cytoplasm and endoplasmic reticulum, and the inner layer, which is composed of membrane and is in turn in contact with chromatin and the nuclear elements. The two layers regularly join at the nuclear pores which are shown in cross section and on-end in Fig. 11. These structures are not simply holes in the nuclear wall (like holes in a whiffle ball) but rather have been shown to contain a number of elements arranged in a highly ordered form (Franke and Scheer, 1974). Many studies are in progress on the nuclear envelope in the hope of discerning more about its semipermeable character with respect to substances being added to the nucleus and the mechanism of penetration of large particles and other elements out of the nucleus into the cytoplasm. While the nucleus is continuously "sensing" cytoplasmic activity, its response is in the form of large particles that must pass through the "retaining wall" of the nuclear envelope. Presumably the nuclear pores serve the function of permitting such large "packages" to migrate out of the nucleus into the cytoplasm. Some electron microscope pictures support this suggestion (Fig. 12).

Chromatin is a complex of nuclear DNA, its associated proteins, RNA, and small molecules (Busch *et al.*, 1975). Chromatin is the interphase state of the chromosomes (Figs. 13 and 14); it has enormous complexity

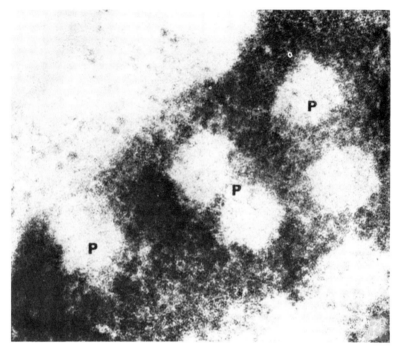

Fig. 11 Vertical section through the nuclear envelope at the nuclear pores (P). (From Franke and Scheer, 1974.)

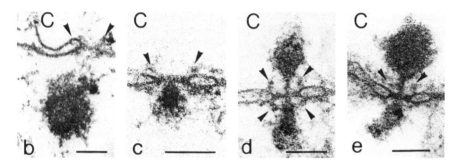

Fig. 12 In (b-e) the possible sequence of events is shown for penetration of the pore complexes (some annular granules are denoted by arrowheads): the large globule approaches the pore complex and becomes connected to it by thin filaments; it then reaches the pore center (b) and elongates into a 100 to 150-Å broad rod; the material passes the pore center in this rodlike form, transitorily assuming a typical dumb-bell-shaped configuration (c); then the material rounds into a spheroid particle (d) and is deposited by the cytoplasmic side, for some time still revealing fibrillar connections. C, Cytoplasmic side. (A) ×83,000. (B) ×135,000. (C) ×110,000. (D) ×100,000. Scale bars in (A–D) indicate 0.1 μm. (From Franke and Scheer, 1974.)

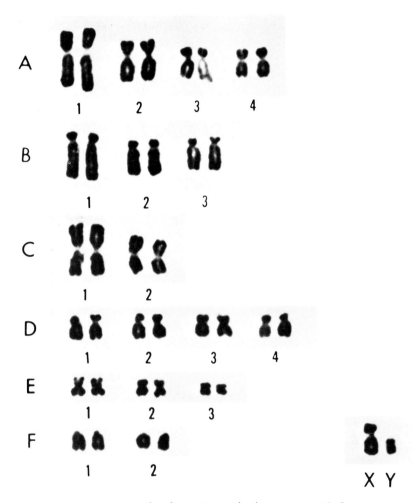

Fig. 13 Normal karyotype showing metacentric chromosomes (A, C, and E), achrocentric chromosomes (B, D, and F), and chromosomes X and Y.

and unusual properties. The basic problems in the manipulation of chromatin relate to the difficulties in handling chemical evaluations of molecules of such enormous size as DNA, which are now generally believed to be as long as chromatids.

The task of sorting out a specific DNA cistron in an intact form from such structures has challenged many investigators and, except for rare cases, such as the amplified and segregated ribosomal DNA (rDNA) found in some satellites, individual DNA species have not been isolated from chromatin.

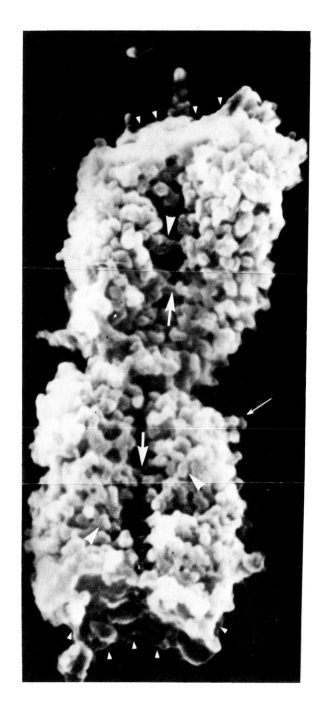

The histones in chromatin are approximately equal in weight to the DNA and, further, DNA is closely associated with histones in somatic cells. Accordingly, it appeared that the histones had a critical structural or stabilizing role, particularly since the number of positive charges on the histones were roughly equal to the number of negative charges on the DNA.

This very interesting equivalence has been subjected to much reappraisal in recent years by virtue of the demonstration that there were significant interactions between histones that were sufficient in themselves to produce small nuclear bodies referred to as nu bodies (Olins and Olins, 1974). These nu bodies are apparently composed of histone subunits, i.e., two molecules each of histones 2A, 2B, 3, and 4 and, further, they may be related to structures also containing histone 1. Nu bodies were originally reported to be "beads on a string" (Fig. 15) in extended chromatin structures. Many studies have led to development of the model (Fig. 16) showing that nu bodies are composed of one and one-half DNA turns surrounding the core octamer of the four histones noted above (Pardon and Richards, 1979).

The role of the nu bodies is undefined. There is a random distribution of nu bodies in both transcribed and untranscribed chromatin. Moreover, virtually all liver sequences transcribed into mRNA are present in nu body-associated DNA. Accordingly, nu body formation is random with respect to DNA sequence, and the nu bodies in any specific DNA region do not restrict transcription.

C. Nonhistone Nuclear Proteins

The definition of nuclear proteins, although apparently obvious, has been the subject of considerable methodological evaluation. Needless to say, what is called a nuclear protein is dependent upon the technique employed for isolation of the nuclei (Fig. 17). It is well recognized that most nuclear proteins (if not all) are synthesized in the cytoplasm and must be present there in small amounts at some point (Comings and Tack, 1973). The early controversy involving "contractile" proteins reported to be present in the cell nucleus (LeStourgeon et al., 1975; Douvas et al., 1975)

Fig. 14 Scanning electron micrograph of whole-mount isolated Chinese hamster ovary metaphase chromosome 2. Membranous platelike structures (small arrowheads) connect both chromatids only at their distal ends. Multiple interchromatidal connections (large arrows) are seen in the interchromatidal furrow. Highly coiled topical "microconvules" (large arrowheads) and axial coilings (small arrows) are present. × 65,000. (From Daskal et al., 1976.)

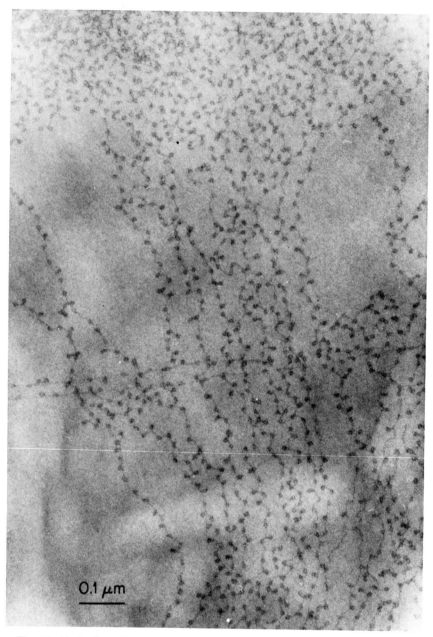

Fig. 15 Nu bodies. Chromatin fibers streaming out of a rat thymus nucleus. The spheroid chromatin units (nu bodies) exhibit local variations in arrangement and separation, possibly due to differential stretching of the fibers. Negative stain, 0.5% ammonium molybdate, pH 7.4 ×326,000. (From Busch *et al.,* 1975.)

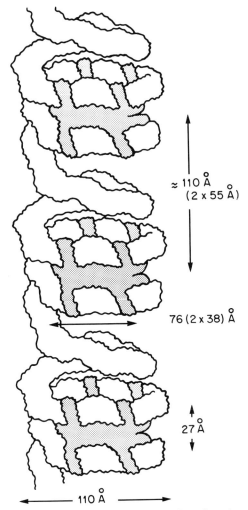

Fig. 16 Diagrammatic representation of interrelation of nucleosomes in chromatin (Pardon and Richards, 1979).

had arisen from the failure of some groups to isolate nuclei in a satisfactory form. As a result, proteins limited to the cytoplasm have been reported to be present in nuclei. The failure to employ satisfactory procedures for nuclear isolation (Busch and Smetana, 1970) results in preparations that confuse the complex problems of nuclear protein chemistry (Comings and Harris, 1975).

It became clear in 1963 (Steele and Busch, 1963) that nonhistone pro-

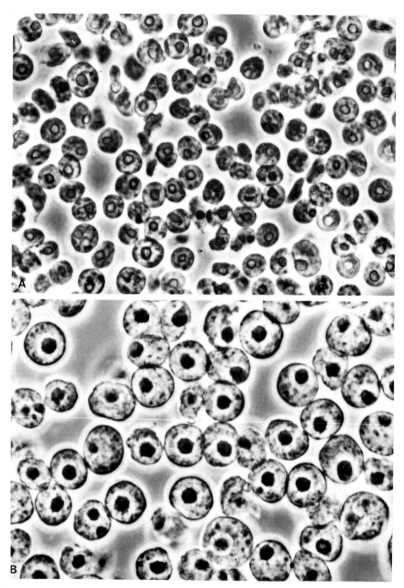

Fig. 17 Phase microscopy of a preparation of isolated nuclei of Morris hepatoma 9618. (A) × 600. (B) × 1100. (From Busch and Smetana, 1970.)

teins were a very heterogeneous series of molecular species, including proteins of the nuclear envelope, nuclear sap, chromatin, and nucleolus (Table III). In each of these groups there are a number of important subgroups that include various enzymes, phosphoproteins, processing enzymes, and transport elements (Busch *et al.*, 1975; Busch, 1965).

The greatest interest in recent years has centered on proteins that are

TABLE III
Nuclear Nonhistone Proteins[a]

Nuclear membrane proteins
  Structural proteins
  Transport proteins
  Processing enzymes
  Nuclear pore proteins
Nuclear sap proteins
  Cytonucleoproteins
    Receptors, normal and modified
    RNP particle proteins
      Small U1 and U2 RNA
      Samarina particles
    Informosomes
  Phosphoproteins
  Enzymes
Chromatin-bound proteins
  Solubility classification
    Acid-soluble
      Acid-soluble
      Acid-insoluble
        Solubilized by DNase
        DNase residue
    Soluble in dilute NaCl
    Solubility in concentrated NaCl
      Soluble in 2 M NaCl
      Soluble in 3 M NaCl 7 M urea
  Soluble in phenol
  Soluble in SDS
  Structural proteins
  Gene control proteins
  Phosphoproteins
  Enzymes
Nucleolar proteins
  Ribosomal precursor proteins
  Structural proteins
  rDNA control proteins
  Phosphoproteins
  Enzymes

[a] From Busch *et al*, 1975.

chromatin-associated, largely because of the finding of Paul and Gilmour (1966a,b, 1968) and subsequently many other workers that gene control proteins were present in these fractions (Table IV). Evidence that gene control proteins were in chromatin was obtained by preextraction of "citric acid" nuclei with a dilute salt solution (0.15 M NaCl–0.1 M Tris) followed by distilled water to swell the chromatin. Following these extractions the residue, called chromatin, was demonstrated to exhibit fidelity of transcription by analysis of products produced after incubation with RNA polymerase and appropriately labeled nucleoside triphosphates. The products formed were then hybridized in competition studies with the RNA of specific tissues.

The key demonstration was that, on reconstitution of the chromatin initially disassociated with high salt (2 M NaCl, 5 M urea, 0.01 M Tris, pH 8.3) and reconstitution with histones, DNA, and nonhistone products in interrupted gradients of salt and urea, the RNA readouts were characteristic of the tissue or origin of the nonhistone proteins and not of the DNA or the histones. Many subsequent findings have supported and extended these conclusions (Table IV).

TABLE IV
Evidence for Specificity of Nonhistone Proteins [a]

Test system [b]	References
Organ-specific transcription of chromatin	Paul and Gilmour (1966a,b, 1968)
Tissue-specific restriction of DNA	Richter and Sekeris (1972); Kamiyama et al. (1972)
Tissue-specific binding of progesterone receptor	Steggles et al. (1971)
Mechanism of action of female sex hormones	Jensen and DeSombre (1972)
NHPs in chromatin—organ specificity	Gilmour and Paul (1970)
Tumor transcriptional specificity, regenerating liver specificity	Kostraba and Wang (1972a,b, 1973); Kadohama and Turkington (1973)
Tissue specificity of NHPs	Barrett and Gould (1973); Orrick et al. (1973); Yeoman et al. (1973a,b)
Antigenic specificity of chromatin	Chytil and Spelsberg (1971); Spelsberg et al. (1971a–d); Zardi et al. (1973)
Specificity of mitotic proteins	Rovera and Baserga (1971); Rovera et al. (1971); Stein et al. (1972)
Phosphoproteins in gene regulation	Teng et al. (1971)
Stimulation of synthesis by phytohemagglutinin	Levy et al. (1973); Pogo and Katz (1974)

[a] From Busch et al. (1975).
[b] NHPs, Nonhistone proteins.

The studies on binding of hormones to nonhistone proteins have been most interesting in this respect. The work of Jensen and his associates (Jensen and DeSombre, 1972) on estrogen–receptor interaction initiated the series of studies in this field. The recent studies (O'Malley and Schrader, 1976) of O'Malley's group (O'Malley and Means, 1974) have shown a relationship between the steroid hormone–receptor complex and the production of special mRNA related to oviduct proteins.

Nonhistone proteins serve very important enzymic functions (Table V), and some have interesting nuclear localizations as suggested by Vorbrodt (1974). Evidence that some of these proteins bind to mRNA has been accumulating.

TABLE V

Nuclear Enzymes[a]

RNA synthesis and processing
RNA polymerases A, B, and so on
RNA modification enzymes; methylases, formation of modified bases
RNA trimming or special cleavage enzymes
RNases; exo-and endonucleolytic
DNA synthesis
True synthetases
Ligases
Excision enzymes
Terminal addition enzymes
DNases
Modification enzymes; methylases, and so on.
Other modification and synthetic enzymes
Histone phosphokinases, methylases, acetylases, deacetylases, proteases
Nonhistone protein kinases and methylases
Nucleoside kinases
NAD pyrophosphorylase
Dehydrogenases
Steroid dehydrogenase
Cytochrome oxidase
Glycerol-3-phosphate dehydrogenases
Glyceraldehyde-3-phosphate dehydrogenase
Succinate, malate, isocitrate, lactate, NADH, NADPH, glucose 6-phosphate, phosphogluconate
Transferases: glycosyl for glycogen phosphorylases and branching enzymes
Enzymes of uncertain function
ATPases
Carboxylesterases
Phosphatases
5'-Nucleotidases
Phosphodiesterase

[a] From Busch et al. (1975).

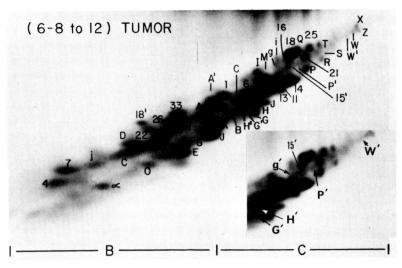

Fig. 18 Two-dimensional polyacrylamide gel electrophoresis patterns of chromatin proteins (G. I. Busch *et al.*, 1974). The horizontal dimension is on 8% acid–urea gel, and the vertical dimension is 8.12% sodium dodecyl sulfate (SDS) gel.

D. Links between Nonhistone Proteins and Histones

Two-dimensional gel electrophoresis methods for nuclear proteins (Figs. 18–20) have led to the unequivocal demonstration that there are very large numbers of these molecules, i.e., in excess of 400 species (G. I. Busch *et al.*, 1974; Orrick *et al.*, 1973; Peterson and McConkey, 1967a,b; Yeoman *et al.*, 1973a,b). Continuing efforts to isolate and identify individual nuclear proteins have led to the demonstration of new high-mobility group (HMG) proteins by Goodwin *et al.* (1975, 1978). A particularly interesting protein, A24 (Fig. 19), named on the basis of its migration on two-dimensional gel electrophoresis, is a conjugated form of histone 2A, with ubiquitin bound to it in an isopeptide linkage (Goldknopf *et al.*, 1977; Olson *et al.*, 1976).

Although the functional role of this protein is not yet known, it seems possible that the nonhistone arm (ubiquitin) may be cleaved from the 2A histone in the course of gene activation (Fig. 21).

The functions of nonhistone proteins have not yet been completely evaluated. Important developments in this area include two-dimensional

Fig. 19 Composite picture of the separation of acid-soluble nucleolar proteins by two-dimensional gel electrophoresis (Orrick *et al.*, 1973); 10% acid–urea horizontal dimension, 12% SDS vertical dimension.

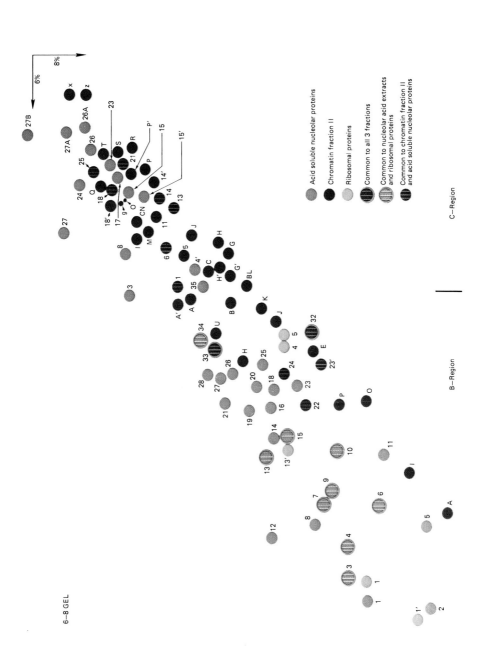

6–8 GEL

6%

8%

27B

x
z
26A
27A
23
26
T
S
R
P'
25
27
Q
24
18
17
18'
g
O
15
P
15'
8
I
M
CN
14'
14
11
6
13
J
5
4'
H
A'
1
35
C
G
A
H'
G'
B
BL
K
3
J
34
U
32
33
26
H
5
28
25
4
E
27
20
24
23'
21
18
23
19
16
22
P
O
14
15
10
11
13
13'
I
12
9
8
7
6
A
4
5
3
1
1'
1
2

● Acid soluble nucleolar proteins

● Chromatin fraction II

● Ribosomal proteins

◉ Common to all 3 fractions

⊜ Common to nucleolar acid extracts and ribosomal proteins

⊟ Common to chromatin fraction II and acid soluble nucleolar proteins

C—Region

B—Region

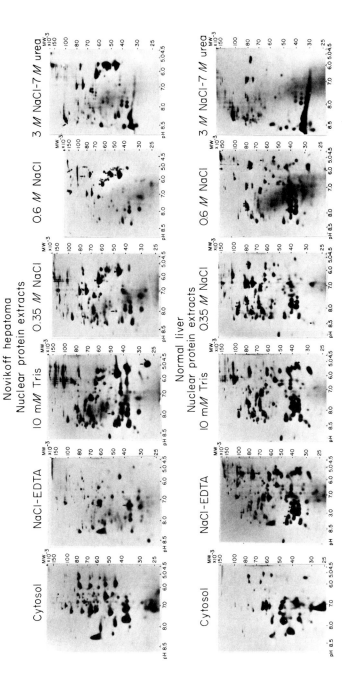

Fig. 20 Composite of two-dimensional gel electrophoresis of the proteins of various nuclear fractions obtainable by salt fractionation using the two-dimensional gel electrophoresis procedure of Hirsch *et al.* (1978) as developed by Takami and Busch (1979). First dimension, 4% isoelectric focusing gel; second dimension, 8% SDS gel.

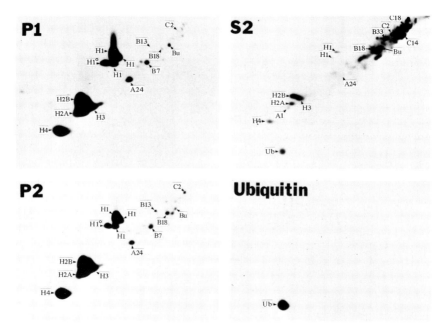

Fig. 21 Two-dimensional polyacrylamide gel electrophoretic fractionation of 500 μg each of 0.4 N H₂SO₄-soluble proteins and 25 μg of ubiquitin. The gels were obtained using proteins from pellet (P1 and P2) and supernatant (S2) chromatin fractions, as well as known samples of purified ubiquitin (lower right). Electrophoresis was from right to left in the first dimension and from top to bottom in the second. Courtesy of Dr. I. L. Goldknopf.

gel electrophoresis using diagonal systems, which show the presence of unique proteins in experimental tumors (Fig. 18, inset arrows), and extended studies on the system differentiated among histones, extranucleolar nuclear proteins, ribosomal proteins, and proteins of chromatin fraction 2 (Fig. 19).

More recently, using another two-dimensional technique (Hirsch *et al.*, 1978), it has been possible to separate over 400 nuclear proteins (Fig. 20) of various cells (Takami and Busch, 1979). The proteins have been separated in part by salt fractionation of the nuclei.

Additional techniques such as labeling with ³²P have permitted identification and demonstration of separable tumor phosphoproteins (Fig. 22).

E. The Nucleolus

The portion of the nucleus that synthesizes about 85% of all cellular RNA is the nucleolus (Fig. 23), which plays an essential role in the production of new ribosomes (Busch and Smetana, 1970). The nucleolus is

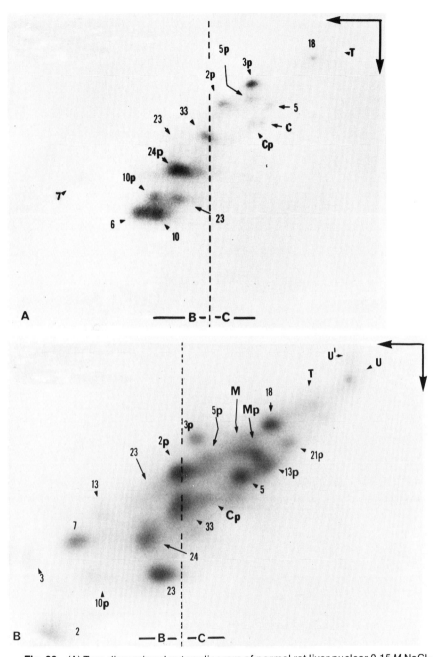

Fig. 22 (A) Two-dimensional autoradiogram of normal rat liver nuclear 0.15 M NaCl-soluble proteins. Samples were run in the first dimension on 9.5-cm tube gels of 6% acrylamide: 4.5 M urea–0.9 N acid at 120 V for 5.5 hours. The second dimension was 8% acrylamide–0.1% SDS–0.1 M phosphate (pH 7.1) slab gel. Gels were stained with Coomassie brilliant blue R after 15 hours of electrophoresis at 50 mA/slab. After destaining, the gels were subsequently dried under vacuum and exposed to X-ray film for 5–15 days. After development, the stained spots were matched with spots on the film. Numbers followed by "p" indicate radioactive spots that do not comigrate with stained spots. (B) Two-dimensional autoradiogram of Novikoff hepatoma nuclear protein soluble in 0.15 M NaCl–0.01 M Tris – 0.001 M phenylmethylsulfonyl fluoride.

the product of nucleolus organizer regions (NORs) of chromatin (Fig. 24), which apparently contain the rDNA and the specific sites of structural organization for interlocking nucleolar protein and RNA products.

The nucleolus is the sole cellular location of very specific cellular and nuclear components (Table VI). One of the most remarkable facets of nucleolar function is production of the enormous nucleotide chains (MW 12,000) of 45 S rRNA which are synthesized by RNA polymerase I (Chambon *et al.*, 1974; Roeder and Rutter, 1969, 1970) with great rapidity on repetitive genes and, in addition, are methylated, cleaved, and modified as the molecules are formed. In addition, the nucleolus is a site of protein binding to the newly synthesized RNA to form the nucleolar granular elements (Fig. 9). These granular elements are the RNP products of the nucleolus (Fig. 9), which after isolation by various procedures have been shown to contain modified long pre-rRNA chains and, in addition, proteins that migrate to cytoplasmic ribosomes and others that do not.

Further maturation of nucleolar products is believed to occur in the nuclear RNP network (Busch and Smetana, 1970) which may provide the locus for joining additional ribosomal and polysomal proteins to these preribosomal elements to complete the fully matured polysomes.

The fibrillar elements of the nucleolus (Fig. 9) apparently provide the matrix composed of rDNA, RNA polymerase I, and juxtaposed enzymes which produce the éarliest stages of synthesis of pre-RNA.

F. rDNA

Beginning with the demonstration of the NOR by Heitz (1933) and the extended studies of McClintock (1934, 1961), further studies have been made on nucleolar DNA in a wide variety of species (Busch and Smetana, 1970). The secondary constrictions or NOR in chromosomes have been described earlier (Fig. 24). The presence in the nucleolus of several classes of DNA has been demonstrated by light and electron microscope techniques and special stains (Fig. 24B). Some DNA regions can be geographically segregated into perinucleolar chromatin and intranucleolar chromatin. rDNA can (Fig. 25) also be subfractioned into condensed and dispersed nucleolar chromatin. In essence, the precise coding chromatin for nucleolar rDNA has not yet been defined in these geographical entities.

Electron microscope analysis has been made (Busch and Smetana, 1970) of DNA within the nucleoli after specific types of digestion. The "Miller pictures" (Fig. 26), prepared using the spreading technique of Kleinschmidt (1968), have shown rRNA in the nucleolar cores of *Xenopus* and other species (Miller and Beatty, 1969). The results support the concept of tandem redundant rDNA genes transcribed simultaneously. Although these products have still not been related to chemical entities, the concept of progressive growth of chains fits well with very long final products of pre-RNA and the associated RNP.

With the development of improved hybridization techniques, attempts have been developed to establish specific information on localization of

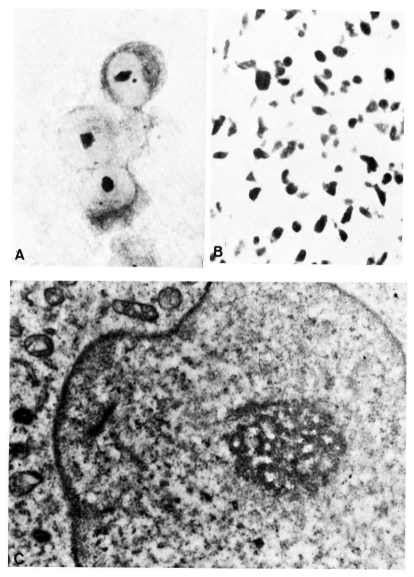

Fig. 23   (Continued)

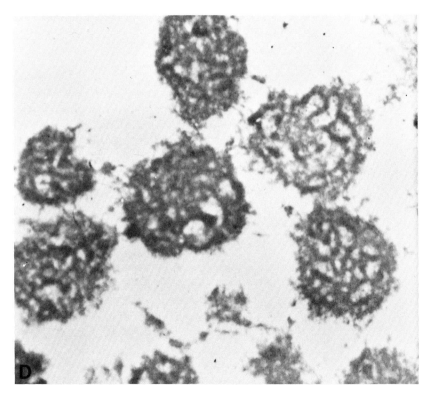

Fig. 23 (A) Smear of nuclear preparations from Walker tumor stained with toluidine blue. The nucleoli and the cytoplasmic basophilic structures are stained intensely. × 1600. (B) Smear of isolated nuclei from Walker tumor stained with toluidine blue after hydrolysis with 1 *N* HCl. Chromatin-containing structures are stained. The nucleolus is not stained, but the perinucleolar nucleolus-associated chromatin is stained. × 1600. Courtesy of Professor K. Smetana. (C) Electron micrograph of liver nuclei showing a magnified nucleus. (D) Isolated liver nucleoli showing morphological similarities to nucleolus in (C).

Fig. 24 (A) Chromosomes of a number of species with secondary constrictions. The arrows represent the positions of the constrictions. (a) *Spilogale putorius* (spotted skunk); (b) *Mephitis mephitis* (striped skunk); (c) *Mustela putorius* (ferret); (d) *Felis catus* (domestic cat); (e) *Cervus canadensis* (elk); (f) *Sus scorfa* (domestic pig); (g) *Carollia perspicillata* (fruit bat); (h) *Pipistrellus subflavus* (Eastern pipestrelle); (i) *Tamiasciurus hudsonicus* (red squirrel); (j) *Chinchilla laniger* (chinchilla); (k) *Tupaia glis* (tree shrew); (l) *Alouatta caraya* (black howler); (m) *Homo sapiens* (human). Courtesy of Professor T. C. Hsu, M. D. Anderson Hospital, Houston, Texas. (B) Silver-stained Novikoff hepatoma cells showing nucleus in metaphase containing NOR doublets. Another nucleus contains rows of three or more of nucleolar dense granules (see Smetana and Busch, Chapter 3). Arrowheads, doublets on NOR's; arrows, rows of granules.

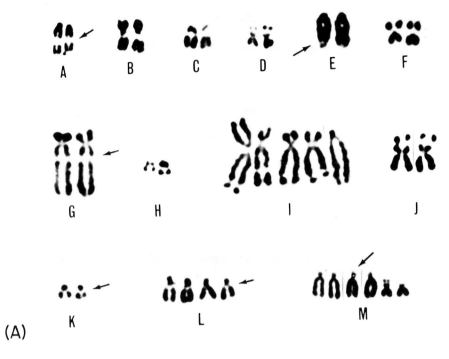

(A)

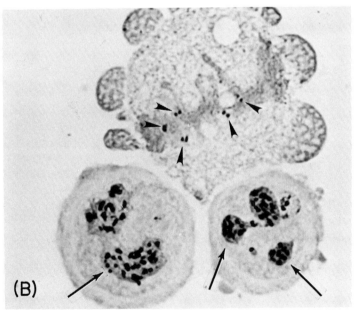

(B)

TABLE VI

Specific Nucleolar Components

rDNA
U3 low-molecular-weight RNA
Specific elements
  Fibrillar elements
  Granular elements
  Interelement spaces
Proteins
  C23—Silver stained
  B23—Silver stained

the rDNA genes. Studies in our laboratory (Sitz *et al.*, 1973) showed that the concentration of rDNA in the nucleolus of Novikoff hepatoma ascites cells was 10 times that of the rDNA throughout the remainder of the nucleus. Accordingly, it appears that the nucleoli contain 90% or more of the total rDNA.

G. Products of Nucleolar RNA

The initial RNA product of the nucleolus is 45 S pre-RNA and oligomers of sedimentation coefficients up to 85 S. By a series of unique, specific endonucleolytic cleavages, these giant nucleolar RNAs are cleaved into three major ribosome species—28, 18, and 5.8 S rRNA (Busch and Smetana, 1970).

H. Nucleolar Proteins and Control of Nucleolar Function

Nucleolar proteins can be divided into (1) structural elements including (a) histones, (b) special proteins of the preribosomal particles, and (c) ribosomal proteins; (2) enzymes of RNA synthesis (RNA polymerase I) and processing (exonucleases and endonucleases); and (3) gene control proteins.

Gene control of nucleolar function may reside in specific elements that are either phosphoproteins (see below) or other specific types of nonhistone proteins. Participation of the nucleolus in important regulatory and phase-specific events indicates that its controls are commonly more responsive than those for special mRNA species.

With the improved methods for isolation of rDNA and various binding proteins, it has now become possible to achieve a more satisfactory approach to the isolation and analysis of proteins involved in the promotion or derepression of rDNA and DNA_{r-prot}. Such studies are of great impor-

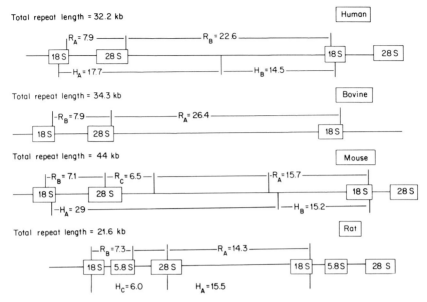

Fig. 25.   Restriction maps of rDNA: human, bovine, and mouse.

tance in understanding both the production of most cellular RNA and the specific controls on a major gene set.

At one time, the nucleolus was considered a simple structure with a small number of elements. The development of technology for determination of the numbers and types of these constutuents has led to the view that the nucleolus contains approximately 200 species of proteins (Orrick *et al.*, 1973). Two-dimensional polyacrylamide gel electrophoresis (Fig. 27) has established that, in addition to all the varieties of histones, approximately 90 nonhistone proteins are extractable from nucleoli with $0.4\ N\ H_2SO_4$. Another group of proteins is acid-insoluble but is extractable under conditions that require solvents that dissociate hydrogen bonds and destroy hydrophobic molecular interactions. The RNA polymerase I that is uniquely localized to the nucleolus accounts for several polypeptides which are presumably enzyme subunits. There are also many proteins that are elements of the nucleolar RNPs of the granular elements and the ribosomes.

Of the nuclear phosphoproteins (Stein *et al.*, 1972; Stein and Kleinsmith, 1975), one is specifically localized to the nucleolus, i.e., protein C18, a recently described nucleolus-specific phosphoprotein (Fig. 28) which apparently accounts for the bulk of ^{32}P incorporated into nucleolar proteins (Olson *et al.*, 1974, 1975). This protein may be related to silver

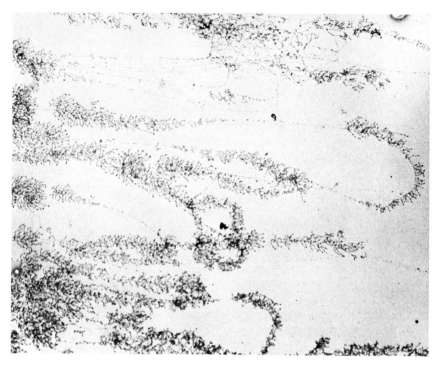

Fig. 26 Miller picture of "Christmas trees" of nucleolar rRNA readouts, synthesized preribosomal RNP elements. Courtesy of Dr. O. L. Miller.

staining of the C23 nucleolus and its granules (Smetana and Busch, 1979; Busch *et al.*, 1979).

1. Silver-Stained Nucleolar Proteins

Recently, a rapid silver staining technique specific for NORs, nucleoli, and nucleolar satellites was developed to provide cytochemical analysis of argyrophilic nucleolar structures and to analyze quantitative changes in highly argyrophilic nucleolar elements in hepatocytes and other cells (Smetana and Busch, 1979). Quantitative analysis of the numbers of dense highly argyrophilic granules in the nuclei and nucleoli of cells with varying nucleolar function and growth rate indicated that the largest numbers of grains (21 per nucleolus) were in rapidly dividing tumor cells and the smallest numbers were in mature lymphocytes (1.3 per nucleolus). In the normal liver there were 4.2 grains per nucleolus, and this number increased to 7.8 and 13.7 in the regenerating liver 6 and 18 hours posthepatectomy.

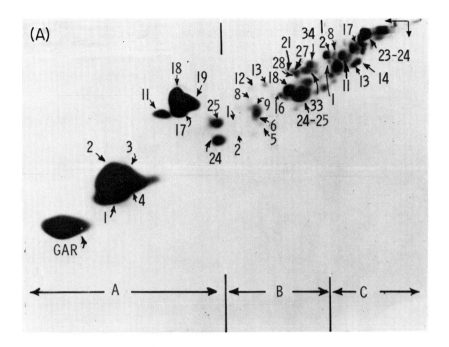

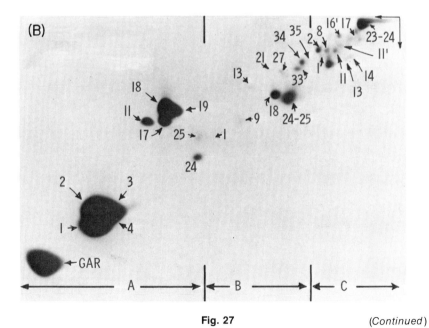

Fig. 27   (Continued)

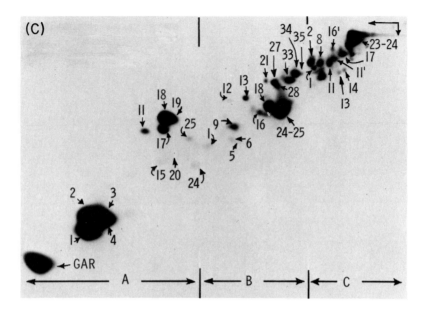

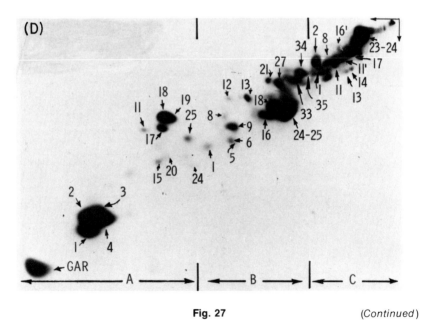

Fig. 27   (Continued)

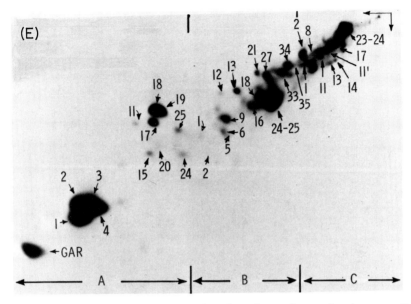

Fig. 27 Two-dimensional gel electrophoretic patterns of normal and regenerating liver nucleolar proteins (Orrick *et al*, 1973). Marked changes were found in the concentration of proteins A11, A24, C13, and C14 from the normal levels (A), 4 hour (B), 8 hour (C), 24 hour (D), and 48 hour (E) of regenerating liver.

In Novikoff hepatoma, KB, and HeLa cells, some of the arrays of nucleolar argyrophilic granules consisted of linearly arranged discrete granules, and others were in two to three rows each containing three to five granules (Fig. 29A). Corresponding formations were not found in either normal or regenerating liver nucleoli. The liver nucleoli contained an argyrophilic network in which the dark argyrophilic granules were associated with the less dark fibrils of the reticulum. Interestingly, the nucleolar argyrophilic granules were readily identifiable in the separated nuclei of the tumor daughter cells in telophase, suggesting that the increased nucleolar activity of the G_1-phase began in these cells even before cell division was completed (Fig. 29B).

I. Morphological Correlates of Increased rRNA Production

The synthetic reactions of the nucleolus are catalyzed by RNA polymerase I, a specific polymerase localized to the nucleolus. The activity in synthesis of pre-rRNA varies greatly with the state of the nucleolus and the cell. In a cell such as the circulating lymphocyte there is a very small nucleolus, and the amount of rRNA produced is correspondingly very

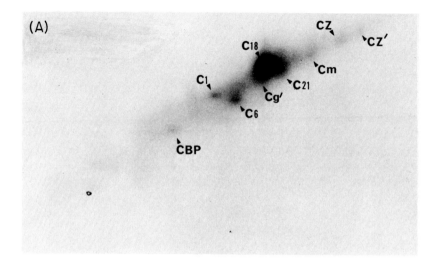

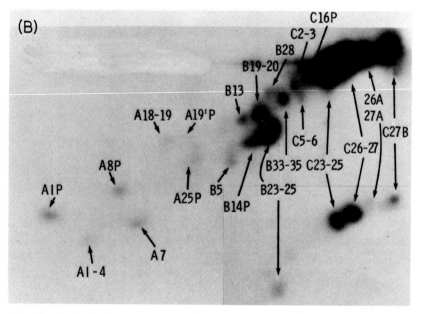

Fig. 28 Nucleolar phosphoproteins of Novikoff hepatoma ^{32}P labeled nuclear preparations chromatin showing the dense spot C18 (A) and the nucleolar extract showing dense spots of proteins C23–C25 and C26–C27 (B).

limited. The number of granular elements produced by these nucleoli is very small, and the rate of ribosome replacement is correspondingly very limited (Busch and Smetana, 1970).

The nucleolus of a normal liver is also a rather small structure; i.e., it contains relatively large amounts of fibrillar elements and relatively small amounts of granular elements. In the normal liver, the rate of production of 45 S pre-rRNA is approximately 3–5 fg/minute per nucleolus.

The nucleoli with the highest rates of production of ribosomes are the large nucleoli of rapidly growing tissues including malignant tumors, regenerating liver, "activated" lymphocytes, and nucleoli of some drug-treated cells. In thioacetamide-treated cells and in some malignant tumors, the rate of 45 S pre-rRNA biosynthesis is 40–45 fg/minute per nucleolus (Busch and Smetana, 1970).

1. Nucleolar Antigens

Nucleoli of tumor cells have been shown to differ from those of normal cells by several techniques. Morphologically, nucleoli in most neoplastic cells are larger and more irregularly shaped than those in normal cells, and such morphological differences have been diagnostically useful.

In previous work in this laboratory, nucleolus-specific antibodies were produced in rabbits immunized with whole nucleoli. Antigens (such as NoAg-1) were found in the nucleolar chromatin of Novikoff hepatoma

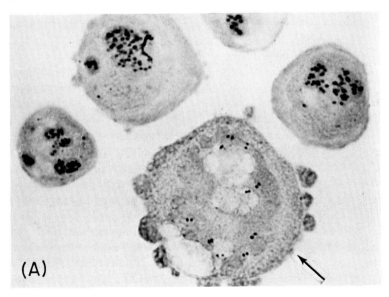

(A)

Fig. 29 (Continued)

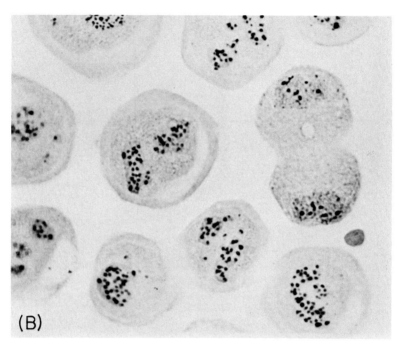

Fig. 29 (A) Silver-stained Novikoff hepatoma cells showing a large cell containing doublets of NOR spots and interphase cells with three or more granules in a row in the nucleoli. (B) Two Novikoff hepatoma cells in telophase showing many granules in the nuclei and nucleoli. These formations suggest that the G_1-phase may begin in these cells before the completion of mitosis.

ascites cells but not in those of normal liver cells; the converse was also true (Busch and Busch, 1977) (Fig. 30).

In studies designed to purify nucleolar antigens first by differential solubilization of nucleolar proteins, antigens soluble in Zubay–Doty buffer (0.075 M NaCl, 0.025 M EDTA), 10 mM Tris–HCl, and 0.6 M NaCl were isolated from normal liver and Novikoff hepatoma nucleoli and compared by Ouchterlony double immunodiffusion and immunoelectrophoresis (Davis *et al.*, 1978).

The various extracts differed both in the number of antigenic species precipitated and in the density of the immunoprecipitin bands. Four precipitin bands were found between the antiliver nucleolar antiserum (AbLi) and liver nucleolar extracts (Fig. 31). Seven distinct antigenic species were precipitated in extracts from Novikoff nucleoli by antitumor nucleolar antiserum (AbTu; Fig. 31). Some of these, such as the middle precipitin band in the RNP and chromation (Chr) fractions were found in more than one fraction.

Studies were done to determine whether antigens were mainly present in normal liver (Li), Novikoff hepatoma (Tu) nucleoli, or extracts of fetal liver nuclei (Fe) (Table VII). As shown in Table VII, one antigen was present in the tumor only, and two were present in the tumor and fetal liver and may be referred to as oncofetal antigens.

Corresponding studies on immunofluorescent nucleolar antigens have now been performed (Davis *et al.*, 1979) with a variety of human tumor and nontumor tissues, as shown in Table VIII. With antisera to HeLa cell nucleoli, positive fluorescence was obtained in each of the tumors studied. On the other hand, the nontumor tissues, except for the slowly growing WI-38 cell culture, did not exhibit positive immunofluorescence. This result is a potentially important indication of antigenic differences between nucleolar proteins of human cancer cells and of other human tissues; the implications of this result may be far-reaching.

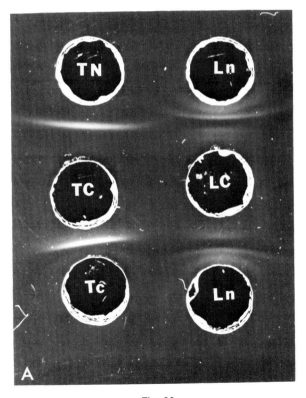

Fig. 30   (*Continued*)

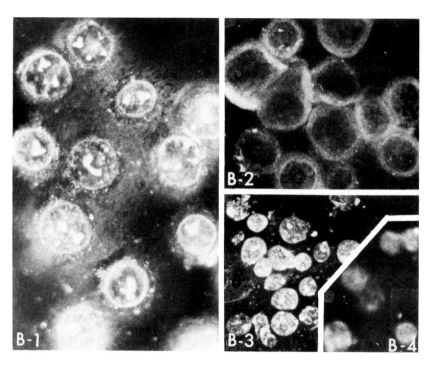

Fig. 30 (A) Immunoprecipitin bands showing that antibodies to tumor chromatin (TC) and liver chromatin (LC) formed specific immunoprecipitates with liver (Ln) and tumor (TN) nucleolar extracts. Only one dense band was found for the tumor, whereas three (or four) were found for the liver. There was no cross-immunoreactivity in these preparations (Busch and Busch, 1977). (B) Immunofluorescence of cells reacted with preabsorbed anti-nucleolar antisera. Preabsorbed antitumor nucleolar antiserum and Novikoff hepatoma cells (B-1) or normal liver cells (B-4); preabsorbed anti-liver nucleolar antiserum with Novikoff hepatoma cells (B-2) or normal liver cells (B-3). (C) Fluorescent nucleoli in HeLa cells. Acetone-treated HeLa cell smears were first incubated with rabbit immunoglobulin in the Tris extract of HeLa cell nuclei and then incubated with fluorescein-labeled goat antirabbit antibodies. (D) Nucleolar fluorescence in nuclear preparations preextracted with 0.075 M NaCl–0.025 M EDTA. TC, antibodies to tumor chromatin; TN, tumor nucleolar antigen; Tc, tumor chromatin antigen; Ln, liver nucleolar antigen; LC antibodies to liver chromatin. All photomicrographs × 1800. (Davis et al., 1978).

J. Coupled Synthesis of rRNA and mRNA$_{prot}$

In a variety of bacterial systems, evidence has been presented for coassociated ribosomal protein and rRNA synthesis (Jaskunas *et al.*, 1975; Lindahl *et al.*, 1975; Watson *et al.*, 1975). This coupling has been based in part on gene proximity, as well as on the obvious need for correlated or simultaneous synthesis. In eukaryotic cells, the synthesis of rRNA and r-proteins is only now coming under study with respect to temporal simi-

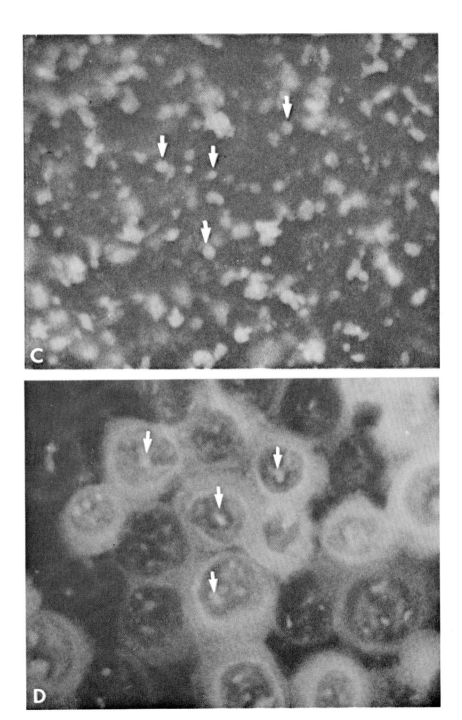

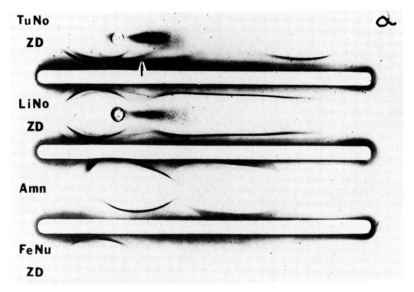

Fig. 31 Immunoelectrophoretic profile of liver, tumor, and fetal Zubay–Doty extracts and amniotic fluid. A precipitin arc in the extract from Novikoff nucleoli which is not detected in the other fractions is marked with an arrow. TuNo, tumor nucleolis; LiNo, liver nucleoli; Amn, amniotic fluid; FeNu, fetal liver nuclei. (Davis *et al.*, 1978).

larity; i.e., the likelihood that the two are made together has now been supported by evidence for increases in both products during liver regeneration (Wu *et al.*, 1977).

Although the genes for rRNA are clustered and tandomly related, the r-protein genes are not identified, and the suggestion has been made that the corresponding mRNAs are derived from a broad group of genes on various chromosomes. If this is the case, the "triggers" for their synthesis must be capable of affecting a very broad range of genes throughout

TABLE VII
Antigens Detected by Antitumor Nucleolar Antiserum

	Number of antigens found in extract[a]						
Extract	L only	T only	F only	L + T only	L + F only	T + F only	L + T + F
ZD	0	1	0	0	0	0	2
Tris	0	0	0	0	0	0	3
RNP	0	1	0	0	0	0	2
Chromatin	0	0	0	0	0	2	3
Residue	0	0	0	0	0	2	2

[a] L, Liver; T, tumor; F, fetal.

TABLE VIII

Nucleolar Immunofluorescence of Human Tissues with Antihela Nucleolar Antibodies

Positive	Negative
Carcinomas	Normal tissue
Prostatic adenocarcinoma (2)	Thyroid
Thyroid carcinoma (2)	Liver
Adenocarcinoma of the colon (3)	Kidney
Metastasis to liver (1)	Marrow hemoblastic lines (5)
Squamous cell carcinoma (10)	Normal lymphocytes (2)
Met spine	Lung (adjacent to tumor)
Met lymph node	Skin
Eccrine gland carcinoma	Placenta
Carcinoma of the esophagus	Buffy coat—blood
Carcinoma of the lung (2)	Benign growing tissues
Adenocarcinoma	Thyroid adenomas (3)
Oat cell	Prostatic hypertrophy
Basal cell carcinoma (2)	PHA-stimulated lymphocytes
Transplantable colon carcinoma	Goiter
(GW-39)	Inflammations
Sarcomas	Bullous pemphigus
Myoblastoma: primary, metastasis	Fibrosed granuloma normal lung
Osteogenic sarcoma (2)	Cirrhotic liver
Synovioma	Chronic hepatitis
Hematological neoplasms	Lupus profundus (mammary skin)
Leukemia	Glomerulonephitis
Hairy cell (spleen)	Cultures
CLL	WI-38 embryonic fibroblasts
Hodgkins' disease (Reed Sternberg,	Breast fibroblasts
lymphocytes)	False Negative
Multiple myeloma	Adenocarcinoma:
Cultures	Met brain
Carcinoma of breast	
HeLa	
Prostate carcinoma (3)	
HEp-2	
Squamous cell (3)	
Colon carcinoma	
Isolated HeLa nucleoli	

the genome. To establish the mechanisms of these activations will require extensive study, because of the numbers and types of genes that must be involved.

K. mRNA

In a sense, mRNA synthesis is the most specific function of the nucleus. The biosynthetic reactions involve complex events in enzymic and structural chemistry. Through interaction of specific nonhistone proteins with the genome, specific mRNA species are produced and transported to the cytoplasm (Fig. 32).

Many individual mRNA species have been isolated including mRNA for hemoglobin, histones, globin, ovalbumin, and insulin. The polysomes that ultimately translate mRNA into proteins are associated with a host of initiation and elongation factors (Busch *et al.*, 1976a).

L. Synthesis of mRNA

The processes involved in mRNA synthesis are apparently very similar to those for rRNA synthesis. The enzyme RNA polymerase II catalyzes

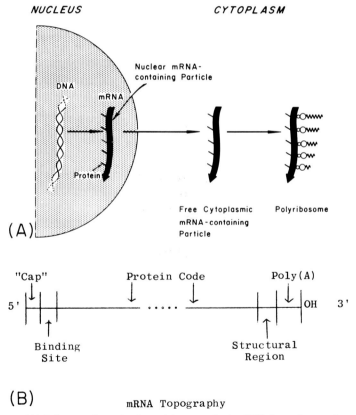

Fig. 32 (A) Scheme of synthesis and transport of mRNA from the nucleus to the cytoplasm where it functions as part of the polyribosome complex. (Courtesy of Dr. Edgar C. Henshaw, Harvard University Medical School.) (B) Topography of mRNA.

the readout of mRNA as a consequence of availability of open gene complexes. This enzyme and its associated factors link nucleoside triphosphates covalently into 3′,5′-phosphodiester bonds of mRNA. There are critical elements of the initiation reactions involved in starting these gene readouts as well as termination factors that are incompletely understood. Termination occurs when appropriate triplet codons are encountered by RNA polymerase II, but recognition proteins are apparently important to the termination process. Although mRNA is linearly synthesized in the nucleus, critical modification reactions are known to occur at each end of mRNA (Fig. 31). A large portion of the mRNA molecule becomes polyadenylated; i.e., an oligomer of approximately 200 adenylic residues is added to the 3′-end by poly(A) polymerase reactions (Busch *et al.*, 1976a,b).

Virtually all functional mRNA must contain 5′-cap structures to be active in protein synthesis (Fig. 32B). The 5′-cap is added by a series of reactions involving guanylyl transferases and methylating enzymes that form the $m^7G(5')ppp(5')Y^mpZ^mp$ cap. The formation of this cap (Busch, 1976b) occurs mainly in the nucleus and partly in the cytoplasm. The 5′-cap

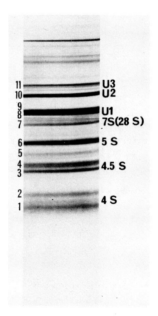

Fig. 33 Polyacrylamide gel (12%) electrophoresis of LMWN RNA from Novikoff hepatoma cell nuclei. Electrophoresis was carried out for 50 hours with a current of 40 mA at a voltage of 300 V in a buffer containing 0.02 *M* Tris–HCl (pH 7.2), 0.02 *M* NaCl, and 0.04 *M* EDTA (Ro-Choi and Busch, 1974a,b).

serves as an allosteric binding site for proteins involved in the initiation of protein synthesis or for mRNA binding directly to special ribosomal proteins (Busch *et al.*, 1975, 1976a). The specific enzyme RNA polymerase II is involved in the transcription of mRNA or DNA templates. It must be closely associated in these transcriptional events with the methylases, pyrophosphorylases, and poly(A) polymerases responsible for synthesis of the completed mRNA. In addition, there are important initiation factors and termination factors that have been identified in both bacterial and eukaryotic systems. For detailed studies on the transcription of a specific mRNA, much more sharply defined systems must be developed.

M. Low-Molecular-Weight Nuclear RNA

Special interest from both the structural and functional points of view has been recently directed to special low-molecular-weight nuclear (LMWN) RNA (Fig. 33) which differs markedly in structure from other types of cellular RNA (Busch *et al.*, 1971; Busch, 1976b; Hellung-Larsen, 1978). Studies on these molecules first revealed the remarkable 5'-cap of RNA species (Busch, 1976b). The 5'-cap of these molecules is different from the 5'-cap of mRNA by virtue of the presence of the base $m^{2,2,7}$-trimethylguanosine rather than the m^7G of mRNA in the 5'-terminal nucleotide. The presence of this base apparently eliminates the possibility that translational systems in the cytoplasm can utilize these LMWN RNA species as mRNA.

Of the three major species of LMWN RNA, one (U3 RNA) is specifically localized to the nucleolus. It does not appear to be present in any other site in the cell. Accordingly, it has been reasoned that this RNA may serve an important role in transcription of the rRNA from the rDNA templates. The number of U3 RNA molecules in the nucleolus is approximately 200,000 (0.3 attamoles or 0.2 pg/nucleolus) which is in large excess over the rDNA genes or the numbers of polymerase molecules. It is possible these are regulatory, since many kinds of control elements are present in large excess over the number of genes with which they interact; e.g., the estrogen receptors in the cell nucleus are in large excess (20,000- to 100,000-fold) over the number of gene sites available for specific readouts.

Among the suggestions for the function of the U3 RNA and other LMWN RNA are: (1) to maintain stable open gene complexes, (2) to act as critical components of the nucleolar fibrillar elements which are the presumed sites of transcription of rDNA; and (3) to form a RNP complex with subunits of RNA polymerases which transcribe RNA. Little is known about the overall sequence of the U3 RNA because the methods used to label it *in vivo* have not yielded sufficient amounts of isotope for complete structural analysis. The structure of U3 RNA is tentatively defined as:

^{2,2,7}CH$_3$G—Am—A—G—U—G—A—C—U—A—U—A—C—U—U—U—C—A—G—G—G—A—U—C—A—U—U—U—
                              10   20   30
C—U—A—U—A—G—U—C—U—G—U—U—A—C—U—A—G—A—G—A—A—G—U—U—U—C—U—C—U—G—
                              40   50   60
A—C—U—G—U—G U—A—G—A—G—C—U—G—C—C—A—C—C—G—A—G—A—C—G—A—A—A—C—A—
                              70   80   90
C—C—G—G—A—G—A—C—A—U—A—G—C—G—U—C—C—C—C—U—C—C—U—G—A—G—C—G—U—G—
                              100   110   120
A—A—G—C—C—G—G—C—U—C—U—A—G—G—U—G—C—U—G—C—U—U—C—U—G—G—A—U—G. C—
                              130   140   150
C—U—A—U—U—G, U—G, U—C—G, C—U—C—U—A—G—U—U—C—U—U—C—U—C—U—C—C—U—U—
                              160   170   180
G—G—G—G—G—G—G—U—C—A—G—A—G—G—G—A—G—G—G—A—A—C—G—C—A—G—U—U—C—G—
                              190   200   210
A—G . . . . G—A—U$_{OH}$
                              215

III. Summary

Although the pace of development of new information on gene control systems in cancer cells has been steadily increasing, there are urgent needs which have not yet been fulfilled. The factors responsible for the crucial mechanisms for initiation of the G$_1$-phase in cancer cells are not yet defined nor are the roles of the new nucleolar antigens found in nucleoli of neoplastic cells. The question is unanswered whether there are specific "on" mechanisms produced in excess in tumors or whether there are losses in these cells of either degradative or blocking elements responsible for the inhibition of special activation reactions. The increased complement of proteins staining with silver and the presence of special antigens in tumors suggest that these activation events are the resultant of gene activation systems which were inactivated or repressed in earlier stages of development and cell function prior to either oncogenesis or cell transformation. The need for isolation and analysis of the factors involved is clear and provides the hope that more specific and meaningful targets for cancer chemotherapy will soon be defined.

Acknowledgments

These studies were supported by the cancer research grant CA-10893 awarded by the National Cancer Institute, Department of Health, Education, and Welfare, the Bristol-Myers Fund, the Pauline Sterne Wolff Memorial Fund, and a generous gift from Mrs. Jack Hutchins.

References

Barrett, T., and Gould, H. J. (1973). *Biochim. Biophys. Acta* **294**, 165.

Bouteille, M., Laval, M., and Dupuy-Coin, A. M. (1974). *In* "The Cell Nucleus" (H. Busch, ed.), Vol. 1, pp. 3–71. Academic Press, New York.

Busch, G. I., Yeoman, L. C., Taylor, C. W., and Busch, H. (1974). *Physiol. Chem. Phys.* **6**, 1–10.

Busch, H. (1965). "Histones and Other Nuclear Proteins." Academic Press, New York.

Busch, H., (1974). *In* "The Molecular Biology of Cancer" (H. Busch, ed.), pp. 1–39. Academic Press, New York.

Busch, H. (1976a). *Cancer Res.* **36**, 4291–4294.

Busch, H. (1976b). *Perspect. Biol. Med.* **19**, 549–567.

Busch, H., ed. (1978a). "The Cell Nucleus, Chromatin A," Vol. 4. Academic Press, New York.

Busch, H., ed. (1978b). "The Cell Nucleus, Chromatin B," Vol. 5. Academic Press, New York.

Busch, H., ed. (1978c). "The Cell Nucleus, Chromatin C," Vol. 6. Academic Press, New York.

Busch, H., and Smetana, K. (1970). "The Nucleolus." Academic Press, New York.

Busch, H., Ro-Choi, T. S., Prestayko, A. W., Shibata, H., Crooke, S. T., El-Khatib, S. M., Choi, Y. C., and Mauritzen, C. M. (1971). *Perspect. Biol. Med.* **15**, 117–139.

Busch, H., Ballal, N. R., Olson, M. O. J., and Yeoman, L. C. (1975). *Methods Cancer Res.* **11**, 43–121.

Busch, H., Choi, Y. C., Daskal, Y., Liarakos, C. D., Rao, M. R. S., Ro-Choi, T. S., and Wu, B. C. (1976a). *Methods Cancer Res.* **8**, 101–197.

Busch, H., Hirsch, F., Gupta, K. K., Rao, M., Spohn, W., and Wu, B. (1976b). *Prog. Nucleic Acids Res.* **19**, 39–61.

Busch, H., Daskal, Y., Gyorkey, F., and Smetana, K. (1979). *Cancer Res.* **39**, 857–863.

Busch, R. K., and Busch, H. (1977). *Tumori* **63**, 347–357.

Chambon, P., Gissinger, F., Kedinger, C., Mandel, J. L., and Meilhac, M. (1974). *In* "The Cell Nucleus" (H. Busch, ed.), Vol. 3, pp. 270–308. Academic Press, New York.

Chytil, F., and Spelsberg, T. (1971). *Nature (London), New Biol.* **223**, 215.

Comings, D. E., and Harris, D. C. (1975). *Exp. Cell Res.* **96**, 161–179.

Comings, D. E., and Tack, L. O. (1973). *Exp. Cell Res.* **82**, 175–191.

Daskal, Y., Mace, M. L., Jr., Wray, W., and Busch, H. (1976). *Exp. Cell Res.* **100**, 204–212.

Davis, F. M., Busch, R. K., Yeoman, L. C., and Busch, H. (1978). *Cancer Res.* **38**, 1906–1915.

Davis, F. M., Gyorkey, F., Busch, R. K., and Busch, H. (1979). *PNAS* **76**, 892–896.

Douvas, A. S., Harrington, C. A., and Bonner, J. (1975). *Proc. Natl. Acad. Sci. U.S.A.* **72**, 3902–3906.

Elgin, S. C. R., and Weintraub, H. (1975). *Annu. Rev. Biochem.* **44**, 725–774.

Fidler, I. (1979). *Methods Cancer Res.* **15**, 399–439.

Fishman, W. H., and Busch, H., eds. (1979). *Methods Cancer Res.* **18**, Academic Press, New York.

Fishman, W. H., and Sells, S. (1976). "Onco-Developmental Gene Expression." Academic Press, New York.

Franke, W. W., and Scheer, U. (1974). *In* "The Cell Nucleus" (H. Busch, ed.), Vol. 1, pp. 220–347. Academic Press, New York.

Furth, J., and Kahn, M. C. (1937). *Am. J. Cancer* **31**, 276–282.

Gilmour, R. S., and Paul, J. (1970). FEBS (Fed. Eur. Biochem. Soc.) Lett. **9**, 242.

Goldknopf, I. L., French, M. F., Musso, R., and Busch, H. (1977). *Proc. Natl. Acad. Sci. U.S.A.* **74**, 5492–5495.

Goodwin, G. H., Nicolas, R. H., and Johns, E. W. (1975). *Biochim. Biophys. Acta* **405**, 280–291.

Goodwin, G. H., Walker, J. M., and Johns, E. W. (1978). *In* "The Cell Nucleus, Chromatin C" (H. Busch, ed.), Vol. 6, pp. 182–219. Academic Press, New York.

Gurdon, J. B. (1974). *In* "The Cell Nucleus" (H. Busch, ed.), Vol. 1, pp. 471–489. Academic Press, New York.

Heitz, E. (1933). *Z. Zellforsch. Mikrosk. Anat.* **19**, 720–742.

Hellung-Larsen, P. (1978). "Low Molecular Weight RNA Components in Eukaryotic Cells." FADL's Forlag, Copenhagen.

Hirsch, F. W., Nall, K. N., Busch, F. N., Morris, H. P., and Busch, H. (1978). *Cancer Res.* **38**, 1514–1522.

Hosokawa, K. (1950). *Gann* **41**, 236–237.

Illmensee, K., and Mintz, B. (1976). *Proc. Natl. Acad. Sci. U.S.A.* **73**, 549–553.

Ishibashi, K. (1950). *Gann* **41**, 1–14.

Jaskunas, S. R., Burgess, R., Lindahl, L., and Nomura, M. (1975). *Nature (London)* **257**, 458–462.

Jensen, E. V., and DeSombre, E. R. (1972). *Annu. Rev. Biochem.* **41**, 203–230.

Kadohama, N., and Turkington, R. W. (1973). *Cancer Res.* **33**, 1194.

Kamiyama, M., Dastugue, B., Defer, N. and Kruh, J. (1972). *Biochim. Biophys. Acta* **277**, 576.

Kleinschmidt, A. K. (1968). *In* "Nucleic Acids" (L. Grossman and K. Moldave, eds.), *Methods in Enzymology*, Vol. 12, Part B, pp. 361–377. Academic Press, New York.

Kostraba, N. C. and Wang, T. Y. (1972a). *Biochim. Biophys. Acta* **262**, 169.

Kostraba, N. C., and Wang, T. Y. (1972b). *Cancer Res.* **32**, 2348.

Kostraba, N. C., and Wang, T. Y. (1973). *Exp. Cell Res.* **80**, 291.

LeStourgeon, W. M., Forer, A., Yang, Y.-Z., Betram, J. S., and Rusch, H. P. (1975). *Biochim. Biophys. Acta* **379**, 529–552.

Levy, R., Levy, S., Rosenberg, S. A., and Simpson, R. T. (1973). *Biochemistry* **12**, 224.

Lindahl, L., Jaskunas, S. R., Dennis, P., and Nomura, M. (1975). *Proc. Natl. Acad. Sci. U.S.A.* **72**, 2743–2747.

McClintock, B. (1934). *Z. Zellforsch. Mikrosk. Anat.* **21**, 294–328.

McClintock, B. (1961). *Am. Nat.* **95**, 265–328.

Miller, O. L., Jr., and Beatty, B. R. (1969). *Science* **164**, 955–957.

Montgomery, T. H. (1898). *J. Morphol.* **15**, 265–564.

Olins, A. L., and Olins, D. E. (1974). *Science* **183**, 330–332.

Olson, M. O. J., Orrick, L. R., Jones, C., and Busch, H. (1974). *J. Biol. Chem.* **249**, 2823–2827.

Olson, M. O. J., Ezrailson, E. G., Guetzow, K., and Busch, H. (1975). *J. Mol. Biol.* **97**, 611–619.

Olson, M. O. J., Goldknipf, I. L., Guetzow, K. A., James, G. T., Hawkins, T. C., Mays-Rothberg, C. J., and Busch, H. (1976). *J. Biol. Chem.* **251**, 5901–5903.

O'Malley, B. W., and Means, A. R. (1974). *In* "The Cell Nucleus" (H. Busch, ed.), Vol. 3, pp. 380–416. Academic Press, New York.

O'Malley, B. W., and Schrader, W. T. (1976). *Sci. Am.* **231**, 32–43.

Orrick, L. R., Olson, M. O. J., and Busch, H. (1973). *Proc. Natl. Acad. Sci. U.S.A.* **70**, 1316–1320.

Pardon, J. F., and Richards, B. M. (1979). *In* "The Cell Nucleus, Chromatin, Part D" (H. Busch, ed.), Vol. 7. Academic Press, New York. 371–412.

Paul, J., and Gilmour, R. S. (1966a). *J. Mol. Biol.* **16**, 242–244.

Paul, J., and Gilmour, R. S. (1966b). *Nature (London)* **210**, 992–993.
Paul, J., and Gilmour, R. S. (1968). *J. Mol. Biol.* **34**, 305–316.
Peterson, J. L., and McConkey, E. H. (1967a). *J. Biol. Chem.* **251**, 548–554.
Peterson, J. L., and McConkey, E. H. (1967b). *J. Biol. Chem.* **251**, 555–558.
Pogo, B. G. T. and Katz, J. R. (1974). *Cell Differentiation* **2**, 119.
Richter, K. H., and Sekeris, C. E. (1972). *Arch. Biochem. Biophys.* **148**, 44.
Ro-Choi, T. S., and Busch, H. (1974a). *In* "Molecular Biology of Cancer" (H. Busch, ed.), pp. 241–276. Academic Press, New York.
Ro-Choi, T. S., and Busch, H. (1974b). *In* "The Cell Nucleus" (H. Busch, ed.), Vol. 3, pp. 152–211. Academic Press, New York.
Roeder, R. G., and Rutter, W. J. (1969). *Nature (London)* **224**, 234–237.
Roeder, R. G., and Rutter, W. J. (1970). *Biochemistry* **9**, 2543–2553.
Rovera, G., and Baserga, R. (1971). *J. Cell Physiol.* **77**, 201.
Rovera, G., Farber, J., and Baserga, R. (1971). *Proc. Nat. Acad. Sci. US* **68**, 1725.
Sandberg, A. A., and Sakurai, M. (1974). *In* "The Molecular Biology of Cancer" (H. Busch, ed.), pp. 81–106. Academic Press, New York.
Sato, S., and Sugimura, T. (1974). *Methods Cancer Res.* **12**, 259–315.
Sitz, T. O., Nazar, R. N., Spohn, W. H., and Busch, H. (1973). *Cancer Res.* **33**, 3312–3318.
Smetana, K., and Busch, H. (1979). Chapter 3, This Volume, pp. 89–105.
Spelsberg, T. C., Hnilica, L. S., and Ansevin, A. T. (1971a). *Biochim. Biophys. Acta* **228**, 550.
Spelsberg, T. C., Steggles, A. W., and O'Malley, B. W. (1971b). *J. Biol. Chem.* **246**, 4188.
Spelsberg, T. C., Steggles, A. W., and O'Malley, B. W. (1971c). *Biochim. Biophys. Acta* **254**, 129.
Spelsberg, T. C., Wilhelm, J. A., and Hnilica, L. S. (1971d). *In* "Sub-cellular Biochemistry" (B. D. Roodyn, ed.), p. 1. Plenum, New York.
Steele, W. J., and Busch, H. (1963). *Cancer Res.* **23**, 1153–1163.
Steggles, A. W., Spelsberg, T. C., and O'Malley, B. W. (1971). *Biochem. Biophys. Res. Commun.* **43**, 20.
Stein, G. S., and Kleinsmith, L. J., eds. (1975). "Chromosomal Proteins and Their Role in the Regulation of Gene Expression." Academic Press, New York.
Stein, G. S., Chaudhuri, S., and Baserga, R. (1972). *J. Biol. Chem.* **247**, 3918–3922.
Sugimura, T. (1976). "Control Mechanisms in Cancer." Raven New York.
Takami, H., and Busch, H. (1979). *Cancer Res.* **39**, 507–518.
Teng, C. S., Teng, C. T., and Allfrey, V. G. (1971). *J. Biol. Chem.* **246**, 3597.
Vorbrodt, A. (1974). *In* "The Cell Nucleus" (H. Busch, ed.), Vol. 3, pp. 309–344. Academic Press, New York.
Watson, R. J., Parker, J., Fiil, N. P., Flaks, J. G., and Friesen, J. D. (1975). *Proc. Natl. Acad. Sci. U.S.A.* **72**, 2765–2769.
Weinhouse, S. (1972). *Cancer Res.* **32**, 2007–2016.
Wu, B. C., Rao, M. S., Gupta, K. K., Rothblum, L. I., Mamrack, P. C., and Busch, H. (1977). *Cell Biol. Int. Rep.* **1**, 31–44.
Yeoman, L. C., Taylor, C. W., and Busch, H. (1973a). *Biochem. Biophys. Res. Commun.* **51**, 956–966.
Yeoman, L. C., Taylor, C. W., Jordan, J. J., and Busch, H. (1973b). *Biochem. Biophys. Res. Commun.* **53**, 1067–1076.
Zardi, L., Lin, J.-C., and Baserga, R. (1973). Nature (London), *New Biol.* **245**, 211.

3

Studies on Silver-Stained Nucleolar Components

KAREL SMETANA AND HARRIS BUSCH

I. Introduction

Recently, a simple silver staining technique for the demonstration of nucleolar organizer regions (NOR), nucleoli, and nucleolar satellites was used to facilitate cytochemical analysis of argyrophilic nucleolar structures and to analyze quantitative changes in highly argyrophilic nucleolar particular elements in hepatocytes and other cells at the light microscope level. Quantitative analysis of the numbers of dense, highly argyrophilic granules in the nucleoli of cells with varying nucoeolar function and

EFFECTS OF DRUGS ON THE CELL NUCLEUS

growth rate indicated that the largest numbers of grains (21 per nucleolus) were in rapidly dividing tumor cells. In the normal liver there were 4.4 grains per nucleolus, and this number increased to 7.8 and 15.3 in the regenerating liver 6 and 18 hours posthepatectomy. The effects of staining with $AgNO_3$ after digestion with RNase A, DNase I, trypsin, or pepsin, and extraction with HCl, H_2SO_4, and NaOH were essentially the same as reported earlier by others for silver staining in chromosomal NOR regions. In addition, it was found that nuclei of investigated cells contained small, highly argyrophilic bodies which may represent micronucleoli, since they showed a remarkable similarity to the nucleoli characteristic of cytochemical and staining procedures.

Recent studies on a great variety of cells clearly indicate that the NOR is characterized by a high affinity for silver salts (Gimenez Martin *et al.*, 1977; Goodpasture and Bloom, 1975; Howell, 1977; Howell *et al.*, 1975; Hubbel and Hsu, 1977; Schwarzacher *et al.*, 1978). This affinity is apparently due to the presence of a unique nonhistone protein, because the silver reaction can be blocked by pretreatment with proteases and NaOH but not by nucleases or acids (Goodpasture and Bloom, 1975; Howell, 1977; Howell *et al.*, 1975; Schwarzacher *et al.*, 1978). The affinity of interphase nucleoli for silver salts is less well defined, although numerous reports on this subject have been published since the end of the last century (Estable and Sotelo, 1951; Gimenez Martin *et al.*, 1974, 1977; Gonzalez Ramirez, 1961; Paweletz *et al.*, 1967; Ruzicka, 1899) mainly on neurocytes, plant cells, and cultured cells. Under defined conditions, silver salts localize in nucleolar granules of fibrils, in nucleolonemas, or in a relatively amorphous material (Das, 1962; Das and Alfert, 1963; Estable and Sotelo, 1951; Fernandez Gomez *et al.*, 1970; Gimenez Martin *et al.*, 1974, 1977; Goldblatt and Trump, 1965; Gonzalez Ramirez, 1961; Izard and Bernhard, 1962; Lettre *et al.*, 1966; Marinozzi, 1961; Paweletz *et al.*, 1967; Schwarzacher *et al.*, 1978; Tandler, 1959).

The present study was undertaken to compare the silver deposits in interphase nucleoli with those associated with the NOR of mitotic chromosomes in neoplastic cells and nontumor cells with varying rates of synthesis of nucleolar pre-rRNA. Under defined conditions in Novikoff hepatoma cells and rat hepatocytes, the cytochemical properties of highly argyrophilic nucleolar granular elements are similar to those of the NOR of mitotic chromosomes. The number of highly argyrophilic particles is related to nucleolar biosynthetic activity resulting in the production of nucleolar pre-rRNA. In addition, it was found that nuclei of hepatocytes and Novikoff hepatoma cells contained a small, argyrophilic body which may represent a micronucleolus.

II. Materials and Methods

Nucleoli of Novikoff ascitic hepatoma cells and hepatocytes from adult male albino rats weighing 250 gm (Holtzman, Madison, Wisconsin) were investigated in smears prepared by the usual cytological procedures. Transcription of the nucleolar RNA in hepatocytes was stimulated by partial hepatectomy, and the nucleoli were examined 6, 12, and 18 hours later (Higgins and Anderson, 1931; Muramatsu and Busch, 1965). To eliminate the interference of various cell components and to control the cytochemical experiments, nucleoli were isolated from liver and Novikoff hepatoma cells by the sonication method described previously (Busch and Smetana, 1970).

Dry smears were stained for RNA with toluidine blue (0.05%) at pH 5 without previous fixation (Smetana *et al.*, 1969). DNA was demonstrated by the Feulgen reaction and toluidine blue staining after fixation with Carnoy's fluid (methanol–acetic acid, 3 : 1) for 10 minutes and hydrolysis with 0.1 N HCl for 10 minutes at 60°C (Busch and Smetana, 1970; Pearse, 1972; Smetana *et al.*, 1967). The specimens fixed in Carnoy's fixative for 10 minutes were also digested with RNase A (Worthington, Freehold, New Jersey) and DNase (Worthington) for 30, 60, and 90 minutes at 37°C. The proteins were digested with trypsin (Sigma, St. Louis, Missouri) and pepsin (Sigma) for 10, 15, and 20 minutes at the same temperature (Howell *et al.*, 1975; Matsui and Sasaki, 1973). RNase A (1 mg/1 ml) was dissolved in distilled, autoclaved water, DNase I (RNase-free) in 0.003 M magnesium acetate (1 mg/1 ml), pepsin in 0.1 N HCl (1.0 and 0.1 mg/1 ml), and trypsin in distilled and autoclaved water (1.0 and 0.1 mg/1 ml). For controls for the specificity of the enzymatic extractions, parallel smears were incubated in the same media without the enzymes. Basic nuclear proteins were extracted with 0.1 N HCl and 0.2 N H_2SO_4 (Howell *et al.*, 1975), and acidic nuclear proteins were extracted with 0.1 N NaOH (Busch and Smetana, 1970, Howell *et al.*, 1975). All extraction procedures were carried out at room temperature on smears fixed in Carnoy's fluid, washed in running water, and dried.

The silver impregnation procedure (Goodpasture and Bloom, 1975; Howell, 1977; Howell *et al.*, 1975; Peters, 1955) was modified for smears to provide standard results in a relatively short period of time. The dry smears were fixed in Carnoy's solution for 10 minutes, washed with running water, and dried again. Then the smears were impregnated with the concentrated $AgNO_3$ solution (1 gm/1 ml) for 5–7 minutes. After pouring off the $AgNO_3$ solution (without washing), the smears were covered with developer consisting of 37% formaldehyde containing 15% methanol as a

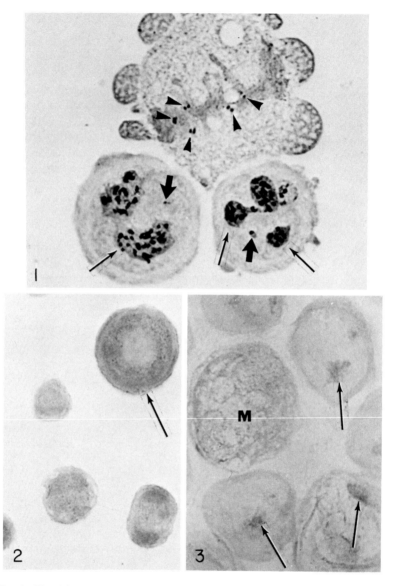

Fig. 1   Fixed Novikoff hepatoma cells stained with AgNO₃. Nucleoli (thin arrows) contain distinct argyrophilic granules which are in a matrix of less argyrophilic material. Note the presence of very small nucleoli (thick arrows). The mitotic cell contains five pairs of argyrophilic granules associated with the metaphase plate (arrowheads). × 2100.

Fig. 2   Fixed Novikoff hepatoma cells predigested with trypsin and then stained

preservative (Fisher, Houston, Texas) mixed with $AgNO_3$ (1 gm/ml) in the ratio 1:1 and usually kept for 3–5 minutes at 40°–50°C on a warm plate. To prevent the formation of precipitates, development was terminated by a thorough wash in running water followed (without drying) by staining with May–Grünwald solution (1.6 gm of methylene blue eosinate per liter of methanol) (Curtin Matheson Co., Houston, Texas) diluted 1:1 with distilled or tap water for 1 minute. After a thorough wash in running water, the smears were air-dried in a vertical position to prevent the formation of precipitates and then examined in a light microscope under oil immersion. The $AgNO_3$ solution should not be kept more than 2 days, and the developer prepared just prior to use.

III. Results

A. Novikoff Hepatoma Cells

The stained nucleoli had an amorphous, yellow-tan background and contained distinct dark-brown particles (Fig. 1). Although these particles were similar in some respects to those of the NOR of mitotic chromosomes in dividing Novikoff hepatoma cells (Fig. 1), they were frequently larger.

When the smears were predigested with trypsin, neither the argyrophilic granules nor the yellow-tan, amorphous background could be detected (Fig. 2; Table I). Preextraction of smears with 0.1 N NaOH also prevented the particles from being impregnated, but the amorphous background was still lightly stained with the silver, as was the rest of the cell (Fig. 3; Table I). Digestion of smears with DNase I (Fig. 4) and RNase A (Fig. 5) or extraction with 0.1 N HCl or 0.2 N H_2SO_4 (Fig. 6) did not affect the silver staining of the granules or the amorphous background (Table I).

The argyrophilic granules associated with the mitotic chromosomes in dividing Novikoff hepatoma cells were also unstained after pretreatment with trypsin and NaOH (Figs. 2 and 3), and they were also resistant to pretreatment with acids and nucleases (Figs. 4–6; Table I).

The resistance of argyrophilic granules in isolated nucleoli to treatment

---

with silver. Argyrophilic structures were not found either in interphase or presumably in mitotic (arrow) cells. × 1800.

Fig. 3 Fixed Novikoff hepatoma cells in interphase and mitosis (M) were extracted with NaOH and then stained with $AgNO_3$. The highly argyrophilic granules were not present, but the less dense argyrophilic material of the nucleolus (arrows) was still visible. The contrast was increased by printing. × 2000.

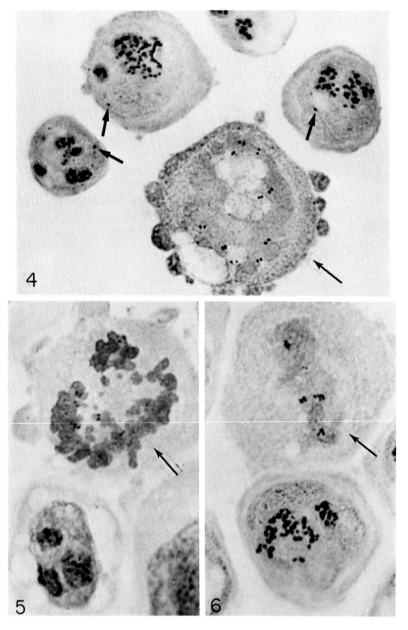

Fig. 4 Fixed Novikoff hepatoma cells predigested with DNase I and stained with AgNO₃. The nucleoli contain numerous highly argyrophilic granules. Note the presence of solitary silver grains in the nuclei (arrows). In the mitotic cell (thinner arrow), 10 pairs of highly argyrophilic granules are present. × 2000.

TABLE I

The Effect of Extraction Procedures on the Argyrophilic Components of Nucleoli in Novikoff Hepatoma Cells

Extraction	Time of extraction (min)	Argyrophilic granules[a]	Amorphous material[a]	Chromosomal (NOR) granules[a]
Control	—	+ + +	+ +	+ +
0.1 N HCl	20	+ + +	+ +	+ + +
0.2 N H$_2$SO$_4$	20	+ + +	+ +	+ + +
0.1 N NaOH	20	0	+	0
Trypsin				
0.1 mg/ml	15	0	0	0
1.0 mg/ml	15	0	0	0
RNase A[b]	90	+ + +	+ +	+ + +
DNase I[c]	90	+ + +	+ +	+ + +

[a] + + +, Argyrophilic structure present and intensely stained; + +, argyrophilic structure present and stained; +, argyrophilic structure present and faintly stained; 0, argyrophilic structure absent.

[b] The basophilic properties of the nucleolus and cytoplasm disappeared when stained for RNA with toluidine blue at pH 5. The control incubation in distilled water did not alter the silver impregnation and staining for RNA.

[c] The nuclear chromatin did not stain positively with the Feulgen reaction. The control incubation in 0.003 M magnesium acetate at pH 7.3 did not alter the positive silver stain or the Feulgen reaction.

with nucleases (Figs. 7 and 8) and acids (Fig. 9) was similar to that of nucleoli *in situ* (Tables I and II). The argyrophilic granules disappeared after digestion with trypsin (Fig. 10) or pepsin (Fig. 11) and extraction with 0.1 N NaOH (Fig. 12). The argyrophilic properties of the amorphous matrix were slightly reduced by extraction with trypsin (Fig. 10), pepsin (Fig. 11), or NaOH (Fig. 12).

B. Hepatocytes

The stained liver nucleoli contained granular structures which appeared to be associated with less argyrophilic trabecular structures, presumably nucleolonemas. Digestion with nucleases or extraction with H$_2$SO$_4$ did

Fig. 5 Argyrophilic granules associated with mitotic chromosomes (arrow) and nucleoli of fixed Novikoff hepatoma cells digested with RNase A before staining with AgNO$_3$. The cytoplasm was not stained with either silver or the May–Grünwald stain. × 2220.

Fig. 6 Resistant highly argyrophilic granules associated with chromosomes (arrow) and in nucleoli of Novikoff hepatoma cells which were extracted with H$_2$SO$_4$ before staining with AgNO$_3$. × 2200.

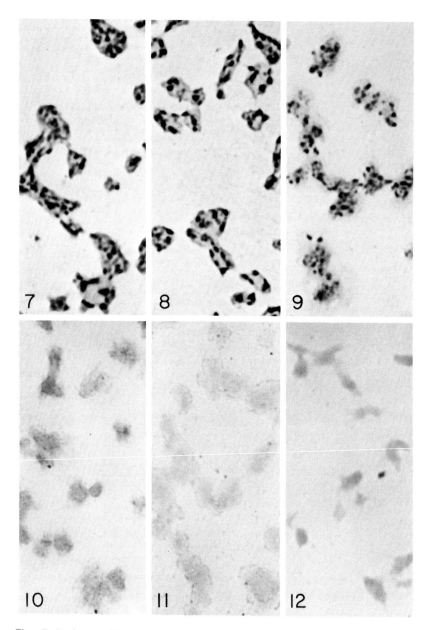

Figs. 7–9 Argyrophilic granules in fixed isolated nucleoli from Novikoff hepatoma cells extracted with RNase A (Fig. 7), DNase I (Fig. 8), and H_2SO_4 (Fig. 9) before staining with AgNO$_3$. Fig. 7. ×2700. Fig. 8. ×2800. Fig. 9. ×2400.

Figs. 10–12 Trypsin (Fig. 10), pepsin (Fig. 11), and NaOH (Fig. 12) pretreatment before staining with AgNO$_3$ destroyed the positive staining of argyrophilic granules. Fig. 10. ×2300. Fig. 11. ×2300. Fig. 12. ×2000.

TABLE II

The Effect of Extraction Procedures on the Argyrophilic Granules in Isolated Nucleoli of Novikoff Hepatoma Cells[a]

Extraction	Time of extraction (min)	Argyrophilic granules
Control	—	+++
0.1 N HCl	20	+++
0.2 N H_2SO_4	20	+++
0.1 N NaOH	20	0
Pepsin	15	0
Trypsin		
0.1 mg/ml	15	0
1.0 mg/ml	15	0
RNase A	90	+++
DNase I	90	+++

[a] See Table I for details.

not prevent the reaction of these nucleolar components with silver (Table III; Figs. 13 and 14). In contrast, the tryptic digestion eliminated the argyrophilic properties of the nucleolar components (Fig. 15). When extracted with 0.1 N NaOH, the very highly argyrophilic deposits on the trabecular structures were more resistant than those in hepatoma nucleoli (Figs. 3 and 16). In addition, the less argyrophilic trabecular nucleolar structures had more resistance to such treatment, like the argyrophilic nucleolar amorphous material of the hepatoma cells (Fig. 16).

C. Small Nuclear Argyrophilic Bodies

In addition to the characteristic nucleoli, very small but distinct satellite argyrophilic bodies were found in nuclei of Novikoff hepatoma cells (Figs. 1 and 4) and hepatocytes (Figs. 13 and 14). The number of these bodies usually ranged between one and two per nucleus, and their presence was noted in 80–100% of the hepatocytes. These highly argyrophilic bodies in hepatocytes had properties similar to those of the highly argyrophilic particles of nucleoli. Thus their affinity for $AgNO_3$ was not prevented by nucleases (Figs. 13 and 14; Table III), and extraction with NaOH abolished their argyrophilic properties (Fig. 16). Tryptic digestion did not aid in identification of the small argyrophilic nuclear bodies, since small silver deposits appeared in nuclei after such treatment.

Like the larger characteristic nucleoli, the small highly argyrophilic nu-

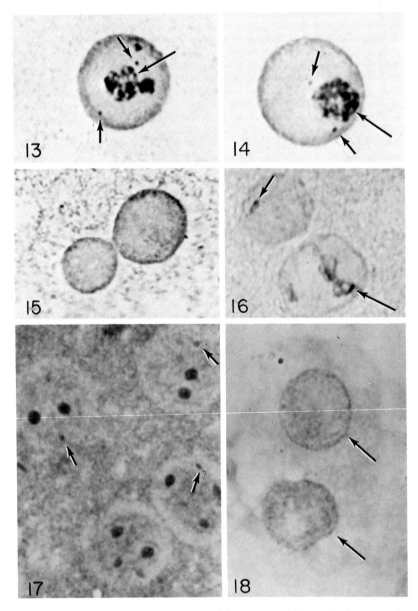

Fig. 13 Highly argyrophilic particles and less argyrophilic nucleolonemas (long arrow) in nucleoli of a hepatocyte; these nuclei contain two very small nuclear argyrophilic bodies (short arrows). The fixed cells were digested with RNase A before staining with AgNO$_3$. × 2500.

Fig. 14 Argyrophilic nucleolar particles and less argyrophilic trabecular structures

TABLE III

Properties of Small Satellite Nucleoli and Characteristic Nucleoli in Rat Hepatocytes

Procedure	Characteristic nucleoli	Satellite nucleoli[a]
RNA staining[b]	$+++$[c]	$++$
Nucleolus-associated chromatin[d]	$++$	?
Silver impregnation	$+++$	$+++$
RNase digestion, RNA stain	0[e]	0
RNase digestion, silver stain[f]	$+++$	$+++$
DNase digestion, Feulgen stain	0[g]	?
DNase digestion, silver stain[f]	$+++$	$+++$
Tryptic digestion, silver stain[f]	0	?

[a] ?, Could not be evaluated—see text.

[b] Staining with toluidine blue at pH 5 without previous fixation.

[c] Intensely stained.

[d] Feulgen reaction and staining with toluidine blue after fixation in Carnoy's fluid and hydrolysis in 1 N HCl at 60°C for 10 minutes.

[e] Completely digested.

[f] For silver stain densities, see Table I.

[g] The nucleolar body was undigested.

clear bodies also stained for RNA, and this was blocked by predigestion with RNase A (Table III; Figs. 17 and 18). The Feulgen reaction and the staining for DNA with toluidine blue did not contribute to the identification or classification of these bodies, since they could not be distinguished from multiple small chromocenters (Fig. 19). The number of chromo-

---

(nucleolonemas) in fixed regenerating liver 6 hours after partial hepatectomy. The sample was pretreated with DNase I. This nucleus also contains two very small argyrophilic bodies (short arrows); long arrow, silver stained nucleolar reticulum. × 2500.

Fig. 15 After predigestion with trypsin before staining with AgNO$_3$, the argyrophilic nucleolar structures were no longer found in normal hepatocytes. × 2400.

Fig. 16 Extraction of fixed hepatocytes with 0.1 N NaOH before staining with AgNO$_3$ removed most of the highly argyrophilic particles. The less argyrophilic trabecular structures and a few associated highly argyrophilic particles (arrows) were visible. × 2500.

Fig. 17 Hepatocytes stained with toluidine blue for the demonstration of RNA. Small basophilic bodies (arrows) were similar to those stained by AgNO$_3$ (Fig. 13 and 14) in the nucleus. The contrast of the picture was slightly reduced by printing to show clearly the positive cytoplasmic staining. × 2500.

Fig. 18 The same specimen as Fig. 17 digested with RNase A before staining with toluidine blue. The cell components containing the RNA were not stained. The density of the intact DNA-containing nuclear structures (arrows) with toluidine blue and the "shadows" of the cytoplasm were increased by printing. × 2400.

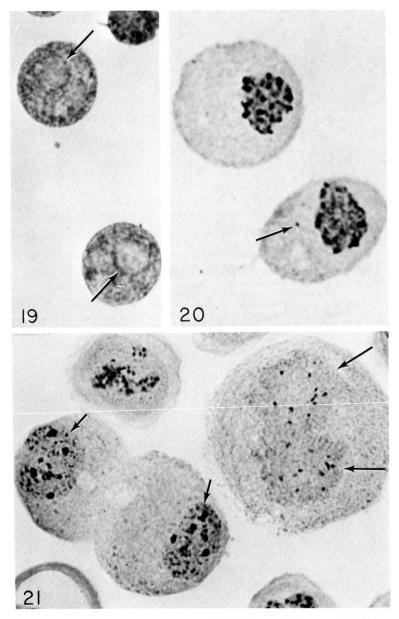

Fig. 19 Feulgen reaction demonstrating DNA in the nucleolus-associated chromatin (arrows) and nuclear chromatin in hepatocytes 6 hours after partial hepatectomy. × 2000.

centers was always higher than that of the small highly argyrophilic nuclear bodies (Figs. 13, 14, 19, and 20).

D. The Number of Highly Argyrophilic Particles in Nucleoli of Investigated Hepatoma and Liver Cells

Starting with anaphase, there was an increasing number of highly argyrophilic particles (associated with the chromosomes) with the progress of mitotic division of the hepatoma cells (Fig. 21). The greatest number was found in telophase (Fig. 21).

In interphase nucleoli of hepatoma cells (Table IV), the number of highly argyrophilic granules averaged 21. In hepatocytes, the number of highly argyrophilic particles per nucleolus averaged 4.4. This number increased to 7.8 at 6 hours after partial hepatectomy (Table IV) and to 15.3 at 18 hours after partial hepatectomy (Fig. 20). The number of these particles in regenerating liver was less than that found for the hepatoma cells (Table IV).

TABLE IV

The Number of Highly Argyrophilic Grains in Nucleoli of Novikoff Hepatoma Cells and Hepatocytes[a]

Cells	Per nucleus	Per nucleolus
Novikoff hepatoma	53.0 ± 7.5	21.0 ± 0.1
Hepatocytes	13.1 ± 1.9	4.4 ± 0.3
Partial hepatectomy hepatocytes		
6 hours after	25.1 ± 1.0	7.8 ± 0.6
18 hours after	33.4 ± 1.7	15.3 ± 0.9

[a] Fifty to 100 nucleoli were evaluated in each sample. Mean and standard deviation are given.

Fig. 20 Two hepatocytic nuclei with numerous highly argyrophilic particles in enlarged nucleoli 18 hours after partial hepatectomy. × 2400.

Fig. 21 Mitotic Novikoff hepatoma cells stained with $AgNO_3$. In one entering anaphase (long arrows), single, dense granules are noted in the chromosomal figure; in the telophase cell containing two newly formed nuclei (short arrows), there is an increased number of highly argyrophilic granules of differing sizes in each nucleus. A defined nucleolus had not yet formed. × 2000.

IV. Discussion

The present study confirmed previous reports that the high affinity of the NOR for silver salts was due to acidic nonhistone proteins as shown by cytochemical digestion and extraction procedures (Goodpasture and Bloom, 1975; Howell, 1977; Howell *et al.*, 1975; Hubbel and Hsu, 1977; Matsui and Sasaki, 1973; Schwarzacher *et al.*, 1978). As in previous reports, the argyrophilic grains associated with the mitotic chromosomes of Novikoff hepatoma cells could not be detected after extraction with trypsin or NaOH but were present after treatment with dilute acids, RNase A, or DNase I. The highly argyrophilic granules of interphase nucleoli of the Novikoff hepatoma cells exhibited similar sensitivity to treatment with NaOH or trypsin and resistance to pretreatment with dilute acids, RNase A, or DNase I. The present observations suggest that similar proteins might be present both in the NOR of mitotic chromosomes (Goodpasture and Bloom, 1975; Howell, 1977; Howell *et al.*, 1975; Hubbel and Hsu, 1977) and interphase nucleoli of Novikoff hepatoma cells. The presence of such proteins was suggested by the cytochemical extraction experiments on isolated nucleoli from the same cells to eliminate interference from other cellular, particularly nuclear, components. In addition, the highly argyrophilic nucleolar granules in cells such as human fibroblasts (Schwarzacher *et al.*, 1978) and rat hepatocytes (in the present study) were also sensitive to digestion with pepsin but resistant to treatment with trichloroacetic acid, HCl, or nucleases.

Since it is generally accepted at present that silver stain preferentially detects acidic nonhistone proteins associated with rDNA sites in the NOR of mitotic chromosomes (Goodpasture and Bloom, 1975; Howell, 1977; Howell *et al.*, 1975; Hubbel and Hsu, 1977; Schwarzacher *et al.*, 1978), the present results suggest that silver stains such proteins at active rDNA sites in the interphase nucleoli of Novikoff hepatoma cells or hepatocytes. The large number of these highly argyrophilic nucleolar granules in Novikoff hepatoma cells in comparison to hepatocytes, and the greater number of such particles in hepatocytes after partial hepatectomy than in normal liver, may relate to higher nucleolar activity in these cells. Biochemical studies in this and other laboratories have clearly shown that nucleolar rRNA synthesis is 9–15 times greater in Novikoff hepatoma cells than in hepatocytes and that nucleoli of hepatocytes in regenerating liver are 3–5 times more active than those in normal liver (Busch and Smetana, 1970). The greater number of highly argyrophilic granules can be also noted in human lymphocytes stimulated with phytohemagglutinin (Schwarzacher *et al.*, 1978). After partial hepatectomy these stimulated lymphocytes and hepatocytes are characterized by a marked increase in rRNA synthesis in comparison with resting or normal unstimulated cells (Busch and Smetana, 1970; Smetana, 1974; Smetana and Busch, 1974).

The relationship between highly argyrophilic granules and classical nucleolar components is not clear at present, and more studies are required in this direction. However, electron microscope studies (Izard and Bernhard, 1962; Paweletz et al., 1967; Schwarzacher et al., 1978) show that silver is deposited in the fibrillar regions of the nucleolus which contain newly transcribed RNA (Busch and Smetana, 1970; Smetana and Busch, 1974). The relationship of the highly argyrophilic nucleolar granules to the nucleolini (Love, 1966) cannot be established because the nature of these structures is also not clear (Smetana and Busch, 1974). On the other hand, some studies indicate that the number and morphology of nucleolini depend on the functional activity of genetic expression of the chromatin in nucleoli of interphase cells (Love, 1966).

Some differences in nucleoli of Novikoff hepatoma cells and normal hepatocytes have been already detected by biochemical and immunological procedures (Busch and Busch, 1977; Davis et al., 1978; Rothblum et al., 1977), but a direct comparison of the cytochemical, biochemical, and immunological results is not possible at present. Moreover, a possibility exists that the relative resistance of the highly argyrophilic nucleolar particles of hepatocytes as compared with Novikoff hepatoma cells also depends on their accessibility to the extractions and on the spatial organization or position within other nucleolar components. In contrast to Novikoff hepatoma cells, the particles in nucleoli of hepatocytes seem to be part of a highly organized trabecular structure of nucleolonemas which in these cells are distinct even in the light microscope. Analysis of the silver staining of nucleolar fractions on two-dimensional gels has indicated that proteins B23 and C23 are the major nucleolar silver-staining proteins (Mamrack et al., 1977, 1978; Olson et al., 1974; Lischne et al., 1979).

When the smeared hepatocytes and Novikoff hepatoma cells were stained with silver, small highly argyrophilic bodies appeared in their nuclei in addition to the argyrophilic components of characteristic nucleoli. Since the cytochemical investigation demonstrated that these argyrophilic bodies in hepatocytes contained RNA, the possibility exists that they represent the small accessory nucleoli. Unfortunately, the cytochemical procedures for the demonstration of DNA and the digestion with trypsin, as well as the extraction with NaOH, did not provide satisfactory results for identification of these nuclear structures. Electron microscope examination, which would show whether the argyrophilic bodies are real nucleoli, is also limited because in ultrathin sections these bodies are easily confused with the peripheral portions of the characteristic nucleoli as suggested for micronucleoli in other cell types (Smetana, 1974). Nevertheless, the possibility that the small argyrophilic nuclear bodies represent nucleoli is supported by observations on micronucleoli of other cells. Micronucleoli may contain ribosomal cistrons (Pardue *et al.*, 1970) which can be detected by the reaction of associated proteins with silver (Goodpasture and Bloom, 1975; Howell, 1977; Howell *et al.*, 1975; Hubbel and Hsu, 1977; Schwarzacher *et al.*, 1978).

Acknowledgments

These studies were supported by cancer research grant CA-10893, awarded by the National Cancer Institute, Department of Health, Education, and Welfare, the Pauline Sterne Wolff Memorial Foundation, the Davidson Fund, and the Bristol-Myers Fund.

References

Busch, H., and Smetana, K. (1970). "The Nucleolus," pp. 59–114, 239–243. Academic Press, New York.
Busch, R. K., and Busch, H. (1977). *Tumori* **63**, 347.
Das, N. K. (1962). *Exp. Cell Res.* **26**, 428.
Das, N. K., and Alfert, H. (1963). *Ann. Histochim.* **8**, 109.
Davis, F. M., Busch, R. K., Yeoman, L. C., and Busch, H. (1978). *Cancer Res.* **38**, 1906.
Estable, C., and Sotelo, J. R. (1951). *Publ. Inst. Invest. Sci. Biol.* **1**, 105.
Fernandez Gomez, M. E., Risueno, M. C., Gimenez Martin, G., and Stockert, J. C. (1970). *Protoplasma* **74**, 103.
Gimenez-Martin, G., de la Tore, C., Fernandez Gomez, E., and Gonzalez Fernandez, A. (1974). *J. Cell Biol.* **60**, 502.
Gimenez-Martin, G., de la Torre, C., Lopez Suez, J. F., and Espona, P. (1977). *Cytobiologie Z. Exp. Zellforsch.* **14**, 421.
Goldblatt, P., and Trump, B. F. (1965). *Stain Technol.* **40**, 105.
Gonzalez Ramirez, (1961). *J. Bol. Inst. Estud. Med. Biol. (Univ. Nac. Auton. Mex.)* **19**, 195.
Goodpasture, C., and Bloom, S. E., (1975). *Chromosoma* **53**, 37.
Higgins, G. M., and Anderson, R. M. (1931). *Arch. Pathol.* **12**, 186.
Howell, M. W. (1977). *Chromosoma* **62**, 361.
Howell, M. W., Denton, T. E., and Diamond, J. R. (1975). *Experientia* **31**, 260.
Hubbel, H. R., and Hsu, T. C. (1977). *Cytogenet. Cell Genet.* **19**, 185.
Izard, J., and Bernhard, W. (1962). *J. Microsc. (Paris)* **1**, 421.
Lettre, R., Siebs, W., and Paweletz, N. (1966). *Natl. Cancer Inst., Monogr.* **23**, 107.
Love, R. (1966). *Natl. Cancer Inst., Monogr.* **23**, 167.
Mamrack, M. D., Olson, M. O. J., and Busch, H. (1977). *Biochem. Biophys. Res. Commun.* **76**, 150.
Mamrack, M. D., Olson, M. O. J., and Busch, H. (1978). *Fed. Proc., Fed. Am. Soc. Exp. Biol.* **37**, 1786.
Marinozzi, V. (1961). *J. Biophys. Biochem. Cytol.* **9**, 121.
Matsui, S., and Sasaki, M. (1973). *Nature (London)* **246**, 148.
Muramatsu, M., and Busch, H. (1965). *J. Biol. Chem.* **240**, 10.
Olson, M. O. J., Orrick, L. R., Jones, C., and Busch, H. (1974). *J. Biol. Chem.* **249**, 2823.

Pardue, M. L., Gerbi, S. A., Eckhardt, R. A., and Gall, J. G. (1970). *Chromosoma* **29**, 268.
Paweletz, N., Siebs, W., and Lettre, R. (1967). *Z. Zellforsch. Mikrosk. Anat.* **76**, 577.
Pearse, A. G. E., (1972). "Histochemistry, Theoretical and Applied." Churchill, London.
Peters, A. (1955). *Q. J. Microsc. Sci.* **96**, 84.
Rothblum, L. I., Mamrack, P. M., Olson, M. O. J., and Busch, H. (1977). *Biochemistry* **16**, 4716.
Ruzicka, V. (1899). *Anat. Anz.* **16**, 557.
Schwarzacher, H. G., Mikelsaar, A. V., and Schnedl, W. (1978). *Cytogenet. Cell Genet.* **20**, 24.
Smetana, K. (1974). *In* "Present Problems in Hematology" (J. Libansky and L. Donner, eds.), p. 185. Excerpta Med. Found., Amsterdam.
Smetana, K., and Busch, H. (1974). *In* "The Cell Nucleus (H. Busch, ed.), Vol. 1, p. 73. Academic Press, New York.
Smetana, K., Lejnar, J., and Potmesil, M. (1967). *Folia Haematol.* **88**, 305.
Smetana, K., Lejnar, J., and Potmesil, M. (1969). *Folia Haematol.* **91**, 381.
Tandler, C. J. (1959). *Exp. Cell Res.* **17**, 560.

Drug Effects on Nucleolar and Extranucleolar Chromatin

Y. DASKAL

I. Introduction

Of the numerous potential targets for drug action in the cell nucleus, only a limited number of such sites have been recognized, and even a fewer number characterized and studied in any detail; among these are the nucleolus, the nuclear pores, metaphase chromatin, and the mitotic apparatus. Few or no morphological or biochemical data are available on the interaction of drugs with extranucleolar chromatin, perichromatinic and interchromatinic granules or complexes, nuclear bodies, and nuclear matrix components. Although these nuclear components have been described as ultrastructural entities of the eukaryotic cell nucleus, no precise data are available on the composition and functions of many of these organelles. Therefore monitoring specific ultrastructural lesions induced by various drugs not only provides valuable information on the particular mode of action of the drug, structure–activity relationships, and even pharmacokinetics, but also provides a powerful probe for elucidation of

EFFECTS OF DRUGS ON THE CELL NUCLEUS

the functional-physiological aspects of a particular nuclear organelle in question.

II. The Nucleolus as a Target for Drug Action

The normal interphase nucleolus (Fig. 1) consists of both fibrillar and granular elements that represent nucleolar chromatin and preribosomal

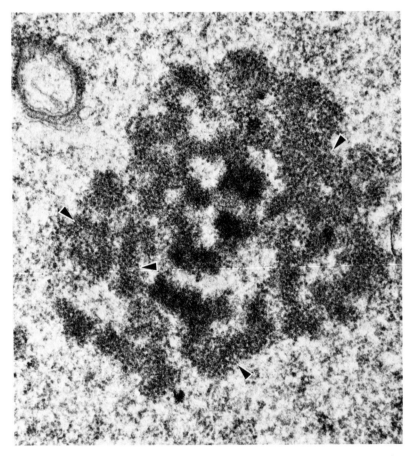

Fig. 1 Normal untreated liver cell nucleolus. The granular components are intertwined with the fibrillar elements. In the center of the nucleolus some fibrillar components of higher electron density can be seen. The combined fibrillar and granular components (arrowheads) are the presumptive sites where active transcription within the nucleolus occurs.

particles (Marinozzi and Bernhard, 1963), respectively. (For historical aspects of the elucidation of the structure and function of the nucleolus, see Busch and Smetana, 1970; Bernhard and Granboular, 1969).

When cells are treated with antimetabolites capable of binding, intercalating, or cross-linking DNA and thereby interfering with its template activity in RNA synthesis, nucleolar segregation occurs (Fig. 2; Reynolds *et al.*, 1964). This is the ultrastructural manifestation of the inhibition of rRNA synthesis. Such drugs, among others, are actinomycin D, anthracyclines, nogalomycin, echinomycin, chromomycin, ethidium bromide, alkylating agents such as mitomycin C, and at relatively high concentrations *cis*-platinum.

In the segregated nucleolus, the individual components become distinct and physically separated from each other. These are the fibrillar (Fig. 2f), the granular Fig. 2g), and the nucleolar organizer components (Fig. 2n). As illustrated by Schoefl (1964), it appears that as soon as "the synthetic processes are blocked, the ordered framework collapses. The specific mechanism of the block is apparently of secondary importance" (Schoefl, 1964).

However, when nucleolar RNA synthesis is blocked by agents such as actinomycin D at high concentrations (Unuma and Busch, 1967; Goldblatt and Sullivan, 1970), marcellomycin, rudolphomycin, or mitomycin C (Daskal *et al.*, 1978a; Daskal and Crooke, 1979), a slight variation in the segregation pattern is evident (Fig. 3) in the form of the presence of microspherules. These microspherules seem to represent sequestered segments of nucleolar fibrillar structures of high electron density that are physically extruded from the nucleolar body into the nucleoplasm (Fig. 3). Treatment of cells with class I anthracyclines such as adriamycin and carminomycin under identical experimental conditions yields segregated nucleoli but without microspherules (Merski *et al.*, 1976; Lambertenghi-Deliliers *et al.*, 1976; Daskal *et al.*, 1978a). Neither the composition, precise origin, or function of these microspherules is known (Recher *et al.*, 1973). Moreover, the relationship between nucleolar segregation as seen *in situ*, the presence of microspherules, and the organization of rDNA cistrons is not clear at present (Figs. 4 and 5) (Miller and Beatty, 1969; Franke *et al.*, 1976, 1979; Scheer *et al.*, 1975).

Examination of a partially spread nucleolus (Fig. 4) shows that the appearance of granular and fibrillar components is a result of the close packing of individual active transcriptional units with the lateral fibrils and their terminal beads forming what appears to be the granular components, while the axial DNA region and the polymerase molecules represent the fibrillar component (Fig. 4, inset).

Upon the inhibition of nucleolar transcription with actinomycin D

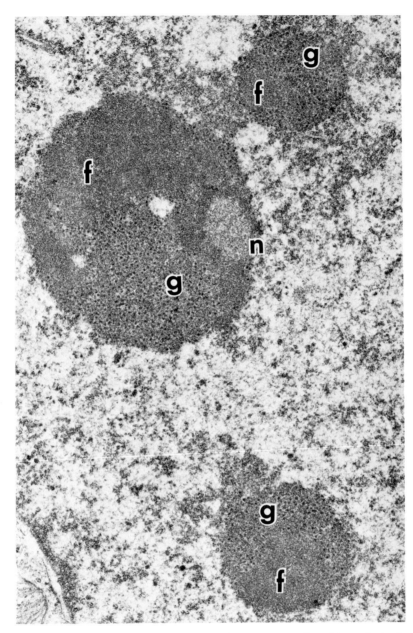

Fig. 2 Novikoff hepatoma cell nucleolus after treatment with adriamycin (a class I anthracycline) for 1 hour (1 μg/ml). The nucleolus has segregated into granular (g), fibrillar (f), and nucleolar organizer components (n). Frequently, nucleolar fragmentation occurs. Like the original nucleolus, even the resulting nucleolar fragments are segregated.

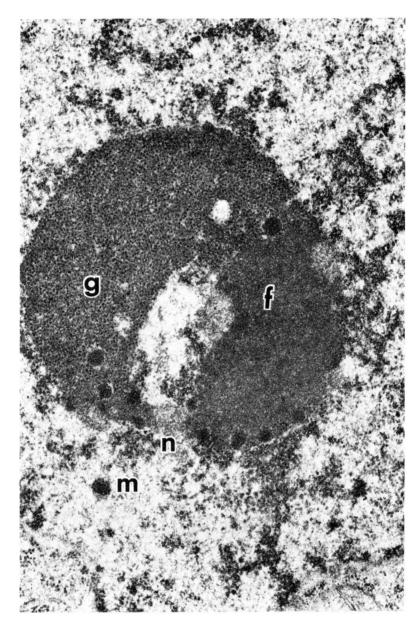

Fig. 3 Nucleolus of Novikoff hepatoma cell after treatment with 0.5 µg/ml for 1 hour with marcellomycin (a class II anthracycline). In addition to segregation of the nucleolar components as described for Fig. 2, nucleolar microspherules (m) are present at the precise boundary between the granular (g) and fibrillar (f) elements or occasionally even extrude from the main nucleolar body.

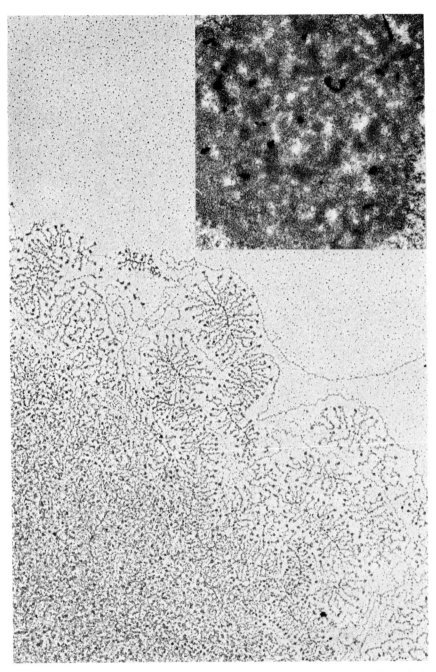

Fig. 4 A partially spread nucleolus of *Pleurodeles waltii* (newt) oocytes demostrating the mode of packaging of nucleolar components into the nucleolus. An active nucleolus as evidenced by the distribution of [³H]uridine over the fibrillar components is shown for comparison (inset).

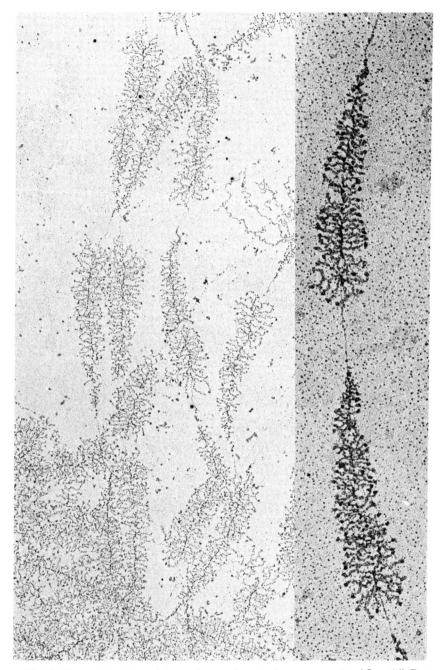

Fig. 5 The substructure of the well-spread nucleolar components of *P. waltii*. Tandemly arranged nucleolar cistrons are separated by regular spacer regions. From the axial fiber (right) the lateral filaments representing nascent ribosomal RNP increase in length, representing the progressive transcription of the rDNA template from the 5′-end (shortest fibers) toward the 3′-end of the DNA. The terminal beads on the lateral fibers represent partially packaged RNP structures.

(Scheer *et al.*, 1975) or class II anthracyclines, the characteristic structure of the transcriptional unit (Fig. 5) is altered (Fig. 6c–e) in that gaps are formed between the lateral fibrils as a result of the detachment of the growing nascent pre-rRNA-containing lateral fibrils. As expected, lateral fibril detachment is related to both the duration and concentration of the drug treatments. Fifteen minutes after treatment with 0.5 μg/ml rudolphomycin (Fig. 6c), less than 50% of the ribosomal transcriptional units were affected. However, even after 60 minutes of drug treatment where 80% of all transcripts were damaged (Figs. 6d and e and 7), some intact transcripts could be still found. Thus, in addition to the cessation of any transcriptional activity, the actual stability of the newly synthesized product on the template is affected. At higher magnifications (Fig. 7), it can be seen that the loss of lateral fibrils after class II anthracycline treatments need not be accompanied by a detachment of polymerase molecules from the templates. Thus it seems that the interaction between the lateral fibril (the nascent RNP) and the polymerase I molecules is preferentially affected by these drugs rather than the interaction between the template and the polymerase molecules proper (Fig. 7a–e).

As described by Scheer *et al.* (1975) with respect to the effects of actinomycin D, the effects of class II anthracyclines on the ribosomal transcriptional unit also were quite heterogeneous in relation to either the initiation or termination sites along the transcript. Based on these observations, it may become possible to reinterpret the morphology of the segregated nucleolus within the context of the structure of the rRNA cistron as demonstrated diagrammatically in Fig. 8. Upon inhibition of transcription, release of the nascent chains occurs, and these accumulate in the form of granular components (Fig. 8). Accumulation of granular components in the segregated nucleolus is evidence that processing of pre-rRNA occurs, since in nucleoli treated with toyocamycin, an adenosine analog (Monneron *et al.*, 1970) that inhibits pre-rRNA processing specifically, no nucleolar segregation occurs but rather nucleolar fragmentation takes place. On the other hand, the remaining denuded axial filament (rDNA) folds on its own and may represent the fibrillar component of the nucleolus.

The main difficulty still rests with interpretation of the origin and function of microspherules. Their presence in the precise interphase between the segregated granular and fibrillar elements (Fig. 3) suggests that they may still be related to the axial rDNA. Three possibilities must be considered as to the possible origin of microspherules: (1) They represent aggregates of polymerase I molecules eventually released from the template; (2) sequential to deactivation of the transcriptional unit the axial DNA becomes reorganized into nucleosomes, and these nucleosomal superstruc-

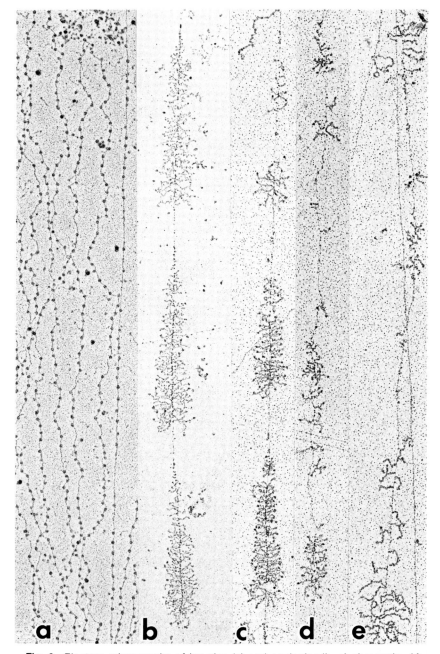

Fig. 6 Electron micrographs of inactive (a) and nucleolar (b–e) chromatin. After the treatment of normal nucleolar chromatin (b) with marcellomycin (5 μg/ml) for 15 minutes (c) or 1 hour (d and e), gaps are formed within the transcriptional unit.

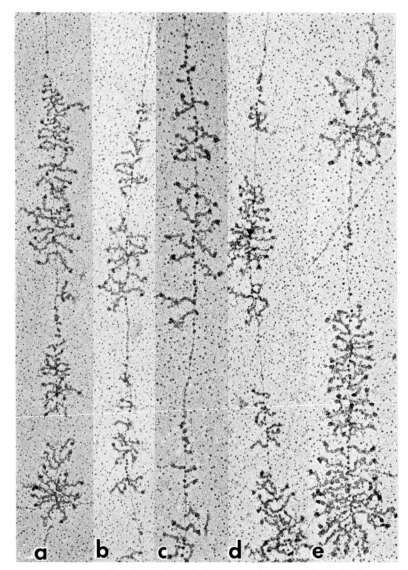

Fig. 7 Higher magnifications of nucleolar transcriptional units as in Fig. 6 after treatment with marcellomycin. No specific regions of lateral fibril deletions were found. RNA polymerase I molecules seen as large, dense spheres on the axial filamets are retained after drug treatment, despite loss of the corresponding lateral (nascent transcript) RNP fibrils.

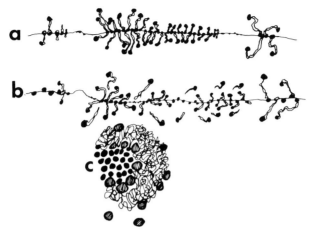

Fig. 8 Diagrammatic representation of the events leading to the segregation of nucleolar components after drug treatments within the context of the rRNA transcriptional unit. (a) Untreated; (b) loss of lateral fibrils after treatment; (c) folding of the transcriptional units into the nucleolus.

tures are then extruded or rearranged within the nucleolus; (3) they represent incomplete transcriptional products and are therefore discarded from the nucleolar body. The use of non-microspherule-producing drugs such as class I anthracyclines in similar experimental systems should provide more insight into the nature and origin of nucleolar microspherules.

III. Extranucleolar Chromatin as a Target for Drug Action

As previously described by Bouteille, perichromatin granules (PCGs), first reported by Watson (1962), are a universal component of the eukaryotic cell nucleus. The precise structure, function, origin, and composition of PCGs are uncertain. Their numbers have been reported to increase after exposure of the cells to supranormal temperature, lasiocarpine, aflatoxin (Monneron and Bernhard, 1969), cortisol (Moyne *et al.*, 1977), α-amanitin (Petrov and Sekeris, 1971), cycloheximide (Daskal *et al.*, 1975), and mitomycin C (Daskal and Crooke, 1979) (Fig. 9). Because of the ultrastructural similarity of PCGs to Balbiani granules, as well as ultracytochemical data, Vasquez-Nin and Bernhard (1971) suggested that PCGs may contain nuclear heterogeneous RNA (hnRNA). However, no direct evidence such as labeling kinetics of PCGs is available to establish the relationship between hnRNA synthesis and the biogenesis of these

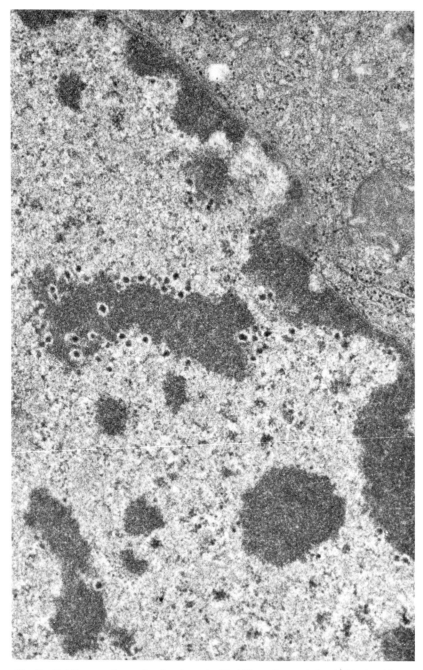

Fig. 9 Rat liver nucleus after treatment with 100 mg/kg cycloheximide for 4 hours. In addition to chromatin condensations into chromocenters, a dramatic increase (approximately threefold) in PCGs occurs. The PCGs are usually found in association with heterochromatin near the nuclear envelope and other chromocenters.

granules. To obtain more information on the structure and function of PGCs as well as the possible mechanisms by which the various drugs induce changes in PCG populations, their isolation was undertaken. Following the isolation procedure (Fig. 10), the nuclear extract was fractionated on a 8–45% sucrose density gradient into three main peaks (Fig. 11). The first main peak of the gradient contained granules approximately 350–400 Å in diameter whose morphology was similar to that of PCGs seen *in situ* (Fig. 12a and b). In addition to PCGs, peak 1 of the sucrose gradient contained an abundance of nucleosomes (Fig. 12, arrowheads). Although optimal yields of PCGs were obtained when the nuclear lysate was di-

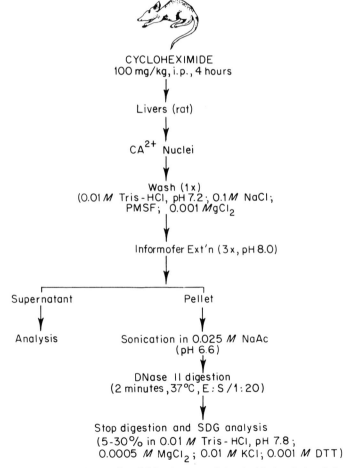

Fig. 10 Isolation scheme for PCGs from cycloheximide-treated rat livers; SDG, sucrose density gradient; DTT, Dithiothriethol. (Daskal *et al.* (1975). *Expt. Cell Res.* **93**, 395.)

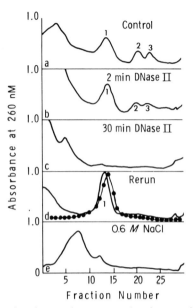

Fig. 11 Analysis of nuclear lysates by sucrose density centrifugation. (a) Fractionation of total undigested nuclear lysate. (b) Fractionation of nuclear lysate after DNase II digestion; the PCGs are concentrated in peak 1 (see Fig. 12). (c) The effects of prolonged DNase II digestion on the sedimentation characteristics of peak 1. (d) The purification and cosedimentation of the isolated PCGs with small ribosomal subunits (40 S); the PCGs sedimented in close proximity to the labeled ribosomal subunits (approximately 35 S). (e) The effects of salt extraction (0.6 *M* NaCl) on sedimentation of the PCGs. After salt treatment the PCGs sedimented approximately at 1–12 S [see (d)].

gested for 2 minutes with DNase II E/S =1:20) (Fig. 11b), extended digestions caused the loss of peak 1 (Fig. 11c). This was confirmed by electron microscopy (Fig. 12e) that showed only nucleosomal complexes in the gradient rather than intact PCGs. Cytochemical studies using Bernhard's preferential bleaching proceduees for RNAs (Bernhard, 1969) suggested that the PCGs consisted of RNP elements, since the granules were not bleached with EDTA (Fig. 12c) while the surrounding DNA-containing structures were completely bleached out.

To determine the sedimentation value of the isolated PCGs, 40 S rat liver, ^{32}P-labeled, purified ribosomal subunits were cosedimented with a partially purified PCG preparation. Accordingly, the sedimentation value of the PCGs was approximately 32–35 S (Fig. 11d). This sedimentation characteristic of the PCGs was highly dependent on the divalent ion concentration of the medium as well as the ionic strength of the buffers used. When the MgCl$_2$ concentration of the buffers was increased to 2 m*M*, the PCGs sedimented in the heavier region of the gradient. Increasing the

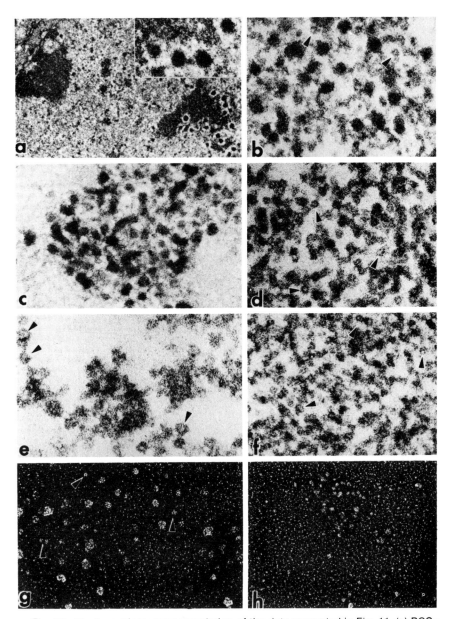

Fig. 12 Electron microscope correlation of the data presented in Fig. 11. (a) PCGs *in situ* after cycloheximide treatment (100 mg/kg, 4 hours). (b) Micrograph of material pelleted from peak 1; compare the structural characteristics of the *in situ* particles (a) and those in the isolated peak; arrowheads indicate hn RNP's. (c) Isolated PCGs after Bernhard's preferential EDTA procedure; the PCGs retained electron staining, suggesting that they contain RNPs. (d) PCGs after a 30-minute digestion with DNase II;

(Continued)

ionic strength to 0.6 M NaCl resulted in a large shift of peak 1 from the 40 S region to approximately 10–12 S (Fig. 11e).

Electron microscope examination of the 0.6 M NaCl-extracted PCGs (Fig. 12h) showed extended filaments with what appeared to be attached particles. A group of selected relaxed PCG complexes is shown in Fig. 13. An average of five particles associated with filaments was seen, however, some longer complexes consisting of up to nine particles were observed.

Data obtained from these studies suggest that PCGs represent a higher order of RNP packing, namely, a physiological-functional assembly of superbeads (Hozier *et al.*, 1977; Zentgraf *et al.*, 1978; Muller *et al.*, 1978). Although the bleaching procedure suggested PCG ribosomal RNP-containing structures, it should be considered that the PCGs are highly compact complexes not amenable to EDTA penetration (Bernhard, 1969; Komaromy *et al.*, 1978; Daskal *et al.*, 1978b).

What is the possible relationship between cycloheximide and other antimetabolites and the increase in the number of nuclear PCGs? It has been shown that newly synthesized chromatin DNA, in the presence of cycloheximide or another protein synthesis inhibitor, has an altered protein composition. In addition, the maturation of DNA intermediates into high-molecular-weight DNA is impaired (Seale and Simpson, 1975). Thus the effective inhibition of protein synthesis by cycloheximide, for example, perturbs the biosynthesis and assembly of both DNA and histones (Weintraub and Holtzer, 1972) by essentially uncoupling the coordinate DNA–protein replicative system (Seale and Simpson, 1975; Robbins and Borun, 1967). Therefore, rather than the PCGs representing accumulating, incompletely processed RNP structures as proposed by Moyne *et al.* (1977), it seems possible that the increase in PCG numbers under conditions of interference with either DNA or protein synthesis represents accumulating incomplete chromatin complexes prior to their final assembly or processing into mature RNP particles, which are temporarily extruded from the main active chromatin mass.

Further studies using other specific antimetabolites (Goldblatt *et al.*, 1969) of both RNA and protein synthesis should clarify whether microspherules and PCG formation represent general or specific reactions of nucleolor and nuclear chromatin, respectively, to an interference in

---

note that the dense and large granules have disappeared. (e) Higher magnification of overdigested PCGs; note the presence of particles within the PCG complex (arrowheads). (f) PCGs after extraction with 0.6 M NaCl. Only what appears to be nucleosomes are present after this extraction (arrowheads). (g and h) PCGs before (g) and after (h) 0.6 M NaCl extraction; shadowed preparations; arrowheads indicate nucleosomes.

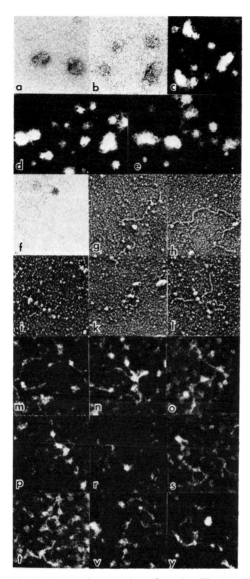

Fig. 13 Selected electron micrographs of native (isolated) and dissociated perichromatin granules, using several techniques for their visualization. (a–e) PCGs examined after deposition on the grid and examined with bright-field electron microscopy after negative staining (a–b) and dark-field electron microscopy (c–e). (f–y) Dissociated PCG complexes after 0.6 M NaCl extractions. (f) Bright-field electron microscopy positive. (g–l) Shadowed preparations (platinum–palladium). (m–y) Dark-field electron microscopy. In all instances, free nucleosomes or even free filaments were observed in the background. After the salt extractions complexes containing five to eight particles were observed. The most frequently observed complex consisted of five nucleosome-like structures associated with distinct filaments. All magnifications are × 150,000 = 10%.

coordinate synthetic processes and their effect on specific steps of the transcription process.

Acknowledgments

The author wishes to acknowledge the collaboration of Drs. U.Scheer and H. Spring of the German Cancer Research Institute, Heidelberg, West Germany, in the study on the effects of anthracyclines on transcriptional units, and of Dr. L. Komaromy in the studies related to the isolation of perichromatin granules; and the excellent technical assistance of Mr. C. Woodard. These studies were supported by cancer research grant CA-10893 P5 (Baylor College of Medicine, Department of Pharmacology, E.M. Unit) and the Bristol-Myers Fund.

References

Bernhard, W. (1969). *J. Ultrastruct. Res.* **27**, 250–265.
Bernhard, W., and Granboulan, N. (1969). *In* "The Nucleus" (A. J. Dalton and F. Haguneau, cds.), pp. 81–149. Academic Press, New York.
Busch, H., and Smetana, K. (1970). "The Nucleolus." Academic Press, New York.
Daskal, Y., and Crooke, S. T. (1979). *In* "Mitomycin C—Current Status and New Developments, Bristol–Myers Symposium." (S. K. Carter and S. T. Crooke, eds.). Academic Press, New York, pp. 41–46.
Daskal, Y., Merski, J. A., Hughes, J. B., and Busch, H. (1975). *Exp. Cell Res.* **93**, 395–401.
Daskal, Y., Woodard, C., Crooke, S. T., and Busch, H. (1978a). *Cancer Res.* **38**, 467–473.
Daskal, Y., Komaromy, L., and Busch, H. (1978b). *J. Cell Biol.* **79**, Part 2, 122 (No. 654).
Franke, W. W., Scheer, U., Trendelenburg, M. F., Spring, H., and Zentgraf, H. (1976). *Cytobiologie Z. Exp. Zellforsch.* **13**, 401–434.
Franke, W. W., Scheer, U., Spring, H., Trendelenburg, M. L., and Zentgraf, H. (1979). *In* "The Cell Nucleus" (H. Busch, ed.), Vol. 7. Academic Press, New York. In press.
Goldblatt, P. J., and Sullivan, R. J. (1970). *Cancer Res.* **30**, 1349–1359.
Goldblatt, P. J., Sullivan, R. J., and Farber, E. (1969). *Cancer Res.* **30**, 1349–1356.
Hozier, J., Renz, M., and Nehls, P. (1977). *Chromosoma* **62**, 301–317.
Komaromy, L., Daskal, Y., and Busch, H. (1978). *Proc. Am. Soc. Cancer Res.* **19**, 359.
Lambertenghi-Deliliers, G., Zanon, P. L., Pozzoli, E. F., and Bellini, O. (1976). *Tumori* **62**, 517–528.
Marinozzi, V., and Bernhard, W. (1963). *Exp. Cell Res.* **32**, 595–598.
Merski, J. A., Daskal, Y., and Busch, H. (1976). *Cancer Res.* **36**, 1580–1584.
Miller, O. L., and Beatty, B. R. (1969). *Science* **164**, 955–957.
Monneron, A., and Bernhard, W. (1969). *J. Ultrastruct. Res.* **27**, 266–268.
Monneron, A., Burglen, J., and Bernhard, W. (1970). *J. Ultrastruct. Res.* **32**, 370–389.
Moyne, G., Nash, R. E., and Puvion, E. (1977). *J. Biol. Cell.* **30**, 5–16.
Muller, U., Zentgraf, H., Eicken, I., and Keller, W. (1978). *Science* **201**, 406–415.
Petrov, P., and Sekeris, C. E. (1971). *Exp. Cell Res.* **36**, 842–860.
Recher, L., Chan, H., and Sykes, J. A. (1973). *J. Ultrastruct. Res.* **44**, 347–354.
Reynolds, R. C., Montgromery, P. O. B., and Huges, B. (1964). *Cancer Res.* **24**, 1269–1278.
Robbins, E., and Borum, T. W. (1967). *Proc. Natl. Acad. Sci. U.S.A.* **57**, 409–416.
Scheer, U., Trendelenburg, M. F., and Franke, W. (1975). *J. Cell Biol.* **65**, 163–179.

Schoefl, G. I. (1964). *J. Ultrastruct. Res.* **10**, 224–243.

Seale, R. L., and Simpson, R. T. (1975). *J. Mol. Biol.* **94**, 479–501.

Unuma, T., and Busch, H. (1967). *Cancer Res.* **27**, 1232–1242.

Vasquez-Nin, G., and Bernhard, W. J. (1971). *J. Ultrastruct. Res.* **36**, 842–860.

Watson, M. L. (1962). *J. Cell Biol.* **13**, 162–167.

Weintraub, H., and Holtzer, H. (1972). *J. Mol. Biol.* **66**, 13–35.

Zentgraf, H., Keller, W., and Muller, U. (1978). *Philos. Trans. R. Soc. London, Ser. B* **283**, 299–303.

5

Biochemical Effects of Drugs on the Cell Nucleus

STANLEY T. CROOKE

I. Introduction

In this chapter an overview of the types of effects drugs may have on the cell nucleus are discussed. Other chapters in this volume discuss most of the mechanisms in more detail. The discussion is organized by the type of effects drugs may have on the cell nucleus rather than chemical or pharmacological classifications. Since many (perhaps most) drugs induce multiple effects on the cell nucleus, and it is often difficult to determine the effect responsible for cytotoxicity, many of the agents must be considered as existing in more than one class. Moreover, since it is not possible with limited space to discuss all the agents that induce effects on the cell nucleus, only a few representative agents are considered.

II. Drugs That Affect DNA

Among the nuclear constituents, DNA of course is the component that is of highest concentration and importance, and many agents induce cytotoxic effects by interacting with DNA. The types of effects produced vary from DNA degradation to modifications which interfere with the function of nuclear DNA.

A. Compounds That Degrade DNA

During the past several years an increasing number of compounds have been shown to be able to degrade DNA under a variety of experimental conditions. However, it has been established for only a few agents that direct degradation of DNA is a major factor in their cytotoxicity. Certainly, to consider DNA degradation a principal part of the mechanism of action of an agent, at a minimum it should be demonstrated that (1) the agent degrades various types of isolated purified DNA, (2) degradation of isolated purified DNA occurs at concentrations approximating concentrations necessary for cytotoxicity, (3) degradation of isolated DNA occurs under conditions which approximate physiological conditions, and (4) intracellular DNA degradation can be demonstrated at concentrations and times compatible with the concept that DNA degradation is related causally to cell death.

Ideally, the cytotoxicity of a series of analogues should be related to their DNA degradative activity. Clearly, there are fewer compounds which fulfill these criteria for inclusion in this group of agents. Nonetheless, there are several.

1. Bleomycin and Its Analogues

Perhaps most clearly demonstrated to induce DNA degradation, and to be cytotoxic as a result of DNA degradative activity, are bleomycin and its analogues. Bleomycin was isolated, purified, and characterized initially by Umezawa and colleagues (Umezawa *et al.*, 1966). The original and the recently modified structures of bleomycin are shown in Fig. 1 (Umezawa, 1974; Takita *et al.*, 1978). Also shown in Fig. 1 is the structure of tallysomycin, the first bleomycin analogue that differs significantly from bleomycin in the bleomycinic acid portion of the molecule (Konishi *et al.*, 1977). However, since the structural proof of tallysomycin was based on the previous characterization of bleomycin, it is likely that the structure of tallysomycin will be modified in a manner analagous to the modification of the bleomycin structure.

All the active analogues of bleomycin have been shown to degrade DNA isolated from various sources in a reaction enhanced by a variety of reducing and oxidizing agents, and ferrous ions (Nagai *et al.*, 1969a,b; Haidle, 1971; Muller *et al.*, 1972; Strong and Crooke, 1978). Figure 2 shows the concentration-dependent degradation of PM-2 DNA by bleomycin A_2 and tallysomycin as detected by the decrease in fluorescence of ethidium bromide in several buffers.

Bleomycin and its analogues have been shown to result in the release of free bases and produce alkali-labile sites, single-strand breaks, and double-strand breaks (which cannot be accounted for by the clustering of sin-

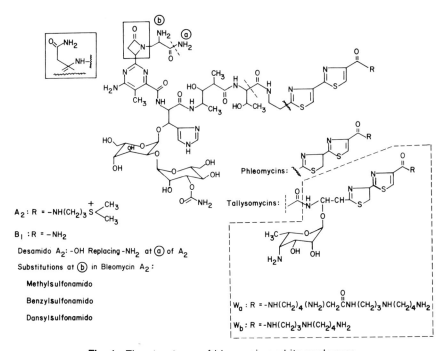

Fig. 1 The structures of bleomycin and its analogues.

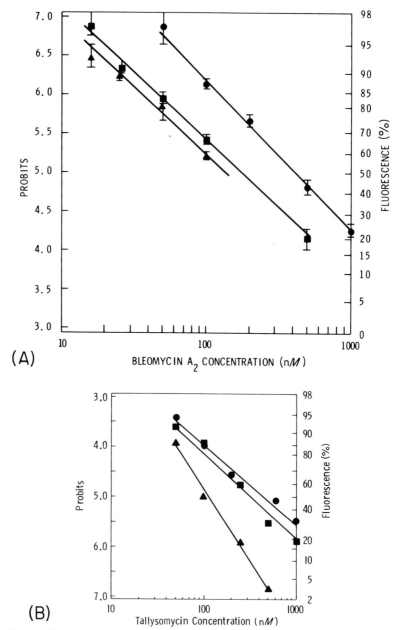

(A)

(B)

Fig. 2 Concentration-dependent degradation of PM-2 DNA by bleomycin A₂ and tallysomycin A. Covalently closed circular PM-2 DNA was incubated with varying concentrations of bleomycin A₂ and tallysomycin A as previously described for 30 minutes. (A) Bleomycin A₂ in borate buffer (▲), CHES buffer (■), and Tris buffer (●). (B) Tallysomycin in the same buffers.

gle-strand breaks in DNA) (Povirk *et al.*, 1977; Haidle *et al.*, 1972; Muller *et al.*, 1972; Strong and Crooke, 1978). Figure 3 shows that both bleomycin A_2 and tallysomycin produce single- and double-strand breaks in PM-2 DNA as determined by agarose gel electrophoresis.

The degradation of DNA by bleomycin and its analogues appears to be related to the ability of these agents to bind to ferrous ions, facilitate the oxidation of ferrous ions, and generate free radicals which may be the proximal degradative compounds (Lown and Sim, 1977; Sausville *et al.*, 1976). Certainly bleomycin and its analogues bind a number of divalent cations (Dabrowiak *et al.*, 1978), and the site at which binding occurs has been defined. More recently, additional studies in our laboratory have shown that semisynthetic derivatives of bleomycin which bind various divalent cations, but do not facilitate the oxidation of ferrous ions, are unable to degrade DNA although they continue to bind to it avidly. Thus these studies confirm that DNA degradation induced by bleomycin is dependent on the oxidation of ferrous ions.

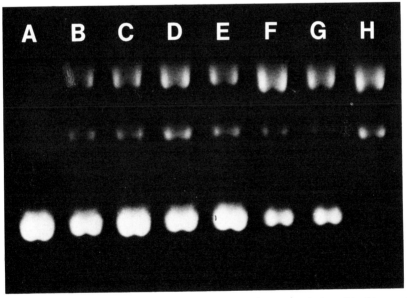

Fig. 3 Agarose gel electrophoresis of PM-2 DNA fragments induced by bleomycin A_2 (BLM) and tallysomycin A (TLM). Covalently closed circular m-2 DNA was incubated with varying concentrations of the drugs and then electrophoresed on 1% agarose gels under neutral conditions as previously described. (A) control; (B) 100 nM TLM; (C) 250 nM TLM; (D) 500 nM TLM; (E) 1 μM TLM; (F) 100 nM BLM A_2; (G) 250 nM BLM A_{2_1}; (H) 1 μM BLM A_2.

2. Macromomycin

Macromomycin is a polypeptide antibiotic which has been shown to have *in vivo* antitumor activity and an approximate molecular weight of 12,000 (Chimura *et al.*, 1968; Im *et al.*, 1978, Yamashita, *et al.*, 1976). The amino acid analysis and preliminary sequence of the first 30 amino acids determined in our laboratory are shown in Table I and Fig. 4, respectively (Sawyer *et al.*, 1979).

Although it has been proposed that macromomycin is not absorbed and induces its antitumor effects by immunological effects and from activities at the cell surface (Coronetti and Lippman, 1976; Lippman and Abbott, 1973; Kunimoto *et al.*, 1972), studies in our laboratory have demonstrated that macromomycin degrades isolated DNA and intracellular DNA at concentrations comparable to those that are cytotoxic (Sawyer *et al.*, 1979).

TABLE I
Amino Acid Composition of Macromomycin

Amino acid	This study (mole %)	Yamashita *et al.* (1976) (mole %)
Asx	6.4	6.3
Thr	15.2	13.5
Ser	7.2	7.9
Glx	7.2	6.3
Pro	4.0	4.0
Gly	14.4	16.7
Ala	15.2	15.1
Cys	2.4	3.2
Val	13.6	13.4
Ile	2.4	2.4
Leu	4.0	3.2
Tyr	1.6	1.6
Phe	2.4	1.6
Lys	2.4	2.4
His	1.6	1.6
Trp	0.8	0.8

[a] Duplicate 10-μg macromomycin samples were hydrolyzed *in vacuo* at 110°C in 5.7 *N* HCl for 22 hours. Samples were analyzed on a Beckman 121M amino acid analyzer with a single-column program. Corrections were made for destruction or time-dependent release. Tryptophan was determined in duplicate 10-μg samples hydrolyzed with 3 *N* mercaptoethanesulfonic acid for 22 hours at 110°C.

H$_2$N-Ala-Pro-Gly-Val- Thr-Val-Thr-Pro-Ala- Thr-
              5   10

Gly-Leu-Ser-Asn- Gly-Glu-Thr-Val-Thr- Val-
11   15   20

Ser-Ala-Thr-Gly-Leu-Thr-Pro-Gly-Thr- Val
21   30

Fig. 4 Partial sequence of macromomycin.

3. Neocarzinostatin

Neocarzinostatin is a polypeptide with a molecular weight of 10,700, the primary sequence of which has been determined (Meienhofer *et al.*, 1972). Although neocarzinostatin has been shown to degrade DNA by a number of investigators (Beerman and Goldberg, 1974), it induces predominantly single-strand breaks, and it is stimulated by reducing agents.

4. Hedamycin

Recently, studies in our laboratory have demonstrated that hedamycin binds to DNA and degrades it. That it results in a decrease in fluorescence due to ethidium bromide binding to PM-2 DNA is shown in Fig. 5.

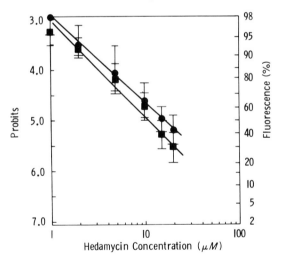

Fig. 5 Effects of hedamycin on the binding of ethidium bromide to covalently closed circular PM-2 DNA. Hedamycin was prepared as a 1 m*M* stock solution in 50% dimethyl sulfoxide (DMSO). PM-2 DNA was incubated with different concentrations of hedamycin for 30 (●) and 60 (■) minutes. The final concentrations of DMSO in the incubation mixture were from 0.1 to 1%. No effects on fluorescence due to DMSO was demonstrated at these concentrations.

Agarose gel electrophoresis showed that hedamycin produced a diffuse staining pattern typical of intercalating agents. However, alkaline sucrose density centrifugation showed that, in addition to intercalation, hedamycin degraded PM-2 DNA as demonstrated by alkaline sucrose density gradient centrifugation.

B. Other Agents

A number of other agents have been reported to degrade DNA under a variety of conditions, and in concentrations which may be different from those operant *in vivo*.

1. Alkylating Agents

Agents which alkylate a variety of subcellular components have been of interest for many years, and numerous agents have been studied. In general, these compounds are capable of alkylating a variety of nuclear substituents, but it is thought that the activity most closely correlated with cytotoxicity is the alkylation of DNA. Clearly, a variety of chemotypes may alkylate DNA, but all alkylating agents are either electrophilic or generate electrophilic compounds *in vivo*.

Many of the activating reactions of alkylating agents are relatively complex. Cyclophosphamide, for example, is metabolized by liver microsomal enzymes to a circulating intermediate, 4-hydroxycyclophosphamide (Hill *et al.*, 1972), and then is subsequently converted to the most cytotoxic derivative, phosphoramide mustard (Colvin *et al.*, 1976). Similarly, mitomycin C is inactive in its native state and undergoes reductive activation to become a di- or trifunctional alkylating agent (Iyer and Szbalski, 1964).

The site of initial attack on DNA by alkylating agents may vary depending upon the agent studied, the type of polynucleotide, and reaction conditions. Certainly the 7-position in guanosine is a sensitive site, but numerous other sites have recently been defined, such as the 0-6 position in guanosine, as important sites (Loveless, 1969; Lawley, 1966; Ludlum, 1977). The ramifications of alkylation also vary from simple alkylation to inter- and intrastrand cross-linking to DNA breakage.

The effects subsequent to modification of DNA also vary, and the effects primarily responsible for cytotoxicity are not clearly defined for any of the alkylating agents. Clearly inhibition of DNA synthesis has been reported to occur at times and concentrations compatible with the concept that it is related causally to cytotoxicity. However, effects on transcription may also be significant.

2. Intercalating Agents

A variety of agents have been shown to intercalate in DNA, and many agents usually classified in other groups, e.g., bleomycin, a DNA-breaking agent, interact with DNA by intercalation. Certainly actinomycin D and its analogues interact with DNA by intercalation, and this results in interference with a variety of functions of DNA (Busch and Smetana, 1970). The site at which actinomycin D intercalation occurs has been proposed to be between adjacent GC base pairs, which results in the cyclic peptides residing in the minor groove of DNA, thus potentially accounting for the preferential inhibition of nucleolar RNA synthesis (Sobell, 1973). Actinomycin D, of course, affects many other cellular functions as well (Hollstein, 1974).

Another group of interesting intercalative agents is the anthracyclines. These agents have been shown to bind preferentially to double-stranded DNA via strong intercalative bonds and weaker ionic bonds (Zunino *et al.*, 1977). However, unlike actinomycin D, studies have failed to demonstrate base pair specificity but have shown that some anthracyclines may bind preferentially to AT-rich DNA species (DiMarco *et al.*, 1975).

TABLE II

Class I Anthracyclines: Structural Modifications in the Adriamycin–Daunomycin Class of Anthracyclines

General structure of the adriamycin–daunomycin class of anthracyclines

Compound	R_1	R_2	R_3	R_4	X
Adriamycin	OCH_3	CH_2OH	H	H	O
Daunomycin	OCH_3	CH_3	H	H	O
Carminomycin	OH	CH_3	H	H	O
Rubidazone	OCH_3	CH_3	H	H	$NNHCCC_6H_5$
AD-32	OCH_3	$CH_2OCOC_4H_9$	H	$COCF_3$	O
AD-41	OCH_3	CH_2OH	H	$COCF_3$	O

   Recent studies in our laboratory have shown that anthracyclines may be fractionated into two classes. Class I anthracyclines include anthracyclines such as adriamycin, carminomycin, and pyrromycin (Table II). Class II anthracyclines include marcellomycin, rudolfomycin, musettamycin, and aclacinomycin (Table III). Class I anthracyclines were shown to inhibit nucleolar RNA synthesis and DNA synthesis at equivalent concentrations. Class II anthracyclines were shown to inhibit nucleolar RNA synthesis at concentrations 200 to 1500-fold lower than those required to inhibit DNA synthesis (Table IV). Structure–activity relationship studies have demonstrated that the length of the glycosidic side chain, and the carbomethoxy group on C-10, are the critical determinants of nucleolar DNA synthesis specificity (Table V) (Crooke *et al.*, 1978; Duvernay *et al.*, 1978). Moreover changes in the glycosidic side chain and the carbomethoxy group of class II anthracyclines markedly affect DNA-binding prop-

TABLE III

Class II Anthracyclines: Structural Modifications in the Cinerubin A–Aclacinomycin Class of Anthracyclines[a]

General Structure of the cinerubin A–aclacinomycin class of anthracyclines

Compound	R_1	$R_2{}^a$	R_3
Pyrromycin	OH	H	H
Musettamycin	OH	DF	H
Marcellomycin	OH	DF-DF	H
Cinerubin A	OH	DF-C	H
Aclacinomycin	H	DF-C	H

[a] The abbreviations DF and C correspond to the sugars 2-deoxyfucose and cinerulose, respectively.

TABLE IV

Nucleic Acid Synthetic Inhibitory Activities of Class I and Class II Anthracyclines

Anthracycline	IC_{50} no RNA (μM)	IC_{50} DNA / IC_{50} whole-cell RNA	IC_{50} DNA / IC_{50} no RNA
Adriamycin	6.0	1.89	1.02
Carminomycin	13.06	1.64	1.12
Pyrromycin	6.15	1.26	0.93
Marcellomycin	0.009	6.53	1256
Musettamycin	0.014	6.66	714
Aclacinomycin	0.037	7.65	170

erties (Duvernay *et al.*, 1978). However, the nucleolar RNA synthetic specificity of class II anthracyclines cannot be explained by DNA sequence specificity, since all the anthracyclines studied bind preferentially to AT-rich DNA (Duvernay and Crooke, unpublished data).

Many other compounds have been shown to interact with DNA by intercalation, including interesting antibiotics such as echinomycin which appears to behave as a double intercalating agent (Waring and Wakelin, 1974), various dyes such as the acridines (Lerman, 1961), and some potentially useful new chemical agents such as M-AMSA.

III. Drugs That Affect Enzymes Involved in Nucleic Acid Metabolism

A. Purine Antagonists

Purine antagonists have been reviewed extensively by several authors (LePage, 1977). Consequently I will deal with them very briefly. Although numerous purine antagonists have been synthesized, 6-mercaptopurine (6-MP) has proven the most useful agent. As with most nucleoside analogues, 6-MP requires "lethal synthesis" for activity (Elion *et al.*, 1963). Once activated, 6-MP acts as a negative feedback inhibitor of *de novo* purine synthesis and inhibits the conversion of orotic acid to xanthylic and adenylic acid (Brockman, 1963; Elion, 1967).

A number of other purine antagonists, such as 6-thioguanine, have been studied and shown to inhibit various steps in DNA synthesis (LePage, 1977). Glutamine analogues such as azaserine also inhibit DNA synthesis by inhibiting purine biosynthesis, but also have other activities such as alkylation (Bennett, 1975).

TABLE V

Effect of Removal of 10-Carbomethoxy Antitumor Activity, Cytotoxicity, and Nucleic Acid Synthetic Activities of Marcellomycin and Rudolfomycin

	In vitro IC$_{50}$ values (μM)				In vivo antitumor activity in L-1210 leukemia (mg/kg/in)
	DNA synthesis	RNA synthesis	No RNA synthesis	Cell viability	
Marcellomycin (MCM)	13.52	3.03	0.014	0.75	0.20
10-Descarbomethoxymarcellomycin (D-MCM)	18.99	4.07	2.56	3.80	4.0
D-MCM/MCM	1.40	1.34	183	5.10	20
Rudolfomycin (RDM)	69.70	3.65	0.29	0.31	0.20
10-Descarbomethoxyrudolfomycin (D-RDM)	18.37	7.24	9.13	>5.0	16.0
D-RDM/RDM	0.264	1.98	31	>16	80

B. Pyrimidine Antagonists

Similar to the purine antagonists, numerous pyrimidine antagonists have been developed, and many extensive reviews are available (Maley, 1977). In general they have been shown to inhibit one or more steps in DNA synthesis as a primary mechanism of action, and produce other effects, e.g., incorporation into DNA and RNA; several have been demonstrated to have modest clinical utility.

C. Folate Antagonists

Amethopterin and other folate antagonists have been shown to produce cytotoxicity because of inhibition of dihydrofolate reductase, and subsequent inhibition of DNA synthesis and other cellular processes (Chabner and Johns, 1977). Additional studies have shown that an excess of amethopterin relative to the intracellular concentration of dihydrofolate reductase is essential (Chabner *et al.*, 1972; Goldman *et al.*, 1975).

IV. Drugs That Affect RNA and RNA Metabolism

A number of drugs that affect RNA and RNA metabolism have been reported. Drugs could conceivably result directly in degradation of RNA, inhibition of RNA synthesis, alteration of processing, or catabolism of RNA. Although several drugs have been reported to degrade DNA, no active compounds have been shown to degrade RNA as a primary mechanism. However, numerous agents have been reported to affect the synthesis of a variety of types of RNA.

Actinomycin D has clearly been shown to inhibit RNA synthesis, and to inhibit selectively nucleolar RNA synthesis at low concentrations, and a new group of anthracyclines has also been shown to produce similar effects as discussed in a previous section. Furthermore, other intercalating agents such as proflavin induce similar effects.

Inhibition of processing of pre-rRNA has been reported to be induced by several agents. Intercalating agents including proflavin, ethidium, and ellipticine have been shown to inhibit the conversion of 45 S RNA to 32 S RNA (Snyder *et al.*, 1971). Toyocamycin, an adenosine analogue, has been shown to inhibit conversion of 45 S RNA to 32 S RNA, by being incorporated into 45 S RNA and inhibiting processing (Tavitian *et al.*, 1969). The processing of nuclear hnRNA has been reported to be inhibited by cordycepin (Penman *et al.*, 1971). It has been suggested that this effect is due to interference with the synthesis and addition of the poly(A) segment to putative mRNA, resulting in interference with the processing of pre-mRNA species (Darnell *et al.*, 1973).

There are no well-characterized examples of drugs that appear to induce cytotoxicity as a result of affecting processes such as methylation, specific cleavage reactions, or nonspecific catabolism. However, given the ubiquitous yet specific nature of many of these reactions, these may be fruitful targets for new drug development.

V. Drugs That Affect Nuclear Proteins

A number of agents have been reported to affect a variety of nuclear proteins. Nitrosoureas have been reported to carbamoylate selectively histones with no carbamoylation of acidic nuclear proteins detected (Woolley *et al.*, 1976; Schmall *et al.*, 1973). Dibromodulictol was shown to bind to acidic nuclear proteins to a greater degree than to histones (Institoris and Hokzinger, 1976).

There arc also a number of drugs that affect nuclear enzymes, many of which have been considered in previous sections. However additional examples deserve discussion. Cytosine arabinoside 5'-triphosphate, for example, has been reported to inhibit selectively a DNA polymerase thought to be involved in DNA repair (Lynch *et al.*, 1972). Bleomycin has been shown to stimulate repair DNA synthesis; however, this is probably an indirect effect due to induction of DNA degradation (Sartiano *et al.*, 1973; Sartiano, personal communication).

VI. Drugs That Affect the Mitotic Apparatus

Several drugs have been shown to inhibit mitosis by disruption of the mitotic apparatus. These drugs include colcichine, vinca alkaloids, podophyllotoxins, and griseofulvin (Creasey, 1977). Each of these agents binds, usually reversibly, to various structures necessary for spindle formation, and results in dissolution.

VII. Drugs That Affect the Nuclear Membrane

Although the nuclear membrane is a possible target for cytoxic drug activity, there are no examples of agents that are active primarily as a result of this mechanism. Moreover, there are no examples of drugs that affect nuclear cytoplasmic transport as a primary mechanism of action.

VIII. Conclusions

In this chapter an overview, with emphasis on several new areas of research, of the possible effects of cytotoxic drugs on the cell nucleus has been presented. Obviously this is an immense topic, and many areas could be discussed only superficially, or not at all (e.g., hormones). Nonetheless, this chapter has demonstrated that the cell nucleus is an important target for cytotoxic compounds.

References

Beerman, T. A., and Goldberg, I. H. (1974). *Biochem. Biophys. Res. Commun.* **59**, 1254–1258.

Bennett, L. L., Jr. (1975). *In* "Antineoplastic and Immunosuppressive Agents II" (A. S. Sartorelli and D. G. Johns, eds.), Springer-Verlag, New York, 1975.

Brockman, R. W. (1963). *Cancer Res.* **23**, 1191–1199.

Busch, H., and Smetana, K. (1970). "The Nucleolus." Academic Press, New York.

Chabner, B. A., and Johns, D. G. (1977). *In* "Cancer, a Comprehensive Treatise" (F. F. Becker, ed.), Vol. 5, Plenum, New York.

Chabner, B. A., Chello, P. L., and Bertino, J. R. (1972). *Cancer Res.* **32**, 2114–2119.

Chimura, H., Istinzuka, M., Hamada, M., Hori, S., Kimura, K., Iwanage, J., Takeuchi, T., and Umezawa, H. (1968). *J. Antibiot.* **21**, 44–49.

Colvin, M., Brudrett, R. B., Kan, M. N., Jardine, I., and Fenselau, C. (1976). *Cancer Res.* **36**, 1121–1126.

Coronetti, E., and Lippman, M. M. (1976). *J. Natl. Cancer Inst.* **56**, 1275–1277.

Creasey, W. A. (1977). *In* "Cancer, a Comprehensive Treatise" (F. F. Becker, ed.), Vol. 5, Plenum, New York.

Crooke, S. T., Duvernay, V., Galvan, L., and Prestayko, A. W. (1978). *Mol. Pharmacol.* **14**, 65–73.

Dabrowiak, J. C., Greenaway, F. T., Longo, W. E., VanHusen, M., and Crooke, S. T. (1978). *Biochim. Biophys. Acta* **517**, 517–526.

Darnell, J. E., Jelineck, W. R., and Molloy, G. R. (1973). *Science* **181**, 1215–1221.

DiMarco, A., Arcamone, F., and Zunino, F. (1975). *In* "Antibiotics III. Mechanism of Action of Antimicrobial and Antitumor Agents" (J. W. Corcoran, ed.), Springer-Verlag, Berlin and New York.

Duvernay, V. H., and Crooke, S. T. (1978). *Proc. Int. Cancer Congr., 12th, Buenos Aires* pp. 272–273,

Duvernay, V. H., Essery, J. M., Doyle, T. D., Bradner, W. T., and Crooke, S. T. (1978). *Mol. Pharmacol.*

Elion, G. B. (1967). *Fed. Proc., Fed. Am. Soc. Exp. Biol.* **26**, 898–903.

Elion, G. B., Callahan, S., Rundles, R. W., and Hitchings, G. H. (1963).*Cancer Res.* **23**, 207–1212.

Goldman, I. D., White, J. C., and Loftfield, S. (1975). *Mol. Pharmacol.* **11**, 287–296.

Haidle, C. W. (1971). *Mol. Pharmacol.* **7**, 645–652.

Haidle, C. W., Kuo, M. T., and Weiss, K. K. (1972). *Biochem. Pharmacol.* **21**, 3308–3312.

Hill, D. L., Laster, W. R., Jr., and Struck, R. F. (1972). *Cancer Res.* **32**, 658–662.

Hollstein, U. (1974). *Chem. Rev.* **35**, 3027–3038.

Im, W. B., Chaing, C. K., and Montgomery, R. (1978). *J. Biol. Chem.* **253**, 3259–3264.

Inst, E., and Hokzinger, L. (1976). *Chem.-Biol. Interact.* **12**, 241–250.

Iyer, V. N., and Szbalski, W. (1964). *Science* **145**, 55–57.

Joel, P. B., and Goldberg, I. (1970). *Biochim. Biophys. Acta* **224**, 361–365.

Konishi, M., Saito, K., Numota, K., Tsuno, T., Asama, K., Tsukuira, H., Naito, T., and Kawaguchi, H. (1977). *J. Antibiot.* **30**, 789–805.

Kunimoto, T., Hori, M., and Umezawa, H. (1972). *Cancer Res.* **32**, 1251–1256.

Lawley, P. D. (1966). *Prog. Nucleic Acid Res. Mol. Biol.* **5**, 89–101.

LePage, G. A. (1977). *In* "Cancer, a Comprehensive Treatise" (F. F. Becker, ed.), Vol. 5, Plenum, New York.

Lerman, L. S. (1961). *J. Mol. Biol.* **3**, 18–30.

Lippman, M. M., and Abbott, B. J. (1973). *Cancer Chemother. Rep.* **57**, 501–503.

Loveless, A. (1969). *Nature (London)* **223**, 206–209.

Lown, J. W. (1979). *In* "Mitomycin C: Current Status and New Developments" (S. K. Carter and S. T. Crooke, eds.). Academic Press, New York. In press.

Lown, J. W., and Sim, S. (1977). *Biochem. Biophys. Res. Commun.* **77**, 1150–1156.

Lown, J. W., Sim, S., Majumdar, K. C., and Chang, R. C. (1976). *Biochem. Siophys. Res. Commun.* **76**, 705–709.

Ludlum, D. B. (1977). *In* "Cancer, a Comprehensive Treatise" (F. F. Becker, ed.), Vol. 5, Plenum, New York.

Maley, F. (1977). *In* "Cancer, a Comprehensive Treatise" (F. F. Becker, ed.), Vol. 5, Plenum, New York.

Meienhofer, J., Maeda, H., Glaser, C. B., Czombos, J., and Kuromiz, K. (1972). *Science* **178**, 875–877.

Muller, W. E. G., Yamazaki, Z., Breter, H., and Zahn, R. K. (1972). *Eur. J. Biochem.* **31**, 518–525.

Nagai, K., Yamaki, H., Suzuki, H., Tanaka, N., and Umezawa, H. (1969a). *Biochim. Biophys. Acta* **179**, 165–171.

Nagai, K., Suzuki, H., Tanaka, N., and Umezawa, H. (1969b). *J. Antibiot.* **22**, 624–628.

Penman, S., Rosbach, M., and Penman, M. (1971). *Proc. Natl. Acad. Sci. U.S.A.* **67**, 1878–1881.

Povirk, I. V., Wubker, W., Kohnlein, W., and Hutchinson, F. (1977). *Nucleic Acids Res.* **4**, 3573–3580.

Sartiano, G. P., Winkelstein, A., Lynch, W., and Boggs, S. S. (1973). *J. Antibiot.* **26**, 437–443.

Sausville, E. A., Peisch, J., and Horwitz, S. B. (1976). *Biochem. Biophys. Res. Commun.* **73**, 814–822.

Sawyer, T. H., Prestayko, A. W., and Crooke, S. T. (1979). *Cancer Res.* (in press).

Snyder, A. L., Kahn, H. E., and Kohn, K. W. (1971). *J. Mol. Biol.* **58**, 555–565.

Sobell, H. M., (1973). *Prog. Nucleic Acid Res. Mol. Biol.* **13**, 153–173.

Strong, J. E., and Crooke, S. T. (1978). *Cancer Res.* **38**, 3322–3326.

Takita, T., Muraoka, Y., Nakatani, T., Fujii, A., Umezawa, Y., Naganawa, H., and Umezawa, H. (1978). *J. Antibiot.*

Tavitian, A., Uretsky, S. C., and Acs, G. (1969). *Biochim. Biophys. Acta* **179**, 50–58.

Umezawa, H. (1974). *Fed. Proc. , Fed. Am. Soc. Exp. Biol.* **33**, 2296–2301.

Umezawa, H., Surhara, X., Takita, T., and Maeda, K. (1966). *J. Antibiot., Ser. A* **19**, 210–219.

Waring, M. J., and Wakelin, L. P. G. (1974). *Nature (London)* **252,** 653–657.

Woolley, P. V., Dion, R. L., Kohnk, and Bono, V. H., Jr. (1976). *Cancer Res.* **36,** 1470—1474.

Yamashita, T., Naoi, N., Watanabe, K., Takeuchi, T., and Umezawa, H. (1976). *J. Antibiot.* **29,** 415–423.

Zunino, F., Gambetta, R., DiMarco, A., Valeich, A., Zaccaro, A., Quadrifoglis, F., and Crescenzi, V. (1977). *Biochim. Biophys. Acta* **476,** 38–46.

Drug Interactions with DNA

HENRY M. SOBELL

During the past few years, important advances have taken place in understanding the molecular basis of drug–DNA interactions. For the most part, these advances reflect the technique of X-ray crystallography in determining the three-dimensional structures of a large number of drug–nucleic acid crystalline complexes and additional supporting data concerning the binding of these drugs and dyes to DNA. This chapter reviews our current understanding of drug–DNA interactions and, in addition, describes concepts of the dynamic nature of DNA structure that gives rise to drug intercalation. The subject of drug intercalation into DNA may be related more broadly to understanding a large number of

EFFECTS OF DRUGS ON THE CELL NUCLEUS
Copyright © 1979 by Academic Press, Inc.
All rights of reproduction in any form reserved.
ISBN 0-12-147654-5

protein–DNA interactions, many of these occurring in the organization of DNA in chromatin within the cellular nucleus. We describe these in this chapter.

I. Dynamic Nature of DNA Structure

An important dynamic aspect of DNA in solution is the presence of coupled motions in its structure that involve bending, stretching, shearing, and unwinding components. We have postulated these motions to arise from wave propagation in the polymer, excited through impulses generated by the random, continuous bombardment of DNA by solvent molecules along its length. This gives rise to structural distortions in DNA that result in DNA breathing and in drug intercalation (Sobell *et al.*, 1976, 1977a,b, 1978; Sobell, 1978; Lozansky *et al.*, 1979).

Figure 1 shows Corey–Pauling–Koltun (CPK) space-filling molecular models of DNA undergoing wave propagation in its structure. We envision low-amplitude (elastic) traveling waveforms in DNA to be right-handed superhelices containing approximately 10 base pairs per turn and having a pitch of about 35 Å (cf. Fig. 1B and C). Such structures balance the unwinding in the helix with right-handed superhelical writhe to keep the linkage invariant (Fuller, 1971), a feature that creates minimal perturbation in DNA structure. Higher-amplitude (elastic) traveling waveforms (shown in Fig. 1D), however, could contain somewhat more than 10 base pairs per turn, and their presence may contribute to the apparent net unwinding of DNA observed in solution [i.e., recent studies of superhelical DNA in solution indicate that DNA has, on the average, approximately 10.4 base pairs per turn (J. C. Wang, personal communication)].

At small amplitudes of oscillation, DNA behaves as an elastic body that accumulates strain energy in its structure through small changes in torsional angles that define the geometry of the sugar-phosphate backbone. These changes are localized primarily in the furanose rings of alternate deoxyribose sugar residues (normally, the puckering of the furanose ring in B DNA is C2'-*endo*; however, the effect of introducing strain energy into the helix is to alter the magnitude and direction of this puckering).

Fig. 1 DNA undergoing wave propagation in its structure. (A) B DNA, drawn by computer graphics. (B) Corey–Pauling–Koltun (CPK) space filling model of B DNA. (C) A low-amplitude elastic wave form in B DNA. (D) A larger-amplitude elastic wave form in B DNA. (E) β-kinked DNA structure, formed by a transient high-energy normal-mode oscillation in DNA structure. (F) β-kinked DNA, drawn by computer graphics. See text for discussion.

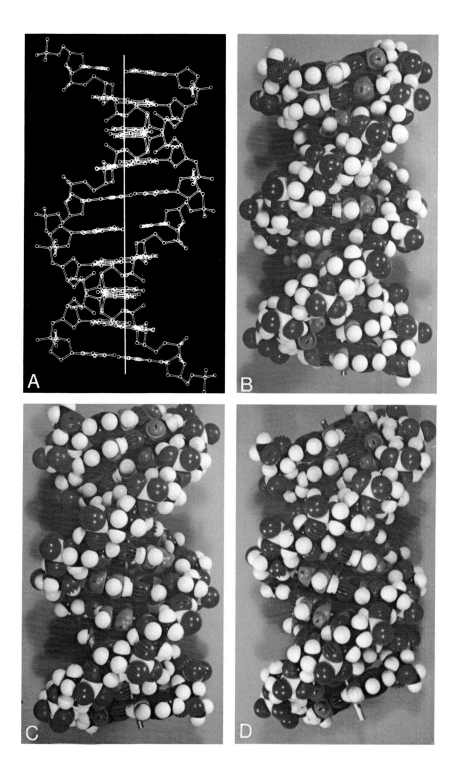

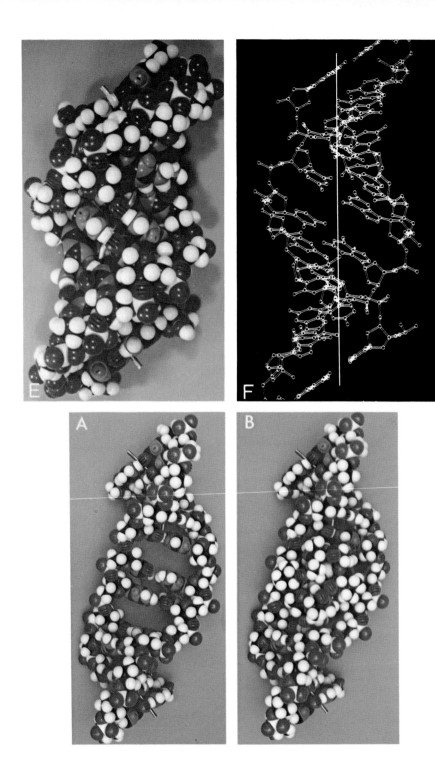

At larger amplitudes of oscillation, the enhanced strain energy in the sugar-phosphate chains begins to flatten out the furanose ring. Finally, at some critical oscillation amplitude, alternate sugars "snap into" a C3′ *endo* sugar conformation with a concommitant partial unstacking of base-pairs (see Plate 16E). This structure (denoted β kinked DNA) corresponds to an inelastic distortion in DNA structure and arises from a transient high energy normal mode oscillation in the helix localized at a specific site. (see Fig. 1E). Such a structure would remain fixed to this site and— through further capture of mechanical wave energy—could be activated to still higher-energy structural intermediates involved in DNA breathing and in drug intercalation.

These dynamic concepts of DNA structure are summarized schematically in Fig. 2. The activated β-kinked DNA structure that gives rise to DNA breathing and drug intercalation is shown with CPK space-filling molecular models in Fig. 3A.

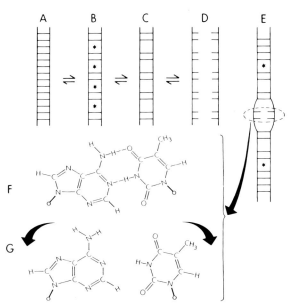

Fig. 2 Schematic illustration of dynamic concepts of DNA structure involved in DNA breathing and in drug intercalation.

Fig. 3 CPK space-filling models of the activated β-kinked DNA structure (A) and this structure with the bis intercalating antibiotic echinomycin in place (B). See text for discussion.

II. Bis Intercalation—A Probe for β-Kinked Structural Distortions in DNA?

An important class of intercalative drugs and dyes that has received considerable attention in recent years are bis intercalators—bifunctional intercalating agents that have two chromophore groups separated by about 10.2 Å (Wakelin and Waring, 1976; Ughetto and Waring, 1977; Le Pecq *et al.*, 1975; Butour *et al.*, 1978; Dervan and Becker, 1978). These molecules intercalate into DNA in a neighbor-exclusion mode (i.e., the intercalative chromophore groups are separated by two base pairs when binding to DNA). One example is echinomycin, a polypeptide-containing antibiotic that binds to DNA and inhibits RNA synthesis. This molecule has two quinoxaline ring systems connected to an octapeptide through amide linkages (see Fig. 4) and probably possesses a pseudodyad axis of symmetry that plays an important role in its structural interactions with DNA (see Fig. 3B). The presence of these two intercalative chromophore groups held 10.2 Å apart by the rigid octapeptide chain suggests that echinomycin recognizes a naturally occurring structural intermediate in RNA synthesis. We have postulated this intermediate to be β-kinked DNA, a key intermediate in DNA unwinding (Sobell, 1978; Sobell *et al.*, 1978). It is of interest that echinomycin is about four to five times more potent than actinomycin in its ability to inhibit RNA synthesis, a feature that makes it an extremely potent antitumor agent. Unfortunately, however, its enhanced cytotoxicity limits its clinical usefulness.

Drugs containing two intercalative chromophore groups have been syn-

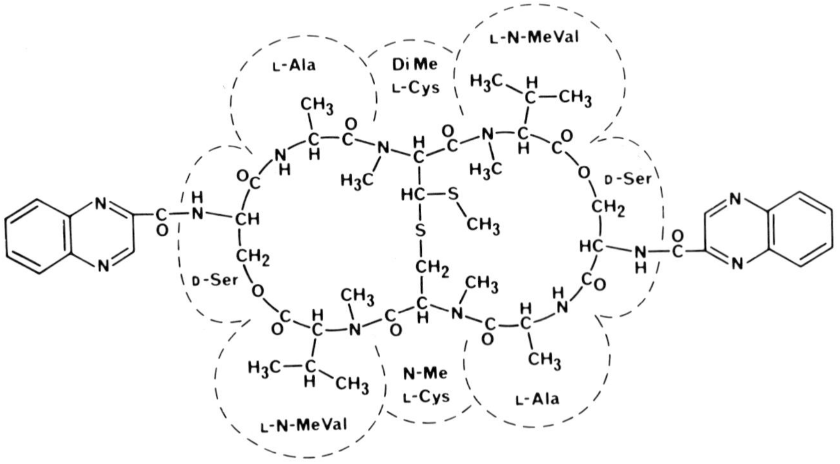

Fig. 4 Chemical structure of echinomycin.

thesized in recent years (Le Pecq *et al.*, 1975; Dervan and Becker, 1978). These include bisacridine and bisethidium (as well as mixed ethidium–acridine) polyintercalating agents. These molecules bind DNA very tightly (i.e., binding constants approaching 10^9 liters/mole have been observed for bisacridine intercalators). Although there are no data as yet concerning the kinetic rate constants for these associations, our model predicts the rate constants for monofunctional and bifunctional intercalation to be very similar (since we postulate β-kinked DNA to be the common structural intermediate), and this can be tested in future years.

III. Actinomycin–DNA Binding

Actinomycin (see Fig. 5) forms a $1:2$ stoichiometric complex with deoxyguanosine, and the stereochemical information provided by this structure has led us to propose a model for actinomycin–DNA binding (Sobell *et al.*, 1971; Jain and Sobell, 1972; Sobell and Jain, 1972). The model involves intercalation of the phenoxazone ring system between base pairs in the DNA double helix and the utilization of specific hydrogen bonds, van der Waals forces, and hydrophobic interactions between the pentapeptide chains on actinomycin and chemical groups in the minor

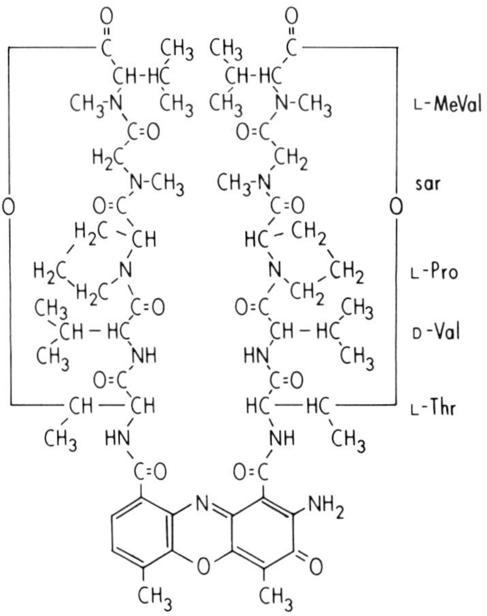

Fig. 5 Chemical structure of actinomycin D.

groove of the DNA helix. Important elements in the recognition of actinomycin for DNA are the guanine specificity and the use of symmetry in the
interaction. These predict a base sequence binding preference of the type
dGpC in actinomycin–DNA binding, which has been verified in model
dinucleoside monophosphate solution binding studies and in synthetic
polymer-binding studies (Krugh, 1972; Wells and Larson, 1970).

Although we believe that the general features of our actinomycin–DNA
binding model are correct, we have presented a slightly modified version
of this model which utilizes many of the insights afforded by the ethidium
and aminoacridine dinucleoside monophosphate crystal studies (Sobell *et
al.*, 1977a). The major features of our revised actinomycin–DNA model
are (see Fig. 6):

1. Intercalation of the phenoxazone ring system between base-paired
dGpC sequences accompanied by a helical screw axis dislocation of about
-0.4 Å (this value was about -1.5 Å in our previous model, because we
attempted to use the precise configuration observed in the actinomycin–
deoxyguanosine crystalline complex; subsequent study has shown,
however, that the polymer backbone imposes stereochemical constraints
which limit this dislocation to about -0.4 Å).

2. A departure from *exact* twofold symmetry in the complex. This reflects the asymmetry of the phenoxazone ring system and the inability of
both pentapeptide chains to interact simultaneously with (or span) guanine residues on opposite chains because of the smaller magnitude of this
helical screw axis dislocation.

3. An additional bending distortion in DNA on both sides of the intercalation site to accommodate the steric bulk of the pentapeptide chains on
actinomycin. This gives rise to a kinked-type DNA structure (helical axes
for B DNA sections on either side of this bend form an angle of about 40°
and are displaced by about -1.6 Å) which could partly explain the anomalous viscosity effects that accompany actinomycin–DNA binding (Gellert *et al.*, 1965; Müller and Crothers, 1968).

The ability of actinomycin to interfere specifically with DNA-dependent RNA polymerase activity almost certainly reflects intercalation by
the phenoxazone ring system into DNA and the presence of the two pentapeptide side chains in the minor groove of the DNA helix. Equally
important are the slow "on" and "off" rate constants observed for actinomycin–DNA binding (Müller and Crothers, 1968; Bittman and Blau,

---

Fig. 6 The actinomycin–DNA binding model. I thank Richard Feldman for supplying these and other computer-generated CPK pictures.

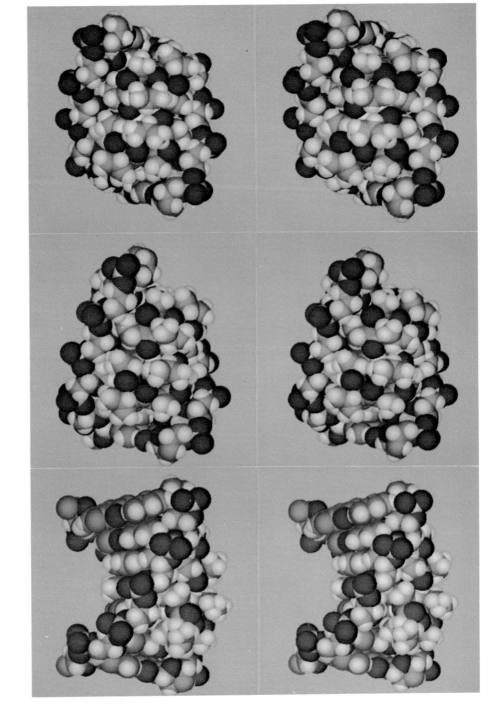

1975). A more precise understanding of the pharmacological activity for actinomycin, however, must await a detailed understanding of the three-dimensional structure of the polymerase enzyme and clarification of its processive catalytic mechanism.

IV. Ethidium–DNA Binding

Ethidium (see Fig. 7) forms two crystalline complexes with the self-complementary dinucleoside monophosphates 5-iodouridylyl(3'-5')adenosine (iodoUpA) and 5-iodocytidylyl(3'-5')guanosine (iodoCpG) (Tsai *et al.*, 1977; Jain *et al.*, 1977). These structures demonstrate intercalative binding between the phenathridinium ring system and the nucleic acid components. A common feature in these structures is the stereochemistry of the sugar–phosphate chains—they can be described by the following pattern of mixed sugar puckering: C-3' endo (3'-5') C-2' endo. This change (as well as additional small but systematic changes in torsional angles that describe the sugar–phosphate chains) allows base pairs to separate 6.8 Å and gives rise to the observed twist angle between base pairs above and below the intercalative drug. We have used this information to understand the general nature of intercalative drug binding to DNA.

To construct the ethidium–DNA binding model, we have added B DNA to either side of an idealized (deoxyribose-containing) configuration common to both the ethidium–iodoUpA and ethidium–iodoCpG structures (see Fig. 8). This is done easily and without steric difficulty. An important realization that immediately emerges is the concept that drug intercalation into DNA is accompanied by a helical screw axis displacement (or dislocation) in its structure (for ethidium intercalation, we estimate that helical axes for B DNA on either side of the phenathridinium ring system are displaced approximately + 1.0 Å). Base pairs in the immediate region are twisted by 10° (this value has been estimated by projecting the interglycosidic carbon vectors on a plane passing midway between base pairs and then measuring the angle between them). This gives rise to an angular unwinding of − 26° at the immediate site of drug

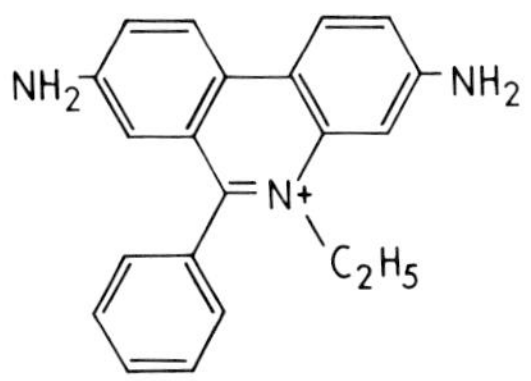

Fig. 7 Chemical structure of ethidium.

intercalation. We have also observed that intercalated base pairs are tilted relative to one another by about 8° in both ethidium crystal structures. This results in a small residual kink of 8° at the intercalation site, and it has been included in our ethidium–DNA binding model.

The magnitude of angular unwinding predicted by our ethidium–DNA binding model is in good agreement with Wang's estimate of ethidium–DNA angular unwinding based on alkaline titration studies of superhelical DNA in cesium chloride density gradients (Wang, 1974). Moreover, the C-3' endo (3'-5') C-2' endo mixed sugar puckering necessarily predicts that intercalation be limited to every *other* base pair at maximal drug–nucleic acid binding ratios (i.e., a neighbor-exclusion model). We have examined the stereochemistry of this model carefully. The effect of having a helical screw axis displacement every other base pair combined with an 8° kink is to give rise to a maximally unwound DNA structure that possesses a slow right-handed superhelical writhe. This structure is shown in Fig. 9.

V. Aminoacridine–DNA Binding

9-Aminoacridine, acridine orange, and proflavine (see Fig. 10A–C, respectively) form crystalline complexes with iodoCpG, and we have solved these structures to atomic resolution (Sakore *et al.*, 1977, 1979; Reddy *et al.*, 1979). Although each structure demonstrates intercalative binding, there are several important differences between them. These have been summarized in Fig. 11.

Acridine orange forms an intercalative structure with iodoCpG in much the same manner as ethidium, except that the acridine nucleus lies asymmetrically at the intercalation site (Fig. 11A). Base pairs above and below the drug are separated about 6.8 Å and are twisted about 10°; this reflects the stereochemistry of the sugar–phosphate chains (i.e., characterized by the C-3' endo (3'-5') C-2' endo mixed sugar puckering pattern). We postulate therefore that acridine orange binds to DNA in much the same manner as ethidium, except that, whereas ethidium binds from the minor groove of the helix, acridine orange binds from the wide groove.

Proflavine, on the other hand, demonstrates symmetric intercalation

---

Fig. 8 The ethidium–DNA binding model.

Fig. 9 Neighbor-exclusion structure for ethidium–DNA binding at maximal drug–DNA binding ratios. This structure is a maximally elongated, unwound DNA molecule possessing a slow right-handed superhelical writhe. An alternating sugar puckering pattern [i.e., C-3' endo (3'-5') C-2' endo (3'-5') C-3' endo, and so on] is postulated to exist in this structure, giving rise to neighbor exclusion.

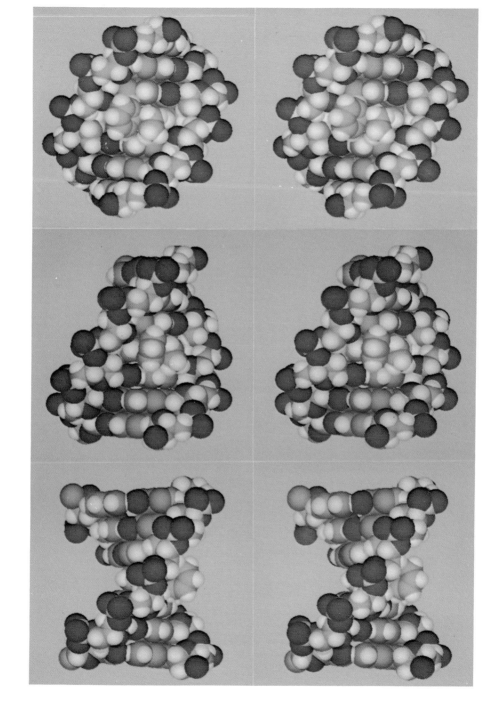

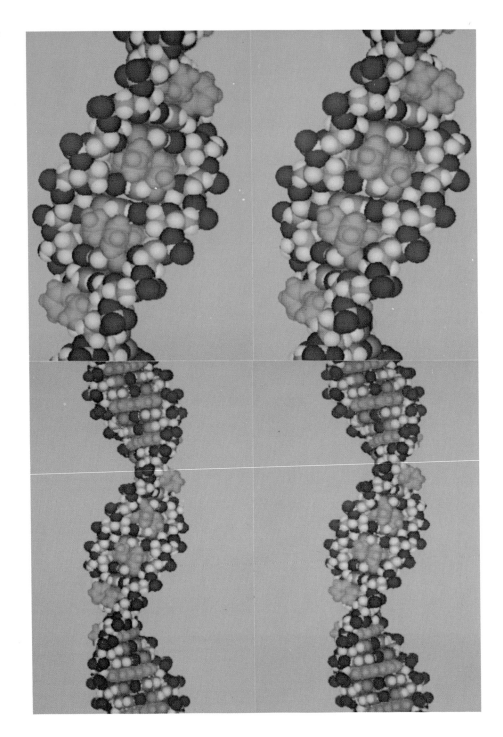

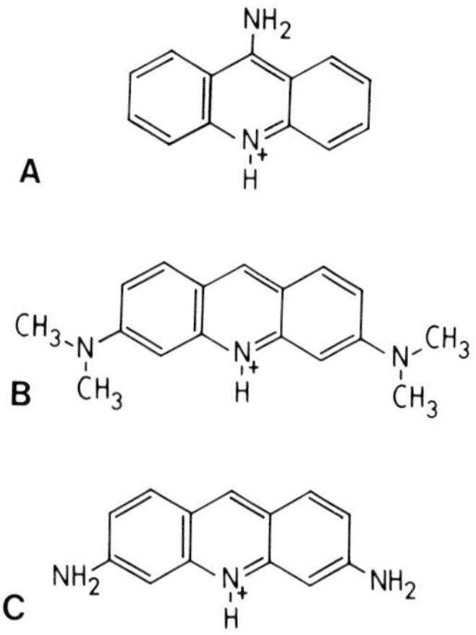

A

B

C

Fig. 10 Chemical structure of 9-aminoacridine (A), acridine orange (B), and proflavine (C).

with iodoCpG (Fig. 11B). Hydrogen bonds connect amino groups on proflavine with phosphate oxygen atoms on the dinucleotide. In contrast to the ethidium and acridine orange crystalline complexes, however, base pairs above and below the intercalative drug are twisted about 36°. This primarily reflects the sugar puckering pattern that is observed: C-3' endo (3'-5') C-3' endo. Since proflavine is known to unwind DNA in much the same manner as ethidium and acridine orange (Waring, 1970), one cannot use the information obtained from this model system to understand how

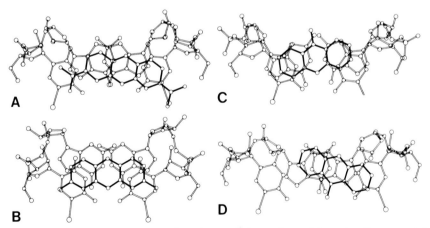

A

C

B

D

Fig. 11 Intercalative geometries observed for aminoacridines by X-ray crystallographic studies. (A) Acridine orange–iodoCpG. (B) Proflavine–iodoCpG. (C) 9-Aminoacridine–iodoCpG (pseudosymmetric). (D) 9-Aminoacridine–iodoCpG (asymmetric).

proflavine binds to DNA (i.e., it is possible that the hydrogen bonding observed between proflavine and iodoCpG alters the intercalation geometry in this model system). Although there is as yet no direct information concerning this, we have proposed a model for proflavine–DNA binding in which proflavine lies asymmetrically at the intercalation site (characterized by the C-3′ endo (3′-5′) C-2′ endo mixed sugar puckering pattern) and forms only *one* hydrogen bond to a neighboring phosphate oxygen atom. Our model for proflavine–DNA binding therefore is very similar to the acridine orange–DNA binding model described above.

9-Aminoacridine demonstrates *two* different intercalative binding modes and, along with these, two slightly different intercalative geometries (Fig. 11C and D). The first of these is very nearly symmetric, the 9-amino group lying in the narrow groove of the intercalated base-paired nucleotide structure. The second shows grossly asymmetric binding to the dinucleotide, the 9-amino group lying in the wide groove of the structure. Associated with these two different intercalative binding modes is a difference in the geometry of the structures. Although both structures demonstrate the C-3′ endo (3′-5′) C-2′ endo mixed sugar puckering pattern (with a corresponding twist angle between base pairs of about 10°), they differ in the magnitude of the helical screw axis dislocation accompanying intercalation. In the pseudosymmetric intercalative structure, this value is about +0.5 Å, whereas in the asymmetric intercalative structure it is about +2.7 Å. These conformational differences are best described as a "sliding" of base pairs on the intercalated acridine molecule. Although the pseudosymmetric intercalative structure can be used in 9-aminoacridine–DNA binding, the asymmetric intercalative structure cannot, since it would pose stereochemical difficulties in connecting neighboring sugar–phosphate chains to the intercalated dinucleotide. It is possible, however, that the asymmetric binding mode is related to the mechanism of 9-aminoacridine-induced frameshift mutagenesis (Sakore *et al.*, 1977, 1979).

VI. Ellipticine– and Tetramethyl-*N*-methylphenanthrolinium–DNA Binding

Ellipticine and tetramethyl-*N*-methylphenanthrolinium (see Fig. 12A and B) also form crystalline complexes with iodoCpG (Jain *et al.*, 1979). These structures demonstrate intercalative binding (see Fig. 13A and B) and in all respects are similar to the ethidium and acridine orange structures. The conformation of the sugar–phosphate chains is C-3′ endo (3′-5′) C-2′ endo, with similar twist angles relating base pairs (i.e., both are

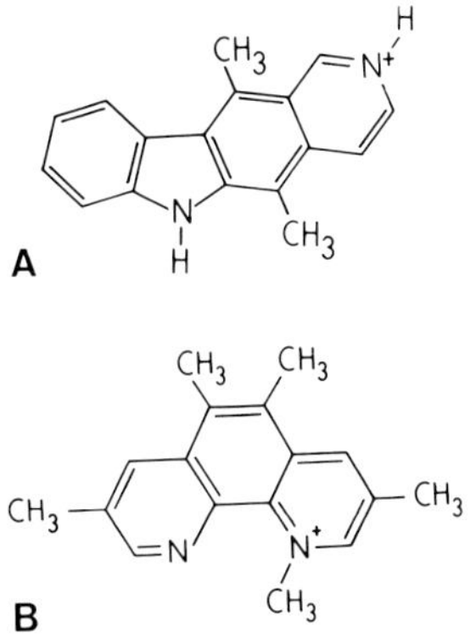

Fig. 12 (A) Chemical structure of ellipticine. (B) 3,5,6,8-Tetramethyl-*N*-methylphenanthrolinium.

about 12°). We have therefore proposed these drugs to interact with DNA much like ethidium and acridine orange (see previous sections).

VII. Irehdiamine–DNA Binding

Irehdiamine A (see Fig. 14) is a sterioidal diamine that binds tightly to DNA (Mahler *et al.*, 1968). Although the precise interaction is unknown, many aspects of the irehdiamine–DNA binding reaction suggest an intercalative-type binding mode. Thus, for example, irehdiamine A unwinds

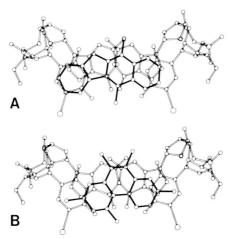

Fig. 13 Intercalative geometries observed for ellipticine–iodoCpG (A) and 3,5,6,8-tetramethyl-*N*-methylphenanthrolinium–iodoCpG (B) complexes.

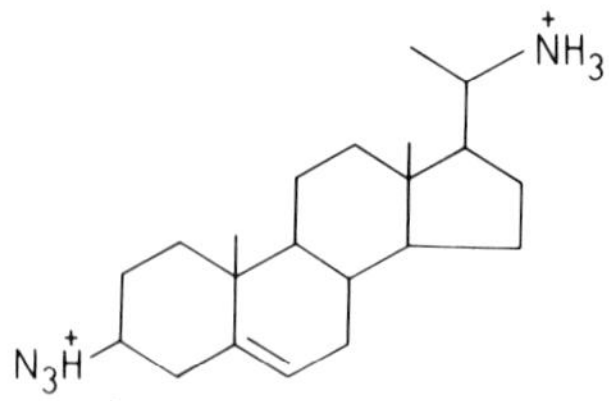

Fig. 14 Chemical structure of irehdiamine A.

superhelical DNA as evidenced by its ability to produce a fall and rise in the sedimentation coefficient of covalently circular supercoiled DNA molecules (Waring, 1970; Waring and Chisholm, 1972; Waring and Henley, 1975). These studies have also indicated that, on a molar basis, irehdiamine unwinds DNA roughly half as much as ethidium. Moreover, at maximal drug–nucleic acid binding ratios, the molecule demonstrates an upper binding limit of one irehdiamine to every four nucleotides (Mahler *et al.*, 1968). Finally, although irehdiamine produces hydrodynamic effects in DNA solutions different from most intercalative drugs or dyes (i.e., there are no clear viscosity or sedimentation changes associated with irehdiamine–DNA binding), it is possible that irehdiamine mimics intercalative drug binding by binding to the kink in DNA (Sobell *et al.*, 1977a,b).

This is shown in Fig. 15. The van der Waals surface of the irehdiamine molecule resembles a triangular wedge whose overall shape allows it to fit into the kink in DNA. Forces stabilizing the complex include electrostatic, van der Waals, and hydrophobic forces. Our model predicts an effective unwinding of $-10°$ associated with irehdiamine–DNA binding. It also predicts a neighbor-exclusion structure, at saturating concentrations of irehdiamine, whose axial repeat length is similar to that of B DNA. This structure (denoted β-kinked DNA) is shown in Fig. 16.

VIII. β-Kinked DNA—Conformation of DNA in Active Genes?

In a previous section, we explained how the presence of mechanical wave energy in DNA could give rise to a conformational change in the

---

Fig. 15 The irehdiamine–DNA binding model.

Fig. 16 Neighbor-exclusion structure for irehdiamine–DNA binding at maximal drug–DNA binding ratios. This structure (denoted β-kinked DNA) contains approximately 10 base pairs per turn of the helix and has an axial pitch of about 34 Å. We postulate this structure to be the structure of the promoter, as well as the conformation of DNA present in active genes. See text for discussion.

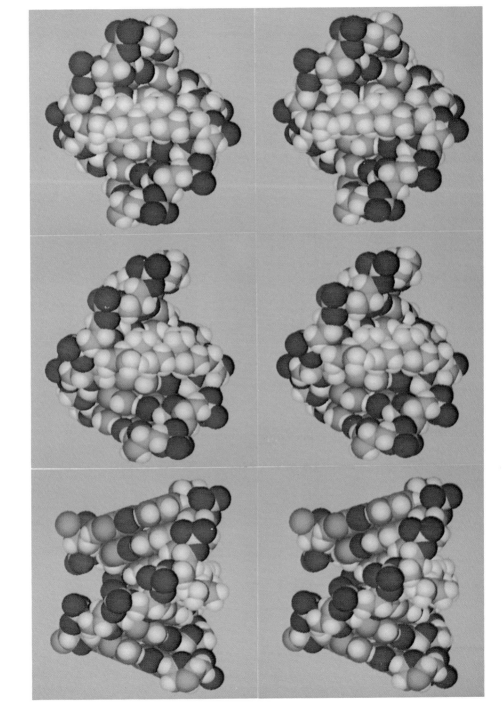

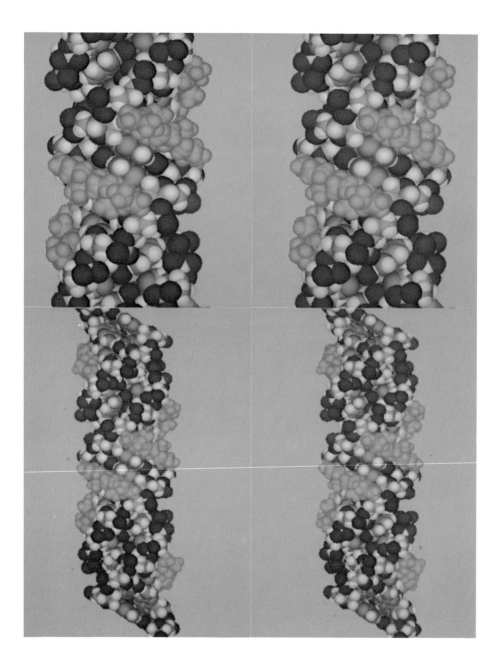

polymer (i.e., β-kinked DNA) that then leads to DNA breathing and to drug intercalation. In addition to these transient structural changes along the polymer, there may, in addition, be specific regions of DNA that remain permanently β-kinked; this corresponds to a second-order phase transition in the polymer, different regions of DNA undergoing this transition at different temperatures. We have postulated these (freely breathing) regions to correspond to promoters (Sobell *et al.*, 1978; Sobell, 1978; Lozansky *et al.*, 1979).

Transcriptionally active chromatin has been shown to be particularly sensitive to pancreatic DNase digestion, active genes being digested between four and five times faster than inactive genes (Weintraub and Groudine, 1976; Garel and Axel, 1977; Flint and Weintraub, 1977). DNA in active genes appears to remain bound to histones, as evidenced by staphylococcal nuclease limit digest studies (Camerini-Otero *et al.*, 1977) and measurements of the thickness of chromatin fibers actively undergoing transcription (about 70 Å wide) (Foe *et al.*, 1976). There is no evidence for a beaded structure in transcriptionally active chromatin; rather, the structure appears to be an extended one in which the DNA exists in a state particularly sensitive to pancreatic DNase.

We have wondered whether this state is β-kinked DNA. If pancreatic DNase recognized kinks in DNA (see below), then it would digest this structure approximately five times faster than κ-kinked DNA (the conformation of DNA we postulate to exist in inactive chromatin). Since β-kinked DNA has the same axial repeat as B DNA, the chromatin fiber could be extended about the same length as that predicted assuming B DNA in these regions. Finally, gene activation could be achieved along the lines originally suggested by Weintraub *et al.* (1976) in which the histone–DNA complex exists as a linear structure (active chromatin) or a helical structure (inactive chromatin). The flip-flop interconversion of these forms could convert the left-handed superhelical writhe in the κ-helix into unwinding in the β-helix, this unwinding being localized at the kinks. Such a mechanism could allow control of premelting changes in DNA necessary for RNA transcription.

IX. κ-Kinked DNA—Conformation of DNA in Inactive Genes?

Inactive chromatin is now established to consist of a beaded structure in which DNA is complexed to each of the four histones (H2a, H2b, H3, and H4). Each bead is an octamer of histones complexed to 140 base pairs, wound, most likely, as a left-handed superhelix around the periphery of the histone core (see, e.g., "Chromatin," *Cold Spring Harbor Symp. Quant. Biol.* **42,** 1977). An important observation concerns the pancreatic DNase digestion patterns reported for inactive chromatin; it demonstrates periodicities of approximate integral multiples of 10 nucleotide bases (i.e., fragments of 10, 20, 30, . . ., 300 bases have been observed), suggesting the presence of nuclease-sensitive sites periodically located every 10 base pairs.

We have postulated these sites to be kinks. A kink could serve as a substrate for both pancreatic DNase and splenic acid DNase II (these nucleases could partially intercalate into DNA), positioning these enzymes along the dyad axis of the kink to effect staggered cleavage about this symmetry axis. A kink placed every 10 base pairs in DNA gives rise to a left-handed superhelical structure with approximately the same dimensions as the nucleosome. We have postulated this structure (as well as higher-order superhelical variants of this structure) to exist in the organization of DNA in inactive chromatin (Sobell *et al.,* 1978; Sobell, 1978).

X. Concluding Remarks

The subject of drug intercalation is a multidimensional one in that it concerns itself with understanding the dynamic nature of the DNA double helix and the structural nature of its flexibility. Our X-ray crystallographic studies on drug intercalation have led us to propose the existence of phonon (wave) energy in DNA structure. This concept allows us to understand the origin of premelting changes in DNA structure that lead to DNA breathing and to drug intercalation. Such premelting phenomena may also be related to understanding the nature of a large number of protein–DNA interactions.

Thus promoters are envisioned to be permanently premelted DNA breathing regions recognized (in part) through partial or complete intercalation by the RNA polymerase enzyme. Histones may have evolved to control this DNA activation process through a flip-flop mechanism in which inactive DNA (κ-kinked B DNA) is converted into active DNA (β-kinked DNA) through the use of topological constraints. Nucleases may have evolved to see kinks in DNA, perhaps by partially (or, in some cases, completely) intercalating aromatic side chains into DNA.

We can therefore expect major advances in future years in our understanding of how proteins bind to DNA and recognize specific structural features in its base sequence. Almost certainly, these advances will be provided by X-ray crystallography, the most powerful tool we now have to understand the structure of biological macromolecules.

Acknowledgments

This work was supported by grants from the National Institutes of Health, the American Cancer Society, and the Department of Energy (DOE). This paper has been assigned report no. UR 3490–1572 at the DOE, the University of Rochester.

References

Bittman, R., and Blau, L. (1975). *Biochemistry* **14**, 2138–2145.
Butour, J. L., Delain, E., Couland, D., Le Pecq, J. B., Barbet, J., and Roques, B. P. (1978). *Biopolymers* **17**, 873–886.
Camerini-Otero, R. D., Sollner-Webb, B., Simon, R. H., Williamson, P., Zasloff, M., and Felsenfeld, G. (1977). *Cold Spring Harbor Symp. Quant. Biol.* **42**, 43–56.
Dervan, P., and Becker, M. M. (1978). *J. Am. Chem. Soc.* **100**, 1968–1970.
Flint, S. J., and Weintraub, H. M. (1977). *Cell* **12**, 783–794.
Foe, V. E., Wilkinson, L. E., and Laird, C. D. (1976). *Cell* **9**, 131–146.
Fuller, B. F. (1971). *Proc. Natl. Acad. Sci. U.S.A.* **86**, 815–818.
Garel, A., and Axel, R. (1977). *Cold Spring Harbor Symp. Quant. Biol.* **42**, 701–708.
Gellert, M., Smith, C. E., Neville, D., and Felsenfeld, G. (1965). *J. Mol. Biol.* **11**, 445–457.
Jain, S. C., and Sobell, H. M. (1972). *J. Mol. Biol.* **68**, 1–20.
Jain, S. C., Tsai, C.-C., and Sobell, H. M. (1977). *J. Mol. Biol.* **114**, 317–331.
Jain, S. C., Bhandary, K. K., and Sobell, H. M. (1979). *J. Mol. Biol.* (in press).
Krugh, T. R. (1972). *Proc. Natl. Acad. Sci. U.S.A.*, **69**, 1911–1914.
Le Pecq, J. B., Le Bret, M., Barbet, J., and Roques, R. P. (1975). *Proc. Natl. Acad. Sci. U.S.A.* **72**, 2915–2919.
Lozansky, E., Sobell, H. M., and Lessen, M., (1979). *In* "Stereodynamics of Molecular Systems" (R. H. Sarma, ed.) Pergamon Press, Inc., Oxford, New York, Frankfurt, Paris, pp. 265–270.
Mahler, H. R., Green, G., Goutarel, R., and Khuong-Huu, Q. (1968). *Biochemistry* **7**, 1568–1582.
Müller, W., and Crothers, D. M. (1968). *J. Mol. Biol.* **35**, 251–290.
Reddy, B. S., Seshadri, T. P., Sakore, T. D., and Sobell, H. M. (1979). *J. Mol. Biol.* (in press).
Sakore, T. D., Jain, S. C., Tsai, C.-C., and Sobell, H. M. (1977). *Proc. Natl. Acad. Sci. U.S.A.* **74**, 188–192.
Sakore, T. D., Reddy, B. S., and Sobell, H. M. (1979). *J. Mol. Biol.* (in press).
Sobell, H. M. (1978). *In* "Biological Control Mechanisms" (R. F. Goldberger, ed.), Vol. 1, pp. 171–199. Plenum, New York.
Sobell, H. M., and Jain, S. C. (1972). *J. Mol. Biol.* **68**, 21–34.
Sobell, H. M., Jain, S. C., Sakore, T. D., and Nordman, C. E. (1971). *Nature (London)* **231**, 200–205.
Sobell, H. M., Tsai, C.-C., Gilbert, S. G., Jain, S. C., and Sakore, T. D. (1976). *Proc. Natl. Acad. Sci. U.S.A.* **73**, 3068–3072.
Sobell, H. M., Tsai, C.-C., and Jain, S. C. (1977a). *J. Mol. Biol.* **114**, 333–365.
Sobell, H. M., Reddy, B. S., Bhandary, K. K., Jain, S. C., Sakore, T. D., and Seshadri, T. P. (1977b). *Cold Spring Harbor Symp. Quant. Biol.* **42**, 57–76.
Sobell, H. M., Lozansky, E., and Lessen, M. (1978). *Cold Spring Harbor Symp. Quant. Biol.* **43**, 11–15.

Tsai, C.-C., Jain, S. C., and Sobell, H. M. (1977). *J. Mol. Biol.* **114,** 333–365.
Ughetto, G., and Waring, M. J. (1977). *Mol. Pharmacol.* **13,** 579–584.
Wakelin, L. P. G., and Waring, M. J. (1976). *Biochem. J.* **157,** 721–740.
Wang, J. C. (1974). *J. Mol. Biol.* **89,** 783–801.
Waring, M. J. (1970). *J. Mol. Biol.* **54,** 247–279.
Waring, M. J., and Chisholm, J. W. (1972). *Biochim. Biophys. Acta* **262,** 18–23.
Waring, M. J., and Henley, S. M. (1975). *Nucleic Acids Res.* **2,** 567–586.
Weintraub, H., and Groudine, M. (1976). *Science* **193,** 848–856.
Weintraub, H., Worcel, A., and Alberts, B. (1976). *Cell* **9,** 409–417.
Wells, R. D., and Larson, J. E. (1970). *J. Mol. Biol.* **49,** 319–342.

7

Effects of Microbial Products on Nuclear DNA-Synthesizing Enzyme Systems

WERNER E. G. MÜLLER

Nuclei from eukaryotic cells contain three DNA polymerases: DNA polymerases α and β, and one terminal deoxynucleotidyl transferase (TdT). The activity of these enzymes in intact nuclei is controlled by a series of epigenetic enzymic systems (e.g., polyamine synthesis, changes in the chromosomal proteins, alterations in the cell membrane). Consequently nuclear DNA synthesis can be affected either by directly acting microbial products or by indirectly acting agents.

The directly acting agents are subdivided into three classes: (1) template inactivators, which inhibit not only nuclear DNA but also nuclear RNA synthesis; (2) enzyme poisons, which noncompetitively reduce DNA polymerase activity (DNA polymerase α: rifamycin, bleomycin, neocarzinostatin; DNA polymerase β: bleomycin; TdT: streptolydigin); and (3) antimetabolites, which inhibit the enzyme reaction competitively and with a high selectivity (DNA polymerase α: araTTP, α-araATP, araUTP, β-araATP; DNA polymerase β: β-araATP, araTTP, araUTP; TdT: β-araATP, 3'dATP).

Four classes of indirectly acting microbial agents are known: (1) inhibitors of polyamine–DNA formation (edeines); (2) inhibitors of poly ADP ribosylation (formycin B), (3) ionophores (A23187), and (4) cell surface enzyme inhibitors (bestatin). The last-mentioned class is of some interest because at least one member of it, bestatin, stimulates DNA synthesis in T-lymphocytes most likely via an induction of DNA polymerase α.

I. Introduction

Microbial products have become of increasing interest in medicine because some of them are (1) inhibitors of growth of microorganisms (antibiotics), (2) inhibitors of virus production (antiviral agents), (3) inhibitors of proliferation of eukaryotic cells (cytostatic and antitumor agents), and (4) enhancers of cell-mediated immunity (immune stimulators). In addition some microbial products are tools both for cell biologists to determine the role of a particular reaction in complex biological processes and for molecular biologists to explore the characteristics of an isolated enzyme system.

It is the task of this chapter to describe the mode of action of the microbial products that interfere, with an at least relative specificity, with nuclear DNA-synthesizing enzyme systems. Only compounds with such a specificity are of interest for use in studies to dissect the individual steps of cellular DNA synthesis on the cell biological and molecular biological levels. Microbial products can modulate nuclear DNA synthesis either directly by affecting DNA-synthesizing enzyme systems or indirectly by altering enzymic mechanisms that precede DNA synthesis (Fig. 1).

A. Target Enzymes

Nuclei from eukaryotic cells are provided with maximally three DNA polymerases: DNA polymerase α, DNA polymerase β, and TdT. These

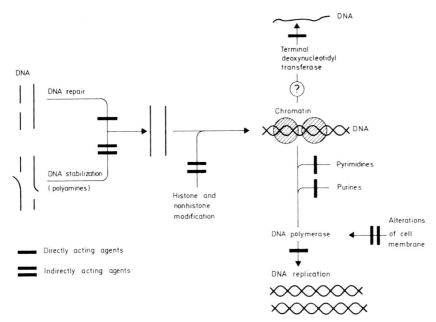

Fig. 1 Effect of directly and indirectly acting agents on DNA synthesis (scheme).

three enzymes were discovered, purified, and characterized by Bollum and co-workers (Bollum, 1975): DNA polymerase α (Bollum and Potter, 1957), TdT (Bollum, 1960), and DNA polymerase β (Chang and Bollum, 1971). First, DNA polymerase α is the DNA-replicating enzyme; its molecular weight ranges from 110,000 to 220,000. This enzyme is present in both cytoplasm and nuclei (Bollum, 1979). The biology of this enzyme is of current interest, since the level of this activity varies with the proliferation rate of cells; its activity is highest during S-phase (Bollum, 1975) and is low or even not present during the other phases (Müller *et al.*, 1978a). Second, DNA polymerase β seems to be essential for DNA repair; its molecular weight has been estimated to be about 45,000. This enzyme is found predominantly in the nucleus. The total amount of DNA polymerase β in eukaryotic cells appears to be relatively constant during the different phases of the cell cycle. Third, TdT is a DNA polymerase with the unique ability to polymerize deoxynucleotides onto a primer in the absence of a template. The enzyme appears to be restricted to the thymus and bone marrow cells. The molecular weight was determined to be 32,000, and the enzyme was found to be associated with the nuclear membrane.

B. DNA Synthesis-Controlling Systems

A small number of microbial products are known which affect nuclear DNA synthesis indirectly via an influence on the enzymic mechanisms that precede or limit DNA synthesis in the narrow sense.

1. DNA stabilization by polyamines (Cohen, 1971): It is well established, that diamines and polyamines stabilize and protect DNA structure against thermal denaturation, mechanical shearing, and irradiation. Increased polyamine (especially spermidine) synthesis is a prerequisite for both DNA synthesis and cell division.

2. Enzymic changes in chromosomal proteins: Among the four main enzymic reactions, which cause stage- and cell cycle-dependent modifications of histones and nonhistones (methylation, phosphorylation, acetylation, and poly ADP ribosylation), at present the last-mentioned is the only reaction which can be influenced by microbial products. Some experimental evidence is available showing that poly ADP-ribose transfer reactions to chromosomal proteins may be correlated with the diversity of the structure and function of chromatin when engaged in DNA replication and DNA repair (Hilz and Stone, 1976).

3. Alterations in the cell membrane: Since the studies of Abercrombie and Heaysman (1953), it has been known that cell surface events control genetic activity. Three types of cell surface alterations may cause changes in gene activity: (a) alteration of the chemical composition of the cell membrane, (b) alteration of the structural arrangements of the cell surface molecules, and (c) alteration of the activity of cell surface enzymes (Müller *et al.*, 1978a; Pressman and Guzman, 1974; Aoyagi *et al.*, 1976). Microbial products are now available that influence the last two cell surface events—ionophores and cell surface enzyme inhibitors.

II. Directly Acting Agents

The different inhibitors of DNA-synthesizing systems are usually subdivided according to their molecular mode of action into the following classes (Müller, 1975). First is the class of compounds that inactivate the DNA template for the programmed syntheses of DNA. These agents can form complexes with DNA either by covalent linkages, as are produced by alkylating agents, or by noncovalent interactions. The group of agents interacting noncovalently with DNA includes the subgroup of adducing agents, which interact via ion binding and hydrogen bonding, and the subgroup of intercalating agents, which form complexes with DNA via hydrogen bonding and van der Waals contact with the nucleo-base pairs above and below. This class of inhibitors can act only in template-dependent DNA-synthesizing systems (DNA polymerases α and β) and not in the template-independent DNA-synthesizing terminal transferase system. Second, some inhibitors have been discovered that interact with enzyme proteins, i.e., DNA polymerases, at sites not identical with the DNA template- or substrate-binding site. These enzymes are termed enzyme poisons. Third, a class of compounds called antimetabolites, which have a structure chemically related to the substrates of the polymerase reaction; they are analogues of deoxyribonucleoside triphosphates.

A. DNA Polymerase α

1. *Template Inactivators*

Generally speaking, no template inactivator of microbial origin (whether an alkylating agent, intercalating agent, or adducing agent) is known which inhibits DNA synthesis with some selectivity. Therefore in the following discussion such compounds are listed that inhibit DNA synthesis to the same extent as RNA synthesis. On the other hand, some antibiotics are known that inhibit RNA synthesis with some selectivity (e.g., actinomycin D; Sobell, 1973).

Mitomycin C was isolated from *Streptomyces caespitosus;* it causes cross-links in double-stranded DNA (for review, see Kersten and Kersten, 1974). Mitomycin C does not react *in vitro* with purified DNA. Prior to cross-linking of DNA, mitomycin C must be metabolically activated by a reductase and NADPH. Mitomycin C treatment of eukaryotic cells results in an immediate suppression of nuclear DNA synthesis; after a lag phase RNA synthesis is also blocked. In one study (Müller and Zahn, 1979a) it was shown that, in the isolated DNA polymerase α system, mitomycin C-treated DNA acted as a competitive inhibitor with respect to the untreated template DNA. From this *in vitro* finding (Müller and Zahn, 1979a) and the *in vivo* observation showing that mitomycin C causes depolymerization of DNA (Kersten and Kersten, 1974) it must be concluded that inhibition of cellular DNA synthesis by mitomycin C is caused by its direct effect on DNA.

Distamycin A is an antibiotic produced by *Streptomyces distallicus;* it binds to poly (dA-dT)-rich regions of DNA through hydrogen bonding and van der Waals forces (Kersten and Kersten, 1974). Distamycin A is a strong inhibitor of cell proliferation; e.g., in the L5178y cell system, the compound reduces cell growth to 50% at a concentration of 13 μM (Müller *et al.*, 1974). This inhibition is most likely due to inactivation of the DNA template for the DNA- as well as the RNA-synthesizing enzyme system (Müller *et al.*, 1974). Distamycin A inhibits a variety of DNA-dependent DNA as well as RNA polymerases (all of them to the same high extent), while inhibition of enzymic RNA-dependent nucleic acid synthesis amounts to only 1.5% (Müller *et al.*, 1974). Kinetic studies reveal that the inhibition is of the competitive type with respect to the template DNA; the template activity of native DNA is more sensitive to the antibiotic than that of denatured DNA (Kersten and Kersten, 1974).

Sibiromycin, produced by *Streptosporangium sibiricum*, forms a complex with native DNA but not with single-stranded DNA or RNA (Kersten and Kersten, 1974). The antibiotic inhibits proliferation of prokaryotic as well as eukaryotic cells as a consequence of the suppression of nucleic acid synthesis. In studies with isolated polymerase systems it was established that inactivation of the template activity of DNA was the biochemical reason for the observed inhibition of the polymerization rate.

The last inhibitor mentioned in this section is streptonigrin, which is a metabolite of *Streptomyces flocculus* (Kersten and Kersten, 1974). Streptonigrin binds to DNA with some preference for denatured DNA. Evidence is available demonstrating that single-strand breaks are formed in streptonigrin-treated DNA. The antibiotic inhibits both *in vivo* as well as in isolated enzyme systems, affecting DNA and RNA synthesis to the same extent.

2. Enzyme Poisons

Three microbial products are described in the literature as enzyme poisons of DNA polymerase α: rifamycin (Yang *et al.*, 1972), bleomycin (Müller and Zahn, 1977), and neocarzinostatin (Kappen and Goldberg, 1977).

Rifamycin is a fermentation product of *Streptomyces mediterranei;* chemically it is an ansa compound, i.e., a compound containing an aromatic system spanned by a long aliphatic bridge. Many rifamycin derivatives have been synthesized by chemical modification of the fundamental molecule. Seven semisynthetic derivatives were found to inhibit DNA polymerase α (Yang *et al.*, 1972); all of them were obtained by substitution at position 3 of the naphthalene ring. Fifty percent inhibition of DNA polymerase α activity is observed at relatively high inhibitor concentrations of about 50 μg/ml. Inhibition of the polymerase by the rifamycin derivatives turned out to be unspecific, because it was found later that these compounds also inhibited other DNA polymerases, RNA polymerase, and RNase H (Wehrli and Staehelin, 1975).

Bleomycin is an antibiotic that inhibits nuclear DNA-synthesizing systems (mediated by DNA polymerases α and β) with some specificity. This microbial product was isolated by Umezawa *et al.* (1966) from cultures of

Streptomyces verticillus. Bleomycin consists of five amino acids, L-gulose, 3-O-carbamoyl-D-mannose, and a terminal cation moiety. Bleomycin inhibits DNA polymerase reactions in a noncompetitive way (Müller, 1977a). This inhibition is not caused by a direct effect of the antibiotic on the enzyme protein but is a result of the influence of the bleomycin-modified DNA (formed in the polymerase assay) on the polymerase. Umezawa's group first reported that bleomycin caused single-strand scissions in native DNA. During this reaction free bases are released, and after that free aldehyde groups can be detected at the nonglycosidic sugar sites. DNA modified by the bleomycin action causes inhibition of a variety of DNA-dependent DNA and RNA polymerase systems (Müller and Zahn, 1977; Müller, 1977a). The sites on the bleomycin-modified DNA responsible for inhibition are the aldehyde groups; after reduction of these aldehyde groups present in bleomycin-modified DNA, by sodium borohydride, the inhibitory potency is almost completely abolished (Müller and Zahn, 1977; Table I). Pretreatment of DNA polymerase α with bleomycin does not cause a reduction in the enzyme activity; after separation of DNA polymerase from bleomycin, the activity of the enzyme is not reduced (Table I). These findings indicate that bleomycin does not affect the enzyme itself but inhibits the polymerase reaction indirectly by modification of the DNA template. The reaction sequence leading to the inhibition of DNA polymerase in an *in vitro* system can be described as follows: (1) modification of native DNA by bleomycin, resulting in the production of

TABLE I

Influence of Bleomycin and Bleomycin-Modified DNA on the Activity of DNA-Dependent DNA polymerase α^a

Bleomycin (μg/ml)	Untreated polymerase (units/ml)	Bleomycin-treated polymerase (units/ml)	Untreated (OD/ml)	Bleomycin-modified (OD/ml)	Enzyme activity (%)
0	1.5	—	2	—	100
5	1.5	—	2	—	57
—	—	1.5	2	—	102
—	1.5	—	2	Nonreduced form, 0.01	48
—	1.5	—	2	Nonreduced form, 0.1	7
—	1.5	—	2	Reduced form, 0.01	95
—	1.5	—	2	Reduced form, 0.1	84

^{a} DNA polymerase α was isolated and assayed as described (Müller, 1977a). The procedures for preparation of bleomycin-modified DNA (nonreduced and reduced forms) was given earlier (Müller, 1977a). DNA polymerase α was treated with bleomycin as follows: 0.5 units of the enzyme preparation was added to a reaction mixture (100 μl) containing 1 μg bleomycin, 5 mM dithiothreitol, 5 mM MgCl$_2$, and 40 mM Tris–HCl, pH 7.8. The assay was incubated for 60 minutes at 2°C; subsequently DNA was used as template for the polymerase reaction. The concentration of DNA added is indicated in OD (optical density)/ml.

free aldehyde groups, and (2) inhibition of DNA polymerase by the modified DNA.

The bleomycin inhibition studies with isolated polymerase systems revealed no pronounced specificity; both a series of DNA-dependent DNA polymerases and several DNA-dependent RNA polymerases are inhibited by almost the same bleomycin concentration. However, in intact cell systems the compound inhibits selectively DNA synthesis (during the S-phase), while RNA and protein synthesis is not diminished (Müller *et al.*, 1975c; Müller and Zahn, 1977). This selectivity of bleomycin action in intact cells is most likely due to an altered histone composition during S-phase. This conclusion stems from the finding that DNA in the chromatin complex isolated from nongrowing cells is more resistant toward bleomycin than DNA in the chromatin complex from rapidly growing cells. It remains to be determined by which mechanism the bleomycin-induced inhibition of DNA synthesis in intact cells is caused, e.g., by a possible noncompetitive inhibition of DNA-dependent DNA polymerase via the aldehyde group present at the strand scissions or by a reduction in the binding affinity of the enzyme for the drug-modified DNA. In this connection one observation (Sartiano *et al.*, 1975) is of interest which shows that after incubation of rat liver nuclei from nonproliferating tissue with bleomycin the activity of the endogeneous DNA polymerase α increases. This finding supports the assumption that, in intact nuclei, bleomycin selectively affects the activity of the endogenous DNA polymerase α.

Like bleomycin, neocarzinostatin, an antibiotic obtained from the culture filtrate of *Streptomyces carzinostaticus* (Meienhofer *et al.*, 1972), causes strand scissions of DNA both *in vitro* and *in vivo* (Kappen and Goldberg, 1977). This microbial product is an acidic polypeptide with a molecular weight of about 9000. Neocarzinostatin was found to inhibit DNA polymerase by a mechanism similar to that described for bleomycin, i.e., by indirect action via a mechanism of DNA modification (Kappen and Goldberg, 1977). In intact mammalian cells, the antibiotic selectively inhibits DNA synthesis (Sawada *et al.*, 1974); it is not yet known whether this selectivity is also due to alterations of the histone composition of the chromatin complex during S-phase.

3. Antimetabolites

Microbial products, acting as selective inhibitors for DNA synthesis in eukaryotic cells are rare. Among them, arabinosyl nucleosides are those most thoroughly studied. 9-β-Arabinofuranosyladenine (β-araAdo) is an antibiotic produced by *Streptomyces antibioticus* (Anderson and Suhadolnik, 1973). The two other naturally occurring arabinosyl nucleosides identified were 1-β-D-arabinofuranosylthymine (araThd) and 1-β-D-arabinofuranosyluracil (araUrd); both compounds were isolated from the sponge *Cryptotethya crypta* (Bergmann and Burke, 1955). It has not yet been determined whether the latter two compounds are produced by the sponge cells or are of bacterial origin; it is well known that at least some sponge species contain specific bacterial flora (Jakowska and Nigrelli, 1960). These three antimetabolites are found to be selective inhibitors both for nuclear DNA synthesis and in the triphosphate state for DNA polymerases α and β (Müller, 1977b; Müller and Zahn, 1979b).

Only β-D-sugar nucleosides have been found naturally. Therefore it was of interest to clarify whether arabinosyl nucleosides in a different isomeric form exerted biological activity. Among the derivatives synthesized, 9-α-D-arabinofuranosyladenine (α-araAdo) gained some interest in regard to selective control of DNA synthesis of eukaryotic cells.

Intracellularly the four nucleosides are metabolically activated to the triphosphates β-araATP (Müller, 1979), α-araATP (Müller, 1979), araTTP (Müller *et al.*, 1978b), and araUTP (Müller and Zahn, 1979b). In this form the triphosphates selectively inhibit DNA synthesis; RNA, poly(A), and poly ADP-ribose synthesis is not affected (Müller *et al.*, 1975a, 1978e,f; Müller and Zahn, 1979b). β-AraAdo, which has been studied most thoroughly, was found to inhibit cell growth during S-phase (Müller *et al.*, 1977a). From the studies on the mode of action of the other three nucleoside analogues it is most likely that the most sensitively affected stage in the cell cycle is the S-phase. This does not exclude the possibility that the compounds exert in addition an effect on DNA repair. From the studies with β-araAdo (Müller *et al.*, 1977a) it is known that this compound exerts in intact cells no effect on the changes both in the dATP pool size and in DNA and RNA polymerase activities, which occur during the transition from G_1- to S-phase. The first hint indicating that β-araAdo inhibits DNA synthesis during S-phase via DNA polymerase came from the observation that, in response to an increase in the intracellular dATP pool size, the cell proliferation inhibitory potency of β-araAdo was diminished.

The common feature of the arabinosyl nucleoside triphosphates in isolated enzyme systems is the fact that they are without effect on the RNA, poly(A), and poly ADP ribose polymerases (Müller, 1976; Müller *et al.*, 1975a, 1978e; Müller and Zahn, 1979b; Furth and Cohen, 1968). β-AraATP, α-araATP, araTTP, and araUTP were found to inhibit DNA polymerase α in a competitive way with respect to their natural substrates dATP and dTTP (Table II). As a measure of the relative affinities of the enzyme for inhibitor and substrate in competitive inhibition, the ratio K_i/K_m can be adopted; the lower this ratio, the higher the potency of the inhibitor in

TABLE II

Influence of β-araATP, α-araATP, araTTP, and araUTP on DNA Polymerases α and β[a]

Enzyme	Michaelis constant (μM)	Inhibitor constant (μM)	K_i/K_m
DNA-dependent DNA polymerase α	dATP, 6.4	β-araATP, 7.4	1.2
	dATP, 6.4	α-araATP, 3.1	0.5
	dTTP, 10.1	araTTP, 2.3	0.2
	dTTP, 10.1	araUTP, 7.8	0.8
DNA-dependent DNA polymerase β	dATP, 14.3	β-araATP, 5.6	0.4
	dATP, 14.3	α-araATP, —	—
	dTTP, 11.9	araTTP, 9.0	0.8
	dTTP, 11.9	araUTP, 12.2	1.0

[a] Data are from Müller (1979), Müller et al. (1978b), and Müller and Zahn (1979b).

reducing the enzyme activity. The highest affinity is observed in the case of araTTP, while the affinities for α-araATP, araUTP, and β-araATP are lower (Table II).

B. DNA Polymerase β

1. Template Inactivators

No template inactivators of microbial origin are known that inhibit either the activity of the isolated DNA polymerase β or the cellular DNA repair synthesis. On the contrary, template inactivators can even stimulate the DNA repair synthesis after their binding to DNA. This phenomenon has been shown in a clear-cut way for the DNA repair mechanism in rat fibroblasts treated with mitomycin C (Bozhkov et al., 1978).

2. Enzyme Poison

No specific enzyme poison of microbial origin for DNA polymerase β is known. As mentioned above, bleomycin inhibits not only DNA polymerase α but also the β enzyme (Müller, 1977a) with the same sensitivity. However, the endogenous DNA polymerase β activity in isolated nuclei is not affected at all by the antibiotic (Sartiano et al., 1975).

3. Antimetabolites

As in the case of DNA polymerase α, only the triphosphates of the microbial products β-araAdo, araTTP, and araUTP are inhibitors of DNA polymerase β (Table II); they exert no inhibitory effect on other nucleic acid-polymerizing enzyme systems. It is interesting that α-araATP, which has been shown to be a potent inhibitor of DNA polymerase α, has no effect on the DNA polymerase β reaction (Müller et al., 1978e). As outlined in Table II, β-araATP is the most potent inhibitor of DNA polymerase β; this nucleotide inhibits the β enzyme three times more sensitively than the α enzyme. AraTTP and araUTP also affect DNA polymerase β effectively, but the values for their relative affinities are higher in comparison to the values found with DNA polymerase α; this means that the inhibitory effect of these triphosphates on DNA polymerase β is somewhat lower than on DNA polymerase α. From the experiments with isolated enzyme systems, we conclude that β-araAdo is a promising agent for inhibiting DNA repair synthesis in intact cell systems via DNA polymerase β (Fig. 2). As outlined above, there is no doubt that cell proliferation is inhibited by β-araAdo during S-phase via a reduction of DNA polymerase α activity. Exact data are lacking on the influence of β-araAdo on DNA repair in intact cells. Only one paper (Nichols, 1964) has reported that β-araAdo causes DNA breakage in human leukocytes. This finding is an indirect hint that β-araAdo may also affect DNA repair synthesis, since it is known from a series of studies (Müller et al., 1975a, 1977c) that during DNA replication β-araAMP is incorporated into DNA in internucleotide linkage. The incorporation of the analogue does not cause the generation of any detectable single-strand regions in the newly synthesized DNA. Hence the observed DNA breakage induced by β-araAdo (Nichols, 1964) could be the result either of an almost complete inhibition of the DNA polymerase β activity or of the inability of DNA polymerase β to continue DNA synthesis in an incorporated β-araAMP moiety. The latter possibility, the function of β-araAMP as a chain terminator, has already been experimentally established for the herpes simplex virus DNA-replicating system (Müller et al., 1977c).

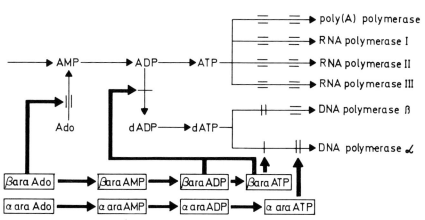

Fig. 2 Sites of inhibition by β-araAdo or α-araAdo and their phosphorylated derivatives. ⸻ , No inhibition; ⸻ , weak inhibition; ⸻ , strong inhibition.

C. Terminal Deoxynucleotidyl Transferase

1. *Enzyme Poisons*

Only one microbial product is known that inhibits terminal TdT: the antibiotic streptolydigin, which was isolated from *Streptomyces lydigus*. Streptolydigin was originally described as a noncompetitive inhibitor of prokaryotic RNA polymerase (Cassani *et al.*, 1971); later it was reported that eukaryotic RNA polymerases I, II, and III (Müller *et al.*, 1978d), as well as eukaryotic DNA polymerases α and β (DiCioccio and Srivastava, 1976), were resistant to its antibiotic action. In this respect, the finding demonstrating streptolydigin to inhibit TdT in a noncompetitive way is of some interest (DiCioccio and Srivastava, 1976). This is because one antibiotic is now available that can be used as a tool for discrimination between the different nuclear DNA-synthesizing systems, catalyzed by either TdT or DNA polymerases α and β.

2. *Antimetabolites*

Very few papers have reported on effects of antimetabolites on the activity of TdT. This enzyme was found to be sensitive toward araATP and 3'dATP (DiCioccio and Srivastava, 1977; Müller *et al.*, 1978c); these nucleosides are antibiotics produced by *Streptomyces antibioticus* or by *Cordyceps militaris*. Both triphosphates inhibit TdT activity competitively with the natural substrate dATP. However, while araATP is not incorporated into DNA during TdT-mediated DNA synthesis, 3'dATP is incorporated into the growing chain and there acts as a chain terminator. The inhibitor constant for araATP ($K_i = 4.9\ \mu M$) in the TdT assay is of the same order of magnitude as those determined for DNA polymerases α and β (Müller *et al.*, 1975a). Of some interest is the observed inhibition of TdT by 3'dATP (Müller *et al.*, 1978c), because DNA polymerases α and β are insensitive toward this analogue (Müller *et al.*, 1977b); only RNA polymerases I, II, and III, as well as poly(A) polymerase and the terminal riboadenylate transferase, are affected by 3'dATP. The K_i value for 3'dATP amounts to 3.4 μM and thus is lower than that for the RNA-synthesizing systems.

III. Indirectly Acting Agents

Understanding DNA replication is more than understanding DNA polymerases. DNA replication in complex cells is discontinuous and is organized into replicons. It is assumed (Bollum, 1975) that the initiation of DNA synthesis starts at a palindromic sequence, which lies at the center of each replicon, because such a DNA structure provides a recognizable site for protein interaction followed by enzyme action. The initiation of DNA synthesis is accomplished by an RNA-synthesizing enzyme; after that, DNA polymerization ensues. Several more protein factors, e.g., unwinding proteins, replicon termination factor, and DNA ligase, are required to complete DNA replication in intact cells. It can be expected that at least some of these protein factors are controlled epigenetically. Because very little is known about these mechanisms, it is not surprising that only a few microbial products are known that influence the enzymic reactions that allow DNA polymerases to work. A brief review of the present state of knowledge on the molecular mechanism of the four classes of agents indirectly acting on DNA synthesis is given in the following section.

A. Inhibitors of Polyamine–DNA Formation

In a basic work, Dion and Cohen (1972) showed that during polyamine depletion in cells both nucleic acid accumulation and cell growth were strikingly inhibited. Transfer of these cells to conditions optimal for polyamine formation, results in a stimulation of both nucleic acid synthesis and cell division. From a series of studies it is known (Cohen, 1971; Stevens, 1967) that there is an optimal length of polyamine molecules (most likely spermidine or spermine) that gives optimal stabilization of the DNA. Hence inhibitors of polyamine formation or polyamine analogues, which have the capability to bind to DNA, can interfere with DNA synthesis. Microbial products, edeines, are known that are structurally related to polyamines and inhibit DNA synthesis in both prokaryotic and eukaryotic cell systems (Kurylo-Borowska, 1975). The major representative of this group is edeine A. Edeines are composed of five amino acid residues and the organic base spermidine (in edeine A). In intact cells, edeine strongly inhibits DNA synthesis, whereas RNA synthesis is slightly stimulated and protein synthesis remains unaffected. Edeine was found to inhibit DNA synthesis only in assays containing membrane-bound DNA polymerase and endogenous template. Even if it is known that edeines bind reversibly to polynucleotide *in vitro,* the final, conclusive proof is missing that the antibiotic causes a disturbance in the natural arrangement of the natural polyamine in the double-stranded DNA.

B. Inhibitors of Poly ADP Ribosylation

Two microbial products are known to act as inhibitors of poly ADP ribosylation in intact cell systems (L5178y mouse lymphoma cells) as well as in isolated enzyme systems: [showdomycin and formycin B (Müller and Zahn, 1975; Müller *et al.*, 1975b)]. The most thoroughly studied are formycin B (Müller *et al.*, 1975b) and its NAD$^+$ derivative nicotinamide formycin dinucleotide (Suhadolnik *et al.*, 1977). Formycin B has been shown to be an inhibitor of poly ADP ribose polymerase isolated from oviduct nuclei of quails. Both the chromatin-bound and the soluble enzyme are inhibited competitively; the relative affinity (K_i/K_m) of formycin B for poly ADP-ribose polymerase is 1.5. The studies on intact L5178y cells revealed that the formation of poly ADP-ribose was reduced with greater sensitivity compared to the biosynthesis of DNA and RNA. In particular the event of polyADP ribosylation of histone subfraction H1 was reduced in the presence of formycin B. This finding was confirmed in part by a later study (Suhadolnik *et al.*, 1977) showing that the formycin derivative nicotinamide formycin dinucleotide reduced the chain length of the poly ADP ribose formation. Because of the well-known fact that NAD$^+$ moieties, which are incorporated into nuclear proteins, are capable of mimicking the enhancement or inhibition of template activity of DNA in the chromosome complex for the DNA polymerase reaction (Suhadolnik *et al.*, 1977; Hilz and Stone, 1976), the observed inhibition of growth of L5178y cells in the presence of formycin B (Müller *et al.*, 1975b) is, at the present stage, thought to be mainly due to an inhibition of poly ADP ribosylation; as a result the inhibition of programmed syntheses is observed.

C. Ionophores

A striking feature of many of cation conductors or ionophores is that they consist of cyclic molecules with lipophilic side chains oriented toward the exterior of the molecule. A large number of ionophores are known, most of which are microbial products. They are usually subdivided into three classes: (1) neutral ionophores, (2) carboxylic ionophores, and (3) channel-forming quasi ionophores (Pressman, 1976). Most of them mediate transmembrane monovalent cation transport with a high selectivity. One antibiotic, produced by fermentation of *Streptomyces chartreusis*, was discovered which has a high selectivity for divalent over monovalent ions: A23187 (Reed and Lardy, 1972). This carboxylic ionophore shows the highest affinity for Ca^{2+} and a somewhat lower one for Mg^{2+} and other divalent cations (Reed and Lardy, 1972). Because of this uniqueness A 23187 was used to study Ca^{2+} transport across biological membranes. The interesting outcome of this study was the fact that the antibiotic activated DNA synthesis both in sea urchin eggs (Steinhardt and Epel, 1974) and in human lymphocytes (Luckasen *et al.*, 1974). These data were explained by the assumption of an increase in Ca^{2+} concentration in the cytoplasm; it was postulated that A23187 induced Ca^{2+} release from either intracellular stores (mitochondria) or the extracellular milieu (Luckasen *et al.*, 1974). However, Ca^{2+} is not the ultimate activator of DNA synthesis but modulates the activity of TMP synthetase (MacManus *et al.*, 1975).

D. Cell Surface Enzyme Inhibitors

Aoyagi *et al.* (1976) discovered a variety of exopeptidases on the cell surface; 13 aminopeptidases have been found to be associated with the cell surface. To determine whether these exopeptidases might serve as modulators or triggers of reactions which take place first on the cell surface and ultimately lead to alteration in the DNA-synthesizing system, Umezawa (Umezawa, 1972; Nishizawa *et al.*, 1977) isolated a variety of inhibitors of proteolytic enzymes from microbial origin. Among them bestatin, which was discovered in culture filtrates of *Streptomyces olivoreticuli*, was found to be a strong competitive inhibitor of aminopeptidase B ($K_i = 6 \times 10^{-8}$) and of leucine aminopeptidase ($K_i = 2 \times 10^{-8}$) (Nishizawa *et al.*, 1977). It was found that bestatin influenced cell-mediated immunity, probably by enhancement of the function of T-lymphocytes (Saito *et al.*, 1977). This working hypothesis was supported by the finding (Saito *et al.*, 1977) that bestatin enhanced *in vitro* T-cell activation caused by concanavalin A; the incorporation of [^{3}H]dThd into DNA was chosen as a parameter for determination of the amount of activation. In a subsequent report it was shown (Müller *et al.*, 1979b) that, in consequence of an increased incorporation rate of dThd into DNA, an up to sixfold increase in polysome assembly occurred. In the present work data are given indicating that DNA polymerases are induced in response to stimulation with bestatin. For these experiments a T-cell lymphoma cell line (L5178y) was used; the cells were passaged into NMRI mice. Lymphoma cells, harvested 12 days after intraperitoneal injection of 2×10^5 cells, were suspended in Fischer's medium and cultivated in suspension (Müller *et al.*, 1975a); the cultures contained, in addition to the L5178y cells, 5% macrophages. The cells were incubated at a density of 5×10^6 cells/ml for 5 hours in the presence of different concentrations of bestatin. During this period of time, the cell number remained constant. After incubation of the cells the two DNA polymerase species, α and β, were extracted and separated (Fig. 3). As shown in Fig. 3, extracts from cells incubated with 5 μg bestatin/ml contained a 1.9-fold higher DNA polymerase α activity than the controls; the activity of DNA polymerase β remained constant. As shown in Fig. 4 the induction of DNA polymerase in L5178y cells is strongly dependent upon the bestatin concentration; at higher concentra-

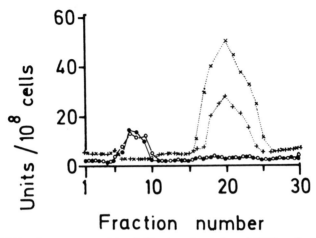

Fig. 3 DNA polymerase α and β activities in extracts from L5178y cells. The extracts were prepared from cells treated with 0 or 5 μg bestatin/ml. Separation of the polymerases was performed in a sucrose velocity gradient (Müller *et al.*, 1977a). The direction of sedimentation is to the right. Treatment with 0 μg/ml: ●, β enzyme; +, α enzyme. Treatment with 5μg bestatin/ml: ○, β enzyme; ×, α enzyme. The ordinate indicates the enzyme activity per fraction; 1 unit of enzyme activity is defined as 1 nmole of radioactive deoxynucleotide incorporated per hour.

tions of the microbial product values are reached that are identical with those for the controls. In analogy to results obtained with other systems (stimulation of DNA polymerase α with phytohemagglutinin or antigens erythropoietin and phenylhydrazine), which revealed a parallelism between the level of DNA polymerase and the rate of both DNA synthesis and cell proliferation, we conclude that bestatin triggers cells from G_0- or

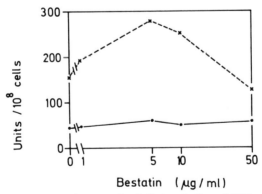

Fig. 4 Alterations in dependence on bestatin incubation of DNA polymerase α and β levels in L5178y cells. ●, β enzyme; ×, α enzyme.

G_1-phase into S-phase. Hence bestatin is the first microbial product acting via inhibition of the activity of a cell surface enzyme on the induction mechanism of DNA polymerase α (Müller *et al.*, 1979a).

Acknowledgments

This work was supported by a grant from the Landesversicherungs-Anstalt, Rheinland-Pfalz, Speyer (Germany).

References

Abercrombie, M., and Heaysman, J. E. M. (1953). *Exp. Cell Res.* **5**, 111.

Anderson, M. M., and Suhadolnik, R. J. (1973). *IUB Int. Congr. Biochem. 9th, Stockholm* Abstr. Book 3r 10.

Aoyagi, T., Suda, H., Nagai, M., Ogawa, K., Suzuki, J., Takeuchi, T., and Umezawa, H. (1976). *Biochim. Biophys. Acta* **452**, 131.

Bergmann, W., and Burke, D.C. (1955). *J. Org. Chem.* **20**, 1501.

Bollum, F. J. (1960). *J. Biol. Chem.* **235**, PC18.

Bollum, F. J. (1975). *Prog. Nucleic Acid Res. Mol. Biol.* **15**, 109.

Bollum, F. J. (1979). *In* "Antiviral Mechanisms for the Control of Neoplasia" (P. Chandra ed.). Plenum, New York. p. 587.

Bollum, F. J., and Potter, R. V. (1957). *J. Am. Chem. Soc.* **79**, 3603.

Bozhkov, V. M., Barskaya, T. V., Fridlyanskaya, I. I., and Tomilin, N. V. (1978). *FEBS Lett.* **86**, 205.

Cassani, G., Burgess, R. R., Goodman, H. M., and Gold, L. (1971). *Nature (London), New Biol.* **230**, 197.

Chang, L. M. S., and Bollum, F. J. (1971). *J. Biol. Chem.* **246**, 5835.

Cohen, S. S. (1971). "Introduction to the Polyamines." Prentice-Hall, Englewood Cliffs, New Jersey.

DiCioccio, R. A., and Srivastava, B. I. (1976). *Biochem. Biophys. Res. Commun.* **72**, 1343.

DiCioccio, R. A., and Srivastava, B. I. S. (1977). *Eur. J. Biochem.* **79**, 411.

Dion, A. S., and Cohen, S. S. (1972). *Proc. Natl. Acad. Sci. U.S.A.* **69**, 213.

Furth, J. J., and Cohen, S. S. (1968). *Cancer Res.* **28**, 2061.

Hilz, H., and Stone, P. (1976). *Rev. Physiol. Biochem. Pharmacol.* **76**, 1.

Jakowska, S., and Nigrelli, R. F. (1960). *Ann. N. Y. Acad. Sci.* **90**, 913.

Kappen, L. S., and Goldberg, I. H. (1977). *Biochemistry* **16**, 479.

Kersten, H., and Kersten, W. (1974). "Inhibitors of Nucleic Acid Synthesis." Springer-Verlag, Berlin and New York.

Kurylo-Borowska, Z. (1975). *In* "Antibiotics" (J. W. Corcoran and F. E. Hahn, eds.), Vol. 3, p. 129. Springer-Varlag, Berlin and New York.

Luckasen, J. R., White, J. G., and Kersey, J. H. (1974). *Proc. Natl. Acad. Sci. U.S.A.* **71**, 5088.

MacManus, J. P., Whitfield, J. F., Boynton, A. L., and Rixon, R. H. (1975). *Adv. Cycl. Nucleotide Res.* **5**, 719.

Meienhofer, J., Maeda, H., Glaser, C. B., Czombos, J., and Kuromizu, K. (1972). *Science* **178**, 875.

Müller, W. E. G. (1975). "Chemotherapie von Tumoren; Biochemische Grundlagen." Verlag Chemie, Weinhaim.
Müller, W. E. G. (1976). *Experientia* **32**, 1572.
Müller, W. E. G. (1977a). *Pharmacol. Ther. A* **1**, 457.
Müller, W. E. G. (1977b). *Jpn. J. Antibiot.* **30**, Suppl., 104.
Müller, W. E. G. (1979). In "Antiviral Mechanisms for the Control of Neoplasia" (P. Chandra, ed.). Plenum, New York. p. 553.
Müller, W. E. G., and Zahn, R. K. (1975). *Experientia* **31**, 1014.
Müller, W. E. G., and Zahn, R. K. (1977). *Prog. Nucleic Acid Res. Mol. Biol.* **20**, 21.
Müller, W. E. G., and Zahn, R. K. (1979a). Submitted.
Müller, W. E. G., and Zahn, R. K. (1979b). *Cancer Res.* **39**, 1102.
Müller, W. E. G., Obermeier, J., Maidhof, A., and Zahn, R. K. (1974). *Chem.-Biol. Interact.* **8**, 183.
Müller, W. E. G., Rohde, H. J., Beyer, R., Maidhof, A., Lachmann, M., Taschner, H., and Zahn, R. K. (1975a). *Cancer Res.* **35**, 2160.
Müller, W. E. G., Steffen, R., Maidhof, A., Lachmann, M., Zahn, R. K., and Umezawa, H. (1975b). *Cancer Res.* **35**, 3673.
Müller, W. E. G., Totsuka, A., Nusser, I., Zahn, R. K., and Umezawa, H. (1975c). *Biochem. Pharmacol.* **24**, 911.
Müller, W. E. G., Maidhof, A., Zahn, R. K., and Shannon, W. M. (1977a). *Cancer Res.* **37**, 2282.
Müller, W. E. G., Seibert, G., Beyer, R., Breter, H. J., Maidhof, A., and Zahn, R. K. (1977b). *Cancer Res.* **37**, 3824.
Müller, W. E. G., Zahn, R. K., Beyer, R., and Falke, D. (1977c). *Virology* **76**, 787.
Müller, W. E. G., Müller, I., and Zahn, R. K. (1978a). "Aggregation in Sponges. Research in Molecular Biology," Vol. 8. Akad. Wiss., Mainz.
Müller, W. E. G., Zahn, R. K., and Arendes, J. (1978b). *Chem.-Biol. Interact.* **23**, 151.
Müller, W. E. G., Zahn, R. K., and Arendes, J. (1978c). *FEBS Lett.* **94**, 47.
Müller, W. E. G., Zahn, R. K., and Falke, D. (1978d). *Virology* **86**, 320.
Müller, W. E. G., Zahn, R. K., Maidhof, A., Beyer, R., and Arendes, J. (1978e). *Biochem. Pharmacol.* **27**, 1659.
Müller, W. E. G., Zahn, R. K., Maidhof, A., Beyer, R., and Arendes, J. (1978f). *Chem.-Biol. Interact.* **23**, 141.
Müller, W. E. G., Zahn, R. K., Arendes, J., Munsch, N., and Umezawa, H. (1979a) *Biochem. Pharmacol.* **28**, in press.
Müller, W. E. G., Zahn, R. K., Maidhof, A., and Umezawa, H. (1979b). *J. Antibiot.* (in press).
Nichols, W. W. (1964). *Cancer Res.* **24**, 1502.
Nishizawa, R., Saino, T., Takita, T., Suda, H., Aoyagi, T., and Umezawa, H. (1977). *J. Med. Chem.* **20**, 510.
Pressman, B. C. (1976). *Annu. Rev. Biochem.* **45**, 501.
Pressman, B. C., and de Guzman, N. T. (1974). *Ann. N.Y. Acad. Sci.* **227**, 380.
Reed, P. W., and Lardy, H. A. (1972). *J. Biol. Chem.* **247**, 6970.
Rohde, H. J., Müller, W. E. G., and Zahn, R. K. (1975). *Nucleic Acids Res.* **2**, 2101.
Saito, M., Aoyagi, T., Umezawa, H., and Nagai, Y. (1977). *Biochem. Biophys. Res. Commun.* **76**, 526.
Sartiano, G. P., Lynch, W., Boggs, S. S., and Neil, G. L. (1975). *Proc. Soc. Exp. Biol. Med.* **150**, 718.
Sawada, H., Tatsumi, K., Sasada, M., Shirakawa, S., Nakamura, T., and Watisaka, G. (1974). *Cancer Res.* **34**, 3341.
Sobell, H. M. (1973). *Prog. Nucleic Acid Res. Mol. Biol.* **13**, 153.
Steinhardt, R. A., and Epel, D. (1974). *Proc. Natl. Acad. Sci. U.S.A.* **71**, 1915.

Stevens, L. (1967). *Biochem. J.* **103,** 811.

Suhadolnik, R. J., Baur, R., Lichtenwalwalner, D. M., Uematsu, T., Roberts, J. H., Sudhakar, S., and Smulson, M. (1977). *J. Biol. Chem.* **252,** 4134.

Umezawa, H. (1972). "Enzyme Inhibitors of Microbial Origin." Univ. of Tokyo Press, Tokyo.

Umezawa, H., Maeda, K., Takeuchi, T., and Okami, Y. (1966). *J. Antibiot.* **19,** 200.

Wehrli, W., and Staehelin, M. (1975). *In* "Antibiotics" (J. W. Corcoran and F. E. Hahn, eds.), Vol. 3, p. 252. Springer-Verlag, Berlin and New York.

Yang, S. S., Herrera, F. M., Smith, R. G., Reitz, M. S., Lancini, G., Ting, R. C., and Gallo, R. C. (1972). *J. Natl. Cancer Inst.* **49,** 7.

A Mechanism for the Degradation
of DNA by Bleomycin

EDWARD A. SAUSVILLE AND SUSAN B. HORWITZ

I. Introduction

Bleomycins are a group of water-soluble, basic glycopeptides originally isolated by Umezawa and collaborators (1966a,b) from *Streptomyces verticillus*. Bleomycin (Blenoxane, Bristol) is a mixture of these compounds currently used in the chemotherapy of neoplastic disease, particularly certain squamous cell carcinomas, lymphomas, and testicular carcinoma. The drug is unique in that myelosuppression does not occur as a consequence of its use, although pulmonary toxicity is a major limiting side effect (Samuels *et al.*, 1976; Aso *et al.*, 1976). Several studies on the action of bleomycin in whole cells indicate that it is through breakage of cellular

EFFECTS OF DRUGS ON THE CELL NUCLEUS
181

DNA that bleomycin damages cells and stops their proliferation (Miyaki et al., 1973; Saito and Andoh, 1973; Iqbal et al., 1976).

The degradation of DNA by bleomycin may be observed with purified DNA under appropriate conditions in vitro. This degradation is known to be most efficient if the drug and DNA are combined in the presence of a reducing agent such as 2-mercaptoethanol, ascorbate, or H_2O_2 (Onishi et al., 1975). Our studies have focused on the mechanism by which these agents act with bleomycin to degrade DNA. We have suggested a model for bleomycin action in vitro in which the drug combines with adventitious Fe(II) while also bound to DNA (Sausville et al., 1978a). We propose that the oxidation of an Fe(II)–bleomycin–DNA complex by molec-

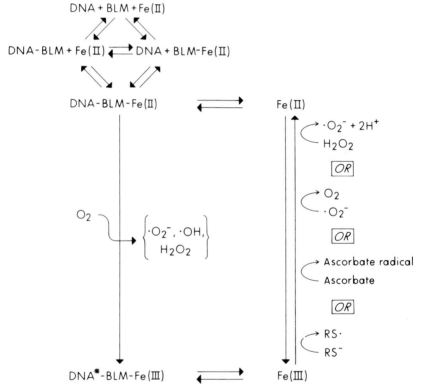

Fig. 1 Model proposed for the degradation of DNA by bleomycin (BLM). The antibiotic complexes with DNA and Fe(II). Oxidation of DNA–BLM–Fe(II) ultimately results in damaged DNA (DNA*). Fe(III) can be reduced to Fe(II) in the presence of a number of reducing agents and thereby take part in many DNA-breaking events. The reduction of Fe(III) shown here does not presuppose a specific site of binding of the metal ion during its reduction to Fe(II). (From Sausville et al., 1978a, reproduced by permission of the American Chemical Society.)

ular oxygen leads to damage of DNA by intermediates of this oxidation. Where the amount of Fe(II) present is limited to that provided by contamination of the reaction mixtures, reducing agents are necessary to allow continued generation of Fe(II) from Fe(III). Our model is summarized in Fig. 1. A significant feature of the action of bleomycin is that it may act by binding simultaneously to DNA and to metal ion, causing degradation of DNA by oxidation of the metal ion in close proximity to DNA. Our goal in this chapter is to present the evidence in recently published work from our laboratory and other laboratories that this mechanism begins to approximate the events that occur when bleomycin causes the degradation of DNA. We also wish to point to the aspects of this field that require further investigation.

A newly revised structure of the bleomycins has recently been proposed (Takita *et al.*, 1978a). Different bleomycins have in common residues I–VI in Fig. 2, as well as the carbohydrate moieties. Bleomycins differ in the residue present at position VII. The clinically used preparation consists of a mixture of approximately 60% bleomycin A_2, where VII is an amine containing a dimethylsulfonium moiety, and about 30% bleomycin B_2, where VII contains a guanidinium function; the remaining 10% is composed of small quantities of other bleomycins. The structure shown in Fig. 2 differs from the previously accepted structure in the absence of a four-membered cyclic amide formerly proposed to exist between residues

BLEOMYCIN A_2

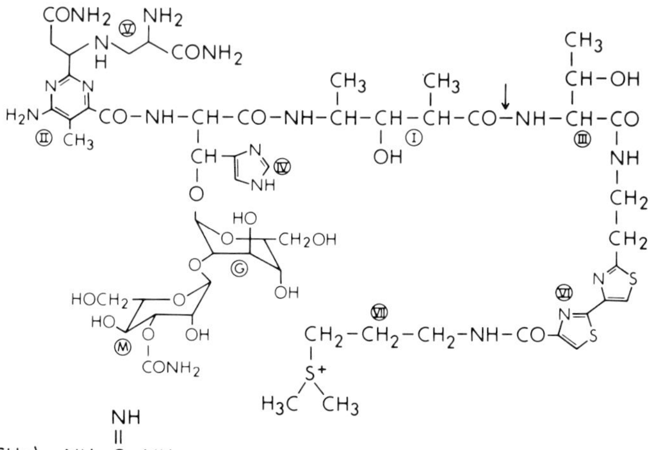

Fig. 2 Structure of bleomycins A_2 and B_2 (Takita *et al.*, 1978a). The arrow indicates the bond hydrolyzed after mild acid treatment. The tripeptide S fragment of bleomycin A_2 consists of residues III, VI, and VII. G = L-glulose; M = 3-O-carbamoyl-D-mannose.

V and II. While the implications of the newly proposed structure for previously published ^{1}H and ^{13}C nuclear magnetic resonance (nmr) assignments (Chen et al., 1977; Dabrowiak et al., 1978b) are not clear, the change in structure does not affect the interpretation of biochemical experiments to be described here nor spectroscopic experiments employing parts of the structure whose chemical basis is certain.

II. The Interaction of Bleomycin with DNA

The binding of bleomycin A_2 and its derivatives to native DNA has been studied under conditions where breakage of DNA does not occur. A study in which binding of the drug to DNA was conclusively demonstrated was conducted in our laboratory (Chien et al., 1977). Quenching of the bithiazole fluorescence of residue VI was used to obtain equilibrium binding data (Table I). The drug has an affinity constant for DNA of about 1×10^5, and the affinity of binding is decreased by increasing ionic strength. The tripeptide S fragment of bleomycin A_2, which consists of residues III, VI, and VII was prepared by mild acid hydrolysis of the parent molecule. We found that this fragment also bound to DNA, and that its affinity for DNA was similar to that of the unaltered drug molecule. These studies revealed that at saturation one molecule of bleomycin binds to every five to six base pairs in DNA. We also studied the interaction of bleomycin with DNA by nmr spectroscopy. In the presence of DNA, absorptions attributed to the methyl groups of residue VII of bleomycin A_2 and of the bithiazole protons of residue VI broaden. This is in contrast to proton absorptions from the β-hydroxyhistidinyl residue IV, which undergo no change on mixing with DNA (Fig. 3). We infer from

TABLE I

Binding of Bleomycin and Tripeptide S to DNA[a]

Ligand	Buffer concentration (mM)[b]	Approximate equilibrium constant, $K \times 10^5$ (M^{-1})	Nucleotides per ligand
Bleomycin	2.5	1.20 ± 0.20	11 ± 1
	25	0.92 ± 0.06	52 ± 4
Tripeptide S	2.5	1.95 ± 0.04	8 ± 0
	25	0.59 ± 0.06	35 ± 4

[a] Measurements of the binding of bleomycin and tripeptide S to DNA are based on fluorescence studies. From Chien et al. (1977). Reproduced by permission of the American Chemical Society.

[b] Tris–HCl, pH 8.4.

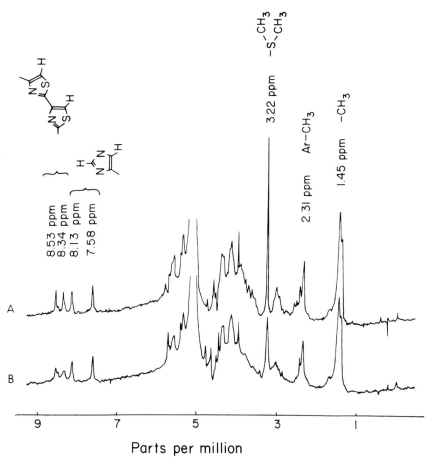

Fig. 3 ^{1}H nmr spectra of bleomycin at 100-MHz resolution. Each spectrum is an average of 512 scans. (A) With 6 mM bleomycin in D_2O at pD 8.4; (B) 6 mM bleomycin and 3.5 mM calf thymus DNA in D_2O, pD 8.4. (From Chien *et al.*, 1977, reproduced by permission of the American Chemical Society.)

these experiments that bleomycin interacts with DNA through close contact of residues VI and VII with the macromolecule, in contrast to the portion of the antibiotic containing residue IV, whose magnetic resonance absorptions are little affected by the binding reaction.

The nature of bleomycin's binding reaction with DNA has recently been studied in greater detail by Povirk *et al.* (1979). These workers have demonstrated that, under conditions where breakage of DNA does not occur, the drug causes relaxation of supercoiled Col El DNA. Continued addition of the drug does not cause rewinding of the DNA supercoils, possibly because the conditions of the experiment require working at near-saturation levels of drug in relation to nucleotide concentration. Most significantly, these workers demonstrate relaxation and rewinding of Col El supercoiled DNA by tripeptide S. These experiments may be taken as evidence that tripeptide S and bleomycin A_2 interact with DNA in a way that is at least partially intercalative in character.

The portion of the antibiotic undergoing intercalation when bleomycin A_2 or tripeptide S binds to DNA is considered to be the bithiazole residue VI, since it is known that the two aromatic rings of this moiety occur in a coplanar conformation (Koyama *et al.*, 1968). The unwinding angle (the dihedral angle through which the DNA is untwisted) of tripeptide S on binding to DNA was found by Povirk *et al* (1979) to be 12° under conditions where bleomycin was known to be active in the degradation of DNA. The latter result was obtained from sedimentation velocity titrations of Col El supercoiled DNA and is taken with reference to the accepted angle of 26° observed for ethidium bromide. The angle between the intercalated bithiazole ring system and the helical axis of DNA was found to be 59°–61°, and the binding of each bleomycin molecule to DNA lengthened the helix by 3.1 Å.

It is clear from these studies that bleomycin can bind to DNA without causing its degradation, and that this binding can proceed in the absence of metal ions. Moreover, substantial evidence has accrued that the bithiazole residue VI binds to DNA via intercalation.

III. The Interaction of Bleomycin with Metal Ions

Bleomycins were originally isolated from bacterial cultures as copper chelates (Umezawa *et al.*, 1966a,b), but the copper is removed prior to their use in chemotherapy. It has since been determined that bleomycin can form chelates with a wide bariety of metal ions (Dabrowiak *et al.*, 1978a). One use of this property has been in the preparation of bleomycin chelates with radioactive isotopes of heavy metals, and in the use of regional scanning techniques to follow the labeled drug into tumor tissues (Kahn *et al.*, 1977). However, the precise way in which metal ions bind to bleomycin and the types of complexes which may be formed have only recently been approached.

The importance of these studies extends from the fact that Fe(II) and bleomycin are capable of causing extraordinarily efficient degradation of DNA. We have proposed (Sausville *et al.*, 1976, 1978a) that this occurs through the formation of an oxygen-sensitive, 1:1 complex of the drug with the metal ion. In Fig. 4, it can be seen that the combination of Fe(II) and bleomycin under anaerobic conditions results in the formation of a 1 : 1 complex with $\lambda_{max} = 476$ nm and $\epsilon_M \approx 3.8 \times 10^2$. The introduction of oxygen is accompanied by the disappearance of this complex and formation of a new species whose absorption extends throughout the near-visible region. If dithionite is added anaerobically to this solution, the complex absorbing at 476 nm is regenerated. This may be taken as evidence that oxygen causes the oxidation of Fe(II)–bleomycin.

The presence of other metal ions, especially Zn(II), Co(II), and Cu(II), in reaction mixtures containing bleomycin and DNA inhibits the degradation of DNA by added Fe(II); but they cannot substitute for Fe(II) in causing efficient DNA degradation. We have previously proposed (Sausville *et al.*, 1978a) that this extends from the binding of the other metal ions by bleomycin with the exclusion of Fe(II). Figure 4C demonstrates that Zn(II) and Fe(II) perturb the ultraviolet (uv) spectrum of bleomycin in a very similar fashion, suggesting that at least one of the ligands binding to the metal ion is the same in both complexes. Dabrowiak and collaborators (1978a) have recently used ^{1}H nmr, electron spin resonance (esr), uv, and visible spectroscopy to approach the question of which ligands bind to the metal ion in Cu(II)– and Zn(II)–bleomycin. Addition of either Cu(II) or Zn(II) to bleomycin shifts a uv absorption attributable to the pyrimidine residue. These workers also attribute the difference spectrum of Zn(II)– bleomycin and bleomycin shown in Fig. 4C (at about 300 nm) to an interaction between the metal ion and the pyrimidine. They interpret the visible and esr spectra of Cu(II)–bleomycin as indicating that four nitrogens, and no oxygen or sulfur atoms, bind to the metal ion. Major shifts in the nmr of protons assigned to the imidazole residue occur upon binding of Zn(II) by the drug, whereas there are very small changes in the nmr signals attributed to protons of the bithiazole residue. These studies implicate the pyrimidine and imidazole groups in binding Zn(II) and probably Cu(II). The similarity of the uv difference spectrum of Zn(II)–bleomycin and that of Fe(II)–bleomycin is evidence for involvement of the pyrimidine residue in binding the metal ion of the latter complex as well.

What is striking in these experiments is the fact that the pyrimidine and the imidazole residues are in a separate portion of the molecule in relation to the bithiazole and the dimethylsulfonium residues of bleomycin A_2. The bithiazole residue has not been implicated in metal binding, but seems to be intimately involved in binding to DNA, as discussed above. It therefore appears that bleomycin A_2 possesses in the same molecule a metal-binding site and a DNA-binding function, although these are apparently localized to distinct parts of the molecule. Clear evidence of this partition of function at the molecular level is given by more recent studies of Dabrowiak *et al.* (1978b), which are shown in Fig. 5. It may be ob-

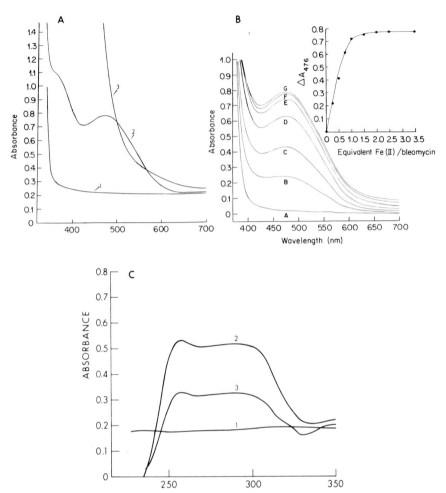

Fig. 4 (A.) Anaerobic spectra of Fe(II)–bleomycin in HEPES buffer. Three milliliters of 2 mM blcomycin in 0.05 M HEPES buffer, pH 7.0, in a Thunberg cuvet was made anaerobic with argon (curve 1). On addition of 60 μl of 0.1 M Fe(II) from the sidearm, curve 2 was observed. On opening the cuvet to air, curve 3 was recorded. The reference sample was H$_2$O. (B) Anaerobic titration of bleomycin with Fe(II) in HEPES buffer. Three milliliters of 2 mM bleomycin in 0.05 M HEPES buffer, pH 7.0, in a Thunberg cuvet was made anaerobic with purified argon. From the sidearm of the cuvette, 5– 8 mg of sodium dithionite was added and an anaerobic solution of Fe(II) was introduced through a rubber septum stopper to the following final molar concentrations: A, O; B, 5×10^{-4}; C, 1×10^{-3}; D, 1.5×10^{-3}; E, 2×10^{-3}; F, 3×10^{-3}; G, 4×10^{-3}, 5×10^{-3}, and 7×10^{-3}. Inset: The observed ΔA_{476} as a function of the ratio of Fe(II) to bleomycin. (C) Difference spectra for Fe(II)–bleomycin, Zn(II)–bleomycin, and bleomycin. In curve 1, the spectrum of 10^{-4} M Fe(II) or 10^{-4} M Zn(II) in 0.05 M HEPES buffer, pH 7.2, versus HEPES buffer is recorded. In curve 2, the optical difference spectrum for a

served that the ^{13}C nmr signals of atoms in the left half of the bleomycin molecule are greatly shifted or disappear on binding of Zn(II) or Cu(II), whereas those occurring in the right half of the molecule (containing the bithiazole residue) are minimally or not at all affected.

While it is true that the structure shown in Fig. 5 does not represent the newly revised structure (see Fig. 2), it does not seem that this revision will alter the validity of the proposal that the bithiazole residue does not have a role in the binding of metal ions examined thus far. Further evidence for this viewpoint is shown in Fig. 6, in which the visible spectrum of phleomycin is examined. Phleomycins are compounds exactly analogous to bleomycins, with the exception that the residue corresponding to the bithiazole of bleomycin has only one thiazole moiety, the other ring existing as a nonaromatic thiazoline moiety (Takita *et al.*, 1978a). It can be seen from Fig. 6 that Fe(II)–phleomycin has a spectrum exactly analogous to that of Fe(II)–bleomycin A$_2$. This argues strongly that the bithiazole portion of both antibiotics does not bind to metal ions, at least to Fe(II).

What is not clear at the present time is the identity of the ligands, in addition to the pyrimidine and imidazole groups, that bind to metals. It has been suggested on the basis of chemical evidence that the amino group of the β-aminoalanine residue V and the carbamoyl group of the mannose group are ligands (Muraoka *et al.*, 1976; Dabrowiak *et al.*, 1978a). However, this viewpoint is not firmly established, especially in view of the recent structural revision involving residue V. While several models have been proposed (Takita *et al.*, 1978b), the important feature that remains true is that, regardless of the eventual structure of the complex, a metal-binding site is located distinct from but in close proximity to an efficient DNA-binding locus.

It has been previously demonstrated (Fig. 4) that, when oxygen is admitted into a solution containing anaerobically prepared Fe(II)–bleomycin, oxidation of the complex occurs with the formation of what is presumed to be some form of Fe(III)–bleomycin. The chemistry of this oxidation, as well as the products formed, are only now becoming known. Dabrowiak and Santillo (1979) have studied the oxidation of bleomycin and its metal derivatives by polarographic techniques. Uncomplexed bleomycin has irreversible reduction waves at -1.22 V (two electrons)

---

solution containing 10^{-4} *M* Fe(II) and 10^{-4} *M* bleomycin versus 10^{-4} *M* bleomycin was studied. All spectra with Fe(II) were obtained in Thunberg cuvets under an argon atmosphere. In curve 3, the optical difference spectrum for a solution containing 10^{-4} *M* ZN(II) and 10^{-4} *M* bleomycin versus 10^{-4} *M* bleomycin was recorded. Both reference and sample solutions were prepared in 0.05 *M* HEPES buffer, pH 7.2. The salts used were Fe(NH$_4$)$_2$(SO$_4$)$_2$·6H$_2$O and ZnCl$_2$.

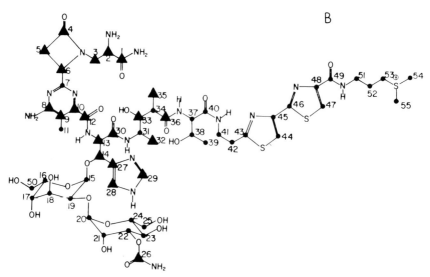

Fig. 5 ¹³C nmr spectra of bleomycin in the presence of Zn(II) and Cu(II). (A) The carbon resonances that shift when Zn(II) binds to bleomycin are indicated (▲) on the structure of bleomycin A₂. (B) The carbon resonances that are missing in the ¹³C nmr spectrum of Cu(II)–BLM are indicated (▲) on the structure of the drug. (From Dabrowiak *et al.*, 1978b, reproduced by permission of the American Chemical Society.)

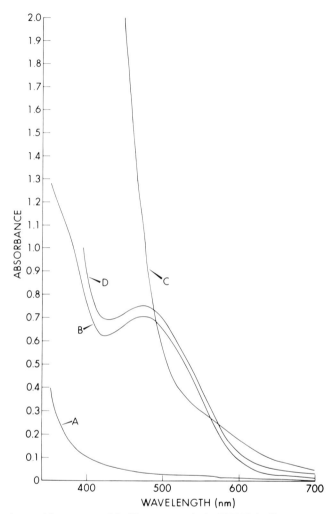

Fig. 6 Anaerobic spectra of Fe(II)–phleomycin in HEPES buffer. Three milliliters of 3.1 mg/ml phleomycin in 0.05 M HEPES buffer, pH 7.2, in a Thunberg cuvet was made anaerobic with argon (curve A). On addition of 60 μl of 0.1 M Fe(II) from the sidearm, cruve B was observed. On opening the cuvet to air, curve C was recorded. The spectrum of curve D was obtained after making the sample anaerobic again and adding sodium dithionite from the sidearm. The reference sample was H_2O.

and -1.48 (multi-electron). The former wave is attributed to the pyrimidine residue and disappears on the addition of Fe(II), Co(II), Zn(II), or Ni(II), thus providing further evidence for the involvement of this residue in the binding of these metal ions. These workers suggest that the polarographic properties of Fe(III)–bleomycin prepared by air-oxidation of

Fe(II)–bleomycin differ from those of the complex prepared by mixing Fe(III) and bleomycin. However, a thorough study on the stoichiometry and optical or other spectra of either proposed Fe(III)–bleomycin has not to date been conducted. Such a study will be necessary to interpret the polarographic experiments more completely.

Caspary *et al.* (1979) have measured the rate of oxygen consumption by Fe(II)–bleomycin. They have found that the consumption of oxygen by solutions of Fe(II) is greatly enhanced by small quantities of bleomycin. They have proposed that bleomycin in this capacity is acting as a ferrous oxidase and have found that 1 mole of bleomycin is capable of oxidizing about 5×10^3 moles of Fe(II)/minute. However, the identity of the products of this oxidation remain to be clearly demonstrated. Previous studies in our laboratory (Horwitz *et al.*, 1979) had indicated that the oxidation of Fe(II) in the presence of bleomycin was accompanied by the uptake of less than stoichiometric amounts of oxygen at apparent completion of the reaction, except at very low concentrations of Fe(II) and bleomycin. One interpretation of these data is that reduced oxygen radical intermediates may also act to oxidize Fe(II)–bleomycin. The importance of future experiments in this area lies in the fact that these intermediates are probably instrumental in the degradation of DNA by Fe(II)–bleomycin.

IV. The Degradation of DNA by Bleomycin, Fe(II), and Oxygen

When bleomycin is added to reaction mixtures containing DNA, breakage of the DNA occurs. In the absence of added reducing agent or metal ion, this breakage occurs to a limited extent and requires high concentrations of bleomycin in relation to the number of breaks actually found (Haidle, 1971; Umezawa *et al.*, 1973). In the presence of reducing agents, the efficiency of the degradation of DNA by bleomycin increases greatly (Umezawa *et al.*, 1973). In no case does the occurrence of DNA-breaking events frankly exceed the number of bleomycin molecules present, as would be expected to occur if bleomycin were acting catalytically to degrade DNA.

The oxidizing and reducing agents observed to stimulate bleomycin's action include 2-mercaptoethanol, dithiothreitol, ascorbate, H_2O_2, NADPH, and $NaBH_4$. The removal of oxygen inhibits the action of bleomycin in the presence of a number of organic reducing agents, as does the addition of aminoethylisothiuronium bromide, a reported free-radical scavenger (Onishi *et al.*, 1975).

Nagai *et al.* (1969) found that Co(II), Zn(II), and Cu(II) inhibited the action of bleomycin in the presence of 2-mercaptoethanol. This early series of experiments measured the ability of bleomycin and 2-mercaptoethanol to cause a decrease in the T_m of DNA. Where breakage of DNA has been followed directly, this result has been confirmed (Shirakawa *et al.*, 1971). It is generally considered that high concentrations of EDTA can inhibit the degradation of DNA in the presence of reducing agents and oxygen (Suzuki *et al.*, 1970; Takeshita *et al.*, 1976; Bearden *et al.*, 1977). Ishida and Takahashi (1975) noted that Fe(II) and Fe(III) increased the degradation of DNA by bleomycin in the presence of 2-mercaptoethanol.

Every DNA substrate thus far examined is a substrate for degradation by bleomycin plus a reducing agent (Umezawa *et al.*, 1973; Müller *et al.*, 1972). It is generally found that single-stranded DNA is degraded with somewhat less efficiency than double-stranded DNA (Onishi *et al.*, 1975). RNA is not a substrate for degradation by bleomycin under any known conditions (Kuo *et al.*, 1977). The DNA of phage PBS-1, containing uracil in place of thymine, is also degraded (Haidle *et al.*, 1972a). The DNA present in a RNA–DNA hybrid is degraded, whereas the RNA is marginally affected (Haidle and Bearden, 1975), although this RNA has not been characterized in detail. Therefore it is proposed that it is the presence of deoxyribose as the nucleic acid sugar which confers sensitivity to bleomycin plus a reducing agent. A correlation has been reported in which DNAs of high AT content are more susceptible to the action of bleomycin than GC-rich DNAs (Müller *et al.*, 1972).

In view of the potent inhibition of DNA degradation by EDTA and the reported stimulation of bleomycin action in the presence of reducing agents by Fe(II) or Fe(III), it occurred to us that Fe(II) could play a role in the degradation of DNA by bleomycin and a reducing agent even when the metal ion was not added to reaction mixtures. We then demonstrated (Sausville *et al.*, 1976) that Fe(II) and bleomycin, but not Fe(III) or other metal ions, could act to cause highly efficient degradation of DNA in the absence of organic reducing agents and that this reaction required the presence of oxygen. These experiments were confirmed by Lown and Sim (1977).

Subsequent studies from our laboratory demonstrated that iron was a significant contaminant of reaction mixtures prepared without its overt addition, that chelating agents inhibited all reactions of bleomycin leading to the breakage of DNA in the absence of added iron, and that Zn(II), Cu(II), and Co(II) inhibited the action of Fe(II) and bleomycin just as they inhibited the degradation of DNA in the presence of organic reducing agents but in the absence of added Fe(II). Most significant was the observation that, in the absence of added Fe(II) but in the presence of 2-mercaptoethanol or 2-mercaptoethanol plus ATP and Mg(II), the degradation of DNA was inhibited by deferoxamine much more efficiently than by EDTA (Sausville *et al.*, 1978a). Deferoxamine is a specific chelator for Fe, in contrast to EDTA which can chelate many metal ions. The result of these studies indicated that, even in reaction mixtures to which the metal ion was not added exogenously, it played an important role as Fe(II) in acting with bleomycin to degrade DNA. To demonstrate that Fe(II) could account for the activity of bleomycin previously described in the degradation of DNA, we studied the products of the degradation reaction (Sausville *et al.*, 1978b). The results of these studies have recently been extended by other workers using newly developed DNA sequencing techniques with DNA substrates of known primary sequence. The following points have been elicited by these studies.

A. Release of Bases

Haidle *et al.* (1972b) demonstrated that, in the presence of high concentrations of bleomycin in relation to DNA and in the presence of 2-mercaptoethanol, the release of all four DNA bases could be detected. These workers also found that base release did not occur if reactions were conducted using nucleosides in place of DNA. Table II shows results from our laboratory in which the release of all four bases from calf thymus DNA was followed by high-pressure liquid chromatography. It can be

TABLE II

Release of Bases during Reaction of DNA with Bleomycin and Fe(II)[a]

Base	Release (%)[b]
Thymine	13.7 ± 1.9
Cytosine	7.8 ± 0.8
Adenine	4.2 ± 0.6
Guanine	2.8 ± 1.2

[a] Reaction mixtures contained in a final volume of 2 ml: $2.4 \times 10^{-4} M$ calf thymus DNA, $2.3 \times 10^{-4} M$ bleomycin, 0.019 M phosphate buffer, pH 7.0, and $2.3 \times 10^{-4} M$ Fe(II). A 20-μl aliquot was analyzed by high-pressure liquid chromatography. From Sausville *et al.* (1978b).

[b] 100 × (moles of base detected)/(moles of base in DNA).

seen that bases are released in a manner different from that expected if random release of bases was occurring. Pyrimidines are more readily released than purines, with $T > C > A > G$ detected. At levels of bleomycin equimolar to DNA nucleotide concentrations, and with equimolar Fe(II), about one base in every four is released following the action of Fe(II) and bleomycin in the presence of oxygen.

Takeshita *et al.* (1978) have examined base release from a reaction mixture containing HeLa cell DNA labeled in different DNA bases and 2-mercaptoethanol, ATP, and $MgCl_2$, but with no added Fe(II). They have found that the order of base release is $T > C > A > G$ and that the extent of total base release is comparable to our reactions, which employed Fe(II) in stoichiometric amounts in the absence of 2-mercaptoethanol. The fact that the products formed in the two systems are comparable is evidence that Fe(II) can be the active species in systems containing organic reducing agents but no added metal ion.

Results analogous to those of Takeshita *et al.* (1978) were demonstrated by Povirk *et al.* (1978). These workers presented evidence that, in addition to the four major bases, altered bases could be detected as minor products of the reaction conducted in the presence of 2-mercaptoethanol and Fe(II), although these substances were not characterized. Chromatography of reaction mixtures in an alkaline medium (pH 11.5) did not alter the amount of base release observed in a less alkaline medium (pH 9.7).

B. Formation of Oligonucleotides

The oligonucleotides resulting from extensive degradation of DNA by bleomycin in the presence of 2-mercaptoethanol were first studied by Kuo *et al.* (1973). These workers found that DNA extensively damaged by the drug consisted of oligonucleotides between 10 and 13 residues in length. Their data may be interpreted to indicate that these species are refractory to the common nucleases and are not sensitive to further degradation by bleomycin. Mononucleotide and dinucleotides were not found as products of reaction mixtures.

We have examined the oligonucleotide products of a limit digest of DNA by bleomycin and Fe(II) by DEAE-cellulose chromatography. The results of these experiments can be seen in Fig. 7, where adenovirus DNA labeled with [^{32}P]- and [^{3}H]-thymine was used. During the reaction shown, 84% of the DNA present as ^{32}P became acid-soluble. The ^{32}P-labeled oligonucleotides derived from the reaction of DNA with bleomycin and Fe(II) elute with a pattern quite distinct from that of the marker nucleotides derived from calf thymus DNA after treatment with pancreatic

DNase. The ^{3}H species present in fractions 10–16 comigrate with thymine using high-pressure liquid chromatography. Fractions with appreciable ^{32}P are present which comigrate with marker oligonucleotides of chain length 5, 6, and 7. An unresolved fraction containing ^{32}P is eluted at greater than 7 residues in length. A significant fraction of the applied label elutes with 2 M NaCl. This latter fraction has been sized by electrophoresis in urea–acrylamide gels and consists of oligonucleotides of greater than 10 but less than 20 residues. From the distribution of ^{32}p label observed in this column, we estimate that the median oligonucleotide produced after incubation of DNA with bleomycin and Fe(II) under these conditions has a size of between 7 and 10 nucleotide residues. In a reaction analogous to that described in Fig. 7, 98% of the ^{32}P label remained in a form that adsorbed to Norit after the reaction of [^{32}P]DNA with bleomycin and Fe(II), thus indicating that free phosphate is not liberated during the reaction. Mono- and dinucleotides are also not found in these products. The material eluting in 2 M NaCl is not a substrate for further action by bleomycin and Fe(II). The results of the experiments summarized in Fig. 7 show that Fe(II) and bleomycin act to degrade DNA in a way that corresponds closely to that described previously wherein bleomycin and 2-mercaptoethanol were allowed to react with DNA in the absence of added metal ions.

Since there is clear preference for release of pyrimidines over purines by bleomycin and Fe(II), it is of interest to determine if breakage of DNA occurs at specific sequence sites. This question has recently been approached by D'Andrea and Haseltine (1978) and by Takeshita et al. (1978), using the DNA-sequencing techniques of Maxam and Gilbert (1977). Comparable results have been obtained by both groups. Breakage of DNA by bleomycin in the presence of either 2-mercaptoethanol or Fe(II) occurs primarily at GT and GC sites in the DNA (Fig. 8). Most significant were their observations that, although Fe(II) in the absence of bleomycin could cause breaks in the DNA, this breakage was not specific and required relatively high concentrations of Fe(II) to generate significant random nicking. Thus these experiments also demonstrate quite clearly that it is the interaction between Fe(II) and bleomycin that leads to specific breakage of DNA, and that this process differs qualitatively and quantitatively from the breakage evoked by Fe(II) alone.

D'Andrea and Haseltine (1978) and Takeshita et al. (1978) observed that nucleotides from DNA treated by bleomycin and Fe(II) or 2-mercaptoethanol migrated with a mobility that differed slightly from that exhibited by marker nucleotides, which have a 3'-phosphate group. In addition, more than one DNA product is observed at some of the cleavage sites. This supports the earlier observation of Kuo and Haidle (1974) that more

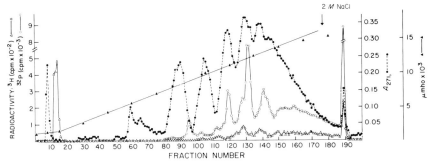

Fig. 7 DEAE-cellulose chromatography of the limit product of Fe(II)–bleomycin degradation of DNA. The reaction mixture contained in a volume of 1.0 ml: 5 mM phosphate, pH 7.0, 22 μM adenovirus-2 [*thymine*-^{3}H, ^{32}P]DNA, 333 μg/ml bleomycin, and 2×10^{-4} M Fe(II). After incubation for 30 minutes at 37°C more bleomycin and Fe(II) were added (to a final concentration of 550 μg/ml and 4.2×10^{-4} M, respectively), and incubation was continued for 30 minutes. The reaction was stopped with 0.01 M EDTA, and 8.8 mg of calf thymus DNA which had been extensively digested with pancreatic DNase was added. After dilution to 0.02 M phosphate buffer and addition of urea to 7 M, the sample was applied to a DEAE-cellulose column and the nucleotides eluted with a 0–0.3 M NaCl gradient (2 liters). Nucleotides not eluted with the gradient were removed by 2 M NaCl in 0.02 M Tris–HCl, pH 7.6, and 7 M urea. A_{271}, μmho, [^{32}P], and ^{3}H in aliquots of column fractions are shown. (From Sausville *et al.*, 1978b, reproduced by permission of the American Chemical Society.)

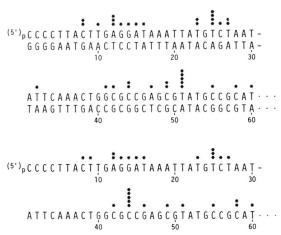

Fig. 8 Release of bases from double- and single-stranded restriction fragments of ϕX DNA by bleomycin. The sequences shown represent a portion of the double- or single-stranded restriction fragment used for analysis of base specificity. Bases released are indicated by asterisks, and the relative intensity of the bands is indicated by the number of symbols. (From Takeshita *et al.*, 1978, reproduced by permission of the National Academy of Sciences.)

than one type of end group was generated after bleomycin damaged DNA, although it is not clear what the structure of these end groups may be. When DNA broken by high concentrations of Fe(II) without bleomycin is examined in these gels, it is found that the labeled DNA fragments have the same mobility as the marker nucleotides. This result indicates that the Fe(II)-treated fragments possess a 3′-phosphate end group.

The nucleotides isolated in the column described in Fig. 7 were examined by digestion with common nucleases. Data presented elsewhere (Sausville *et al.*, 1978b) indicate that these nucleotides are refractory to digestion by venom phosphodiesterase or spleen phosphodiesterase, even with pretreatment by alkaline phosphatase. For example, Fig. 9 shows that, in contrast to full-length adenovirus DNA, Fe(II)–bleomycin-treated DNA fragments are refractory to the action of venom phosphodiesterase with or without pretreatment with pancreatic DNase. These results, coupled with the observation of D'Andrea and Haseltine (1978), suggest that the products of bleomycin's action on DNA may be heterogeneous and differ from the spectrum of products normally obtained after the uncomplicated nucleolytic digestion of DNA.

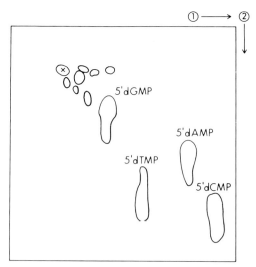

Fig. 9   Thin-layer chromatography of a nuclease digest of Fe(II)–bleomycin-treated DNA. A reaction in a final volume of 1.0 ml contained 21 μM adenovirus [^{32}P]DNA 33 μg/ml bleomycin, and 2.0 × 10^{-4} M Fe(II), in 0.005 M phosphate, pH 7. After incubation for 15 minutes at 37°C, the reaction was stopped with 0.01 M EDTA. The sample was treated with pancreatic DNase and venom exonuclease and then analyzed by thin layer chromatography. The origin (X) is indicated, as are the positions of the four 5′dNTPs obtained after analogous digestion of 21 μM adenovirus [^{32}P]DNA which had not been treated with Fe(II) and bleomycin. The four 5′dNTPs were the only compounds detected in this system after digestion of non-bleomycin-treated DNA.

C. Alkali-Labile Bonds and Double-Strand Breaks

It has been known for many years that apurinic or apyrimidinic regions of DNA are susceptible to scission in an alkaline environment (Tamm *et al.*, 1953). Since bleomycin causes the release of DNA bases, it is of interest to inquire whether this process is always accompanied by strand scission, or whether base release can occur alone. In the latter event, one would expect that the DNA would become labile to alkali.

Ross and Moses (1978) found alkali-labile bonds in DNA treated with bleomycin in the absence of thiol reducing agents and put forth the view that bleomycin action consists only of base release without strand scission. Povirk *et al.*, (1977) found that alkali-labile bonds occurred in the presence of bleomycin and 2-mercaptoethanol. Our interpretation of these experiments is that the action of bleomycin and Fe(II) on DNA can lead to various results. In one case, only base release occurs as a result of breakage of the glycoside bond, and thus the DNA is alkali-labile. In another possible mechanism, the intermediate resulting from the oxidation of Fe(II)–bleomycin causes damage to the deoxyribose portion of the molecule, with resulting liberation of bases at the same time as strand breakage. Another observation of Ross and Moses (1978) was that the alkali lability of bleomycin-treated DNA was not increased by exposure to heat before the addition of alkali. This stands in contrast to the results of studies with alkylating agents, where the alkylated bases were liberated by heat treatment and thus the degree of alkali lability was increased by prior heat treatment. This result indicates that the process leading to base release by bleomycin differs from that associated with alkylating agents.

Povirk *et al.* (1977) presented an intriguing series of results in which it was demonstrated that double-strand breaks occurred in DNA treated with bleomycin and 2-mercaptoethanol to a degree greater than that expected if single-strand breaks occurred randomly. Similar results have been reported by Lloyd *et al.* (1978). The latter workers propose that a dimeric species of bleomycin A_2 is responsible for the occurrence of this phenomenon, although the existence of this species has not yet been demonstrated. We wish to note that other explanations exist for this effect. It is possible that the binding of bleomycin to DNA occurs with a degree of cooperativity such that a fraction of the bleomycin is bound with a locally high concentration of monomeric bleomycin. Alternatively, it is possible that, in the production of radical intermediates by Fe(II), bleomycin, and oxygen, a local chain reaction is established, with radicals being generated either in bleomycin or in DNA, as well as through the expected reduced forms of oxygen. The establishment of such a process could increase the probability of a break in both strands of a DNA helix to which one molecule of bleomycin is bound. Finally, it is possible that the occurrence of double-strand breaks may reflect the generation of more than one cycle of Fe(II)–bleomycin oxidation at a single locus. This is a consideration especially where a reducing agent such as mercaptoethanol is present. An understanding of the reaction sequence leading to a double-strand break is of importance, because such an event would be expected to have lethal consequences for a cell were it to occur *in vivo*.

D. The Production of Aldehyde

Kuo and Haidle (1974) observed that, when DNA was exposed to bleomycin for relatively long periods of time in the presence of 2-mercaptoethanol, a product was formed which reacted with 2-thiobarbituric acid to give a chromophore identical to that observed after the reaction of 2-thiobarbituric acid with malondialdehyde. We have recently demonstrated

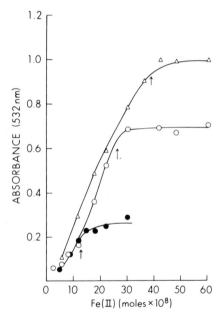

Fig. 10 Generation of a malondialdehyde-like product after the reaction of bleomycin and Fe(II) with DNA. Reactions contained in a volume of 1.3 ml: 0.019 M phosphate, pH 7.0, 2.9×10^{-3} M calf thymus DNA, Fe(II) in the indicated amount, and 155 (0.13 μmole, ●), 310 (0.26 μmole, ○), or 465 μg/ml (0.39 μmole, △) bleomycin. After incubation at 37°C for 15 minutes, an aliquot was removed from each reaction mixture for the determination of malondialdehyde-like material. The arrows indicate the amount of iron approximately equimolar to the bleomycin present in each reaction mixture. (From Sausville *et al.*, 1978b, reproduced by permission of the American Chemical Society.)

that this product is formed with great efficiency by the action of Fe(II) and bleomycin on calf thymus DNA (Sausville *et al.*, 1978b). Figure 10 demonstrates that, in reaction mixtures containing excess DNA in relation to bleomycin, the formation of the product occurs with a stoichiometry of 1 mole of Fe(II) to 1 mole of bleomycin. This experiment demonstrates that the 1:1 Fe(II)–bleomycin complex whose spectrum is shown in Fig. 4 is probably of direct relevance to the degradation of DNA. It should be understood that the unambiguous identification of the aldehyde released after the reaction of Fe(II)–bleomycin with DNA as malondialdehyde has not yet been accomplished, as the thiobarbituric acid derivative may be formed from other aldehydes (see discussion in Sausville *et al.*, 1978b).

V. Summary and Overview

The results described in the preceding sections are entirely consistent with the mechanism for bleomycin action proposed in Fig. 1. What is of particular interest is that this mechanism emphasizes a dual role for bleomycin: The drug binds Fe(II) and DNA in a way that renders the DNA susceptible to damage. As discussed previously, this dual role seems to be compartmentalized into separate portions of the antibiotic molecule.

There seems to be little question that an oxidative event is required for the degradation of DNA by Fe(II)–bleomycin. This is shown most clearly in the experiment in Fig. 11A where it is seen that the highly efficient degradation of DNA to acid-soluble materials requires the presence of oxygen. A question that immediately arises is whether this mechanism is unique to bleomycin. Its essence is that a drug molecule is endowed with the properties of being a free-radical generator in a way that efficiently exposes DNA to the action of these radicals. In the case of bleomycin, this is apparently accomplished by the binding of an oxidizable metal ion close to DNA. It is not clear at the present time if the portion of the bleomycin molecule that binds to metal ions allows some type of unique interaction between the metal ion and DNA which is important in producing degradation of DNA.

Other molecules are known that probably degrade DNA by an oxidative mechanism. Recent studies in our laboratory (Burger *et al.*, 1978) have indicated that neocarzinostatin, an acidic protein of molecular weight 10,700, also requires oxygen to degrade DNA efficiently in the presence of reducing agents (Fig. 11B). Previous studies with this compound (Poon *et al.*, 1977; Beerman and Goldberg, 1977) had indicated that it also released free bases from DNA, as it generated breaks in the DNA, and that thiol compounds were required for its action. However, neocar-

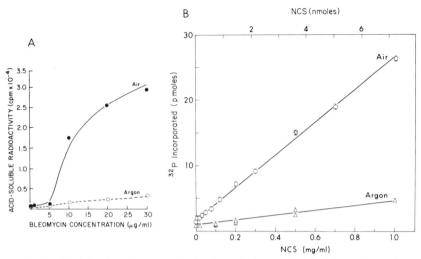

Fig. 11 Participation of oxygen in the degradation of DNA by bleomycin and neocarzinostatin. (A) Bleomycin. Reactions contained in a volume of 1.0 ml: 2.0 μM adenovirus [^{3}H]DNA (49,600 cpm), 0.05 M phosphate, pH 7.0, the indicated concentrations of bleomycin and 1 × 10^{-4} M Fe(II) added from a sidearm after equilibration with argon or air. Reactions were conducted in the presence of argon (○) or air (●) at 22°C for 10 minutes before the addition of a final concentration of 0.05 M anaerobic EDTA. (From Sausville *et al.*, 1978b, reproduced by permission of the American Chemical Society.) (B) Neocarzinostatin (NCS). The final concentration of reactants, after addition of bacteriophage λ DNA and dithiothreitol from the sidearm was 61 μM DNA, 3 mM dithiothreitol, 10 mM Tris–HCl buffer, pH 7.5, and the indicated concentrations of neocarzinostatin in a final volume of 75 μl. Reactions were conducted in the presence of argon or air at 37°C for 30 minutes and terminated by the addition of 0.1 M NaOH. DNA cleavage was determined by a phosphatase–kinase assay. Reversal of anaerobiosis (▽) was effected by replacing the argon with air. (From Burger *et al.*, 1978, reproduced by permission of the American Society of Biological Chemists, Inc.)

zinostatin differs from bleomycin in a number of respects. The requirement for thiol groups is apparently specific, as other reducing agents are not able to cause DNA degradation with the drug. There is no evidence that metal ions are involved in the action of neocarzinostatin, nor is there yet good evidence that the compound binds to DNA. Neocarzinostatin causes breaks in DNA at A and T residues, and the nature of the break is not heterogeneous; product oligonucleotides migrate in a way commensurate with the existence of a 3′-phosphate group at the site of the break (D'Andrea and Haseltine, 1978; Hatayama *et al.*, 1978).

The probability exists that the induction of free radicals at appropriate cellular locations will be seen as a potent mechanism for cytotoxicity induced by antineoplastic drugs. As this process is reflected in the action of bleomycin, however, numerous questions remain. For example, there has not yet been an unambiguous demonstration of the binding of $Fe(II)$–bleomycin to DNA. In addition, the stoichiometry of DNA breakage or base release in relation to bound $Fe(II)$–bleomycin is also not clear. The mechanism presented in Fig. 1 postulates the existence of $Fe(II)$–bleomycin–oxygen, yet the interaction of oxygen with the complex remains to be described in detail.

Additional questions concern the role of bleomycin in the reaction process. Is the drug merely a passive carrier of $Fe(II)$ to a site vicinal to DNA, or does it have an active role in the process either by forming a radical itself or by condensing with aldehyde groups generated in DNA? Examination of this question will require a labeled drug of high specific activity so that its fate during a reaction may be followed. What is the reaction sequence followed? Does base release proceed, follow, or have no relation to strand scission? A major problem in answering these and related questions is that DNA degradation by bleomycin and $Fe(II)$ occurs with extreme rapidity (Sausville *et al.*, 1978b). This most likely reflects the speed or efficiency of the oxidative process. In addition, the possible intermediates active in DNA degradation (including the superoxide anion and hydroxyl radical) have brief lifetimes and are not amenable to analysis by standard chemical techniques. The use of scavenging agents such as superoxide dismutase, catalase, and high concentrations of ethanol to study these questions must be rigorously controlled if the results are to be of value, because the binding of $Fe(II)$ to bleomycin or of the complex may be deleteriously affected by their presence. In addition, since radicals are generated at their site of action, these species need not diffuse and thus be accessible to the actions of the radical scavengers.

Another series of questions pertains to the apparent specificity of $Fe(II)$–bleomycin in causing the preferential release of pyrimidines and breakage at GC and GT sites in DNA. Recent studies by Kasai *et al.*, (1978) have demonstrated that bleomycin binds preferentially to nucleic acid polymers containing guanine. The bithiazole and dimethylsulfonium or polyamine portions of different bleomycins could bind at specific loci in the DNA helix, thus positioning the metal portion of the antibiotic in regions that would be rich in GT and GC sites. The possibility that the intermediates generated in the oxidation of $Fe(II)$–bleomycin may have their own intrinsic specificity for breaking particular types of purine or pyrimidine linkages, independent of the binding of the drug molecule, must be considered. Evidence bearing on these points is at present lacking, but could be obtained using new sequencing techniques and small, synthetic polynucleotides of known structure.

Finally, a most important question concerns the relevance of what is now known of the action of bleomycin *in vitro* to the events occurring in cells exposed to the drug. There is at present no good evidence that Fe(II) is involved in the action of the drug in cells, although the potential for this involvement raises the possibility that tumor resistance to this compound could occur by selective mechanisms of sequestering Fe(II) from use by the antibiotic. Alternatively, it is conceivable that Fe(II)– or Fe(III)– bleomycin is a more efficacious cytotoxic and chemotherapuetic agent than the presently used metal-free bleomycin. Definitive experiments bearing on these points remain to be performed.

Acknowledgments

The authors are indebted to Dr. Jack Peisach for his interest, advice, and assistance. Research that originated in the authors' laboratory was supported in part by United States Public Health Service grant RO1 CA15714.

References

Aso, Y., Yoneda, K., and Kikkawa, Y. (1976). *Lab. Invest.* **35**, 558.
Bearden, J. C., Lloyd, R. S., and Haidle, C. W. (1977). *Biochem. Biophys. Res. Commun.* **75**, 442.
Beerman, T. A., and Goldberg, I. H. (1977). *Biochim. Biophys. Acta* **475**, 281.
Burger, R. M., Peisach, J., and Horwitz, S. B. (1978). *J. Biol. Chem.* **253**, 4830.
Caspary, W. J., Niziak, C., Lanzo, D. A., Friedman, R., and Bachur, N. R. (1979). *Mol. Pharm.* **16**, 256.
Chen, D. M., Hawkins, B. L., and Glickson, J. D. (1977). *Biochemistry* **16**, 2731.
Chien, M., Grollman, A. P., and Horwitz, S. B. (1977). *Biochemistry* **16**, 3641.
Dabrowiak, J. C., and Santillo, F. S. (1979). *J. Electrochem. Soc.* In press.
Dabrowiak, J. C., Greenaway, F. T., Longo, W. E., vanHusen, M., and Crooke, S. T. (1978a). *Biochim. Biophys. Acta* **517**, 517.
Dabrowiak, J. C., Greenaway, F. T., and Grulich, R. (1978b). *Biochemistry* **17**, 4090.
D'Andrea, A. D., and Haseltine, W. A. (1978). *Proc. Natl. Acad. Sci. U.S.A.* **75**, 3608.
Haidle, C. W. (1971). *Mol. Pharmacol.* **7**, 645.
Haidle, C. W., and Bearden, J., Jr. (1975). *Biochem. Biophys. Res. Commun.* **65**, 815.
Haidle, C. W., Kuo, M. T., and Weiss, K. K. (1972a). *Biochem. Pharmacol.* **21**, 3308.
Haidle, C. W., Weiss, K. K., and Kuo, M. T. (1972b). *Mol. Pharmacol.* **8**, 531.
Hatayama, T., Goldberg, I. H., Takeshita, M., and Grollman, A. P. (1978). *Proc. Natl. Acad. Sci. U.S.A.* **75**, 3603.
Horwitz, S. B., Sausville, E. A., and Peisach, J. (1979). *In* "Bleomycin: Chemical Biochemical and Biological Aspects" (S. Hecht, ed.). Springer-Verlag, Berlin and New York. In press.
Iqbal, Z. M., Kohn, K. W., Ewig, R. A. G., and Fornace, A. J., Jr. (1976). *Cancer Res.* **36**, 3834.
Ishida, R., and Takahashi, T. (1975). *Biochem. Biophys. Res. Commun.* **66**, 1432.
Kahn, P. C., Milunsky, C., Dewanjee, M., and Rudders, R. A. (1977). *Am. J. Roentgenol.* **129**, 267.

Kasai, H., Naganawa, H., Takita, T., and Umezawa, H. (1978). *J. Antibiotics* **31**, 1316.

Koyama, G., Nakamura, H., Muraoka, Y., Takita, T., Maeda, K., and Umezawa, H. (1968). *Tetrahedron Lett.* 4635.

Kuo, M. T., and Haidle, C. W. (1974). *Biochim. Biophys. Acta* **335**, 109.

Kuo, M. T., Haidle, C. W., and Inners, L. D. (1973). *Biophys. J.* **13**, 1296.

Kuo, M. T., Auger, L. T., Saunders, G. F., and Haidle, C. W. (1977). *Cancer Res.* **37**, 1345.

Lloyd, R. S., Haidle, C. W., and Robberson, D. L. (1978). *Biochemistry* **17**, 1890.

Lown, J. W., and Sim, S. (1977). *Biochem. Biophys. Res. Commun.* **77**, 1150.

Maxam, A. M., and Gilbert, W. (1977). *Proc. Natl. Acad. Sci. U.S.A.* **74**, 560.

Miyaki, M., Morohashi, S., and Ono, T. (1973). *J. Antibiot.* **26**, 369.

Müller, W. E. G., Yamazaki, Z., Breter, H., and Zahn, R. K. (1972). *Eur. J. Biochem.* **31**, 518.

Muraoka, Y., Kobayashi, H., Fujii, A., Kunishima, M., Fujii, T., Nakayama, Y., Takita, T., and Umezawa, H., (1976). *J. Antibiot.* **29**, 853.

Nagai, K., Yamaki, H., Suzuki, H., Tanaka, N., and Umezawa, H. (1969). *Biochim. Biophys. Acta* **179**, 165.

Onishi, T., Iwata, H., and Takagi, Y. (1975). *J. Biochem. (Tokyo)* **77**, 745.

Poon, R., Beerman, T. A., and Goldberg, I. H. (1977). *Biochemistry* **16**, 486.

Povirk, L. F., Wübker, W., Köhnlein, W., and Hutchinson, F. (1977). *Nucleic Acids Res.* **4**, 3573.

Povirk, L. F., Hogan, M., and Dattagupta, N. (1979). *Biochemistry* **18**, 96.

Povirk, L. F., Köhnlein, W., and Hutchinson, F. (1978). *Biochim. Biophys. Acta* **521**, 126.

Ross, S. L., and Moses, R. E. (1978). *Biochemistry* **17**, 581.

Saito, M., and Andoh, T. (1973). *Cancer Res.* **33**, 1696.

Samuels, M. L., Johnson, D. E., Holoye, P. Y., and Lanzatti, V. J. (1976). *J. Am. Med. Assoc.* **235**, 1117.

Sausville, E. A., Peisach, J., and Horwitz, S. B. (1976). *Biochem. Biophys. Res. Commun.* **73**, 814.

Sausville, E. A., Peisach, J., and Horwitz, S. B. (1978a). *Biochemistry* **17**, 2740.

Sausville, E. A., Stein, R. W., Peisach, J., and Horwitz, S. B. (1978b). *Biochemistry* **17**, 2746.

Shirakawa, I., Azegami, M., Ishii, S., and Umezawa, H. (1971). *J. Antibiot.* **24**, 761.

Suzuki, H., Nagai, K., Akutsu, E., Yamaki, H., Tanaka, N., and Umezawa, H. (1970). *J. Antibiot.* **23**, 473.

Takeshita, M., Grollman, A. P., and Horwitz, S. B. (1976). *Virology* **69**, 453.

Takeshita, M., Grollman, A., Ohtsubo, E., and Ohtsubo, H. (1978). *Proc. Natl. Acad. Sci. U.S.A.* **75**, 5983.

Takita, T., Muraoka, Y., Nakatani, T., Fujii, A., Umezawa, Y., Naganawa, H., and Umezawa, H. (1978a). *J. Antibiot.* **31**, 801.

Takita, T., Muraoka, Y., Nakatani, T., Fujii, A., Iitaka, Y., and Umezawa, H. (1978b). *J. Antibiot.* **31**, 1073.

Tamm, C., Shapiro, H. S., Lipshitz, R., and Chargaff, E. (1953). *J. Biol. Chem.* **203**, 673.

Umezawa, H., Maeda, K., Takeuchi, T., and Okami, Y. (1966a). *J. Antibiot.* **19**, 200.

Umezawa, H., Suhara, Y., Takita, T., and Maeda, K. (1966b). *J. Antibiot.* **19**, 210.

Umezawa, H., Akasura, H., Oda, K., and Hori, S. (1973). *J. Antibiot.* **26**, 521.

Drug-Induced Macromolecular Damage of Nuclear DNA

KURT W. KOHN

The DNA of a typical mammalian chromosome, assuming that it exists as uninterrupted strands, has a single-strand molecular weight of about 5×10^{10}, corresponding to a contour length of about 5 cm. Although it is not certain that all this DNA is in uninterrupted strands, it is safe to say that the continuous strand lengths must be at least $\frac{1}{10}$ of this figure. These extremely long strands, in the form of a double helix, are wound about nucleosomal cores which are themselves arranged in an extended coil. Yet this complicated topology must allow the DNA strands to function in processes such as transcription and replication which require localized or extended unwinding of the strand pairs. In addition, the coiling of the DNA strands may constrain chromatin topology so as to provide a form of functional regulation.

Drug-induced DNA damage can interfere with DNA function in two general, although not mutually exclusive, ways. First, chemical alterations in DNA may affect the direct interactions of the damaged sites with enzymes or other molecules. Typical of this category is DNA base damage. In the second category are changes that affect the topological behavior of the DNA strands. This may be designated macromolecular damage and is exemplified by chain breaks, interstrand cross-links, and DNA–protein cross-links. The first damage category includes actions that lead to mutation and carcinogenesis, while the second category is more prominently associated with cytotoxicity and anticancer activity.

The study of macromolecular DNA damage in mammalian cells has recently been facilitated by the use of filter techniques sensitive to the size of long DNA strands and to the linkage of DNA strands to proteins or other types of molecules that adsorb to certain types of filters (see Kohn, 1978, for review).

This chapter is presented in two parts. The first is a brief review of the current picture of macromolecular DNA lesions produced by various agents; the second is a summary of recent studies on drug effects on mammalian cells using filter elution techniques.

I. Macromolecular DNA Damage in Mammalian Cells

The major classes of macromolecular DNA damage are illustrated in Fig. 1, and the types of effects produced by various drugs are outlined in Table I. The table also should be consulted for references.

A. Single-Strand Breaks

Single-strand breaks can result from chemical damage to DNA (1) as an immediate consequence of the damage, (2) as a delayed consequence of a slow, spontaneous decomposition process, or (3) as a result of enzyme action. Immediate single-strand break production is most prominent for

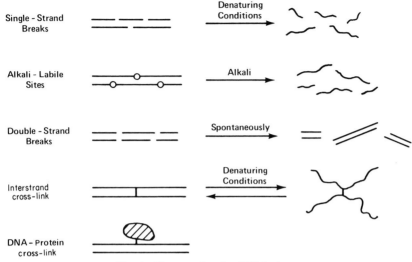

Fig. 1 Macromolecular DNA lesions.

ionizing radiation, which, however, also produces base damage that can lead to enzymic breaks (see Table I for references). Other agents, such as visible light (Bradley *et al.*, 1978) and H_2O_2 (M. O. Bradley and L. C. Erickson, unpublished data), also produce immediate single-strand breaks in mammalian cells. Single-strand breaks by these agents are rapidly repaired and are not a major source of cytotoxicity. The effect of single-strand breaks may, however, be enhanced by the repair-inhibiting action of carbamoylating agents (Kann *et al.*, 1974; Kann, 1978; Erickson *et al.*, 1978a). The chemical details, however, may differ for different types of single-strand breaks, and these lesions may behave differently, depending on how they are produced.

Delayed decomposition leading to strand breakage occurs most notably at base-free sites which result from the chemical or enzymic elimination of a base (Lindahl and Anderson, 1972; Crine and Verly, 1976). Alkylated purines are the major case in which spontaneous base elimination may be of significance (Lawley and Brookes, 1963; Verly, 1974). In addition, bleomycin, which extracts thymine and possibly other bases from DNA, may produce strand breaks by this mechanism (see Table I for references). Delayed decomposition of base-free sites, however, is accelerated in cells because of catalysis by specific enzymes (Verly, 1974; Ljungquist and Lindahl, 1974; Linsley *et al.*, 1977).

Cells contain a variety of enzyme systems that provide a remarkable ability to repair DNA damage. Single-strand breaks occur transiently dur-

TABLE I
DNA Lesions Produced in Mammalian Cells by Various Agents[a]

Agent	SSB		DSB	ISC	DPC	Base damage
	Direct	Enzymic				
X-rays	++		+	−	+	++
Uv light (254 nm)	−	+	−	−	+	++
Bleomycin	++		+	−	−	−
Nitrogen mustards and mitomycin	−[b]			++	++	++
Chloroethylnitrosoureas (BCNU, CCNU, chlorozotocin)	+			++	++	++
Cis-Pt(II)	−[b]			++	++	++
Trans-Pt(II)	−			±	++	++
Adriamycin and other intercalators	+[c]				+[c]	−
Psoralen plus light	−[b]		−	++	±	++

[a] SSB, Single-strand breaks (or alkali-labile sites); DSB, double-strand breaks; ISC, interstrand cross-links; DPC, DNA-protein cross-links.

[b] Not observed, but may be obscured by cross-links.

[c] Protein-associated strand breaks.

References:

X-ray: Ahnström and Edvardsson (1974); Bradley et al. (1976); Coquerelle et al. (1973); Corry and Cole (1973); Dugle et al. (1976); Elkind (1971); Elkind and Chang-Liu (1972); Fornace and Little (1977); Hawkins (1976, 1978); Kohn et al. (1974, 1976); Lafleur et al. (1976); Lange (1974); Lehmann and Stevens (1977); Mattern et al. (1975); Minsky and Braun (1977); Rydberg (1975); Rydberg and Johanson (1975).

Uv light: Cleaver (1974); Dingman and Kakunaga (1976); Fornace et al. (1976); Fornace and Kohn (1976); Han et al. (1975); Hariharan and Cerutti (1977); Smith and O'Leary (1967); Strriste and Rall (1976).

Bleomycin: Bearden et al. (1977); Fujiwara and Kondo (1973); Haidle (1971); Haidle et al. (1972); Iqbal et al. (1976); Kohn and Ewig (1976); Lloyd et al. (1978); Müller et al. (1972); Povirk et al. (1977); Umezawa et al. (1973).

Nitrogen mustards: Chun et al. (1969); Ewig and Kohn (1977, 1978); Golder et al. (1964); Grunicke et al. (1973); Harrap and Gascoigne (1976); Jolley and Ormerod (1974); Klatt et al. (1969); Kohn et al. (1965, 1966); Lawley and Brookes (1967); Ross et al. (1978c); Thomas et al. (1978a); Yin et al. (1973).

Mitomycin: Fornace and Little (1977); Fujiwara and Tatsumi (1977); Lyer and Szybalski (1963).

Chloroethylnitrosoureas: Erickson et al. (1977, 1978c); Ewig and Kohn (1977, 1978); Gutin et al. (1977); Hilton et al. (1977); Kohn (1977); Lown et al. (1978); Thomas et al. (1978b).

Platinum complexes: Filipski et al. (1979); Harder (1975); Munchausen (1974); Pascoe and Roberts (1974); Roberts and Pascoe (1972); Zwelling et al. (1978, 1979).

Intercalators: Bases et al. (1977); Ross et al. (1978a,b).

Psoralen: Ben-Hur and Elkind (1973); Cohen et al. (1979); Ley et al. (1977); Lown and Sim (1978).

ing nucleotide excision repair by the action of specific endonucleases that incise the DNA near the site of a defect (Painter, 1974; Grossman *et al.*, 1975), as well as by enzymes that cleave DNA at base-free sites.

Another class of enzymes that can produce transient single-strand breaks are topoisomerases, so called because they can change the topological winding number of the DNA helix (Pulleyblank *et al.*, 1975). These enzymes produce a single-strand break, permit the helix to wind or unwind, and then close the break.

Although single-strand breaks have not been implicated in cell killing, they may be responsible for a transient inhibition of DNA replication initiation observed following exposure of cells to ionizing radiation and methylating agents (Painter and Young, 1976; Painter, 1977; Povirk, 1977). Single-strand breakage may act by releasing the topological strain in the DNA helix, which may be required for the initiation of new DNA chains. The recovery of DNA synthesis takes significantly longer than the repair of breaks, and this extra time may be required to reestablish the winding strain before the synthesis of new chains can begin.

B. Alkali-Labile Sites

Most of the methods used to detect single-strand breaks in cells require alkaline conditions which can convert certain types of chemical damage to strand breaks. The effect observed therefore is due to a combination of preexisting breaks and breaks generated from alkali-labile sites during assay. Two types of alkali-labile sites have been identified: base-free sites and alkylated DNA phosphate groups (Verly, 1974; Schooter, 1976). In many cases, it is not clear to what degree the single-strand breaks observed following drug treatment reflect preexisting breaks as opposed to alkali-labile sites.

C. Double-Strand Breaks

Probably of greater significance (to cell killing) than single-strand breaks are double-strand breaks. From studies with purified DNA, double-strand breaks are known to be produced by ionizing radiation and by bleomycin (see Table I for references). Although their frequency is less than that of single-strand breaks, their potency in inactivating the biological activity of DNA is much greater. The available methods for measurement of double-strand breaks in cells, however, still present unresolved difficulties. There is, for example, still conflicting evidence on whether or not double-strand breaks are repaired in mammalian cells.

D. Interstrand Cross-links

The significance of cross-links in cytotoxic and antitumor actions has been suspected for more than two decades, since it is apparent that, for alkylating agents, high activity is associated with bifunctionality (Goldacre *et al.*, 1949; Stacey *et al.*, 1958). Interstrand DNA cross-links would prevent the DNA strand separation that must occur during normal DNA replication and transcription. Such cross-links are produced by a variety of bifunctional agents, including nitrogen mustards, mitomycins, and *cis*-Pt(II) complexes (see Table I for references). They also are produced by chloroethylnitrosoureas which, although chemically monofunctional, lead to the formation of an alkylating group at one macromolecular site which can then form a cross-link by reacting with a second site (Kohn, 1977). Another type of cross-linking agent is psoralen, an unsaturated polycycle that intercalates in the DNA helix and can absorb visible light to form photochemical adducts with DNA bases. By the successive absorption of two light quanta, the same psoralen molecule can react twice, once with a base on each DNA strand, thereby forming an interstrand cross-link (see Table I for references).

E. DNA–Protein Cross-Links

With the possible exception of psoralen, all the agents observed to produce interstrand cross-links in cells also produce DNA–protein cross-links. DNA–protein cross-links are repaired in mammalian cells and are not necessarily cytotoxic (Ewig and Kohn, 1977). This is especially clear in the case of *trans*-Pt(II)(NH$_3$)$_2$Cl$_2$, which can generate large numbers of DNA–protein cross-links with little cytotoxic effect (Zwelling *et al.*, 1978, 1979). The identity of the bound proteins, as well as their sites of binding on the DNA, however, may differ for different agents, so that the DNA–protein cross-links, produced for example by ultraviolet (uv) light, may be of greater significance to the cell.

II. Filter Elution Studies of DNA Damage Produced by Various Agents in Mammalian Cells

A. Methods

Alkaline filter methods are based on two phenomena: (1) the strand length dependence of the rate at which long DNA single strands pass through filters, and (2) the adsorption to the filters of proteins to which the DNA may have become linked (for review, see Kohn, 1978).

In the basic procedure (Kohn *et al.*, 1976; Fornace *et al.*, 1976), cells are lysed on a membrane filter by a detergent such as sodium dodecyl sarkosinate at pH 10. Most of the cell protein and RNA are washed through the filter, while the nuclear DNA remains quantitatively on the filter. When it is desired to eliminate the adsorptive effects due to possible DNA –protein cross-linking, the enzyme proteinase-K is included in the lysis solution and a 1-hour incubation at room temperature is allowed (Ewig and Kohn, 1978). The filter is then eluted by slowly pumping through it a solution of tetrapropylammonium hydroxide–EDTA at pH 12, and the kinetics of elution of the DNA from the filter is determined.

The experimental cells are usually labeled for one or more cell doublings with [^{14}C]thymidine. In order to improve quantitation, an internal standard is often used, consisting of ^{3}H-labeled control cells given 150 R of X rays in the cold in order to introduce a convenient frequency of single-strand breaks. The internal standard essentially provides a corrected time scale.

For the measurement of cross-links, it is necessary to introduce single-strand breaks that normally cause the DNA to elute relatively quickly. This is done by irradiating the cells with 300 R in the cold just before the elution assay. Cross-links then have the effect of reducing DNA elution.

B. Ionizing Radiation: Dependence of DNA Elution Kinetics on Strand Size

The effect of X rays on DNA elution is illustrated in Fig. 2. The cells were irradiated on ice so as to prevent repair. At least for the first 10 hours of elution, the loss of DNA from the filter is first-order with respect to time and independent of elution pH from 11.9 to 12.8. These kinetics are also almost independent of cell number, filter type, and extent of protein removal.

The initial rate constant of elution is proportional to the X-ray dose (Fig. 3). Thus a random distribution of strand lengths, produced by randomly placed single-strand breaks by X-rays, gives elution kinetics that are first-order both with respect to time and to break frequency. The inherent assumptions are that X rays produce random breaks at a frequency proportional to the X-ray dose, and that individual strands elute independently of each other, depending only on their length. The independent behavior of strands is supported by the observed independence of elution kinetics of differently labeled DNA from mixtures of cell populations subjected to different X-ray doses. From these considerations, one can deduce the functional dependence of elution kinetics on strand length. One can infer that the elution rate for strands of a given length is constant with

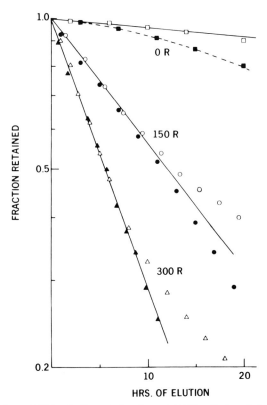

Fig. 2 Kinetics of DNA alkaline elution from L1210 cells irradiated with 0, 150, or 300 R of X rays in the cold. Elution was carried out either at pH 11.96 (open symbols) or at pH 12.82 (solid symbols). (From Kohn *et al.*, 1976.)

time and inversely proportional to strand length, and that elution continues until all the strands of that length have eluted from the filter. The derivation of this deduction is presented elsewhere. From this inference one can predict the elution kinetics for any distribution of strand lengths. Conversely, the strand length distribution can be deduced from the elution kinetics. A proviso here is that any adsorptive effects, such as could be produced by DNA–protein cross-linking, have been eliminated.

C. Bleomycin

Bleomycin produces single- and double-strand breaks, possibly related to the elimination of thymine and perhaps other bases (see Table I for references). In mammalian cells, increases in alkaline elution rates can read-

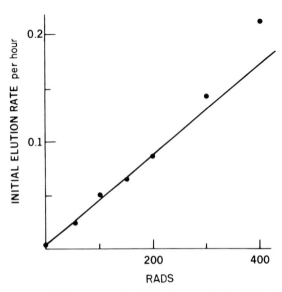

Fig. 3 Dependence of the apparent initial rate constant of DNA elution on X-ray dose. (From Kohn *et al.*, 1976.)

ily be demonstrated and are dependent both on drug concentration and on exposure time (Figs. 4 and 5). In these studies, care must be taken to remove excess bleomycin which otherwise may cause spurious DNA breaks during alkaline assays. On comparing the elution curves following bleomycin with the linear curves produced by X rays (Fig. 4), it is clear that the break distribution produced by bleomycin is nonrandom. It appears that part of the DNA or, alternatively, part of the cell population, is relatively insensitive to the drug.

The action of bleomycin on cells depends on the pH of the medium; the drug is more effective at pH 7.5 than at pH 6.7 (Fig. 5). This pH dependence is observed both in the effect on DNA elution and in the effect on cell survival, so that the two effects bear a consistent relation to each other (Fig. 6).

D. Nitrosoureas: Single-Strand Breaks and Alkali-Labile Sites

1-Methyl-(-nitrosourea (MNU) is a highly active alkylating agent that methylates a variety of sites on DNA bases as well as DNA phosphate (Singer, 1975). Both enzymic breaks and alkali-labile lesions may occur. The formation of alkali-labile sites is suggested by the kinetics of alkaline elution (Fig. 7). As opposed to the linear kinetics exhibited by X rays,

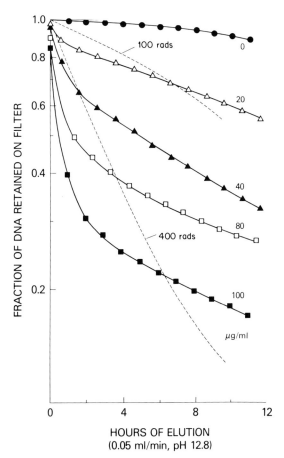

Fig. 4 Alkaline elution of DNA from L1210 cells exposed to the indicated concentrations of bleomycin for 1 hour. Dashed line shows elution from cells exposed to the indicated doses of X rays. (From Iqbal *et al.*, 1976.)

MNU produces elution curves that bend downward. The acceleration in the rate of elution may be due to the continuous conversion of alkali-labile sites to breaks.

1-(2-Chloroethyl)-1-nitrosoureas are much more cytotoxic than MNU, and doses that give comparable cytotoxicity produce much less enhancement elution. The elution patterns also differ from the case of MNU in that no significant downward bending of the curve is apparent (Fig. 8). This suggests that these breaks have an enzymic origin rather than an alkali-labile origin. The breaks disappear within a few hours, suggesting repair.

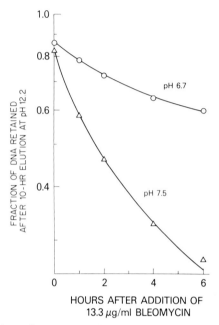

Fig. 5 Effect of time of exposure to bleomycin at pH 6.7 or 7.5 on DNA in L1210 cells. Cells were treated in growth medium buffered at the indicated pH. (From Kohn and Ewig, 1976.)

Although alkaline elution and alkaline sedimentation experiments usually give consistent results, the two methods gave discrepant results for the action of chloroethylnitrosoureas on two human cell lines (Fig. 8). To begin with, the extent of single-strand breakage estimated by sedimentation was much greater than that estimated by elution. Second, sedimentation indicated a greater effect on the normal as opposed to the transformed cell line, whereas the reverse was indicated by elution. Although these results are not definitely explained, they may stem from the higher pH in the sedimentation experiments than in the elution experiments. It may be that the sedimentation conditions reveal a class of alkali-labile sites that do not fully develop under the conditions of elution, which may detect mainly enzymic breaks.

E. Ultraviolet Light: Enzymic Single-Strand Breaks

Uv light produces little or no immediate single-strand breakage. Within a few minutes after exposure to uv light, however, normal human cells

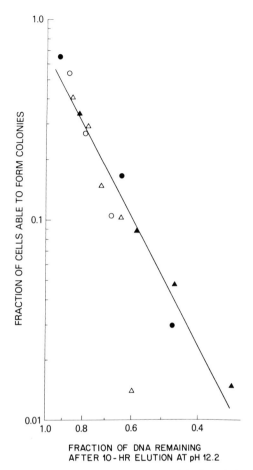

Fig. 6 Effect of bleomycin on colony-forming ability in relation to effect on DNA elution. L1210 cells were exposed to bleomycin in medium buffered at pH 6.7 (▲ and ●) or pH 7.5 (△ and ○). ○ and ●, cells exposed for 1 hour to bleomycin at 0, 10, or 50 μg/ml; △ and ▲, cells exposed to 13.3 μg/ml for 0, 1, 2, 4, or 6 hours. (From Kohn and Ewig, 1976.)

show an increase in alkaline elution indicative of breaks (Fig. 9B). These breaks then disappear with time (Fig. 9C), the rate of disappearance depending on the uv dose. The transient breaks probably represent intermediate states in the process of nucleotide excision repair. Accordingly, xeroderma pigmentosum cells defective in this type of repair do not show the appearance of these breaks (Fig. 9D).

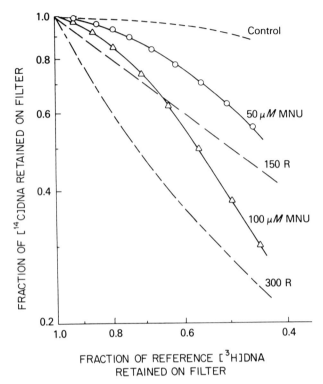

Fig. 7 Accelerated alkaline elution curves from L1210 cells treated with MNU for 1 hour. Dashed lines show comparison with elution curves due to X rays. (From Ewig and Kohn, 1977.)

F. Bifunctional Alkylating Agents, Chloroethyl-1-nitrosoureas, and Pt(II) Complexes: Interstrand Cross-Links and DNA–Protein Cross-Links

The two types of cross-links both reduce the rate of DNA alkaline elution. Interstrand cross-links do so by increasing the effective strand length, and DNA–protein cross-links by linking DNA strands to protein molecules that adsorb to the polyvinylchloride filters. In order to bring out these effects, a suitable frequency of single-strand breaks is introduced by exposing the cells to 300 R of X rays before the alkaline elution assay. The DNA–protein cross-links are selectively removed by incubating the cell lysate with proteinase K before alkaline elution, thereby providing an estimate of the relative magnitudes of the two types of cross-links (Kohn 1978).

Typical results using these assays are shown in Fig. 10 for the case of

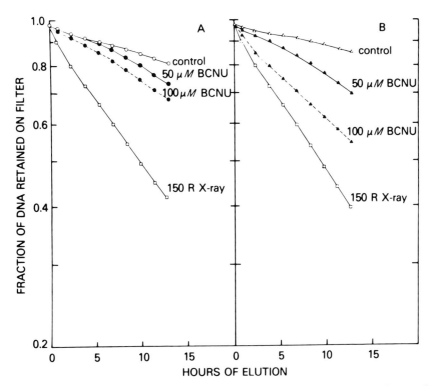

Fig. 8   DNA single-strand breaks produced by BCNU in normal human embryo cell strain WI-38 (A) and in a SV40-transformed derivative, VA-13 (B). Cells were treated with the indicated concentration of BCNU for 1 hour. For reference, elution curves for cells exposed to 150 R are also shown; this X-ray dose generated 4.4 (WI-38) or 4.7 (VA-13) single-strand breaks per 10^{10} daltons of DNA. (From Erickson *et al.*, 1977.)

L1210 cells treated for 1 hour with 1,3-bis(2-chloroethyl)-1-nitrosourea (BCNU). The controls (Fig. 10A) show that proteinase K had little effect on the elution curves, either in the assay without X rays or in the assay using 300 R of X rays. Immediately after treatment (Fig. 10B), two changes can be seen. First, there is an increase in the elution rates in the assays without X rays, signifying the appearance of strand breaks. Second, the assay using 300 R of X rays shows a decrease in elution rate relative to that of the corresponding controls, but this effect is almost completely eliminated by proteinase K. This may be interpreted as indicating DNA–protein cross-links without interstrand cross-links. When the cells were then postincubated for 4.5 hours after removal of the drug (Fig. 10C), the extent of cross-linking was increased and was only partially sensitive to proteinase K. The main conclusion is that interstrand cross-links

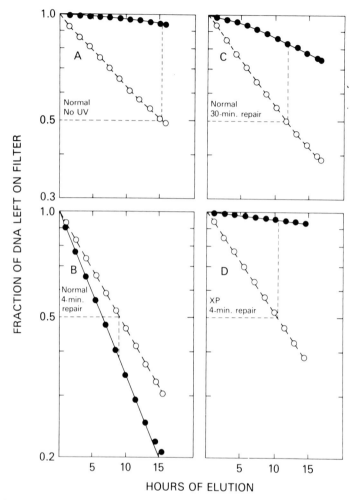

Fig. 9 DNA single-strand breaks in human fibroblasts exposed to UV light (1.5 J/m², 254 nm). Normal cells: (A) control; (B) 4 minutes after uv; (C) 30 minutes after uv. (C) Xeroderma pigmentosum cells (complementation group A) 4 minutes after uv. ●, ¹⁴C-labeled experimental cells; ○, ³H-labeled reference cells (L1210 cells treated with 150 R of X rays). (From Fornace et al., 1976.)

are formed in a slow reaction that can take place after the removal of BCNU, whereas DNA–protein cross-links are formed more rapidly.

The production by chloroethylnitrosoureas of interstrand cross-links and the delay in their formation agree with observations on the effect of these drugs on purified DNA (Kohn, 1977). A possible mechanism, shown in Fig. 11, is that a DNA site (X) becomes chloroethylated and then

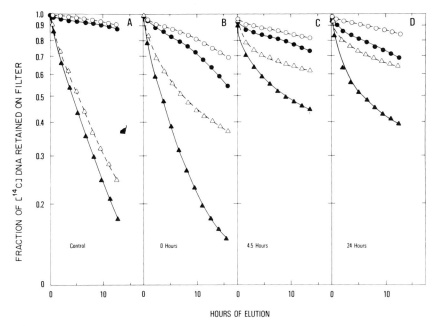

Fig. 10 Effects of BCNU on DNA alkaline elution from L1210 cells. Cells were exposed to 50 μM BCNU for 1 hour and then incubated in the absence of the drug for 0, 4.5, or 24 hours. Cell aliquots were assayed in four ways: ○, without proteinase, no X rays; ●, with proteinase, no X rays; △, without proteinase, 300 R of X rays; ▲, with proteinase, 300 R of X rays. (From Ewig and Kohn, 1977.)

slowly reacts with a second site (Y) on the opposite strand to form an ethylene bridge between the two strands. The identities of X and Y, presently unknown, will hopefully soon be determined by isolation and identification of cross-linked base products.

The rapid formation of DNA–protein cross-links, as compared with interstrand cross-links, also can be rationalized. The chloroethylation of proteins is likely to occur at –SH or –NH$_2$ groups, thereby forming sulfur or nitrogen mustard groups with potent alkylating ability. These protein-bound alkylating groups could react rapidly with strongly nucleophilic DNA sites to form DNA–protein cross-links.

Analogous results have been obtained with cis-Pt(II)(NH$_3$)$_2$Cl$_2$, except that this agent produces little or no strand breakage (Zwelling $et\ al.$, 1978, 1979). Like the chloroethylnitrosoureas, cis-Pt(II) generates both interstrand and DNA–protein cross-links, and the former type appears more slowly than the latter. Both types of cis-Pt(II)-induced cross-links are lost (presumably repaired) over a period of about 20 hours. This repair appears to be more rapid than is the case with chloroethylnitrosoureas.

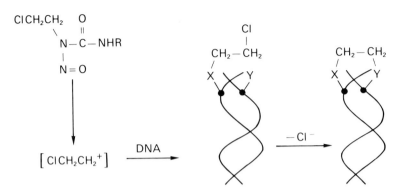

Fig. 11 Proposed mechanism of DNA interstrand cross-linking by chloroethylnitro-soureas. (From Kohn, 1977.)

The delayed formation of cross-links has also been observed with the following bifunctional alkylating agents: melphalan, a 2,5-bisaziridinyl-quinone, a 4-sulfoalkylcyclophosphamide, and phosphoramide mustard (Ross *et al.*, 1978a; Ewig, Erickson, and Ross, unpublished data).

In the case of nitrogen mustard (HN2), however, there is much less delay in the formation of either type of cross-link, and both types of cross-links are repaired (Ewig and Kohn, 1977). The marked difference between HN2 and melphalan in regard to the kinetics of cross-link formation and removal is shown in Fig. 12. Although separate measurements of the two types of cross-links formed by these drugs have not yet been completed, it appears that, for melphalan, interstrand cross-links are repaired more rapidly than DNA–protein cross-links (Ross, unpublished data).

G. Relation between Cross-Linking and Cytotoxicity

In the investigation of possible relationships between DNA damage and cell killing, it is desirable for the DNA damage measurements to be sensitive enough to determine damage at drug dosages that produce pharmacologically reasonable extents of cell kill. This requirement has been found to hold for most of the drugs that have been mentioned for which some form of DNA effect has been shown at dosages that permit 10% or more of the cells to retain the ability to form colonies. The identification of the DNA lesions that have the greatest cytotoxic significance is complicated, however, by the multiple types of DNA damage produced (Table I) and by the need to consider the rates of formation and repair of the lesions. Nevertheless, initial attempts to establish such relationships have been encouraging.

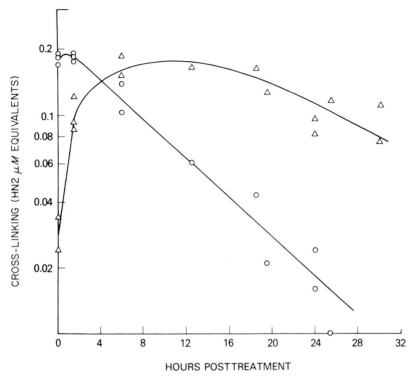

Fig. 12   Total DNA cross-linking as a function of time following a 0.5-hour treatment of L1210 cells with 0.2 μM HN2 (O) or 15 μM melphalan (△). (From Ross *et al.*, 1978a.)

The first case studied in some detail was a comparison between two human colon carcinoma lines that could be propagated in cell cultures and as xenograft tumors in athymic mice. The two tumors had been found to differ in sensitivity to 1-(2-chloroethyl)-3-(4-*trans*-methylcyclohexyl)-1-nitrosourea (MeCCNU) (Thomas *et al.*, 1978b), and the difference was retained in cell culture (Erickson *et al.*, 1978c).

Cross-linking effects were readily detected following MeCCNU treatment, both in the cultured cells and in the xenograft tumors. Typical elution data are shown in Fig. 13 for cultured cells treated for 1 hour with MeCCNU, followed by a 20-hour postincubation. In these studies, only *total* cross-linking was assayed. It can be seen that the more drug-sensitive cell line (BE) showed more cross-linking than the resistant cell line (HT). The time course of the appearance and disappearance of cross-links after a 1-hour treatment of the two cell lines with MeCCNU is shown in Fig. 14. The results are expressed in terms of relative elution rates, so that cross-linking increases with decreasing value of the vertical scale. During

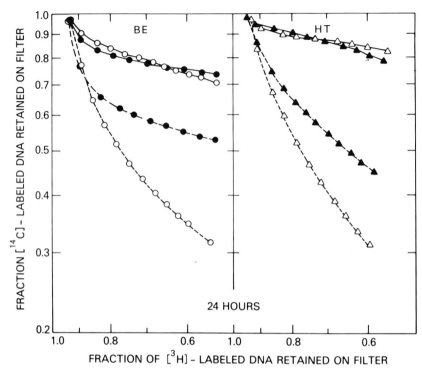

Fig. 13 Differential effect of MeCCNU on DNA in a sensitive (BE) and a resistant (HT) line of human colon carcinoma cells in culture. The cells were exposed to 100 μM MeCCNU for 1 hour and then washed and incubated for 24 hours in the absence of drug. Open symbols, no drug; solid symbols, MeCCNU. Upper two curves (solid line), no X rays; lower two curves (broken line), 300 R of X rays. (From Erickson *et al.*, 1978c.)

the first 5 hours following treatment, cross-linking increased comparably for the two cell lines. At 24 hours, however, the difference already noted (Fig. 13) was reproducible and increased further by 48 hours. The major differential in this experiment appeared to be in the repair of cross-links in the resistant HT cells, as opposed to the lack of repair in the sensitive BE cells.

The two cell types also differed in the xenograft tumor system (Fig. 15). In this case, however, the sensitive BE tumor exhibited more cross-linking at the outset than the resistant HT tumor. [Data are also shown for a tumor (CA) of intermediate drug sensitivity.]

Differences between the sensitive and resistant cell types were thus seen both *in vitro* and *in vivo*, but the apparent mechanism of resistance may differ in the two systems. Resistance in the *in vitro* system was associated with the ability of the cells to remove drug-induced DNA cross-

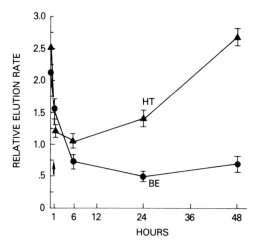

Fig. 14 DNA cross-linking in sensitive (BE) and resistant (HT) human colon carcinoma cells in culture as a function of time following a 1-hour exposure to 100 μM MeCCNU. Total cross-linking was measured by alkaline elution without proteinase in cells given 300 R of X rays. Cross-linking is indicated by reduction in elution rate. (From Erickson *et al.*, 1978c.)

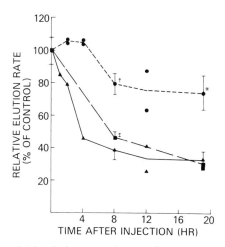

Fig. 15 DNA cross-linking in human colon carcinoma xenografts in athymic mice treated with a single intraperitoneal injection of 18 mg/kg MeCCNU. ▲, MeCCNU-sensitive tumor, BE; ●, resistant tumor, HT; ■, tumor of intermediate sensitivity, CA. Tumors BE and CA were obtained from Dr. B. Giovanella; tumor HT was derived from cell culture line HT-20, obtained from Dr. E. Jensen. (From Thomas *et al.*, 1978b.)

links, whereas *in vivo* resistance was associated with a lower extent of cross-link formation. The significance and generality of these initial findings require further testing.

Differences in DNA cross-linking associated with differences in drug sensitivity have also been observed in a pair of human embryo cell lines. The normal cell strain, IMR-90, was found to be less sensitive to chloroethylnitrosoureas than a SV40-transformed line (VA-13) (Erickson *et al.*, 1978a; M. O. Bradley, unpublished data). Associated differences in DNA cross-linking were more apparent in proteinase-K assays, suggesting that interstrand cross-linking was a more important determinant of cell killing than DNA–protein cross-linking (L. C. Erickson, R. Ewig, and J. Ducore, unpublished data).

Another approach has been to compare the effects of related compounds on given cell lines. A comparison between *cis*- and *trans*-Pt(II)(NH$_3$)$_2$Cl$_2$ was of interest because, although both isomers produce interstrand cross-links in purified DNA (Harder, 1975), the *cis* isomer is an effective antitumor agent while the treans isomer is inactive.

When examined by the alkaline elution method, both isomers produced cross-linking effects in L1210 cells, but there was a marked difference in the sensitivity of the cross-links to proteinase–K (Zwelling *et al.*, 1978, 1979). Whereas only part of the cross-linking effect produced by the *cis* isomer was proteinase-sensitive, almost all the cross-linking produced by the *trans* isomer was reversed by the enzyme. It appears therefore that both isomers produce DNA–protein cross-links in mammalian cells, but that interstrand cross-linking is much more prominent in the case of the *cis* isomer. As in the case of chloroethylnitrosoureas, DNA–protein cross-linking was faster than interstrand cross-linking. Cell survival was similar for the two compounds at dosages yielding similar extents of interstrand cross-links. At dosages giving similar extents of total cross-linking, on the other hand, the *cis* was much more cytotoxic than the *trans* compound. The interstrand cross-linking therefore may be related to cell killing, but the DNA–protein cross-links produced by *trans*-Pt(II) either are nonlethal or are repaired before a potentially lethal effect is expressed.

H. Quantitation of DNA–Protein Cross-Links

DNA–protein cross-links reduce DNA elution because of the adsorption of the linked protein to the filter (Kohn and Ewig, 1979). This is supported by findings that protein adsorption and DNA retention are both reduced by including a detergent in the eluting solution, by digesting the protein with proteinase K, or by using polycarbonate (Nucleopore) filters. The picture can be represented as shown in Fig. 16. A convenient relation

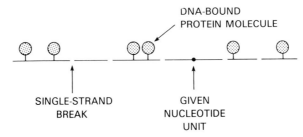

Fig. 16 Model representing randomly distributed single-strand breaks and protein links. Equation (1) (see text) is derived by expressing the probability that a randomly selected nucleotide unit will find itself in a strand segment bearing no cross-links. (From Kohn and Ewig, 1979.)

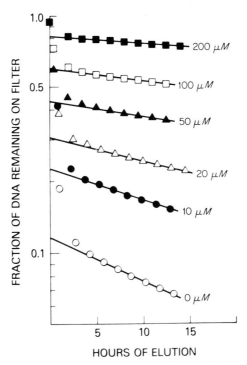

Fig. 17 Alkaline elution of DNA from L1210 cells treated with various concentrations of *trans*-Pt(II)(NH$_3$)$_2$Cl$_2$ for 1 hour and then exposed to 3000 R of X rays. (From Kohn and Ewig, 1979.)

can be derived if we assume (1) that DNA–protein cross-links are randomly distributed with a frequency proportional to the drug concentration, (2) that single-strand breaks are randomly distributed with a frequency proportional to the X-ray dose, and (3) that a DNA single-strand segment will be retained by the filter if and only if it is linked to one or more protein molecules. In order to obtain a clean separation between free and protein-linked DNA strands, the drug-treated cells are exposed to a relatively high dose of X rays (typically 3000 R), which normally causes most of the cell DNA to elute very rapidly. The fraction of the DNA linked to protein is then represented by a component that remains bound to the filter. Under these conditions, the fraction of the DNA retained on the filter (r) is related to the drug concentration (D) and X-ray dose (R) in the following way (Kohn and Ewig, 1979):

$$1(1 - r)^{1/2} = 1 + (k_{cR}/k_{bR}) + (k_{cD}/k_{bR})(D/R) \qquad (1)$$

where k_{cD} is the efficiency of cross-link production by the drug, k_{bR} is the efficiency of single-strand break production by the X rays (determined by independent measurement), and k_{cR}/k_{bR} is the ratio of cross-links to breaks due to X rays.

This model was initially tested using *trans*-Pt(II)(NH$_3$)$_2$Cl$_2$ which had

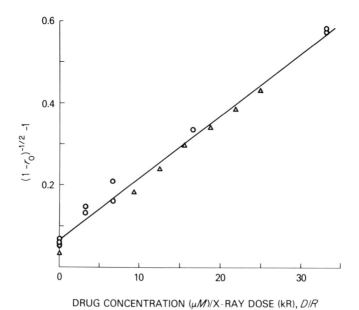

DRUG CONCENTRATION (μM)/X-RAY DOSE (kR), D/R

Fig. 18 Cross-linking data similar to those shown in Fig. 17, plotted according to theory [Eq. (1); see text].

been found to produce DNA–protein cross-links with little or no inter-strand cross-linking or single-strand breakage. Figure 17 shows that, when cells are irradiated with 3000 R, the DNA is clearly separable into rapidly and slowly eluting components, and the magnitude of the slowly eluting component increases with the *trans*-Pt(II) concentration. When the data are plotted according to Eq. (1), the expected straight line is obtained (Fig. 18). A similar linear relationship has been obtained for HN2. The slope of this line estimates the frequency of drug-induced DNA–protein cross-links.

I. Protein Associated Single-Strand Breaks

An unexpected type of DNA alteration was observed in cells treated with adriamycin or other intercalating agents. Although alkaline sedimen-

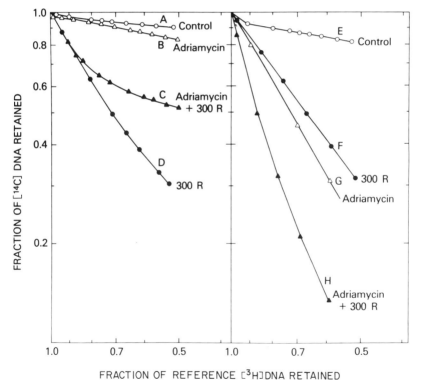

Fig. 19 Effects of adriamycin (2.8 μM for 1 hour) on DNA in L1210 cells. Alkaline elution assays were performed with (right) or without (left) proteinase K, and with or without 300 R of X rays as indicated. (From Ross *et al.*, 1978c.)

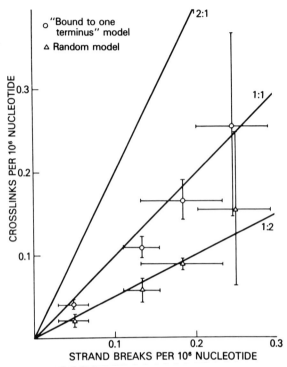

Fig. 20 Relation between DNA–protein cross-link frequency and DNA single-strand break frequency in L1210 cells treated for 1 hour with various concentrations of adriamycin. (From Ross *et al.*, 1978c.)

tation studies had indicated that adriamycin produced single-strand breaks (Schwartz, 1976), alkaline elution at first failed to disclose any breaks (Fig. 19, curve B). When proteinase K was used, however, breaks became apparent (curve G). In addition, DNA–protein cross-links were detected (curve C); the cross-links were reversed by proteinase (curve H). The results suggest that adriamycin produces DNA single-strand breaks, but that the breaks are associated with DNA–protein cross-links (Ross *et al.*, 1978c). A specific relation between the locations of the breaks and cross-links was suggested by the observation that, although the drug-induced breaks were completely hidden by the cross-links (curve B), an equal frequency of X-ray-induced breaks was only partially hidden (curve C). If X rays produce random breaks, adriamycin must produce breaks whose location is in some way correlated with the location of the protein links produced by the same treatment.

An attractive explanation of the preceding results is that protein links occur at the sites of the single-strand breaks, perhaps at one of the strand termini. In that case adriamycin should produce an equal frequency of DNA–protein cross-links and single-strand breaks. The frequency of DNA–protein cross-links was therefore estimated using the method summarized in the previous section. The calculation of cross-link frequencies by Eq. (1), however, is based on the assumption of independent locations of breaks and cross-links. The corresponding equation for the "bound-to-one-terminus" model is

$$1/(1 - r) = [1/(1 - r_0)] + (k_{cD}/k_{bR})(D/R) \qquad (2)$$

where k_{cD} in this case is the frequency of drug-induced protein-associated breaks and r_0 is the fraction of DNA retained in the case of non-drug-treated irradiated cells.

The results summarized in Fig. 20 were calculated both according to the random model [Eq. (1)] and according to the bound-to-one-terminus model [Eq. (2)]. Regardless of which calculation was used, the DNA–pro-

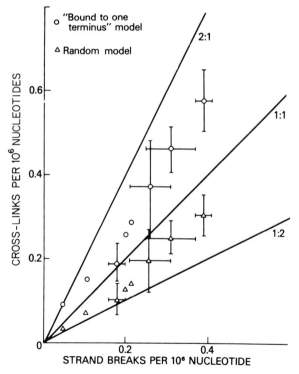

Fig. 21 Same as in Fig. 20 except various concentrations of ellipticine (1–20 μM for 1 hour) were used. (From Ross et al., 1978c.)

tein cross-link frequency was found to be within a factor of 2 of the single-strand break frequency.

A similar equivalence was obtained with ellipticine (Fig. 21), a polycyclic intercalator that binds tightly to DNA (Kohn *et al.*, 1975) but has no quinone function. Ellipticine, however, was much less cytotoxic than adriamycin when L1210 cells were treated with dosages of the two drugs that gave equal frequencies of protein-associated DNA breaks (Ross *et al.*, 1978c). The higher cytotoxicity of adriamycin therefore must be due to some other factor.

Protein-associated DNA breaks were detected in cells treated with a variety of other intercalating agents, including actinomycin, ethidium, and lucanthone (Miracil D). They were not detected in cells treated with the nonintercalative DNA binders anthramycin and chromomycin, or with the antimetabolite cytosine arabinoside.

An attractive hypothesis is that intercalation, by changing the topological winding of DNA in chromatin, stimulates endonuclease action in which the enzyme is covalently linked (perhaps in a reversible reaction) to one terminus of the single-strand break.

III. Conclusions

Anticancer agents produce several types of macromolecular DNA damage, often repairable, in mammalian cells. DNA single-strand breaks, interstrand cross-links, and DNA–protein cross-links are measurable after treatment of cells with pharmacologically relevant dosages using the technique of alkaline elution. Drugs presently amenable to this approach include bifunctional alkylating agents, nitrosoureas, platinum complexes, and bleomycin. The intercalating agents produce a specific effect on DNA —the formation of protein-associated strand breaks—the significance of which, with respect to cell survival, remains to be determined. The relationship between DNA lesions and cell lethality is a complex problem because of the multiplicity of DNA lesions produced and the dependence on the rates of lesion formation and repair. Initial results, however, suggest that these problems can be resolved.

References

Ahnström, G., and Edvardsson, K.-A. (1974). Radiation-induced single-strand breaks in DNA determined by rate of alkaline strand separation and hydroxyapatite chromatography: An alternative to velocity sedimentation. *Int. J. Radiat. Biol.* **26**, 493–497.

Bases, R., Leifer, A., Rozycki, H., Blake, C., Jr., and Neubort, S. (1977). Effects of lucanthone on the sedimentation properties of DNA from HeLa cells. *Cancer Res.* **37**, 2177–2181.

Bearden, J. C., Lloyd, R. S., and Haidle, C. W. (1977). Bleomycin-induced breakage of closed-circular DNA. *Biochem. Biophys. Res. Commun.* **75**, 442–448.

Ben-Hur, E., and Elkind, M. M. (1973). DNA crosslinking in Chinese hamster cells exposed to near ultraviolet light in the presence of 4,5′,8-trimethylpsoralen. *Biochim. Biophys. Acta* **331**, 181–193.

Bradley, M. O., Erickson, L. C., and Kohn, K. W. (1976). Normal DNA strand rejoining and absence of DNA crosslinking in progeroid and aging human cells. *Mutat. Res.* **37**, 279–292.

Bradley, M. O., Erickson, L. C., and Kohn, K. W. (1978). Non-enzymatic DNA strand breaks induced in mammalian cells by fluorescent light. *Biochim. Biophys Acta* **520**, 11–20.

Chun, E. H. L., Gonzales, L., Lewis, F. S., Jones, J., and Rutman, R. J. (1969). Differences in the *in vivo* alkylation and cross-linking of nitrogen mustard-sensitive and -resistant lines of Lettré–Ehrlich ascites tumors. *Cancer Res.* **29**, 1184–1194.

Cleaver, J. E. (1974). Repair processes for photochemical damage in mammalian cells. *Adv. Radiat. Biol.* **4**, 1–75.

Cohen, L., Ewig, R. A. G., Glaubiger, D., and Kohn, K. W. (1979). In preparation.

Coquerelle, T., Bopp, A., Kessler, B., and Hagen, U. (1973). Strand breaks and 5′ end-groups in DNA of irradiated thymocytes. *Int. J. Radiat. Biol.* **24**, 397–404.

Corry, P. M., and Cole, A. (1973). Double-strand rejoining in mammalian cells. *Nature (London), New Biol.* **245**, 100–101.

Crine, P., and Verly, W. G. (1976). A study of spontaneous DNA degradation. *Biochim. Biophys. Acta* **442**, 50–57.

Dingman, C. W., and Kakunaga, T. (1976). DNA strand breaking and rejoining in response to ultraviolet light in normal human and xeroderma pigmentosum cells. *Int. J. Radiat. Biol.* **30**, 55–66.

Dugle, D. L., Gillespie, C. J., and Chapman, J. D. (1976). DNA strand breaks, repair, and survival in X-irradiated mammalian cells. *Proc. Natl. Acad. Sci. U.S.A.* **73**, 809–812.

Elkind, M. M. (1971). Sedimentation of DNA released from Chinese hamster cells. *Biophys. J.* **11**, 502–520.

Elkind, M. M., and Chang-Liu, C.-M. (1972). Repair of a DNA complex from X-irradiated Chinese hamster cells. *Int. J. Radiat. Biol.* **22**, 75–90.

Erickson, L. C., Bradley, M. O., and Kohn, K. W. (1977). Strand breaks in DNA from normal and transformed human cells treated with BCNU. *Cancer Res.* **37**, 3744–3750.

Erickson, L. C., Bradley, M. O., and Kohn, K. W. (1978a). Differential inhibition of rejoining of X-ray-induced DNA strand breaks in normal and transformed human fibroblasts. *Cancer Res.* **38**, 672–677.

Erickson, L. C., Bradley, M. O., and Kohn, K. W. (1978b). Measurements of DNA damage in Chinese hamster cells treated with equi-toxic and equi-mutagenic doses of nitrosoureas. *Cancer Res.* **38**, 3197–3203.

Eickson, L. C., Osieka, R., and Kohn, K. W. (1978c). Differential repair of Me-CCNU-induced DNA damage in 2 human colon tumor cell lines. *Cancer Res.* **38**, 802–808.

Ewig, R. A. G., and Kohn, K. W. (1977). DNA damage and repair in mouse leukemia L1210 cells treated with nitrogen mustard, 1,3-Bis(2-chloroethyl)-1-nitrosourea, and other nitrosoureas. *Cancer Res.* **37**, 2114–2122.

Ewig, R. A. G., and Kohn, K. W. (1978). DNA–protein crosslinking and DNA interstrand crosslinking by haloethylnitrosoureas in L1210 cells. *Cancer Res.* **38**, 3197–3203.

Filipski, J., Kohn, K. W., Prather, R., and Bonner, W. M. (1979). Thiourea reverses cross-links in and restores biological activity Pt(II)-treated DNA. *Science* (in press).

Fornace, A. J., Jr., and Kohn, K. W. (1976). DNA-protein crosslinking by ultraviolet radiation in normal human and xeroderma pigmentosum fibroblasts. *Biochim. Biophys. Acta* **435**, 95–103.

Fornace, A. J., Jr., and Little, J. B. (1977). DNA crosslinking induced by X-rays and chemical agents. *Biochim. Biophys. Acta* **477**, 343–355.

Fornace, A. J., Jr., Kohn, K. W., and Kann, H. E., Jr. (1976). DNA single-strand breaks during repair of UV damage in human fibroblasts and abnormalities of repair in xeroderma pigmentosum. *Proc. Natl. Acad. Sci. U.S.A.* **73**, 39–43.

Fujiwara, Y., and Kondo, T. (1973). Strand-scission of HeLa cell DNA by bleomycin *in vitro* and *in vivo*. *Biochem. Pharmacol.* **22**, 323–333.

Fujiwara, Y., and Tatsumi, M. (1977). Cross-link repair in human cells and its possible defect in Fanconi's anlumia cells. *J. Mol. Biol.* **113**, 635–649.

Goldacre, R. J., Loveless, A., and Ross, W. C. J. (1949). Mode of production of chromosome abnormalities by the nitrogen mustards. The possible role of cross-linking. *Nature (London)* **163**, 667–669.

Golder, R. H., Martin-Guzman, G., Jones, J., Goldstein, N. O., Rotenberg, S., and Rutman, R. J. (1964). Experimental chemotherapy studies. III. Properties of DNA from ascites cells treated *in vivo* with nitrogen mustard. *Cancer Res.* **24**, 964–968.

Grossman, L., Braun, A., Feldberg, R., and Mahler, I. (1975). Enzymatic repair of DNA. *Annu. Rev. Biochem.* **44**, 19–43.

Grunicke, H., Bock, K. W., Becher, H., Gang, V., Schnierda, J., and Puschendorf, B. (1973). Effect of alkylating antitumor agents on the binding of DNA to protein. *Cancer Res.* **33**, 1048–1053.

Gutin, P. H., Hilton, J., Fein, V. J., Allan, A. E., Rottman, A., and Walker, M. D. (1977). *Cancer Res.* **37**, 3761–3765.

Haidle, C. W. (1971). Fragmentation of DNA by bleomycin. *Mol. Pharmacol.* **7**, 645–652.

Haidle, C. W., Weiss, K. K., and Kuo, M. T. (1972). Release of free bases from DNA after reaction with bleomycin. *Mol. Pharmacol.* **8**, 531–537.

Han, A., Korbelik, M., and Ban, J. (1975). DNA to-protein cross-linking in synchronized HeLa cells exposed to UV light. *Int. J. Radiat. Biol.* **27**, 63–74.

Harder, H. (1975). Renaturation effects of *cis* and *trans* Platinum II and IV compounds on calf thumus DNA. *Chem.-Biol. Interact.* **10**, 27–39.

Hariharan, P. V., and Cerutti, P. A. (1977). Formation of products of the 5,6-dihydroxydihydrothymine type by UV light in Hela cells. *Biochemistry* **16**, 2791–2795.

Harrap, K. R., and Gascoigne, E. W. (1976). The interaction of bifunctional alkylating agents with DNA of tumor cells. *Eur. J. Cancer* **12**, 53–59.

Hawkins, R. B. (1976). Measurements of ionizing radiation-induced crosslinkage of DNA and protein in bacteriophage. *Radiat. Res.* **68**, 300–307.

Hawkins, R. B. (1978). **33**, 425–441. Quantitative determination of crosslinkage of bacteriophage DNA and protein by ionizing radiation. *Int. J. Radiat. Biol.*

Hilton, J., Bowie, D. L., Gutin, P. H., Zito, D. M., and Walker, M. D. (1977). DNA damage and repair in L1210 cells exposed to CCNU. *Cancer Res.* **37**, 2262–2266.

Iqbal, Z. M., Kohn, K. W., Ewig, R. A. G., and Fornace, A. J., Jr. (1976). Single-strand scission and repair of DNA in mammalian cells by bleomycin. *Cancer Res.* **36**, 3834–3838.

Iyer, V. N., and Szybalski (1963). A molecular mechanism of mitomycin action: Linking of complementary DNA strands. *Proc. Natl. Acad. Sci. U.S.A.* **50**, 355–362.

Jolley, G. M., and Ormerod, M. G. (1974). The incomplete separation of complementary strands of high molecular weight DNA in alkali. *Biochim. Biophys. Acta* **353**, 200–214.

Kann, H. E., Jr. (1978). Cytotoxic synergism between radiation and various nitrosoureas. *Proc. Am. Assoc. Cancer Res.* **19**, 214.

Kann, H. E., Jr., Kohn, K. W., and Lyles, J. M. (1974). Inhibition of DNA repair by the BCNU breakdown product, 2-chloroethylisocyanate. *Cancer Res.* **34**, 398–402.

Klatt, O., Stehlin, J. S., Jr., McBride, C., and Griffin, A. C. (1969). The effect of nitrogen mustard treatment on the DNA of sensitive and resistant Ehrlich tumor cells. *Cancer Res.* **29**, 286–290.

Kohn, K. W. (1977). Interstrand crosslinking of DNA by 1,3-Bis(2-chloroethyl)-1-nitro-sourea and other 1-(2-haloethyl)-1-nitrosoureas. *Cancer Res.* **37**, 1450–1454.

Kohn, K. W. (1978). DNA as target in cancer chemotherapy: Measurement of macro-molecular DNA damage produced in mammalian cells by anti-cancer agents and carcinogens. *Methods Cancer Res.* **16**, 291–345.

Kohn, K. W., and Ewig, R. A. G. (1976). Effect of pH on the bleomycin-induced DNA single-strand scission in L1210 cells and the relation to cell survival. *Cancer Res.* **36**, 3839–3841.

Kohn, K. W., and Ewig, R. A. G. (1979). DNA–protein crosslinking by *trans*-Pt(II)(NH$_3$)$_2$Cl$_2$ in mammalian cells, a new method of analysis. *Biochim. Biophys. Acta* **562**, 32–40.

Kohn, K. W., Steigbigel, N. H., and Spears, C. L. (1965). Crosslinking and repair of DNA in sensitive and resistant strains of *E. coli* treated with nitrogen mustard. *Proc. Natl. Acad. Sci. U.S.A.* **53**, 1154–1161.

Kohn, K. W., Spears, C. L., and Doty, P. (1966). Interstrand crosslinking of DNA by nitrogen mustard. *J. Mol Biol.* **19**, 266–288.

Kohn, K. W., Friedman, C. A., Ewig, R. A. G., and Iqbal, Z. M. (1974). DNA chain growth during replication of asynchronous L1210 cells. Alkaline elution of large DNA segments from cells lysed on filters. *Biochemistry* **13**, 4134–4139.

Kohn, K. W., Waring, M. J., Glaubiger, D., and Friedman, C. A. (1975). Intercalative binding of ellipticine to DNA. *Cancer Res.* **35**, 71–76.

Kohn, K. W., Erickson, L. C., Ewig, R. A. G., and Friedman, C. A. (1976). Fractionation of DNA from mammalian cells by alkaline elution. *Biochemistry* **15**, 4629–4637.

Lafleur, M. V. M., VanHeuved, M., VanderStroom, H. A., and Loman, H. (1976). Biological relevance of gamma-ray-induced alkali-labile sites in single-stranded DNA in aqueous solution. *Int. J. Radiat. Biol.* **30**, 223–228.

Lange, C. S. (1974). The repair of DNA double-strand breaks in mammalian cells and the organization of the DNA in their chromosomes. *In* "Molecular Mechanisms for Repair of DNA" (P. C. Hanawalt and R. B. Setlow, eds.), Part B, pp. 677–683. New York.

Lawley, P. D., and Brookes, P. (1963). Further studies on the alkylation of nucleic acids and their constituent nucleotides. *Biochem. J.* **89**, 127–144.

Lawley, P. D., and Brookes, P. (1967). Interstrand crosslinking of DNA by difunctional alkylating agents. *J. Mol. Biol.* **25**, 143–160.

Lehmann, A. R., and Stevens, S. (1977). The production and repair of double strand breaks in cells from normal humans and from patients with ataxia telangiectasia. *Biochim. Biophys. Acta* **474**, 49–60.

Ley, R. D., Grube, D. D., and Fry, R. J. M. (1977). Photosensitizing effects of 8-methoxy-psoralen on the skin of hairless mice—I. Formation of interstrand crosslinks in epidermal DNA. *Photochem. Photobiol.* **25**, 265–268.

Lindahl, T., and Anderson, A. (1972). Rate of chain breakage at apurinic sites in double-stranded DNA. *Biochemistry* **11**, 3618–3622.

Linsley, W. S., Penhoet, E. E., and Linn, S. (1977). Human endonuclease specific for apurinic/apyrimidinic sites in DNA. *J. Biol. Chem.* **252**, 1235–1242.

Ljungquist, S., and Lindahl, T. (1974). A mammalian endonuclease specific for apurinic sites in double-stranded DNA. *J. Biol. Chem.* **249**, 1530–1535.

Lloyd, R. S., Haidle, C. W., and Robberson, D. L. (1978). Bleomycin-specific fragmentation of double-stranded DNA. *Biochemistry* **17**.

Lown, J. W., and Sim, S.-K. (1978). Photoreaction of psoralen and other furocoumarins with nucleic acids. *Bioorg. Chem.* **7**, 85–95.

Lown, J. W., McLaughlin, L. W., and Chang, Y.-M. (1978). Mechanism of action of 2-haloethylnitrosoureas on DNA and its relation to their antileukemic properties. *Bioorg. Chem.* **7**, 97–110.

Mattern, M. R., Hariharan, P. V., and Cerutti, P. A. (1975). Selective excision of gamma ray-damaged thymine from the DNA of cultured mammalian cells. *Biochim. Biophys. Acta* **395**, 48–55.

Minsky, B. D., and Braun, A. (1977). X-ray mediated cross-linking of protein and DNA. *Radiat. Res.* **71**, 505–515.

Müller, W. E. G., Yamazaki, Z., Breter, H., and Zahn, R. K. (1972). Action of bleomycin on DNA and RNA. *Eur. J. Biochem.* **31**, 518–525.

Munchausen, L. L. (1974). Chemical of biological effects of cis-dichloradiammine-Pt(II). *Proc. Natl. Acad. Sci. U.S.A.* **71**, 4519–4522.

Painter, R. B. (1974). DNA damage and repair in eukaryotic cells. *Genetics* **78**, 139–148.

Painter, R. B. (1977). *Mutat. Res.* **42**, 299–304.

Painter, R. B., and Young, B. R. (1976). Formation of nascent DNA molecules during inhibition of replicon initiation in mammalian cells. *Biochim. Biophys. Acta* **418**, 146–153.

Pascoe, J. M., and Roberts, J. J. (1974). Interactions Between mammalian cell DNA and inorganic Platinum compounds—I. DNA interstrand crosslinking and cytotoxic properties of Platinum(II) compounds. *Biochem. Pharmacol.* **23**, 1345–1357.

Povirk, L. F. (1977). Localization of inhibition of replicon initation to damaged regions of DNA. *J. Mol. Biol.* **114**, 141–151.

Povirk, L. F., Wübker, W., Köhnlein, W., and Hutchinson, F. (1977). DNA double-strand breaks and alkali-labile bonds produced by bleomycin. *Nucleic Acid Res.*

Pulleyblank, D. E., Shure, M., Tang, D., Vinograd, J., and Vosberg, H.-P. (1975). Action of nicking–closing enzyme on supercoiled and non-supercoiled closed circular DNA: Formation of a Boltzmann distribution of topological isomers. *Proc. Natl. Acad. Sci. U.S.A.* **72**, 4280–4284.

Roberts, J. J., and Pascoe, J. M. (1972). Cross-linking of complementary strands of DNA in mammalian cells by antitumor Platinum compounds. *Nature (London)* **235**, 282–284.

Ross, W. E., Ewig, R. A. G., and Kohn, K. W. (1978a). Differences between melphalan and nitrogen mustard in the formation and removal of DNA crosslinks. *Cancer Res.* **38**, 1502–1506.

Ross, W. E., Glaubiger, D. L., and Kohn, K. W. (1978b). Protein-associated DNA breaks in cells treated with adriamycin and ellipticine. *Biochim. Biophys. Acta* **519**, 23–30.

Ross, W. E., Glaubiger, D., and Kohn, K. W. (1978c). Qualitative and quantitative aspects of intercalator-induced DNA strand breaks. *Biochim. Biophys. Acta* **562**, 41–50.

Rydberg, B. (1975). The rate of strand separation in alkali of DNA of irradiated mammalian cells. *Radiat. Res.* **61**, 274–287.

Rydberg, B., and Johanson, K. J. (1975). Radiation-induced DNA strand breaks and their rejoining in crypt and villous cells of the small intestine of the mouse. *Radiat. Res.* **64**, 281–292.

Schooter, K. V. (1976). The kinetics of the alkaline hydrolysis of phosphotriesters in DNA. *Chem.-Biol. Interact.* **13**, 151–163.

Schwartz, H. S. (1976). Alkali-labile regions and strand breaks in DNA from cells treated with daunorubicin. *J. Med. (Basel)* **7**, 33–46.

Singer, B. (1975). The chemical effects of nucleic acid alkylation and their relation to mutagenesis and carcinogenesis. *Prog. Nucleic Acid Res. Molec. Biol.* **15**, 219–284.

Smith, K. C., and O'Leary, M. E. (1967). Photoinduced DNA–protein crosslinks and bacterial killing: A correlation at low temperatures. *Science* **155**, 1024–1026.

Stacey, K. A., Cobb, M., Cousens, S. F., and Alexander, P. (1958). The reactions of the "radiomimetic" alkylating agents with macromolecules *in vitro. Ann. N.Y. Acad. Sci.* **68**, 682–701.

Strniste, G. F., and Rall, S. C. (1976). Induction of stable protein–DNA adducts in Chinese hamster cell chromatin by UV. *Biochemistry* **15**, 1712–1719.

Thomas, C. B., Kohn, K. W., and Bonner, W. (1978a). Characterization of DNA–protein crosslinks formed by treatment of L1210 cells and nuclei with nitrogen mustard. *Biochemistry* **17**, 3954–3958.

Thomas, C. B., Osieka, R., and Kohn, K. W. (1978b). DNA crosslinking by *in vivo* treatment of sensitive and resistant human colon carcinoma xenografts in nude mice with 1-(2-chloroethyl)-3-(4-methylcyclohexyl)-1-nitrosourea (MeCCNU). *Cancer Res.* **38**, 2448–2454.

Umezawa, H., Asakura, H., Oda, K., and Hori, S. (1973). The effect of bleomycin on SV40 DNA: Characteristics of bleomycin action which produces a single scission in a superhelical form of SV40 DNA. *J. Antibiot.* **26**, 521–527.

Vander Schans, G. P., Bleichrodt, J. F., and Blok, J. (1973). Contribution of various types of damage to inactivation of a biologically active double-stranded circular DNA by gamma radiation. *Int. J. Radiat. Biol.* **23**, 133–150.

Verly, W. G. (1974). Commentary: Monofunctional alkylating sites and apurinic sites in DNA. *Biochem. Pharmacol.* **23**, 3–8.

Yin, L., Chun, E. H. L., and Rutman, R. J. (1973). A comparison of the effects of alkylation on the DNA of sensitive and resistant Lettré–Ehrlich cells following *in vivo* exposure to nitrogen mustard. *Biochim. Biophys. Acta* **324**, 472–481.

Zwelling, L. A., Kohn, K. W., Ross, W. E., and Anderson, T. (1978). The kinetics of formation and disappearance of DNA crosslinks in mouse leukemia L1210 cells treated with *cis*- and *trans*-Pt(II) $(NH_3)_2Cl_2$. *Cancer Res.* **38**, 1762–1768.

Zwelling, L. A., Anderson, T., and Kohn, K. W. (1979). DNA–protein and DNA interstrand crosslinking by *cis* and *trans*-Pt(II)$(NH_3)Cl_2$ in L1210 cells. *Cancer Res.* **39**, 365–369.

10

Studies on the Binding of Nitrosoureas and Nitrosoguanidines to Nuclear Proteins

PAUL V. WOOLLEY, III, AND SETH D. PINSKY

I. Introduction

Nitrosoguanidines and nitrosoureas are compounds that have activity both as carcinogens and as antitumor agents. Chemically they are capable of acting as conventional alkylating agents to modify DNA. However, they possess another pathway of chemical activity as well, by which interaction with protein is possible. Although emphasis has been placed upon the capacity of these compounds to modify DNA in terms of their carcinogenic capabilities, we have been interested in the possibility that reactions with nuclear proteins are relevant in this regard.

241

II. Structure and Reactivity of Nitroso Compounds

The structures of some of the members of this group of compounds are given in Table I. The parent structures are 1-methyl-1-nitrosourea (MNU) and 1-methyl-3-nitro-1-nitrosoguanidine (MNNG). The 1-ethyl derivatives are also potent carcinogens. Several nitrosourea derivatives such as 1,3-bis(2-chloroethyl)-1-nitrosourea (BCNU), 1-(2-chloroethyl)-3-cyclo-hexy-1-nitrosourea (CCNU), 1-(2-chloroethyl)-3-(3-methylcyclohexyl)-1-nitrosourea (methyl CCNU), streptozotocin, and chlorozotocin also possess significant antitumor activity.

The chemistry of these compounds is important in that they undergo two distinct reactions with biological material that produce covalent modification of macromolecules. An understanding of protein modification by these compounds requires consideration of their chemical decomposition into reactive species.

The synthesis of N-methyl-N-nitroso-N'-nitroguanidine was described as a synthetic route to N-aryl-N'-nitroguanidines (McKay and Wright, 1947). The nitrosation of methylnitroguanidine produced MNNG, and this compound was capable of subsequent reaction with other primary amines, which resulted in elimination of the methylamino group to form alkylaminonitroguanidines:

$$CH_3-\underset{\underset{NH}{\|}}{\overset{\overset{H}{|}}{N}}-\overset{\overset{H}{|}}{C}-\overset{\overset{H}{|}}{N}-NO_2 \xrightarrow{HNO_2} CH_3-\underset{\underset{NO}{|}}{\overset{\overset{HN}{\|}}{N}}-\overset{\overset{HN}{\|}}{C}-\overset{\overset{H}{|}}{N}-NO_2 \qquad (1)$$

$$CH_3-\underset{\underset{NO}{|}}{N}-C\,(NH)-\overset{\overset{H}{|}}{N}-NO_2 + RNH_2 \longrightarrow RNH-\underset{\underset{NO_2}{|}}{\overset{\overset{NH}{|}}{C}}-NH + CH_3N-NO \qquad (2)$$

The synthesis of several N-substituted N'-nitroguanidines was possible via these reactions (McKay, 1949). It was subsequently recognized (Henry, 1950) that the methylamino groups lost from MNNG in these reactions with primary amines went on to participate in methylation of compounds such as aniline.

Also of interest was a similar group of reactions that occurred with thiopseudoureas, leading to the formation of substituted primary amines (Fishbein and Gallaghan, 1954):

$$RNH_2 + CH_3-\underset{\underset{NH}{\|}}{\overset{\overset{H}{|}}{S}}-C-NH-NO_2 \longrightarrow RNH-\underset{\underset{NH}{\|}}{C}-NH-NO_2 + CH_2SH \qquad (3)$$

An analogous scheme of decomposition and chemical reactivity occurs for nitrosoureas. MNU decomposes spontaneously in alkaline medium to

TABLE I

Structures of Nitrosoureas

$$\begin{array}{ccc} H & O & NO \\ | & \| & | \\ R_1\!-\!N\!-\!C\!-\!N\!-\!R_2 \end{array}$$

R_1	R_2	Name
H	CH_3	1-Methyl-1-nitrosourea (MNU)
$Cl\!-\!CH_2CH_2$	CH_2CH_2Cl	1,3-Bis(2-chloroethyl)-1-nitrosourea (BCNU)
Cyclohexyl	CH_2CH_2Cl	1-(2-Chloroethyl)-3-cyclohexyl-1-nitrosourea (CCNU)
3-Methyl-cyclohexyl	CH_2CH_2Cl	1-(2-Chloroethyl)-3-(3-methyl-cyclohexyl)-1-nitrosourea (methyl CCNU)
Glucose	CH_3	1-Methyl-3-glucosyl-1-nitro-sourea (streptozotocin)
Glucose	CH_2CH_2Cl	1-(2-Chloroethyl)-3-glucosyl-1-nitrosourea (chlorozotocin)

$$\begin{array}{c} NH \\ \| \\ O_2N\!-\!N\!-\!C\!-\!N\!-\!CH_3 \\ | \qquad | \\ H \qquad NO \end{array}$$ 1-Methyl-3-nitro-1-nitroso-guanidine (MNNG)

produce a cyanate ion and a methylating group (Hecht and Kozarich, 1973). The cyanate ion can react with lysine residues, and the ability of MNU to alkylate DNA is well recognized (Swann and Magee, 1968).

The other nitrosoureas also react in this fashion. CCNU has been particularly well studied. Montgomery *et al.* (1967) showed that CCNU decomposed in aqueous solution by way of an intermediate isocyanate, cyclohexylisocyanate, which is a reactive species capable of forming carbamoylated derivatives with primary amino groups. The chloroethyl group from this compound gives rise to a carbonium ion which acts as an alkylating agent. This scheme is representative of the chemical decomposition of all the nitrosoureas shown in Table I. The substituent at the 3-nitrogen gives rise to an organic isocyanate which can react with protein, while the alkyl group produces a carbonium ion.

III. Reactions with Proteins and Nucleic Acids *in Vitro* and *in Vivo*

The reaction of MNNG with primary amines can also occur with lysine groups in protein in aqueous medium at neutral pH, which extends their importance to biological systems. Saroff and Evans (1959) described conversion of the amino group of some amino acids and of serum albumin into a nitroguanidino group with the use of 2-methyl-1(or 3)-nitro-2-thiopseudourea. There was extensive modification of serum albumin (40 out of 56–60 lysine groups present) when the reaction occurred at pH 9, and there was also a satisfactory reaction with glycine, β-alanine, and δ-aminovaleric acid in alkaline solution. Exposure of albumins to MNNG in aqueous solution at neutral pH also resulted in the modification of ϵ-amino groups to lysine to form nitroguanido groups (McCalla and Reuvers, 1968). This produced an increase in the extinction coefficient of the protein and alteration of its electrophoretic mobility. Of note, however, was the fact that protein modification was demonstrated at an MNNG concentration well in excess of that required for lethal effects upon cells and for the inactivation of transforming DNA. These latter changes appeared at 10 μg/ml, a concentration that did not produce substantial modification of protein. The evidence suggested that damage to protein was not the primary mechanism of the biological effects observed when cells were exposed to MNNG. However, the reaction with protein might have a promoting effect by accelerating production of the alkylating group.

The reaction of MNNG with other proteins, including nuclear histones, has also been examined (Sugimura et al., 1968). Study of these reactions was facilitated by the synthesis of MNNG labeled either in the guanidino group or in the methyl group, so that the relative importance of guanidination and alkylation could be assessed. Interactions with several macromolecules, including histone, cytochrome c, RNase, serum globulin, DNA, RNA, poly(A), and poly(U) were assessed at a MNNG concentration of 250 μg/ml ($\sim$1.9 mM). Progressive reaction of the guanidino group with histone and other proteins was observed over time, to the point that 6.3 moles of guanidino carbon were incorporated per mole of histone at 24 hours. The other three proteins showed values of 2.5–4 moles/mole or protein. The incorporation of guanidino carbon into DNA, RNA, and polynucleotides was negligible, but methylation of DNA as well as RNA was readily demonstrated. Approximately 10 nmoles of methyl carbon were incorporated per 500 μg of DNA in 24 hours.

These experiments have been extended (Nagao et al., 1969) to the interaction of MNNG with ascites hepatoma cells in culture. Following the incubation of cells at a MNNG concentration of 50 μg/ml (2 $\times$ 10^{-4} M), progressive incorporation of radioactivity from both guanidino and methyl labels could be demonstrated in acid-insoluble materials from whole cells. Both guanidination and methylation of whole histone extracts was shown to occur, but fractionation into individual histone species was not performed. On the basis of molar incorporation, guanidination of histones was more important than methylation (0.3 nmoles guanidino carbon/mg of histone and 0.17 nmoles methyl carbon/mg of histone). At the same time there was no incorporation of guanidino carbon into DNA, but 1.1 nmoles of methyl carbon/mg of DNA were measured. The molar quantities of guanidination and methylation of histones were 4 mmoles/mole and 1.2 mmoles/mole, respectively. Thus concurrent guanidination of histones and methylation of DNA was demonstrated in whole cells.

An important subsequent study suggested a correlation between histone modification by MNNG and the carcinogenic activity of the drug (Saito and Sugimura, 1973). It is known that MNNG administered in drinking water or by gastric lavage is a reliable gastric carcinogen, but is less so in other organs, including the liver. When [*guanidino*-^{14}C]MNNG and [*methyl*-^{14}C]MNNG were administered to rats, high levels of radioactivity were found in the stomach, small intestine, liver, and kidney. Levels of methyl carbon were comparable in all tissues, whether or not they were susceptible to carcinogenesis. In contrast, the incorporation of guanidino carbon into acid-insoluble material was highest in the stomach and small intestine and lower in the liver and kidney, which corresponded roughly to the organotropism of the drug. Extraction of histones and DNA from the stomach and liver revealed substantial guanidination of histones in the stomach and methylation of histones and DNA in the stomach, but no guanidination of histones in the liver and much lower levels of methylation of histones and DNA in the liver. Thus the correlation between drug binding and carcinogenicity favored a correlation between high levels of guanidination and methylation.

Studies in our laboratory are presently aimed at expanding these observations. In particular a comparison of the binding of the two carcinogens MNU and MNNG has been undertaken.

MNU has been obtained with either a carbonyl-^{14}C label or a methyl-^{14}C label. Likewise MNNG has been obtained with either a guanidino-^{14}C or a methyl-^{14}C label. An examination of the binding of these compounds to the nuclear proteins of L1210 cells has been made (Pinsky *et al.*, 1979). The data show that, at drug concentrations of 0.038–3.8 mM, modification of histones and acid-soluble nonhistones is readily detectable. Results at drug doses of 3.8 mM are given in Table II. MNU produces carbamoylation of H2B and H3 in particular. It also readily alkylates all histones, the highest levels being seen in H2A and H1. Guanidination by MNNG over the same time period of 1 hour is more extensive than carbamoylation by MNU, the modification of H1 being the most important on a molar basis. Methylation by MNNG is much closer to the levels achieved with MNU and, like that produced by MNU, is most notable in H1 and H2A.

As shown in the last line of Table II, drug binding to acid-extractable nonhistones exceeded binding to histones by ratios of 2.1:1 to 8.7:1. Other

TABLE II

MNU and MNNG Binding to L1210 Cell Histones [a]

Histone	[carbonyl-^{14}C] MNU	[guanidino-^{14}C] MNNG	[methyl-^{14}C] MNU	[methyl-^{14}C] MNNG
H1	1.1	332.1	4.8	13.0
H2A	1.3	191.0	6.0	14.0
H2B	8.3	136.4	2.8	7.7
H3	12.7	78.8	3.4	7.7
H4	2.2	55.3	2.3	6.3
Ratio of drug binding of acid-extractable non-histones to that of histones	3.8	8.7	2.1	2.1

[a] Expressed as picomoles of drug per nanomole of histone.

studies, however (Sudhakar *et al.*, 1979), have shown that MNU binding to acid-insoluble protein is relatively low.

These studies can be compared to similar studies with CCNU. As noted above, this compound decomposes to produce an organic isocyanate and a carbonium ion. It was shown by Cheng *et al.* (1972) that the cyclohexyl and chloroethyl groups of CCNU possessed different reactivity and specificity toward different macromolecules. The cyclohexyl group modified proteins such as albumin and histone, and also polylysine, but showed virtually no reactivity toward either DNA or RNA. The chloroethyl moiety showed some capacity to react with protein, albeit only 5–10% that of the cyclohexyl group, but had definite reactivity with DNA and tRNA. On this basis it was suggested that CCNU acted in a dual capacity to modify macromolecules by (1) carbamoylation via cyclohexyl isocyanate and (2) alkylation via a carbonium ion generated from the chloroethyl portion of the molecule. Thereafter Schmall *et al.* (1973) clarified the interaction of the cyclohexyl group with protein, demonstrating that CCNU produced cyclohexyl carbamoylation of lysine residues. Wheeler *et al.* (1975) further showed that the interaction of CCNU with proteins and peptides resulted in carbamoylation of terminal amino groups, as well as ϵ-amino groups of lysine.

These observations originally led us to examine the interaction of CCNU with nuclear proteins (Woolley *et al.*, 1976). A detailed analysis was undertaken of the interaction of CCNU labeled in the cyclohexyl ring or in the chloroethyl group with the histones and acidic nuclear proteins of the L1210 cell. At a concentration of 10^{-5} M CCNU, incorporation of radioactivity from [*cyclohexyl*-^{14}C]CCNU into histones was detectable. The predominant modification was that of H1, to the extent of 10–20 mmoles drug/mole of protein. It was noted that two forms of drug binding were present, one dissociable under mild alkaline conditions and the other stable at pH 8. Under the conditions of this study, which included extensive dialysis of drug-treated proteins at alkaline pH, acidic proteins were not appreciably affected. There was no detectable modification of either group of proteins by the chloroethyl group under these conditions. Thus, at 10^{-5} M CCNU, the predominant modification of nuclear proteins by this agent was the modification of H1 by the cyclohexyl group.

Additional data on this point have been obtained by Sudhakar *et al.* (1979). As part of a study of the chromatin-associated enzyme poly ADP-ribose polymerase, carbamoylation of nuclear proteins in HeLa cells by CCNU was examined. In this case, the CCNU concentration was 3.3 mM, considerably higher than in the previous study. Among the histones, H1, H2A, and H3 were the predominant modified species. However, incorporation of cyclohexyl label into acid-soluble nonhistone proteins was found to exceed incorporation into histones, and measurable modification of a broad spectrum of acid-insoluble nonhistones was found as well. Taken together, these data indicate that, at low CCNU concentrations, H1 and other histones are the predominant species modified by CCNU, while at higher concentrations reactions with high-mobility group proteins and acid-insoluble nonhistones become important.

In summary, these studies indicate the spectrum of reactivity of this entire class of compounds with nuclear material. Since these compounds represent biologically important agents that are important carcinogens, much work remains to delineate the significance of the individual reactions to the overall process of carcinogenesis. Understanding of the relation of protein function to modification by carcinogens is also embryonic. The entire field is one for fruitful research.

Acknowledgment

These studies were supported in part by grant CA19744 from the National Pancreatic Cancer Project, National Institutes of Health.

References

Cheng, C. J., Fujimura, S., Grunberger, D., and Weinstein, I. B. (1972). Interaction of 1-(2-chloroethyl)-3-cyclohexyl-1-nitrosourea (NSC-79037) with nucleic acids and proteins *in Vitro* and *in Vivo*. *Cancer Res.* **32**, 22–27.

Fishbein, L., and Gallaghan, J. A. (1954). The preparation and reactions of 2-alkyl-1 (or 3)-nitro-2-thiopseudourea, Part I. Reaction with amines *J. Am. Chem. Soc.* **76**, 1877–1879.

Hecht, S. M., and Kozarich, J. W. (1973). Mechanisms of the base induced decomposition of *N*-nitroso-*N*-methylurea. *J. Org. Chem.* **38**, 1821–1824.

Henry, R. A. (1950). The reaction of amines with *N*-methyl-*N*-nitroso-*N*'nitroguanidine. *J. Am. Chem. Soc.* **72**, 3287–3289.

McCalla, D. R., and Reuvers, A. (1968). Reaction of *N*-methyl-*N*'-nitro-*N*-nitrosoguanidine with protein: Formation of nitroguanido derivatives. *Can. J. Biochem.* **46**, 1411–1415.

McKay, A. F. (1949). The preparation of *N*-substituted-*N*'-nitroguanidines by the reaction of primary amines with *N*-alkyl-*N*-nitroso-*N*'nitroguanidines. *J. Am. Chem. Soc.* **71**, 1968–1970.

McKay, A. F., and Wright, G. F. (1947). Preparation and properties of *N*-methyl-*N*-nitroso-*N*'-nitroguanidine. *J. Am. Chem. Soc.* **69**, 3028–3030.

Montgomery, J. A., James, R., McCaleb, G. S., and Johnston, T. P. (1967). The modes of decomposition of 1,3-bis (2-chloroethyl)-1-nitrosourea and related compounds. *J. Med. Chem.* **10**, 668–674.

Nagao, M., Yokoshima, T., Hosoi, H., and Sugimura, T. (1969). Interaction of *N*-methyl-*N*'-nitro-*N*-nitrosoguanidine with ascites hepatoma cells *in vitro*. *Biochim. Biophys. Acta* **192**, 191–199.

Pinsky, S. D., Tew, K. D., Smulson, M. E., and Woolley, P. V. (1979). L1210 cell nuclear protein modification by the carcinogens 1-methyl-1-1-nitrosourea and 1-methyl-3-nitro-1-nitrosoguanidine. *Cancer Res.* **39**, 923–928.

Saito, T., and Sugimura, T. (1973). Interaction of *N*-methyl-*N'*-nitro-*N*-nitrosoguanidine with DNA and histone in rat tissues *in vivo. Gann.* **64**, 537–543.

Saroff, H. A., and Evans, R. L. (1959). The conversion of the amino group of amino acids and proteins to the nonbasic nitroguanidino group. *Biochim. Biophys. Acta* **36**, 511–518.

Schmall, B., Cheng, C. J., Fujimura, S., Gersten, N., Grunberger, D., and Weinstein, I. B. (1973). Modification of proteins by 1-(2-chloroethyl)-3-cyclohexyl-1-nitrosourea (NSC-79037) *in vitro. Cancer Res.* **33**, 1921–1924.

Sudhakar, S., Tew, K. D., Schein, P. S., Woolley, P. V., and Smulson, M. E. (1979). Nitrosoureas: Interaction with chromatin and effect on poly (ADP-Ribose) polymerase activity. *Cancer Res.* **39**, 1411–1417.

Sugimura, T., Fujimura, S., Nagao, M., Yokoshima, T., and Hasegawa, M. (1968). Reaction of *N*-methyl-*N'*-nitro-*N*-nitrosoguanidine with protein. *Biochim. Biophys. Acta* **170**, 427–429.

Swann, P. F., and Magee, P. N. (1968). Nitrosamine induced carcinogenesis. The alkylation of nucleic acids of the rat by *N*-methyl-*N*-nitrosourea, dimethyl nitrosamine, dimethyl sulphate and methylmethane sulphonate. *Biochem. J.* **110**, 39–47.

Wheeler, G. P., Bowdon, B., and Struck, R. F. (1975). Carbamoylation of amino acids, peptides and proteins by nitrosoureas. *Cancer Res.* **35**, 2974–2984.

Woolley, P. V., Dion, R. L., Kohn, K. W., and Bono, V. H. (1976). Binding of 1-(2-chloroethyl)-3-cyclohexyl-1-nitrosourea to L1210 cell nuclear proteins. *Cancer Res.* **36**, 1470–1474.

11

Drug Effects on Heterogeneous Nuclear RNA

IGOR TAMM AND PRAVINKUMAR B. SEHGAL

I. Introduction

Heterogeneous nuclear RNA (hnRNA) comprises the bulk of RNA transcribed from DNA by RNA polymerase II in eukaryotic cells (Roeder, 1976). Many but not all of the primary transcripts are processed into mRNA (Darnell, 1978).

Each primary transcription unit has a promoter for the initiation of transcription. In prokaryotes there are controls not only over the initiation of

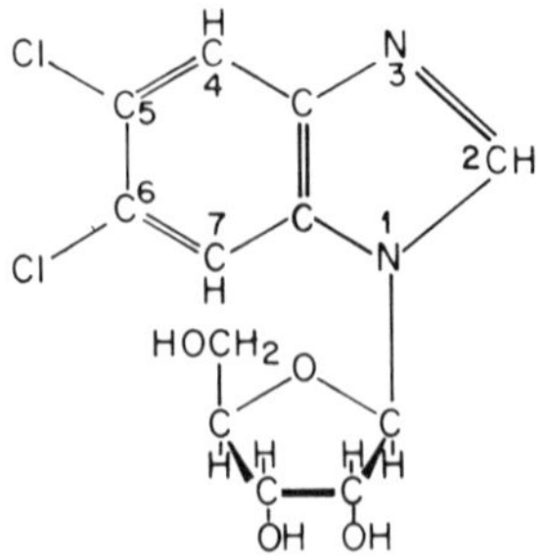

DRB
(5,6 - Dichloro -1 -β - D -
ribofuranosyl benzimidazole)

Fig. 1   The structure of DRB.

transcription at promoters, but also over the termination of transcription in attenuator regions 100–200 nucleotides downstream from promoters (Zurawski *et al.*, 1978; Di Nocera *et al.*, 1978; Barnes, 1978). Much less is known about transcriptional controls in eukaryotes. There are probably controls over initiation at promoters. The topic of this chapter concerns the possibility that transcription units in eukaryotes may also be regulated by attenuation, i.e., control of transcription termination. 5,6-Dichloro-1-β-D-ribofuranosylbenzimidazole (DRB), a halogenated benzimidazole riboside (Fig. 1), appears to be a probe for the exploration of attenuation of RNA transcription in eukaryotes.

DRB selectively inhibits the synthesis of hnRNA in insect, echinoderm, amphibian, avian, and mammalian cells (reviewed in Tamm and Sehgal, 1978; Sehgal and Tamm, 1978). The biological activity of DRB was first detected in studies of virus inhibition by benzimidazole derivatives 25 years ago (Tamm *et al.*, 1954). The sensitivity of certain viruses to DRB is based on the fact that these viruses, e.g., influenza virus and adenovirus, require a fully functioning host cell RNA polymerase II for their replication.

II. Action of DRB on hnRNA and mRNA Synthesis of Mammalian Cells

DRB inhibits hnRNA synthesis in human (HeLa, FS-4) and mouse (L) cells in a dose-dependent manner (Tamm *et al.*, 1976; Sehgal *et al.*, 1975, 1976b). Inhibition is detectable at a 5 μM concentration and is near maximal at 75 μM. The inhibitory effect is promptly reversible upon removal of DRB from the medium after a treatment period of up to a few hours

(Tamm *et al.*, 1976). Recovery takes longer after the treatment of cells for several hours (Sehgal and Tamm, 1976).

In HeLa cells treated with 75 μM DRB there is a progressive decrease in the rate of hnRNA synthesis during the first 5 minutes, and maximal inhibition (about 65%) is reached between 5 and 15 minutes (Fig. 2) (Sehgal *et al.*, 1976b). Cells treated with DRB for 15 minutes or longer show that there is a DRB-resistant fraction of hnRNA which amounts to approximately one-third of total hnRNA synthesis (Tamm *et al.*, 1976; Sehgal *et al.*, 1976a,b). The amount of drug-resistant hnRNA synthesis is approximately the same even after prolonged exposure to DRB.

The fraction of DRB-resistant RNA in HeLa cells is independent of the duration of labeling, which suggests that the metabolic turnover of DRB-resistant hnRNA is similar to that of bulk hnRNA (Sehgal *et al.*, 1976b). Such RNA has been demonstrated by labeling cells with [^{3}H]uridine, [^{3}H]adenosine, and $^{32}PO_4$.

The DRB-resistant one-third of hnRNA in HeLa cells is similar to hnRNA isolated from drug-free control cells in size distribution, poly(A) content, and extent of methylation and capping (Sehgal *et al.*, 1976b;

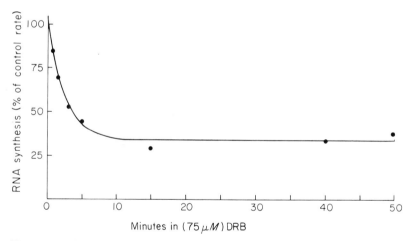

Fig. 2 Inhibition of the rate of hnRNA synthesis in HeLa cells treated with 75 μM DRB for varying periods. Cells were incubated with actinomycin D (0.04 μg/ml) for 25 minutes to inhibit pre-rRNA synthesis. They were then treated with DRB (75 μM) for varying periods and pulse-labeled with [^{3}H]uridine (60–100 μCi/ml) for 30–45 seconds in the continued presence of the drugs. Nuclear RNA was extracted, denatured with 80% dimethyl sulfoxide, and analyzed on sucrose gradients. [^{3}H]uridine incorporation into hnRNA (> 10 S) in the presence of DRB was corrected for the inhibition of [^{3}H]uridine transport into cells and is expressed as percent of incorporation in control cultures. The figure presents the pooled data from several separate experiments. (From Sehgal *et al.*, 1976b.)

Tamm *et al.*, 1976; Tamm, 1977). DRB-resistant RNA in Ehrlich mouse ascites cells is initiated with both ATP and GTP in the presence of DRB (Dreyer and Hausen, 1978b). The continuation of synthesis of DRB-resistant RNA in nuclei isolated from DRB-treated HeLa cells is sensitive to α-amanitin (1 μg/ml) (Tamm, 1977).

DRB-resistant hnRNA (30% of total) continues to be synthesized in HeLa cells in the presence of the drug at the very high concentration of 150 μM (Fig. 3). A comparison of Fig. 3A and C shows that, under steady-state labeling conditions, DRB-resistant hnRNA is distributed over the entire size range of hnRNA. It is apparent from Fig. 3B and D that 150 μM DRB significantly inhibits the synthesis of 45 S pre-rRNA. The selective effect of DRB on hnRNA synthesis is most clearly demonstrable at 10–20 times lower concentrations in L cells (Tamm *et al.*, 1976). At higher concentrations of DRB the synthesis of pre-rRNA is significantly inhibited in L cells as well. Based on similar findings in chick embryo fibroblasts, Granick (1975a,b) proposed that DRB may have a partial inhibitory effect on RNA polymerase I.

DRB reduces the labeling of both hnRNA and nuclear poly(A) by 65–75% (Sehgal *et al.*, 1976b). The residual labeled nuclear poly(A) appears to be of normal length. In contrast, the appearance of labeled cytoplasmic poly(A)-containing RNA and of cytoplasmic poly(A) is inhibited by 95% or more in DRB-treated cells.

A brief (6-minute) treatment of cells with 75 μM DRB inhibits the incorporation of [³H] uridine into poly(A)-containing polysomal RNA by 90% (Sehgal *et al.*, 1976b). Such treatment also inhibits the incorporation of [³H]uridine into total polyribosomal EDTA-releasable 20–70 S ribonucleoprotein (mRNP) by 90%. These findings suggest that DRB inhibits the appearance in the cytoplasm of both poly(A)-containing and poly(A)-lacking mRNA, since it has been estimated that poly(A)-lacking mRNA comprises about 30% of the total mRNA (Milcarek *et al.*, 1974).

The evidence reviewed above indicates that DRB inhibits only two-thirds of hnRNA synthesis but inhibits mRNA labeling by >95%. In the presence of DRB, the DRB-resistant hnRNA contributes <5% to mRNA even though it possesses normal amounts of poly(A), 5'-caps, and internal methylated sites. Does DRB inhibit the posttranscriptional processing of the resistant hnRNA into mRNA?

An attempt was made to test this possibility by using the actinomycin D chase protocol described by Adesnik *et al.* (1972). These investigators reported that, when cells labeled with [³H]uridine for 7.5 minutes were exposed to actinomycin D or to a combination of actinomycin D and 3'-deoxyadenosine (3'dA, cordycepin) for a further 40 minutes, the radioactivity in EDTA-released, 20–70 S mRNP in the actinomycin D and 3'dA-

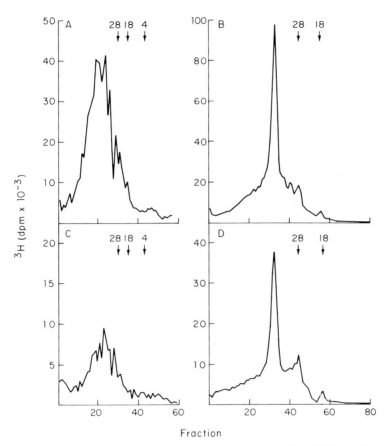

Fig. 3 Inhibition of synthesis of hnRNA and pre-rRNA by 150 μM DRB in HeLa cells *in vivo*. Cells were incubated with DRB for 15 minutes at 37°C and then labeled with [³H]uridine (10 μCi/ml) for 15 minutes in the continued presence of DRB. Actinomycin was not used. The nuclei were isolated and fractionated. RNA was extracted from the nucleoplasmic and nucleolar fractions and analyzed by electrophoresis on gels containing 1.0% polyacrylamide and 1.0% agarose (A and C), or 2.0% polyacrylamide and 1% agarose (B and D), respectively. (A) Nucleoplasmic RNA, control; (B) nucleolar RNA, control; (C) nucleoplasmic RNA, 150 μM DRB; (D) nucleolar RNA, 150 μM DRB. Incorporation of [³H]uridine into RNA in DRB-treated cells was corrected for reduced transport of the precursor.

treated group was much lower than that in the group that received actinomycin D alone. Since it was believed that actinomycin D inhibited RNA synthesis rapidly and completely, these results were interpreted as evidence for a posttranscriptional inhibitory effect of 3′dA. Figure 4 presents the results of a similar experiment using DRB together with the appropriate actinomycin D and 3′dA controls (Sehgal, 1977). It is apparent that

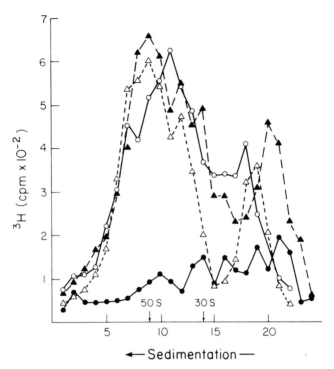

Fig. 4 Does DRB or 3'dA have a posttranscriptional inhibitory effect? Cultures of 5 × 10⁷ HeLa cells were incubated with actinomycin D (0.04 μg/ml) for 30 minutes and labeled with [³H]uridine (1 mCi per culture of 15 ml) for 7.5 minutes. They were then treated with actinomycin D (10 μg/ml) either alone or in combination with 3'dA (100 μg/ml) or DRB (75 μM) for another 40 minutes. Polysomes were prepared as described by Adesnik *et al.* (1972). The polysomes were diluted with 2 volumes of NEB (0.01 *M* Tris, 0.01 *M* NaCl, 0.01 *M* EDTA), layered onto a 20–40% sucrose gradient in NEB, and centrifuged in an SW27 rotor at 27,000 rpm for 18 hours at 4°C. The gradients were fractionated, and trichloroacetic acid-precipitable radioactivity was determined. ●, Zero time (cells labeled for 7.5 minutes only); ○, cells chased in actinomycin D; △, actinomycin D and 3'dA; ▲, actinomycin D and DRB. (From Sehgal, 1977.)

neither 3'dA nor DRB had a posttranscriptional inhibitory effect under conditions where cells were prelabeled for 7.5 minutes with [³H]uridine. The results described by Adesnik *et al.* (1972) could not be reproduced. A detailed analysis of the data in Fig. 4 and of the reagents used for this experiment suggests that the actinomycin D used previously (Adesnik *et al.*, 1972) may have only partially blocked RNA synthesis during the chase.

At present we are unable to design a sound kinetic experiment to evaluate whether DRB has a posttranscriptional inhibitory effect on mRNA synthesis.

The overall effects of DRB can be summarized as follows. DRB inhibits reversibly the synthesis of two-thirds of hnRNA, but mRNA appearance is inhibited by 95% or more under conditions of near-maximal or maximal inhibition. It therefore appears that mRNA may be largely derived from the two-thirds of hnRNA that is sensitive to inhibition by DRB. The one-third of hnRNA that is resistant to DRB may not be a precursor of mRNA, or it may provide only a small fraction of the total cytoplasmic mRNA. Information is not yet available as to whether DRB-resistant RNA contains mRNA coding sequences.

It is of interest to relate the findings concerning the DRB-resistant one-third of hnRNA to the sequence analyses of hnRNA by Greenberg and Perry (1971) and Herman *et al.* (1976). Greenberg and Perry (1971) have examined the hybridzation properties of DNA sequences directing the synthesis of mRNA and hnRNA in L cells and have obtained evidence that there is a fraction of hnRNA (about one-third) transcribed from sequences that are more highly repeated than those from which mRNA is transcribed. This is consistent with the idea that some of the highly redundant sequences in DNA may be used for transcribing RNA that is restricted to the nucleus. Herman *et al.* (1976) have found that at least 30% of the poly(A)-adjacent sequences in hnRNA have no apparent counterparts in the cytoplasm. This result was obtained by hybridizing the complementary DNA copy of isolated poly(A)-containing fragments of alkali-cleaved hnRNA with cytoplasmic mRNA. Complementary DNA prepared from hnRNA sedimenting faster than 45 S under denaturing conditions gave similar results, showing that some of the very large transcripts also may not contain mRNA sequences. The 30% of the poly(A)-containing hnRNA molecules that do not contain mRNA sequences have not been characterized.

III. Termination of Nascent hnRNA Chains of HeLa Cells a Short Distance from Initiation Sites

A. Labeling of RNA in Intact Cells

If DRB acts at or near the sites of initiation of hnRNA chains, then early during inhibition the *relative* amount of label appearing in longer molecules should increase progressively (Egyházi, 1974, 1975, 1976). We have treated HeLa cells with DRB for varying periods and then pulse-labeled the RNA for a very short time to obtain profiles of growing chains (Sehgal *et al.*, 1976a). In these experiments RNA larger than >10 S (>1000 nucleotides) was analyzed by sucrose gradient centrifugation. It was found that brief treatment of cells with DRB preferentially reduced the labeling of shorter RNA molecules, as would occur if DRB acted at or near the site of initiation of new chains. Molecules that had already reached considerable length before DRB was added to the culture continued to elongate, and presumably grew to full size.

More recently several different kinds of experiments have been carried out, the results of which are consistent with the view that DRB does not inhibit the initiation of transcription by RNA polymerase II but causes termination a short distance downstream from initiation sites.

In vivo-labeled nascent RNA was investigated by polyacrylamide gel analysis under conditions which permitted examination of chains shorter than 1000 nucleotides (Tamm, 1979). HeLa cells were treated with 75 μM DRB for 40 minutes and labeled with [^{3}H]uridine for 45 seconds in the continued presence of DRB. We have plotted in Fig. 5 the radioactivity in the RNA of control and DRB-treated samples, and the ratio of the two in groups of corresponding gel fractions. The ratios reveal clearly the varying degree of inhibition of [^{3}H]uridine incorporation into RNA chains of different lengths.

As expected, the synthesis of > 10 S RNA is markedly inhibited, with some lessening of inhibition in the higher-molecular-weight range (> 28 S). The fact that there are substantial amounts of large RNA labeled

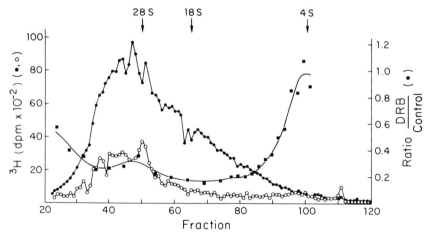

Fig. 5 Profile of nascent hnRNA chains after treatment with DRB. HeLa cells were treated with 75 μM DRB for 40 minutes and labeled for 45 seconds with [^{3}H]uridine (100 μCi/ml) in the continued presence of DRB. Actinomycin D (0.04 μg/ml) was present for 25 minutes before labeling and during labeling. Nuclear RNA was extracted, denatured with 50% formamide, and analyzed on gels of polyacrylamide, (1.5%) plus agarose (1%). Control cells received no DRB. DRB caused 60% inhibition of RNA synthesis as determined after correction of acid-precipitable counts per minute for reduced uptake of [^{3}H]uridine into cells in the presence of DRB. (From Tamm, 1979.)

after a 40-minute treatment with DRB suggests that there may be pauses or slowdowns in the elongation of long chains. If all chains are at all times growing at the estimated overall rate of 3000–6000 nucleotides/minute (Sehgal *et al.*, 1976a), and if the largest hnRNA molecules are ~ 60,000 nucleotides long, then 40 minutes should be more than adequate for the completion of growing chains, and the labeling of large molecules should be limited to the one-third fraction of DRB-resistant hnRNA.

The striking finding is the active labeling of nuclear RNA <300 nucleotides long in DRB-treated cells. Under the conditions of this experiment [i.e., analysis of nuclear RNA after a 45-second labeling in the presence of actinomycin D (0.04 μg/ml)], it is likely that the bulk of the labeling in the 100–300 nucleotide region is due to the labeling of newly initiated hnRNA precursor chains and that other RNA species make only a small contribution.

The results of the *in vivo* labeling experiments agree well with data obtained by the combined *in vivo–in vitro* procedure (Tamm, 1977, 1979) discussed below.

B. Labeling of RNA in Isolated Nuclei

Isolated HeLa cell nuclei are able to synthesize hnRNA molecules over most of the size range of HeLa cell hnRNA (Tamm, 1977). After pretreatment of cells with DRB for 10 or 40 minutes there is a time-dependent reduction in hnRNA synthesis in isolated nuclei. Of special interest is the fact that pretreatment of cells with DRB *in vivo* does not reduce the extent of labeling *in vitro* of chains that reach a mean length of about 400 nucleotides after a 15-minute incubation of isolated nuclei at 26°C *in vitro* (Tamm, 1977). The growth of such chains is sensitive to inhibition by α-amanitin at 1 μg/ml. These findings suggest that putative hnRNA precursor chains can be initiated *in vivo* in the presence of DRB, but that elongation of about two-thirds of the chains is blocked *in vivo* a short distance from the site of initiation (Tamm, 1977).

The question arises as to whether DRB terminates chain growth *in vivo* at sites of no physiological significance or whether it accentuates a mechanism for transcription termination (Tamm, 1977). The profiles of RNA from control cells that have not been treated with DRB also show a minor peak of *in vitro*-labeled molecules in the 100–700 nucleotide range (Tamm, 1977). Thus, after reaching a critical size *in vivo*, some of the putative hnRNA precursor molecules appear to be blocked or delayed in their growth even in the absence of DRB. This results in a molar excess of short chains.

The available evidence indicates that the block which is in place in intact cells is lifted when nuclei are isolated and make RNA *in vitro* in the presence of heparin. Heparin enhances the labeling of RNA chains of varying length (Tamm, 1977), and notably increases the rate of elongation of the abundant short short chains (Tamm, 1979). DRB added to isolated nuclei has no significant effect on RNA transcription (Tamm, 1977, 1979; Dreyer and Hausen, 1978).

Heparin can be used to block RNA chain initiation *in vitro*. In isolated nuclei there is repeated reinitiation of chains of 4.5 S pre-tRNA and 5 S RNA by RNA polymerase III (McReynolds and Penman, 1974). It can be seen in Fig. 6 that in a 15-minute *in vitro* labeling experiment heparin effectively eliminates incorporation of [^{3}H]uridine triphosphate into molecules smaller than about 300 nucleotides and makes possible the clear definition of a subpopulation of molecules which was initiated *in vivo* and which reached a mean size of about 550 nucleotides during the 15 minutes of labeling *in vitro* (Tamm, 1977). It is evident that the labeling of this short RNA *in vitro* is not affected by pretreatment of cells with DRB. Thus DRB treatment of cells does not diminish the subpopulation of the most abundant nascent molecules which can be clearly defined by *in vitro* labeling in the presence of heparin. The synthesis of this RNA is sensitive to inhibition by α-amanitin (1 μg/ml).

Pretreatment of cells with DRB leads to a striking reduction in the labeling of chains longer than those in the clearly resolved subpopulation of DRB-resistant molecules (Fig. 6), which confirms observations based on RNA profiles obtained by *in vitro* labeling in the absence of heparin.

Heparin permits a clear definition of the subpopulation of nascent DRB-resistant RNA chains not only because it prevents initiation of new chains, but also because it enhances the elongation of already initiated chains (Tamm, 1977; Tamm, 1979). Thus heparin permits study of the kinetics of growth *in vitro* of the polymerase II-catalyzed chains that were initiated *in vivo* just before the isolation of nuclei. This can be done over a chain length range of 100–1000 nucleotides in pulse-chase or continuous-labeling experiments. If the newly initiated chains were elongating *in vivo* at a rate of 3000–6000 per minute (Sehgal *et al.*, 1976a), they would reach a length of 1000 nucleotides in 10–20 seconds *in vivo*. It can be estimated that a molecule whose length after a minimal period of *in vitro* labeling is 100 nucleotides was initiated *in vivo* ~1–2 seconds before nuclear isolation.

A kinetic analysis of the *in vitro* elongation of putative pre-mRNA chains indicates that transcription of the DRB-sensitive hnRNA is prematurely terminated by DRB *in vivo* about 100–300 nucleotides from the origins of transcripts (Tamm, 1979). Furthermore, such analysis provides additional evidence that, even in the absence of DRB, many nascent chains

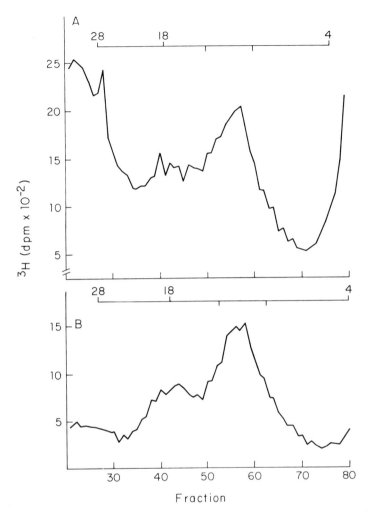

Fig. 6 A subclass of DRB-resistant RNA in HeLa cells defined with the aid of hepa-rin. Cells were treated with DRB (60 μM) for 40 minutes and with actinomycin D (0.04 μg/ml) for 25 minutes at 37°C prior to isolation of nuclei. The isolated nuclei were then incubated for 15 minutes with [³H]uridine triphosphate (100 μCi/ml) in the presence of heparin (2 mg/ml). Control nuclei were obtained from cells which had not been treated with DRB. Radioactivity in the nuclei from DRB-treated cells was 38% of that in nuclei from control cells. RNA extracted from the nuclei was analyzed on 2.2% polyacryla-mide–1.0% agarose gels. (A) Control. (B) DRB. (From Tamm, 1977.)

are delayed or blocked in their growth *in vivo* after reaching a length of ~100–300 nucleotides. The findings are as follows. When the nuclear preparation from control cells is pulse-labeled with [³H]uridine triphosphate for 5 minutes at 26°C immediately after isolation and chased for 5, 10, or 15 minutes, a broad band of labeled molecules can be resolved on 3.5% polyacrylamide gels. The molecules in the broad band undergo an increase in mean size from ~300 to ~700 nucleotides in 20 minutes. In the nuclear preparation from DRB-treated cells, the band of short, abundant molecules is undiminished and may be possibly increased. Extrapolation of the chain elongation curves for these broad bands of the most abundant molecules to zero time for the *in vitro* reaction gives length estimates of 100–300 nucleotides for nascent molecules whose growth is delayed or prematurely terminated *in vivo*.

Capping of 5′-ends of the primary transcripts takes place at the time of initiation of new chains or a short time thereafter (Sommer *et al.*, 1978). If the population of DRB-resistant short chains represents a population of prematurely terminated nascent chains of hnRNA, then it would be expected that RNA made in the presence of DRB would have an above-normal cap content. We have observed in preliminary experiments that DRB inhibits incorporation of methyl label into cap structures to a lesser extent than ³²P or nucleoside incorporation into RNA (Sehgal, 1977; also cited in Tamm and Sehgal, 1978). Incorporation of methyl label into 5′-cap structures during a 30-minute pulse with [³H]methionine was reduced to 53% of the control, whereas treatment of HeLa cells with 75 μM DRB for 40 minutes reduced ³²P or nucleoside incorporation into hnRNA to 30–40% of the control.

IV. Termination of Nascent RNA Chains of Adenovirus a Short Distance from Initiation Sites

In interpretating the data concerning the DRB-resistant synthesis of short RNA chains catalyzed by RNA polymerase II, results obtained in the adenovirus system have played an important role. It has been unequivocally demonstrated in this system that short DRB-resistant adenovirus-specific RNA chains represent transcripts from promoter-proximal regions (Fraser *et al.*, 1978; Sehgal *et al.*, 1979). This has been possible because of the availability of restriction fragments of adenovirus DNA and information concerning the location of the initiation sites for transcription in the adenovirus genome. While the synthesis by RNA polymerase II of short DRB-resistant RNA chains was first detected by a combined *in vivo* –*in vitro* procedure using uninfected HeLa cells (Tamm, 1977), the likely significance of the finding emerged when adenovirus results became available showing that DRB acted on the transcription of specific regions of the adenovirus type 2 (Ad2) genome and caused premature termination of RNA chains (Fraser *et al.*, 1978; Sehgal *et al.*, 1979).

A. Late Ad2 Transcription *in Vivo*

Inhibition through an effect of DRB on the elongation of all growing chains should result in rapid inhibition of the incorporation of [³H]uridine. The action of DRB at or near the site of chain initiation would be expected to inhibit incorporation more gradually, as chains which had already completed the DRB-sensitive step would be able to grow to full length after the addition of DRB.

Figure 7 shows that after the beginning of treatment of infected cells with DRB there is a gradual reduction in the amount of virus-specific nuclear RNA labeled in a 2-minute pulse, with a near-maximal effect in 15–30 minutes. While the kinetics of action of DRB on adenovirus RNA and cellular hnRNA transcription are similar, adenovirus RNA labeling is inhibited 90–95%, while cellular hnRNA labeling is inhibited only ~70%.

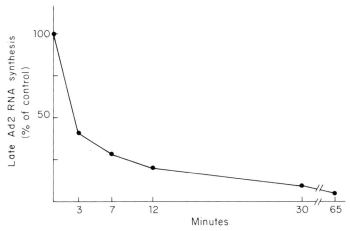

Fig. 7 Inhibition of the rate of late adenovirus-2 transcription in HeLa cells treated with DRB for varying periods. Cells were infected with adenovirus at a multiplicity of ~2000 virus particles per cell. Treatment with 75 µM DRB was begun 16 hours after infection. At intervals thereafter, aliquots of cells were labeled with [³H]uridine (0.4 mCi/ml) for 2 minutes. Nuclear RNA was extracted, and 1/10 part hybridized to nitrocellulose filters containing 2 µg of adenovirus DNA. ³H incorporation in the presence of DRB was corrected for inhibition of [³H]uridine transport into cells. The figure represents data from several experiments. (From Fraser *et al.*, 1978.)

However, the appearance of label in both adenovirus-specific mRNA and cellular mRNA is inhibited >95% (Fraser *et al.*, 1978).

Late in Ad2 infection there is transcribed in the rightward direction a large (>25-kilobase) RNA molecule which represents close to 85% of the genome (Bachenheimer and Darnell, 1975; Ziff and Evans, 1978; Fraser *et al.*, 1979a). The site of initiation of the large late adenovirus transcript has been located at 16.4 map units on the genome (Ziff and Evans, 1978).[1] If DRB acts near, but not at the site of chain initiation, then labeling of RNA sequences complementary to the DNA sequences a short distance downstream from the promoter will be the first to cease, and labeling of RNA sequences most distal to the promoter will continue longest. Labeling of sequences at the initiation site should be resistant to inhibition by DRB.

HeLa cells late in Ad2 infection were treated briefly with DRB and then pulsed with [³H]uridine for 2 minutes. Incorporation of radioactivity into nuclear RNA hybridizing to various DNA restriction fragments that span the large, late transcription unit was determined and was expressed as a fraction of that in control cells not exposed to DRB. Figure 8 shows that DRB causes an ordered, decreasing inhibition of the labeling of nascent virus-specific RNA beginning at 18 and extending to 100 on the physical map of the viral genome (Fraser *et al.*, 1978). The critical finding is that ³H incorporation into RNA complementary to the restriction fragment *Sma*I f (11.6–18.2), which contains the origin of the large transcript, is not inhibited as strongly by DRB as that into RNA transcribed from the adjacent fragment downstream. The graded diminishing inhibition of incorporation across the remainder of the large transcript is consistent with action close to the site of RNA chain initiation.

There is continued transcription in adenovirus-infected DRB-treated cells of a short piece of RNA from the promoter-containing region (11.6–18.2) but not from the neighboring segment downstream (18.8–36.7) (Fraser *et al.*, 1978). A short DRB-resistant RNA transcript has also been found which hybridizes to fragment 3.0–11.0 (*Sma*I e), a region that contains a second adenovirus transcription unit that operates late in infection.

Figure 9 shows that in the control culture the *Sma*I-f-specific (11.6–18.2) RNA that was labeled was both larger and smaller than about 1000 bases, extending down to molecules as short as 100 nucleotides. The promoter for the larger rightward-reading transcript lies in *Sma*I f, but the 2-minute pulse label allowed chains to be synthesized with labeled *Sma*I-f-specific sequences which were as large or larger than 1 kilobase. In the DRB-treated culture essentially all the labeled RNA that hybridized to *Sma*I f was small (7–9 S), and the amount of incorporation into the small RNA was similar to that in the control culture.

---

[1] (One map unit = 350 base pairs; entire genome = 100 units = 35,000 base pairs.)

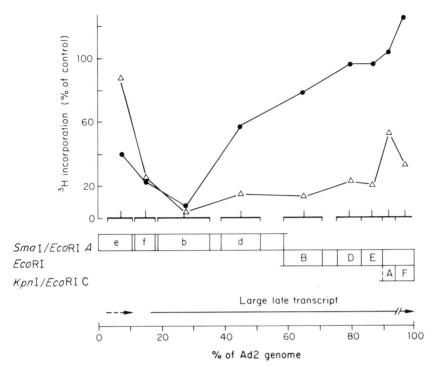

Fig. 8 Hybridization across the Ad2 genome of [³H]uridine pulse-labeled nuclear RNA late in infection after a brief treatment with DRB. Infected cells were treated with DRB (75 μM) for 7 (●) or 40 (△) minutes 16 hours after infection and pulse-labeled with [³H]uridine (0.4 mCi/ml) for 2 minutes. Nuclear RNA was extracted, fragmented by treatment with alkali to a length of ~200–300 nucleotides, and hybridized to restriction fragments of Ad2 DNA. The total radioactivity hybridized was corrected for inhibition of [³H]uridine transport by DRB. (From Fraser et al., 1978.)

The SmaI-b-specific (18.8–36.7) RNA in the control culture was almost all larger than about 1000 bases (the maximum distance from the expected promoter site to the SmaI-b region), and much of the SmaI-b-specific RNA sedimented to the bottom of the sucrose gradient. In the presence of DRB very little SmaI-b-specific RNA was labeled.

Additional experiments confirmed that DRB-resistant, SmaI-f-specific RNA was transcribed from the correct, rightward-reading strand (Fraser et al., 1978). In an attempt to further characterize these molecules we have exposed Ad2-infected HeLa cells to DRB (100 μM) for 0.5–1.0 hour beginning at 12.5–13.0 hours after infection and then labeled these cells with ³²PO₄ for a further 4–5 hours in the continued presence of the drug (Fraser et al., 1979b). Nuclear RNA which hybridized to SmaI f was prepared and fingerprinted. It was observed that DRB-resistant SmaI-f-spe-

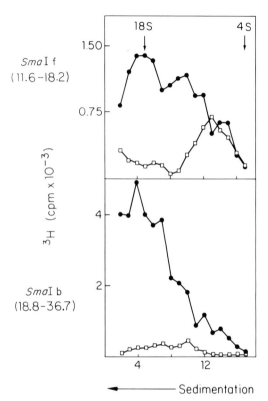

Fig. 9 Size of DRB-resistant *Sma*I-f-specific late Ad2 RNA. Infected cells were exposed to DRB (75 μM) for 60 minutes late in infection (□) and pulse-labeled with [³H]uridine for 2 minutes. An untreated sample of infected cells served as a control (●). The nuclear RNA was extracted and sedimented through a 15–30% sucrose gradient such that 18 S RNA sedimented close to the bottom of the gradient. RNA from each fraction >4 S was broken with alkali and hybridized to Ad2 restriction fragments *Sma*I f (11.6–18.2) or *Sma*I B (18.8–36.7). Incorporation in the presence of DRB was corrected for the reduction of [³H]uridine transport into cells. (From Fraser *et al.*, 1978.)

cific RNA contained all the five large T1 oligonucleotides known to be transcribed from 16.4 to 18.1 (the right half of *Sma*I f). Furthermore, two capped oligonucleotides were observed in the DRB-resistant material in approximately the same proportion to other oligonucleotides, as is observed in *Sma*I-f-specific RNA obtained from control, DRB-free Ad2-infected cells. Similar results were obtained when ³²P-labeled, DRB-resistant *Sma*I-e-specific RNA was fingerprinted. These observations clearly demonstrate that DRB does not interfere with the capping reaction and furthermore is unlikely to interfere with RNA chain initiation per se.

In further experiments *Sma*I-f-specific nuclear RNA (< 18 S in size) prepared from both DRB-treated and from DRB-free Ad2-infected cells late in infection was denatured and analyzed in 5% polyacrylamide gels. It was found that *Sma*I-f-specific RNA obtained from DRB-treated cells was generally smaller than that obtained from DRB-free cells. Furthermore, both the DRB and the control preparations formed a series of well-resolved bands in the size range of 100–800 nucleotides. Though the bands were more prominent in the DRB preparation, the control preparation also revealed bands which generally comigrated with those in the DRB preparation. Since these labeled RNA species were observed after 4–5 hours of labeling with $^{32}PO_4$, we cannot unequivocally conclude that all these bands represent RNA chains generated by termination of transcription. That at least some of them may represent products of transcription termination is suggested by (1) the presence of 5′-capped ends in *Sma*I-f-specific DRB-resistant RNA bands eluted from the gel, and (2) the broad distribution of DRB-resistant *Sma*I-f-specific 7–9 S RNA molecules seen on sucrose gradients even in a 2-minute pulse with [^{3}H]uridine (Fig. 9). It appears that the resolution of the sucrose gradient may be inadequate to resolve individual bands. These data suggest that DRB may accentuate termination at multiple physiological attenuator regions within a single Ad2 transcription unit.

The hypothesis that physiological attenuators exist in the large late Ad2 transcription unit requires that on a molar basis an excess of promoter-proximal RNA should be normally synthesized compared to promoter-distal RNA. That *Sma*I f and, to a lesser extent, *Sma*I b are transcribed in a molar excess compared to the rest of the transcription unit has recently been documented (Fraser *et al.*, 1978; Evans *et al.*, 1979).

These findings establish that DRB does not inhibit RNA chain initiation but causes chain termination close to the promoter. These investigations indicate that DRB may be useful for mapping promoter sites in eukaryotic transcription units and for the accumulation and isolation of RNA sequences near promoter sites.

B. Early Ad2 Transcription *in Vivo*

DRB (150 μM) inhibits the accumulation of early adenovirus-specific nuclear RNA by ~90%, but that of cytoplasmic RNA by >95% (Broötz *et al.*, 1978).

The usefulness of DRB in mapping promoters has been documented by using it to map early adenovirus promoters (Sehgal *et al.*, 1979). The results agree well with and extend those obtained by ultraviolet irradiation mapping and by pulse-labeling of small RNA. There is an accumulation of promoter-proximal labeled RNA chains in DRB-treated cells after a 10-minute [³H]uridine pulse.

Figure 10 summarizes the early mRNA and transcription maps for Ad2. In DRB-treated, infected cells [³H]uridine continues to be incorporated into short (4–10 S) RNA that hybridizes to the following DNA restriction fragments known to contain promoter sites for RNA synthesis: rightward-reading: *Sma*I j (0.0–3.0), *Eco*RI D (75.9–83.4); leftward-reading: *Eco*RI C (89.7–100), *Eco*RI F (70.7–75.9). In addition, in untreated control cells smaller amounts of pulse-labeled RNA have been found to hydridize to leftward-reading *Sma*I f (11.6–18.2) than in the above regions, and labeling of a portion of this RNA also is DRB-resistant. Finally, the 3.0–11.1 region (*Sma*I e) may contain one or more promoter sites for early rightward-reading transcripts. This region may also contain a DRB-resistant transcription unit.

The action of DRB on early transcription may be illustrated by the example of the transcription unit whose promoter is is in fragment *Eco*RI F (70.7–75.9). The 5′-end of the mRNA for the 72,000-dalton DNA-binding protein hybridizes at about 74.9 (reviewed in Flint, 1977). *Eco*RI F (70.7–75.9) is the promoter-containing adenovirus DNA fragment, and *Eco*RI B (58.5–70.7) is its neighbor in the known (leftward) direction of transcription. Figure 11 shows that, in the presence of DRB, small RNA (~400 nucleotides long) complementary to 70.7–75.9 continued to be labeled, whereas essentially no DRB-resistant RNA complementary to 58.5–70.7 was made.

Results of studies on the effects of DRB on the transcription of early and late adenovirus RNA show clearly that DRB causes the termination of transcripts within a few to several hundred nucleotides downstream from promoter sites. It appears that at least some of the small RNAs which continue to be made in the presence of DRB have counterparts in untreated cells. Thus it is possible that DRB may accentuate termination in physiological attenuator regions in the adenovirus genome.

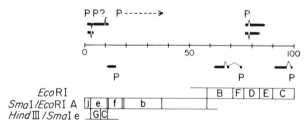

Fig. 10   Early Ad2 mRNA and transcription map. Solid lines denote map locations of the spliced sequences in the abundant mRNA molecules, and P denotes initiation sites for RNA synthesis. (From Sehgal *et al.*, 1979.)

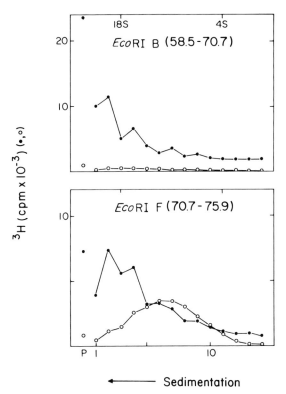

Fig. 11 Size of DRB-resistant early Ad2 RNA. HeLa cells were infected with Ad2 at a multiplicity of ~2000 virus particles per cell. Cells were treated with cycloheximide (25 μg/ml) from 1 to 5 hours after infection to increase labeling of virus-specific RNA and to ensure the absence of late RNA synthesis. At 4 hours after infection, cells were treated with DRB (75 μM) for 50 minutes and then labeled for 10 minutes with [³H]uridine in the continued presence of DRB. Nuclear RNA was extracted and size-fractionated by sucrose gradient centrifugation. RNA from each fraction >4 S was broken with alkali to ~500 nucleotides and hybridized to adenovirus DNA restriction fragments. [³H]uridine incorporation in the presence of DRB was corrected for reduced transport of the precursor. ●, Control; ○, DRB. (From Sehgal et al., 1979.)

V. Approaches to the Biochemical Mechanism of Action of DRB

Figure 12 presents a model for the action of DRB on the transcription of hnRNA in mammalian cells. It may be postulated that attenuator sites exist in the DNA of mammalian cells coding for pre-mRNA, but not in DNA coding for other hnRNA. DRB may then accentuate premature termination of pre-mRNA transcription at the attenuator sites or regions.

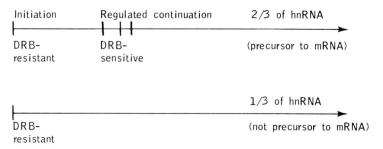

Fig. 12 A model for the action of DRB on the transcription of hnRNA by RNA polymerase II.

The possibility remains open, however, that there is some DRB-resistant pre-mRNA ($<5\%$ of total). Such pre-mRNA could be derived from DNA lacking attenuators.

We use the term "attenuator" (Kasai, 1974; Bertrand *et al.*, 1975) to refer to a region of DNA which acts as an attenuator of transcription by limiting the frequency of complete transcription of a primary transcription unit. Thus the attenuator functions as a termination signal by which the cell governs the fraction of initiated RNA polymerase II molecules that will transcribe the entire transcription unit. While this operational use of the term follows closely the original usage in prokaryotic systems, there is no basis to suggest that the mechanism of attenuation in eukaryotes is either similar to or different from that in prokaryotes. It should be noted that there are significant differences between the eukaryotic and prokaryotic systems in terms of processing of primary transcripts and coordination between transcription and translation. Thus the mechanisms of attenuation in the two systems would not be expected to be necessarily similar.

In considering the enzymic basis of the findings that, while two-thirds of hnRNA synthesis is sensitive, one-third is resistant to DRB, it was suggested that there may be more than one polymerase involved in the synthesis of hnRNA (Tamm *et al.*, 1976). To explain the results indicating that DRB acts not at the point of initiation but a short distance downstream, it was proposed that RNA polymerase II may function in two forms, of which the resistant form initiates transcripts and the sensitive form carries out a specific step in transcription a short distance downstream (Tamm, 1977).

Thus there are two distinct problems, each of which raises the possibility that RNA polymerase II may exist in two functional states. There may be a difference in one of the subunits of the enzyme or in the presence of a cofactor. It is possible to explain the two sets of findings by postulating just two forms of RNA polymerase II (as is implicit in the model in Fig. 12); however, the situation may be more complex. Recently Dreyer and Hausen (1978a) have found that transcription by endogenous RNA polymerase II in lysates of Ehrlich ascites cells exhibits two salt optima; one at 0.025 M and another at 0.3 M ammonium sulfate. It is of interest that preincubation of cells with DRB results in a selective inactivation of RNA polymerase II active at the lower salt concentration (Dreyer and Hausen, 1978a). The possibility should be noted that DRB may not necessarily interact with the RNA polymerase molecule itself, but with a component which plays a regulatory role in RNA transcription.

An understanding of attenuation as a physiological control mechanism operating in animal cells can be expected to provide a basis for identification of the molecular target for DRB. At present, information concerning the molecular mode of DRB action is very limited. However, the important finding has recently been reported that cells do not phosphorylate DRB to a measurable extent (Dreyer and Hausen, 1978b). Thus it is highly unlikely that DRB acts as a metabolic antagonist at the nucleoside triphosphate level. In cell-free systems DRB triphosphate at high concentrations inhibits the activity of RNA polymerase II and, to a lesser extent, that of RNA polymerase I and *E. coli* holoenzyme (Dreyer and Hausen, 1978b). The inhibitor concentrations required for 50% inhibition greatly exceed the concentration of nucleoside triphosphates used as substrates. There is no preferential inhibition of initiation of transcription in the polymerase II assay using poly d(AT) as template. The fact that high concentrations of DRB triphosphate are required to cause *in vitro* inhibition indicates that DRB triphosphate has a low affinity for RNA polymerase II. DRB itself and DRB monophosphate have no effect on transcription in either isolated nuclei or purified polymerase systems (Tamm, 1977; Dreyer and Hausen, 1978b; see also Tamm and Sehgal, 1978).

The outstanding structure–activity relationships are as follows: (1) For highest activity the glycosidic moiety must be the β-linked ribofuranose, which may play a critical role in the binding of inhibitors to the target molecule. (2) The activity of derivatives increases with increased halogenation in the benzenoid ring. (3) The activity of bromo-substituted derivatives is in general higher than that of chloro compounds (reviewed in Tamm and Sehgal, 1978; Sehgal and Tamm, 1978). Much of this information is based on studies of influenza virus multiplication; however, structure–activity relationships of derivatives with respect to their effects on cellular RNA synthesis in influenza virus multiplication, cell proliferation, and superinduction of interferon production are all strikingly similar (Tamm and Sehgal, 1977).

The inhibitory effect of DRB (60–90 μM) on cellular protein synthesis appears to be secondary to the inhibition of mRNA synthesis (reviewed in Tamm and Sehgal, 1978; Sehgal and Tamm, 1978). A treatment period longer than 30 minutes is required to detect inhibition of protein synthesis. Short-term treatment with DRB results only in a minor (20%) reduction in the rate of cellular DNA chain elongation (Hand and Tamm, 1977). As would be expected, treatment for periods longer than 30 minutes causes marked inhibition of DNA replication. These findings are consistent with the view that the primary action of DRB on cellular biosynthesis is its effect on mRNA synthesis.

DRB inhibits nucleoside transport (reviewed in Tamm and Sehgal, 1978; Sehgal and Tamm, 1978). The inhibitory effect of DRB on [^{3}H]uridine uptake in HeLa cells is considerably greater than that in L cells; however, the inhibition of hnRNA synthesis is similar in the two cell types (Tamm et al., 1976). In studies of the inhibitory effects of DRB on nucleic acid synthesis in intact cells it is necessary to correct acid-precipitable radioactivity for reduced transport of nucleosides. Estimates of the effect of DRB on hnRNA synthesis, based on corrected acid-precipitable radioactivity data, agree closely with estimates obtained by using ^{32}P, whose uptake is not affected by DRB (Sehgal et al., 1976b).

VI Summary and Conclusions

Although the precise biochemical mechanism of action of DRB is not yet clear, considerable advances have recently been made in defining its effects on the transcription of cellular and viral DNA by RNA polymerase II.

Kinetic studies of growth of newly started chains of hnRNA have produced evidence that DRB permits the initiation of new chains, but blocks the elongation of such chains 100–300 nucleotides from their initiation site. Moreover, in drug-free cells, too, a fraction of hnRNA chains may be blocked 100–300 nucleotides from their initiation site. Thus mammalian cells appear to be capable of regulating the transcription of hnRNA chains by attenuation.

We propose that DRB blocks the synthesis of approximately two-thirds of hnRNA and >95% of mRNA by accentuating attentuation. If so, and if DRB inhibits hnRNA synthesis by a single mechanism, it follows that the bulk of mRNA precursor molecules are transcribed from DNA containing attenuator regions.

The one-third of hnRNA whose synthesis is resistant to DRB may be transcribed from DNA lacking attenuator regions. Most of this RNA is not a precursor of mRNA; however, the possibility remains open that a small fraction of mRNA may be derived from DRB-resistant hnRNA. The content of mRNA coding sequences in the DRB-resistant RNA has not been determined as yet.

Analysis of Ad2 transcription by hybridization of the products to restriction fragments of the viral genome has established that DRB permits transcription of virus-specific RNA in regions of DNA which contain promoters, but blocks transcription a few to several hundred nucleotides downstream from promoters. With the aid of DRB, two late and several early promoters have been detected and located on the adenovirus genome map. A high-resolution study of the transcription products belonging to the large late transcription unit of adenovirus has provided evidence for the existence of physiological attenuator regions. DRB may accentuate termination in such regions. Thus DRB can be used to map promoters and to accumulate promoter-proximal transcription products for sequence analysis. It remains to be determined whether the sites at which DRB blocks transcription are of any special significance in the process by which intervening sequences are deleted and coding regions joined in the processing of primary transcripts.

Detailed investigation of the mechanism of action of DRB should provide new information about the regulation of transcription in mammalian cells.

Acknowledgments

We thank Drs. James E. Darnell, Jr., and Nigel W. Fraser for helpful discussions, and Miss Toyoko Kikuchi for excellent assistance. We are grateful to Drs. D. Wang and S. Moore for protease-free and RNase-free pancreatic DNase and to Dr. Arthur F. Wagner, Merck Sharp & Dohme Research Laboratories, for DRB used in these studies. Investigations carried out in the authors' laboratory were supported by research grant CA-18608 and program project grant CA-18213 awarded by the National Cancer Institute. P.B.S. is a postdoctoral fellow of the National Cancer Institute (5 F32 CA05900-02).

References

Adesnik, M., Salditt, M., Thomas, W., and Darnell, J. E. (1972). *J. Mol. Biol.* **71**, 21–30.
Bachenheimer, S., and Darnell, J. E. (1975). *Proc. Natl. Acad. Sci. U.S.A.* **72**, 4445–4449.
Barnes, W. M. (1978). *Proc. Natl. Acad. Sci. U.S.A.* **75**, 4281–4285.
Bertrand, K., Korn, L., Lee, F., Platt, T., Squires, C. L., Squires, C., and Yanofsky, C. (1975). *Science* **189**, 22–26.
Brötz, M., Doerfler, W., and Tamm, I. (1978). *Virology* **86**, 516–529.
Darnell, J. E., Jr. (1978). *Prog. Nucl. Acid Res. Mol. Biol.* **22**, 327–352.
Di Nocera, P. P., Blasi, F., De Lauro, R., Frunzio, R., and Bruni, C. B. (1978). *Proc. Natl. Acad. Sci. U.S.A.* **75**, 4276–4280.

Dreyer, C., and Hausen, P. (1978a). *Eur. J. Biochem.* **86**, 241–253.

Dreyer, C., and Hausen, P. (1978b). *Nucleic Acids Res.* **5**, 3325–3335.

Egyházi, E. (1974). *J. Mol. Biol.* **84**, 173–183.

Egyházi, E. (1975). *Proc. Natl. Acad. Sci. U.S.A.* **72**, 947–950.

Egyházi, E. (1976). *Nature (London)* **262**, 319–321.

Evans, R., Weber, J., Ziff, E. and Darnell, J. E. (1979). *Nature (London)* **278**, 367–370.

Flint, J. (1977). *Cell* **10**, 153–166.

Fraser, N. W., Sehgal, P. B., and Darnell, J. E. (1978). *Nature (London)* **272**, 590–593.

Fraser, N. W., Nevins, J. R., Ziff, E., and Darnell, J. E., Jr. (1979a). *J. Mol. Biol.* **129**, 643–656.

Fraser, N. W., Sehgal, P. B., and Darnell, J. E. (1979b). *Proc. Natl. Acad. Sci. U.S.A.* **76**, 2571–2575.

Granick, D. (1975a). *J. Cell Biol.* **65**, 389–417.

Granick, D. (1975b). *J. Cell Biol.* **65**, 418–427.

Greenberg, J. R., and Perry, R. P. (1971). *J. Cell Biol.* **50**, 774–786.

Hand, R., and Tamm, I. (1977). *Exp. Cell Res.* **107**, 343–354.

Herman, R. C., Williams, J. G., and Penman, S. (1976). *Cell* **7**, 429–437.

Kasai, T. (1974). *Nature (London)* **249**, 523–527.

McReynolds, L. and Penman, S. (1974). *Cell* **1**, 139–145.

Milcarek, C., Price, R., and Penman, S. (1974). *Cell* **3**, 1–10.

Roeder, R. G. (1976). *In* "RNA Polymerase" (R. Losick and M. Chamberlin, eds.), pp. 285–329. Cold Spring Harbor Lab., Cold Spring Harbor, New York.

Sehgal, P. B. (1977). Ph.D. Thesis, Rockefeller Univ., New York.

Sehgal, P. B., and Tamm, I. (1976). *Proc. Natl. Acad. Sci. U.S.A.* **73**, 1621–1625.

Sehgal, P. B., and Tamm, I. (1978). *Biochem. Pharmacol.* **27**, 2475–2485.

Sehgal, P. B., Tamm, I., and Vilček, J. (1975). *Science* **190**, 282–284.

Sehgal, P. B., Derman, E., Molloy, G. R., Tamm, I., and Darnell, J. E. (1976a). *Science* **194**, 431–433.

Sehgal, P. B., Darnell, J. E., Jr., and Tamm, I. (1976b). *Cell* **9**, 473–480.

Sehgal, P. B., Fraser, N. W., and Darnell, J. E., Jr. (1979). *Virology* **94**, 185–191.

Sommer, S., Lavi, U., and Darnell, J. E., Jr. (1978). *J. Mol. Biol.* **124**, 487–499.

Tamm, I. (1977). *Proc. Natl. Acad. Sci. U.S.A.* **74**, 5011–5015.

Tamm, I. (1979). In preparation.

Tamm, I., and Sehgal, P. B. (1977). *J. Exp. Med.* **145**, 344–356.

Tamm, I., and Sehgal, P. B. (1978). *Adv. Virus Res.* **22**, 187–258.

Tamm, I., Folkers, K., Shunk, C. H., and Horsfall, F. L., Jr. (1954). *J. Exp. Med.* **99**, 227–250.

Tamm, I., Hand, R., and Caliguiri, L. A. (1976). *J. Cell Biol.* **69**, 229–240.

Ziff, E., and Evans, R. (1978). *Cell* **15**, 1463–1476.

Zurawski, G., Brown, K., Killingly, D., and Yanofsky, C. (1978). *Proc. Natl. Acad. Sci. U.S.A.* **75**, 4271–4275.

12

Drug Effects on tRNA

K. RANDERATH

There are two populations of tRNA in mammalian cells, those coded for by nuclear genes (at least 60 different cytoplasmic tRNA species) and those coded for by mitochondrial genes (20–25 different mitochondrial tRNA species). At the present time, little is known about mammalian mitochondrial tRNAs, except that they have been found by base composition analysis to be rich in adenosine (A) and uridine (U) (Chia *et al.*, 1976), while cytoplasmic tRNAs are rich in guanosine (G) and cytidine (C). No mammalian mitochondrial tRNA has been sequenced thus far, while the structures of about 10 mammalian cytoplasmic tRNAs are known. In drug studies on tRNA, mitochondrial tRNA has usually not been analyzed separately from cytoplasmic tRNA but, in view of the small amount of mitochondrial tRNA in mammalian cells (about 2.5% of the total tRNA) (Chia *et al.*, 1976), this is not expected to affect the results of these studies significantly. Whether drug effects observed for total cellular tRNA also apply to mitochondrial tRNA remains to be investigated.

The major biological function of tRNA is that of an adaptor in protein synthesis, acting at the interface between polynucleotides and polypeptides. tRNA ensures the correct translation of the language of DNA into the language of protein. It interacts with mRNA at its anticodon end, while at the other end it carries the growing polypeptide chain attached to the 3′-terminal adenosine residue. During protein synthesis it is bound to ribosomal components (proteins and RNAs). An intricate mechanism guarantees that each tRNA is charged with its cognate amino acid. In addition to protein synthesis, tRNA is involved in a number of other biological functions, such as the regulation of protein synthesis, the transfer of

EFFECTS OF DRUGS ON THE CELL NUCLEUS

275

amino acids to acceptor molecules in the absence of ribosomes, the initiation of DNA synthesis (shown for RNA tumor viruses), enzyme inhibition, and perhaps other as yet unknown functions (Rich and RajBhandary, 1976; Goddard, 1977).

Drug effects on tRNA may entail the incorporation of drugs or their metabolites into tRNA, thereby altering the sequence of the four major
bases, or affect posttranscriptional modifications, for instance, methylation of tRNA constituents. While in the past the incorporation of drugs
such as purine and pyrimidine analogues into tRNA and other nucleic
acids was recognized as a major effect of these compounds, our laboratory has recently presented evidence for pronounced, sometimes highly
selective effects of drugs on the posttranscriptional modification of tRNA,
as will be discussed in detail later.

The sequences of all tRNAs can be written in the familiar cloverleaf
form (Fig. 1) consisting of several loop and stem areas, the latter consisting mainly of GC and AU base pairs. The planar cloverleaf, though cor-
rectly displaying the loops and stems of a tRNA molecule, does not provide a correct picture of the three-dimensional structure of tRNA. Only
recently, the latter has been elucidated by X-ray crystallographic analysis
(see reviews by Rich and RajBhandary, 1976; Goddard, 1977). Although

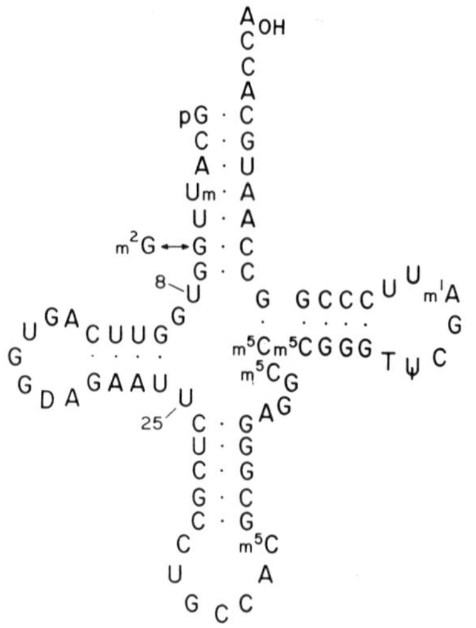

Human placenta tRNA$_{GCC}^{Gly}$

Fig. 1 The structure of human tRNA$_{GCC}^{Gly}$ in the cloverleaf form. (From Gupta et al.,
1979).

only one tRNA species (tRNA[Phe] from yeast) has thus far been analyzed by this technique, other results suggest that the three-dimensional structure of many (perhaps all) other tRNAs is quite similar to that of yeast tRNA[Phe]. X-ray crystallographic studies revealed an unexpected fact: The tRNA molecule has a bent or L-shaped appearance in which the amino acid acceptor and T-loop stems form one leg of the L; the D-stem and anticodon stem form the other leg of the L (Fig. 2). The structure is energetically stabilized by extensive hydrophobic stacking interactions between the bases, as well as by tertiary hydrogen-bonding interactions between base, ribose, or phosphate residues, in addition to the secondary Watson–Crick base pairs of the cloverleaf structure. tRNA constituents that are far apart in the cloverleaf structure are held in close contact by tertiary hydrogen-bonding interactions.

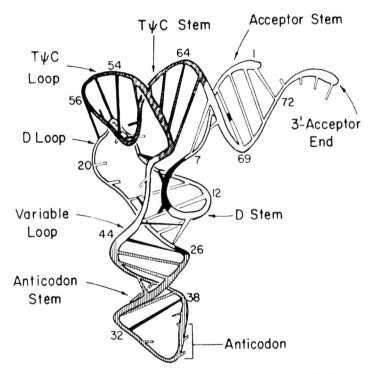

Fig. 2 The folding of the ribose phosphate backbone of yeast tRNA[Phe], determined by X-ray crystallography. The numbers refer to nucleotide residues in the sequence. Hydrogen-bonding interactions between bases are shown as cross-rungs; tertiary interactions between bases are solid black. Bases that are not involved in hydrogen bonding to other bases are shown as shortened rods attached to the backbone. (From Quigley and Rich, 1976, with permission.)

Sequence studies on tRNAs have demonstrated the presence of numerous modified nucleosides. Thus human glycine tRNA (Fig. 1) contains 5-methylcytidine, 5-methyluridine (ribothymidine), 5,6-dihydrouridine, pseudouridine, N^2-methylguanosine, 1-methyladenosine, and 2'-O-methyluridine. The modified nucleosides are formed by the posttranscriptional modification of tRNA precursor molecules which are DNA transcripts and therefore consist of the four major constituents only. The processing of tRNA precursors, which are larger than mature tRNAs, involves trimming steps in addition to posttranscriptional modification (McClain, 1977; O'Farrell et al., 1978). The modification reactions, which appear to take place mainly in the cell nucleus, exhibit an extraordinary degree of specificity. For example, in human glycine tRNA (Fig. 1), ribose methylation of uridine to 2'-O-methyluridine is restricted to the fourth nucleotide residue from the 5'-end of the tRNA; no ribose methylation is found in uridine in the fifth position from the 5'-end. Similarly, base methylation of guanine is detected only in position 6 and not in position 7 (Fig. 1). Sequence studies on tRNA have provided many other examples of the great specificity of its posttranscriptional modification reactions. The great precision characteristic of the numerous modification reactions of tRNA suggests important, as yet poorly defined, functional roles of the modified tRNA constituents (Nishimura, 1972; Feldman, 1977). It is noteworthy that posttranscriptional modification of tRNA has increased during evolution. For example, Escherichia coli tRNA is methylated only half as much as mammalian tRNA, and five methylated constituents of mammalian tRNA (3-methylcytidine, 5-methylcytidine, 1-methyladenosine, N^2-methylguanosine, and N^2,N^2-dimethylguanosine) are not found in E. coli tRNA.

Among the group of tRNA-modifying enzymes, tRNA methyltransferases have been investigated most extensively (see review by Kerr, 1978). These enzymes catalyze the transfer of the methyl group from S-adenosylmethionine to specific positions in the tRNA molecule. Study of the tRNA methyltransferases has attracted attention since elevation of their activities appears to be a general feature of malignant neoplasms (Borek and Kerr, 1972). The increased enzyme activities were found to correlate with tumor growth rates (Sheid et al., 1971). These observations suggest that tRNA methyltransferases might provide potential targets for cancer chemotherapy.

Because of their potential value as anticancer agents, inhibitors of tRNA methyltransferases have been studied in several laboratories. It has long been established that the reaction product of biological transmethylations, S-adenosylhomocysteine, is a potent inhibitor of methyltransferases, including tRNA methyltransferases. In recent years, several analogues of this compound have been synthesized and their inhibitory activity investigated (Hildesheim et al., 1973; Pugh et al., 1977; Hoffman,

1978; Kerr, 1978). The most inhibitory analogue is S-tubercidinylhomo-cysteine which is even more active against tRNA methyltransferases than S-adenosylhomocysteine (Coward *et al.*, 1974; Trewyn and Kerr, 1976). Several other drugs have recently been found to inhibit tRNA methylation *in vitro*. Among these are cytokinins, isopentenyl adenosine, and tuberci-dine (Wainfan and Borek, 1967; Wainfan and Landsberg, 1973), L-dopa, dopamine, and epinephrine (Moller *et al.*, 1977; Miller and Balis, 1977), polysaccharides (Sheid and Wilson, 1970), polyanions (Liau *et al.*, 1973), alkaloids (Lee *et al.*, 1977), and intercalating agents (Liau *et al.*, 1977). However, none of these agents has been shown to reduce the methyl con-tent of mammalian tRNA *in vivo*. Cycloleucine, a competitive inhibitor of ATP:L-methionine S-adenosyltransferase (Lombardini *et al.*, 1970), was reported to inhibit RNA methylation in cultured cells (Caboche and Ba-chellerie, 1977; Amalric *et al.*, 1977), but the methylation of bulk liver tRNA was found to be normal after administration of cycloleucine to mice (Harris and Randerath, 1978, unpublished experiments).

Very few compounds have been shown thus far to cause undermethyla-tion of tRNA *in vivo* after their administration to experimental animals. These include ethionine (Rajalakshmi, 1973; Wainfan *et al.*, 1975; Kerr, 1975; Lu *et al.*, 1976a; Friedman, 1977), 5-azacytidine (Lu *et al.*, 1976b; Lu and Randerath, 1978), 5-fluorouracil (Tseng *et al.*, 1977, 1978), 5-fluorouridine (Lu *et al.*, 1976c), and 5-fluorocytidine (Lu *et al.*, 1978). It is somewhat ironical that none of these compounds is a strong inhibitor of mammalian tRNA methyltransferases *in vitro*, while the great number of compounds capable of inhibiting tRNA methylation in the test tube have not been shown to cause undermethylation of tRNA in animals.

I shall now review the actions on tRNA of compounds that have been shown to cause undermodification of animal tRNA *in vivo*.

I. Ethionine

S-Adenosylethionine, which accumulates in the livers of animals treated with ethionine, the ethyl analogue of methionine, is a very poor substrate for tRNA methyltransferases but a good inhibitor of these en-zymes (Moore and Smith, 1969; Pegg 1971, 1972). Rajalakshmi (1973) re-ported that tRNA exhibiting significant *in vitro* methyl acceptor activity in a homologous assay system could be isolated from the livers of ethionine-treated rats. This work was confirmed and extended by Wainfam *et al.* (1975) and Kerr (1975), who also characterized the undermethylated tRNA by its ability to accept methyl groups *in vitro*. Base composition analysis of tRNA from ethionine-treated mice indicated a reduction in all methylated bases of liver tRNA (Lu *et al.*, 1976a). This effect was dose-dependent and specific for the methylated bases; individual methylated components were found to be affected to different extents (Fig. 3). Possibly in response to tRNA undermethylation, tRNA methyltransferase activities were found to rise substantially after an initial depression during exposure to ethionine (Hancock, 1968; Moore and Smith, 1969; Wainfan *et al.*, 1977). Ethionine-induced methyl-deficient liver tRNA cannot be fully methylated *in vitro* by tRNA methyltransferase preparations from liver (Friedman, 1977; Tseng *et al.*, 1978; Kerr, 1978). It appears that all the methyl-deficient sites are not available for *in vitro* methylation and that even those that are initially accessible become less available after prolonged *in vivo* exposure to ethionine (Friedman, 1977). The reasons for this have not as yet been elucidated. The relationship between the action of ethionine on tRNA and tRNA methyltransferases and its hepatocarcinogenic action is also not clear. Additionally, ethionine causes ethylation of tRNA and, to a much lesser extent, of other nucleic acids (Farber *et al.*, 1967; Rosen, 1968; Ortwerth and Novelli, 1969; Pegg, 1972). Since alkylating agents are powerful carcinogens, the alkylation of nucleic acids following the administration of ethionine may conceivably be involved in the carcinogenic action of this compound.

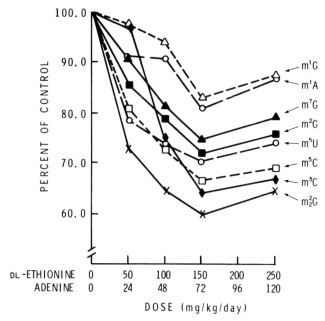

Fig. 3 Effects of DL-ethionine on methylated bases in mouse liver tRNA. (From Lu *et al.*, 1976a).

In *E. coli*, ethionine preferentially inhibits the methylation of uridine in tRNA (Tscherne and Wainfan, 1978).

II. Pyrimidine and Pyrimidine Nucleoside Analogues

Several pyrimidine and pyrimidine nucleoside analogues carrying a modification at the position corresponding to the 5-position of uracil or cytosine (Fig. 4) such as 5-fluorouracil (Tseng *et al.*, 1977, 1978), 5-fluorouridine (Lu *et al.*, 1976c), 5-fluorocytidine (Lu *et al.*, 1979), and 5-azacytidine (Lu *et al.*, 1976b; Lu and Randerath, 1979) were recently found in our laboratory to inhibit the posttranscriptional modification of pyrimidines in tRNA in a highly specific way. This effect was first observed in studies on the effects of 5-fluorouracil on tRNA in a mouse mammary adenocarcinoma (Tseng *et al.*, 1977, 1978). Bulk tRNA isolated from tissues of 5-fluorouracil-treated mice was analyzed by a radioactive derivative method for base composition analysis of RNA developed in our laboratory (Randerath *et al.*, 1972, 1974). As illustrated in Fig. 5, tRNA was first completely degraded enzymically to a mixture of ribonucleosides, which were then converted to ^{3}H-labeled nucleoside trialcohols by successive treatment with sodium metaperiodate and ^{3}H-labeled potassium borohydride. The radioactive nucleoside derivatives were separated by two-dimensional thin-layer chromatography on cellulose, located by low-temperature scintillation fluorography (Randerath, 1970), and assayed by liquid scintillation counting. Because incorporation of ^{3}H-label by this procedure is stoichiometric, the count rates obtained for individual labeled derivatives are directly proportional to the amount of the parent nucleoside in the RNA.

When this procedure was applied to bulk tRNA from 5-fluorouracil-treated tissues (Fig. 6), the following observations were made:

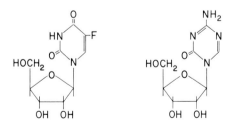

5-FLUOROURIDINE   5-AZACYTIDINE

Fig. 4 The structures of 5-fluorouridine and 5-azacytidine.

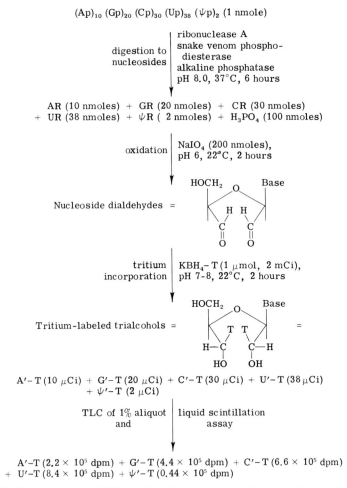

$(Ap)_{10}$ $(Gp)_{20}$ $(Cp)_{30}$ $(Up)_{38}$ $(\psi p)_2$ (1 nmole)

digestion to
nucleosides

ribonuclease A
snake venom phospho-
diesterase
alkaline phosphatase
pH 8.0, 37°C, 6 hours

AR (10 nmoles) + GR (20 nmoles) + CR (30 nmoles)
+ UR (38 nmoles) + ψR (2 nmoles) + H_3PO_4 (100 nmoles)

oxidation

$NaIO_4$ (200 nmoles),
pH 6, 22°C, 2 hours

Nucleoside dialdehydes =

tritium
incorporation

KBH_4– T (1 μmol, 2 mCi),
pH 7-8, 22°C, 2 hours

Tritium-labeled trialcohols =   =

A'– T (10 μCi) + G'– T (20 μCi) + C'– T (30 μCi) + U'– T (38 μCi)
+ ψ'– T (2 μCi)

TLC of 1% aliquot
and

liquid scintillation
assay

A'–T (2.2×10^5 dpm) + G'– T (4.4×10^5 dpm) + C'– T (6.6×10^5 dpm)
+ U'–T (8.4×10^5 dpm) + ψ'– T (0.44×10^5 dpm)

Fig. 5 Base analysis of RNA by digestion to nucleosides and chemical ^{3}H incorporation. (From Randerath *et al.*, 1972.)

1. A spot (FU' in Fig. 6), located in the right-hand lower corner of the chromatogram, was found only in tRNA from 5-fluorouracil-treated animals, not in tRNA from control animals (see also Fig. 10A). This compound cochromatographed with the ^{3}H-labeled trialcohol prepared by treatment of authentic 5-fluorouridine with sodium metaperiodate and potassium borotritide. It was derived from 5-fluorouracil incorporated into tRNA from treated animal tissues and thus allowed us to measure the incorporation of drug into tRNA. Incorporation was found to be dose-dependent.

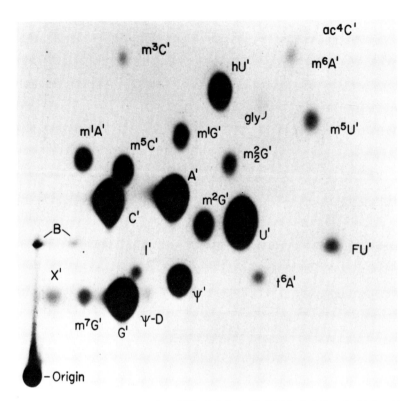

Fig. 6 Fluorogram (Randerath, 1970) of chemically ³H-labeled digest obtained from tRNA from mammary tumor of 5-fluorouracil-treated mice (Tseng *et al.*, 1978). N', a nucleoside trialcohol; B, background spot (not from RNA); ψ-D, decomposition product of pseudouridine; gly, glycerol; X, 3-(3-amino-3-carboxypropyl)uridine.

2. There was no dose-related effect of 5-fluorouracil on purines (major and modified) and cytosine and its derivatives in tRNA.

3. There was a dose-dependent reduction in the amounts of uridine derivatives modified in the 5-position of the pyrimidine ring (5-methyluridine, pseudouridine, and 5,6-dihydrouridine), while the sum of uridine and its derivatives remained unaffected at all doses of 5-fluorouracil examined. Similar observations were made for 5-fluorouridine (Lu *et al.*, 1976c).

The effects of 5-fluorouracil and its derivatives on modified uridine derivatives in tRNA were attributed previously to the incorporation of 5-fluorouridine into positions normally occupied by modified uridine derivatives, which was thought to prevent physically the modification reactions at the 5-position of uridine (see review by Heidelberger, 1975). If the decrease in the amount of each modified uridine derivative were simply due to random incorporation of 5-fluorouridine into the positions of uridine in pre-tRNA during transcription, then the percentage of decrease in each modified uridine derivative would equal the percentage of substitution of total uridine by 5-fluorouridine. However, it was found that in liver and tumor tRNA the percentage of decrease in each modified uridine derivative was much larger than the percentage of substitution at each dose; the decrease was largest for 5-methyluridine (Tseng *et al.*, 1978). Preferential incorporation of 5-fluorouridine into the positions normally occupied by modified uridine derivatives has been suggested to explain the reduction in 5-methyluridine in the tRNA from 5-fluorouracil-treated *E. coli* (Baliga *et al.*, 1969). This mechanism implies that the total decrease in modified uridine derivatives should not exceed the amount of 5-fluorouridine incorporated into tRNA following treatment with any 5-fluorouracil dose. However, it was found that, in tRNA from both normal and tumor tissue, the amount of incorporated 5-fluorouridine was smaller than the decrease in modified uridine derivatives (Fig. 7). Thus these data indicate a probable inhibition by 5-fluorouracil of enzymic modification reactions responsible for converting uridine to 5-methyluridine, pseudouridine, and 5,6-dihydrouridine during tRNA maturation, in addition to a physical replacement of uridine by 5-fluorouridine during tRNA transcription.

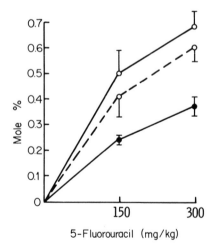

Fig. 7 Effects of a 5-fluorouracil dose on 5-fluorouridine incorporation and the amounts of modified uridine derivatives in tRNA from normal liver isolated 24 hours after treatment with a single dose of 5-fluorouracil. —, Decrease in 5-methyluridine plus pseudouridine plus hydruridine; ----, decrease in pseudouridine plus hydrouridine hU; ●, 5-fluorouridine incorporation; bars indicate. S. D. (From Tseng *et al.*, 1978.)

To obtain direct evidence for an effect of 5-fluorouracil on modifying enzymes, we determined the tRNA methyltransferase activities of extracts from control and drug-treated tissues. With *Mycoplasma hominis* or homologous methyl-deficient tRNA as the substrate, tumor enzyme catalyzed methylation faster than liver enzyme, but both reactions plateaued at the same level in about 60 minutes. Figure 8 shows the distribution of methyl groups accepted by partially methyl-deficient mouse liver tRNA (induced by ethionine treatment) during *in vitro* methylation by enzyme extracts from liver (Fig. 8A) and mammary tumor (Fig. 8B) of 5-fluorouracil-treated mice. ^{3}H-Methyl incorporation into each base was calculated as the percentage of methylation relative to total radioactivity recovered from identified methylated products. Only 5-methyluridine formation showed a sharp dose-dependent reduction, while the other methy-

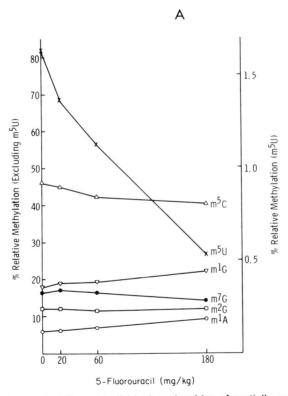

Fig. 8 *In vitro* methylation of individual nucleosides of partially methyl-deficient liver tRNA by enzymes extracted from liver (A) and mammary tumor (B) isolated 24 hours after treatment with single doses of 5-fluorouracil. Values are the average of two assays. (From Tseng *et al.,* 1978.)

(*continued*)

B

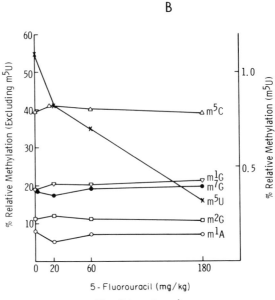

Fig. 8 (continued)

lated bases remained approximately the same. Most of the sites in the tRNA available for methylation were in cytosine and guanine moieties. The degree of methylation for individual nucleosides did not parallel the actual methyl deficiency caused by ethionine treatment. For example, *in vitro* methylation of the most deficient base, N^2,N^2-dimethylguanosine, was not detectable. In contrast, a relatively large amount of the least deficient base, 1-methylguanosine, was formed by *in vitro* methylation. When heterologous *M. hominis* tRNA, which is highly deficient in 5-methyluridine, was used as the substrate for methylation, similar results were obtained (Tseng *et al.*, 1978); again, only 5-methyluridine formation was inhibited in a dose-dependent manner after exposure to 5-fluorouracil.

Figure 9 illustrates the time course of inhibition of tRNA uracil-5-methyltransferase after a single i.p. dose of 5-fluorouracil (180 mg/kg). The enzyme activity in liver and tumor was reduced very rapidly after treatment, and over 90% of the activity was lost 6 hours after treatment. The enzyme activity had recovered very little after 24 hours, indicating prolonged inhibition.

Thus the *in vitro* methylation assays demonstrated a specific, rapid, and prolonged decrease in the activity of tRNA uracil-5-methyltransferase in liver and mammary tumor following treatment with 5-fluorouracil. In addition, base composition analysis of tRNA from 5-fluorouracil-treated tis-

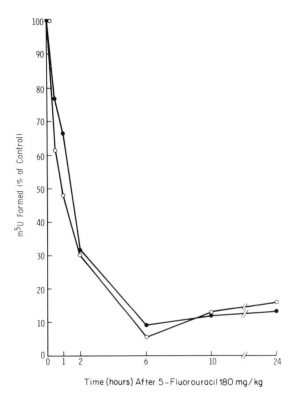

Time (hours) After 5 - Fluorouracil 180 mg / kg

Fig. 9 Time course of inhibition of tRNA uracil-5-methyltransferase in liver (○) and mammary tumor (●) following treatment with a single dose of 5-fluorouracil (180 mg/kg). The 5-methyluridine formed by dialyzed enzyme extracts with *M. hominis* tRNA as the substrate was calculated as a percentage of the control. Values are the average of two assays. (From Tseng *et al.,* 1978.)

sues indicated that the reduction in the amounts of pseudouridine and 5,6-dihydrouridine also was due at least in part to the inhibition of posttranscriptional modification reactions.

We next asked whether a cytidine analogue, 5-fluorocytidine, would exhibit related effects on the posttranscriptional modification of tRNA. Following the administration of this compound, mouse liver tRNA was found to contain both 5-fluorocytidine and 5-fluorouridine (Fig. 10). The presence of the latter suggests the partial *in vivo* conversion of 5-fluorocytidine to 5-fluorouridine derivatives. The decreased methylation of tRNA (Fig. 11) was due to prolonged dose-dependent inhibition of tRNA cytosine-5-methyltransferase and tRNA uracil-5-methyltransferase following treatment with 5-fluorocytidine; tRNA cytosine-5-methyltransferase was strongly inhibited as late as 72 hours after a single dose of 18 mg/kg (Lu *et*

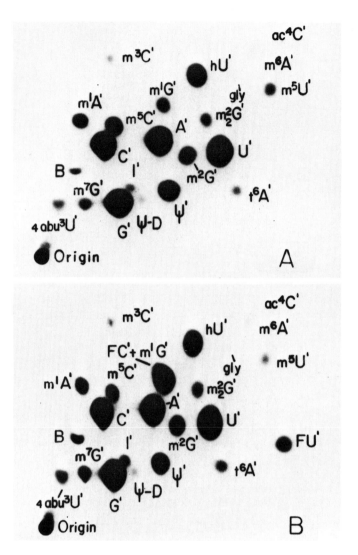

Fig. 10 Fluorograms (Randerath, 1970) of chemically ³H-labeled digests obtained from liver tRNA of control (A) and 5-fluorocytidine-treated (B) mice. For abbreviations, see legend for Fig. 6. (From Lu *et al.*, 1979.)

al., 1979). Inhibition of tRNA uracil-5-methyltransferase probably was a consequence of the *in vivo* conversion of 5-fluorocytidine to 5-fluorouridine derivatives.

The ability to inhibit the modification of pyrimidine bases in tRNA was found not to be restricted to 5-fluoropyrimidines and their nucleosides.

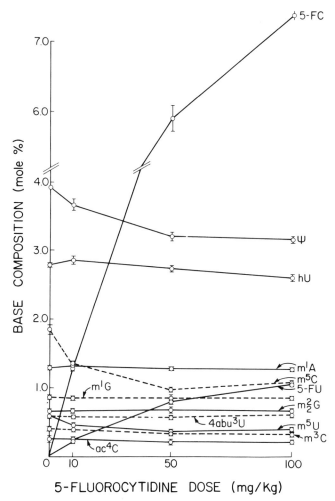

Fig. 11 Dose-dependent effect of 5-fluorocytidine on the base composition of tRNA. Mice were given one daily i.p. injection of the indicated dose of 5-fluorocytidine for four consecutive days. tRNA was isolated 24 hours after the last injection. Data are the means ± S.D. of four chromatographic analyses. 5-FC, 5-fluorocytidine incorporated into tRNA. (From Lu *et al.*, 1979.)

Thus the administration of 5-azacytidine, a nitrogen bioisostere of cytidine (Fig. 4), to mice was shown to cause a marked reduction in the 5-methylcytidine content of liver tRNA (Lu *et al.*, 1976b). This effect was dose-dependent and specific for methylation of the 5-position of cytidine; the drug had no effect on 3-methylcytidine, 4-acetylcytidine, 5-methyluridine, dihydrouridine, pseudouridine, and modified purines (Fig. 12). In

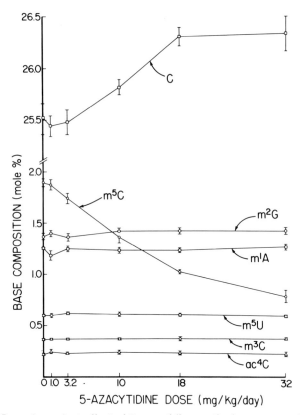

Fig. 12 Dose-dependent effect of 5-azacytidine on the base composition of tRNA. Mice were given one daily i.p. injection of the indicated dose of 5-azacytidine for four consecutive days. tRNA was isolated 24 hours after the last injection. Data are the means ± S.D. of four to six analyses. (From Lu *et al.*, 1976b.)

contrast to 5-fluorouridine and 5-fluorocytidine, 5-azacytidine was not measurably incorporated into mature tRNA, as assayed by the ^{3}H derivative procedure. A calculation showed that the maximum extent of replacement of cytidine by 5-azacytidine was less than 1 in 50 cytidine residues (Lu *et al.*, 1976b). To elucidate the mechanism underlying the effect, tRNA methyltransferases from drug-treated tissues were analyzed. The ability to catalyze the formation of 5-methylcytidine in substrate tRNA *in vitro* was greatly reduced for tRNA methyltransferase preparations from 5-azacytidine-treated liver. The inhibition of tRNA cytosine-5-methyltransferase was dose-dependent (Fig. 13) and prolonged (Fig. 14). The onset of this inhibitory effect was extremely fast; it could be detected as early as 20 minutes after i.p. administration of 18 mg/kg of 5-azacytidine.

Minimum of enzyme activity was found at 4–7 hours, at which time it was barely detectable. While tRNA cytosine-5-methyltransferase activity was inhibited at all time points studied (Fig. 14), during the first 7 hours of exposure the drug appeared to have no effect on tRNA adenine and guanine methyltransferase activities. However, 12 hours after drug administration, 1-methyladenosine, N^2-methylguanosine, and N^2,N^2-dimethylguanosine methyltransferase activities were found to increase rapidly, with a peak at about 24 hours. The increase in the activities of the purine-specific tRNA methyltransferases was also observed during chronic administration of 5-azacytidine (Fig. 13). The mechanism of this increase

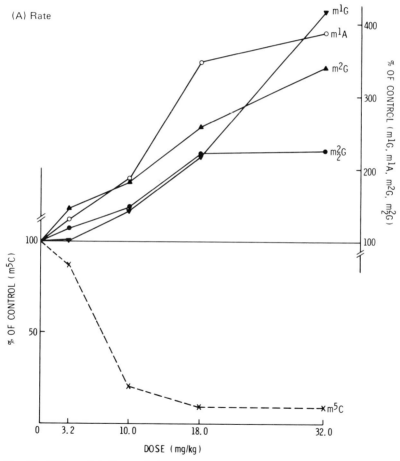

Fig. 13 Differential effects of chronic 5-azacytidine administration (four daily injections of the indicated dose) on activity (A) and capacity (B) of tRNA methyltransferases from mouse liver (See p. 292). (From Lu and Randerath, 1979.)

(*Continued*)

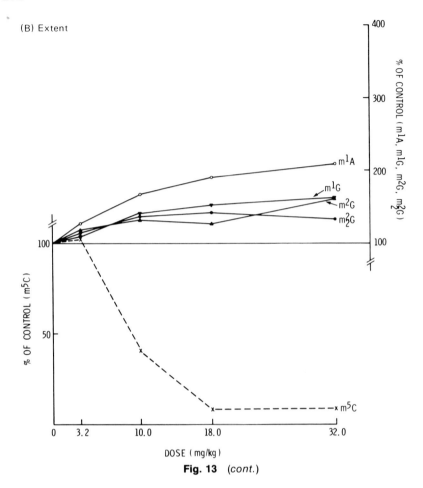

Fig. 13   (cont.)

has not yet been elucidated. It is not likely that the effect represents a response of the cell to tRNA undermethylation, in analogy to the increase in tRNA methyltransferase activities induced by ethionine (see above), because the increase in the activities of the purine-specific methyltransferases was not observed during treatment with 5-fluorocytidine in spite of undermethylation of tRNA caused by this drug (Lu *et al.*, 1979).

Effects of 5-fluorocytidine, 5-fluorouracil, 5-fluorouridine, and 5-azacytidine on tRNA and tRNA modifications are summarized in Table I.

Work currently in progress in our laboratory is directed at elucidating the mechanism(s) underlying the specific effects of the pyrimidine antimetabolites on tRNA modifying enzymes. Because these drugs are inhibitors of RNA and protein synthesis, it was of interest to investigate whether

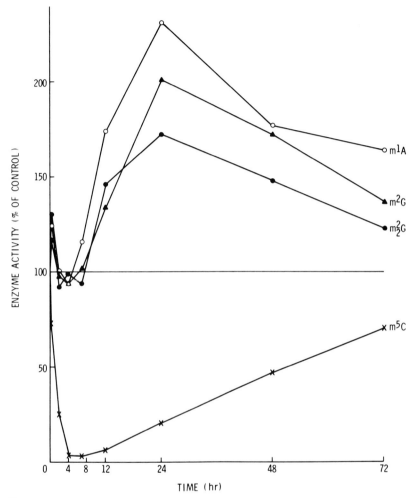

Fig. 14 Activities of mouse liver tRNA methyltransferases after a single i.p. administration of 18 mg/kg of 5-azacytidine as a function of time. (From Lu and Randerath,
1979.)

inhibition of RNA or protein synthesis had any effect on tRNA methyltransferases. Administration of actinomycin D, an inhibitor of RNA synthesis (Fig. 15), or cycloheximide, an inhibitor of protein synthesis (Fig.
16), was without effect on liver tRNA methyltransferases (W.-C. Tseng
and K. Randerath, unpublished data). Thus it appears unlikely that inhibition of RNA or protein synthesis is directly involved in the effects of
the pyrimidine analogues on tRNA modifying enzymes. The addition of

TABLE I

Effects of 5-Fluorocytidine, 5-Fluorouracil, 5-Fluorouridine, and 5-Azacytidine on tRNA and tRNA Modification

Analog[a]	Incorporation	Inhibitory effects on:[b]			
		m^5C	m^5U	ψ	hU
5-FCR	$++++$[c] $++$[d]	$++++$	$+++$	$++$	$+$
5-FU and 5-FUR	$++$	$-$	$++++$	$+++$	$+$
5-AzaCR	N.D.[e]	$++++$	$-$	$-$	$-$

[a] FCR, 5-Fluorocytidine; FU, fluorouracil; FUR, 5-fluorouridine; AzaCR, 5-azacytidine.

[b] m^5C, 5-Methylcytidine; m^5U, 5-methyluridine; ψ, pseudouridine; hU, 5-dihydrouridine.

[c] Incorporation of 5-FCR.

[d] Incorporation of 5-FUR.

[e] Not detected (<1 in 50 cytidine residues).

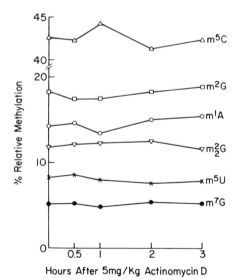

Fig. 15 Activities of tRNA methyltransferases from mouse liver after a single i.p. dose of actinomycin D. (From Tseng and Randerath, 1978, unpublished data.)

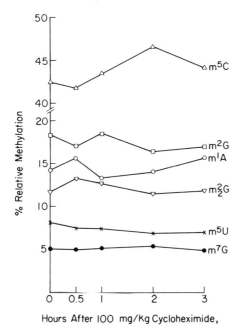

Fig. 16 Activities of tRNA methyltransferases from mouse liver after a single i.p. dose of cycloheximide. (From Tseng and Randerath, 1978, unpublished data.)

5-fluorouracil, 5-fluorouridine, 5-fluorouridine monophosphate, 5-fluorouridine diphosphate (Fig. 17), or 5-fluorouridine triphosphate (Fig. 18) to the enzyme assay had no effect on tRNA methyltransferase activities. It was also found that pretreatment of mice with an inhibitor of RNA synthesis such as actinomycin D or α-amanitin (Fig. 19) reversed the effect of 5-fluorouracil on tRNA uracil-5-methyltransferase. Other inhibitors of RNA synthesis such as D-galactosamine (Keppler, 1977) and 3-deazauridine (McPartland *et al.*, 1974) also exhibited this effect, but inhibitors of protein synthesis did not affect the 5-fluorouracil-induced inhibition of tRNA uracil-5-methyltransferase (W.-C. Tseng and K. Randerath, unpublished work). It thus appears that the inhibitory effect of 5-fluorouracil on this enzyme requires RNA synthesis. Since RNA synthesized during exposure to the drug contains 5-fluorouridine, it may be hypothesized that inhibition of the enzyme is a consequence of drug incorporation into RNA. We are currently screening RNA fractions from drug-treated tissue for inhibitory activities in tRNA methyltransferase assays. In view of the low incorporation of 5-azacytidine into tRNA, it is

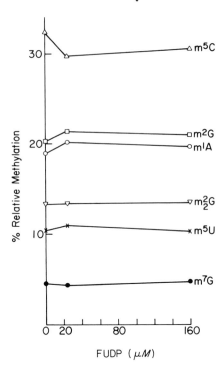

Fig. 17 Assay of tRNA methyltransferases from normal mouse liver in the presence of various concentrations of 5-fluorouridine 5'-diphosphate (FUDP). (From Tseng and Randerath, 1978, unpublished data.)

possible that the mechanism of action of this compound on tRNA cytosine-5-methyltransferase differs from that of 5-fluorouracil on tRNA uracil-5-methyltransferase. However, incorporation of 5-azacytidine into other RNAs in mammalian cells has been reported (Vesely and Cihak, 1978).

The possibility that fraudulent nucleic acids may play an active role in modifying the activities of enzymes involved in normal nucleic acid metabolism deserves further investigation. The functional properties of drug-altered tRNAs also need to be explored. Recent work in our laboratory has shown that 5-methylcytidine-deficient tRNA can be aminoacylated normally (Harris and Randerath, 1978), suggesting that 5-methylcytidine is involved in a different function of tRNA, which has yet to be determined. Drug-altered tRNAs may thus become important tools for probing the functions of modified constituents of tRNAs.

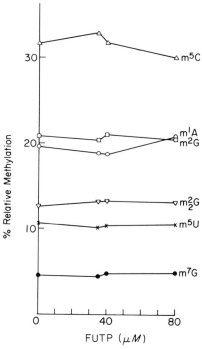

Fig. 18 Assay of tRNA methyltransferases from normal mouse liver in the presence of various concentrations of 5-fluorouridine 5′-triphosphate (FUTP). (From Tseng and Randerath, 1978, unpublished data.)

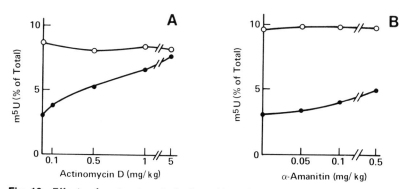

Fig. 19 Effects of pretreatment of mice with actinomycin D (A) and α-amanitin (B) on inhibition of tRNA uracil-5-methyltransferase activity. Mice were given actinomycin D or α-amanitin 1 hour before i.p. injection of 5-fluorouracil (500 mg/kg). tRNA methyltransferases were isolated 2 hours after administration of 5-fluorouracil. (From Tseng and Randerath, 1978, unpublished data.)

Acknowledgments

Work reported from our laboratory was supported by USPHS grants CA-13591, CA-16840, CA-10893(P8), and by a Faculty Research Award from the American Cancer Society (PRA-108).

References

Amalric, F., Bachellerie, J.-P., and Caboche, M. (1977). *Nucleic Acids Res.* **4**, 4357.

Baliga, B. S., Hendler, S., and Srinivasan, P. R. (1969). *Biochim. Biophys. Acta* **186**, 25.

Borek, E., and Kerr, S. J. (1972). *Adv. Cancer Res.* **15**, 163.

Caboche, M., and Bachellerie, J.-P. (1977). *Eur. J. Biochem.* **74**, 19.

Chia, L. S. Y., Morris, H. P., Randerath, K., and Randerath, E. (1976). *Biochim. Biophys. Acta* **425**, 49.

Coward, J. K., Bussolotti, D. L., and Chang, C.-D. (1974). *J. Med. Chem.* **17**, 1286.

Farber, E., McConomy, J., Franzen, B., Marroquin, F., Stewart, G. A., and Magee, P. N. (1967). *Cancer Res.* **27**, 1761.

Feldman, M. Y. (1977). *Prog. Biophys. Mol. Biol.* **32**, 83.

Friedman, S. (1977). *Nucleic Acids Res.* **4**, 1853.

Goddard, J. P. (1977). *Prog. Biophys. Mol. Biol.* **32**, 233.

Gupta, R. C., Roe, B. A., and Randerath, K. (1979). In preparation.

Hancock, R. L. (1968). *Biochem. Biophys. Res. Commun.* **31**, 77.

Harris, J. S., and Randerath, K. (1978). *Biochim. Biophys. Acta* **521**, 566.

Heidelberger, C. (1975). *In* "Handbook of Experimental Pharmacology" (A. C. Sartorelli and D. G. Johns, eds.), Vol. 38/2, p. 193. Springer-Verlag, Berlin and New York.

Hildesheim, J., Hildesheim, R., Blanchard, P., Farrugia, G., and Michelot, R. (1973). *Biochimie* **55**, 541.

Hoffman, J. L. (1978). *J. Biol. Chem.* **253**, 2905.

Keppler, D. O. R. (1977). *Cancer Res.* **37**, 911.

Kerr, S. J. (1975). *Cancer Res.* **35**, 2969.

Kerr, S. J. (1978). *Methods Cancer Res.* **15**, 163.

Lee, J. W., MacFarlane, J. O., Zee-Cheng, R. K. Y., and Chang, C. C. (1977). *J. Pharm. Sci.* **66**, 986.

Liau, M. C., Hunt, J. B., Smith, D. W., and Hurlbert, R. B. (1973). *Cancer Res.* **33**, 323.

Liau, M. C., Lin, G. W., Knight, C. A., and Hurlbert, R. B. (1977). *Cancer Res.* **37**, 4202.

Lombardini, J. B., Coulter, A. W., and Talalay, P. (1970). *Mol. Pharmacol.* **6**, 481.

Lu, L. W., and Randerath, K. (1979). *Cancer Res.* **39**, 940.

Lu, L. W., Chiang, G. H., and Randerath, K. (1976a). *Nucleic Acids Res.* **3**, 2243.

Lu, L. W., Chiang, G. H., Medina, D., and Randerath, K. (1976b). *Biochem. Biophys. Res. Commun.* **68**, 1094.

Lu, L. W., Chiang, G. H., Tseng, W.-C., and Randerath, K. (1976c). *Biochem. Biophys. Res. Commun.* **73**, 1075.

Lu, L. W., Tseng, W.-C., and Randerath, K. (1979). *Biochem. Pharmacol.* **28**, 489.

McClain, W. H. (1977). *Acc. Chem. Res.* **10**, 418.

McPartland, R. P., Wang, M. C., Bloch, A., and Weinfeld, H. (1974). *Cancer Res.* **34**, 3107.

Miller, H. K., and Balis, E. (1977). *Biochim. Biophys. Acta* **474**, 435.

Moller, M. L., Miller, H. K., and Balis, E. (1977). *Biochim. Biophys. Acta* **474**, 425.

Moore, B. G., and Smith, R. C. (1969). *Can. J. Biochem.* **47**, 561.

Nishimura, S. (1972). *Prog. Nucleic Acid Res. Mol. Biol.* **12,** 49.

O'Farrell, P. Z., Cordell, B., Valenzuela, P., Rutter, W. J., and Goodman, H. M. (1978). *Nature (London)* **274,** 438.

Ortwerth, B. J., and Novelli, G. D. (1969). *Cancer Res.* **29,** 380.

Pegg, A. E. (1971). *FEBS Lett.* **16,** 13.

Pegg, A. E. (1972). *Biochem. J.* **128,** 59.

Pugh, C. S. G., Borchardt, R. T., and Stone, H. O. (1977). *Biochemistry,* **16,** 3928.

Quigley, G. J., and Rich, A. (1976). *Science* **194,** 796.

Rajalakshmi, S. (1973). *Proc. Am. Assoc. Cancer Res.* **14,** 39.

Randerath, E., Yu, C.-T., and Randerath, K. (1972). *Anal. Biochem.* **48,** 172.

Randerath, K. (1970). *Anal. Biochem.* **34,** 188.

Randerath, K., Randerath, E., Chia, L. S. Y., and Nowak, B. J. (1974). *Anal. Biochem.* **59,** 263.

Rich, A., and RajBhandary, U. L. (1976). *Annu. Rev. Biochem.* **45,** 805.

Rosen, L. (1968). *Biochem. Biophys. Res. Commun.* **33,** 546.

Sheid, B., and Wilson, S. M. (1970). *Biochim. Biophys. Acta* **224,** 382.

Sheid, B., Wilson, S. M., and Morris, H. P. (1971). *Cancer Res.* **31,** 774.

Trewyn, R. W., and Kerr, S. J. (1976). *In* "Onco-Developmental Gene Expression" (W. H. Fishman, ed.), p. 101. Academic Press, New York.

Tscherne, J. S., and Wainfan, E. (1978). *Nucleic Acids Res.* **5,** 451.

Tseng, W.-C., Medina, D., and Randerath, K. (1977). *Proc. Am. Assoc. Cancer Res.* **18,** 105.

Tseng, W.-C., Medina, D., and Randerath, K. (1978). *Cancer Res.* **38,** 1250.

Vesely, J., and Cihak, A. (1978). *Pharmacol. Ther. A* **2,** 813.

Wainfan, E., and Borek, E. (1967). *Mol. Pharmacol.* **3,** 595.

Wainfan, E., and Landsberg, B. (1973). *Biochem. Pharmacol.* **22,** 493.

Wainfan, E., Moller, M. L., Maschio, F. A., and Balis, M. E. (1975). *Cancer Res.* **35,** 2830.

Wainfan, E., Tscherne, J. S., Maschio, F. A., and Balis, M. E. (1977). *Cancer Res.* **37,** 865.

13

Potentiation by 2'-Deoxycoformycin of the Inhibitory Effects of Cordycepin and Xylosyladenine on Nuclear RNA Synthesis in L1210 Cells

ROBERT I. GLAZER

I. Introduction

A novel approach to cancer chemotherapy has recently been developed in which the tight-binding adenosine deaminase inhibitor 2'-deoxycoformycin (dCF) (Fig. 1) (Agarwal *et al.*, 1977) is used in combination with adenosine analogues. The effectiveness of this chemotherapeutic approach is based on the ability of dCF to prevent catabolism of the anticancer drugs that serve as substrates for adenosine deaminase and whose activity is compromised in target tissues with high levels of the enzyme. Thus dCF has been shown to enhance profoundly the antitumor activity of adenine arabinoside (LePage *et al.*, 1976), as well as cordycepin (3'-

EFFECTS OF DRUGS ON THE CELL NUCLEUS
301

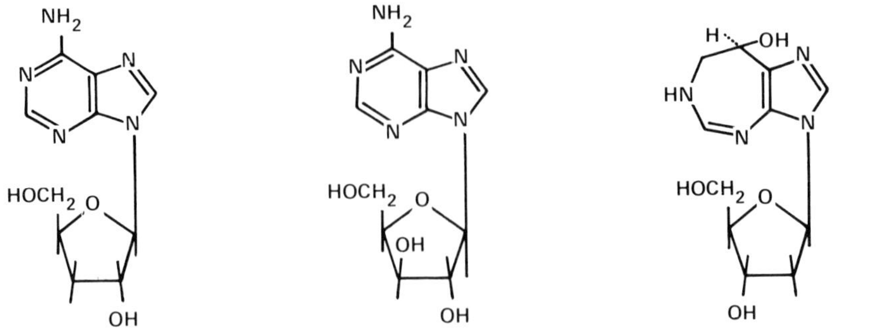

CORDYCEPIN   XYLOSYLADENINE   2'-DEOXYCOFORMYCIN

Fig. 1   Structures of cordycepin, xylosyladenine, and dCF.

deoxyadenosine) and xylosyladenine (Adamson *et al.*, 1977; Johns and Adamson, 1976). dCF also exerts an immunosuppressive action of its own which may be mediated by the decreased catabolism of intracellular metabolites of adenosine in lymphoid tissue (Adamson *et al.*, 1978).

Cordycepin is a potent inhibitor of nuclear RNA (nRNA) synthesis in normal (Glazer, 1975, 1978; Rizzo *et al.*, 1972) and neoplastic tissues (Darnell *et al.*, 1971; Glazer *et al.*, 1978; Kann and Kohn, 1972; Penman *et al.*, 1970; Truman and Frederiksen, 1969). Although its inhibitory effect in tumor cells was shown to be selective for rRNA and poly(A) synthesis (Darnell *et al.*, 1971; Glazer *et al.*, 1978; Kann and Kohn, 1972; Penman *et al.*, 1970; Truman and Frederiksen, 1969), this distinction was not found to pertain to normal or regenerating liver (Glazer, 1975, 1978; Rizzo *et al.*, 1972). That deamination of cordycepin plays a significant role in compromising its pharmacological activity was established by the marked potentiation that dCF exerted on the cytostatic effects of this drug in P388 leukemia cells (Johns and Adamson, 1976).

Another adenosine analogue that is particularly sensitive to deamination is xylosyladenine. The antitumor and growth inhibitory properties of the drug were potentiated by dCF to a degree similar to that observed for cordycepin (Adamson *et al.*, 1977). Although the mechanism of action of xylosyladenine has not been extensively studied, its structure is sterically akin to that of cordycepin (Fig. 1) and therefore might be expected to produce similar alterations in RNA synthesis. Inhibition of *de novo* purine synthesis was previously noted (Ellis and LePage, 1965; Smith and Henderson, 1976). Recent studies of the effect of xylosyladenine on nRNA synthesis have shown it to be approximately 30 times more potent than cordycepin in the absence of dCF, with both drugs being potentiated to a significant extent when deamination is blocked (Glazer *et al.*, 1978; Peale and Glazer, 1978).

This chapter details some of the findings of experiments with cordyce-pin and xylosyladenine designed to assess the influence of deamination on their inhibitory effects. More specifically, the transcription of various species of nRNA, as well as polyadenylylation and methylation of nRNA, were assessed in the absence and presence of dCF.

II. Results

All the studies described were carried out *in vitro* with murine L1210 leukemia cells. Initial experiments were designed to determine the concentration of dCF required to inhibit completely intracellular adenosine deaminase activity (Fig. 2).

dCF completely inhibited adenosine deaminase activity assayed in the 100,000 g supernatant fluid prepared from L1210 cells incubated for 30 minutes with the inhibitor. The ID_{50} for dCF was 4 $10^{-8} M$, but 1 $10^{-6} M$ dCF was used in all further experiments to ensure complete inhibition of the enzyme.

The effects of cordycepin and xylosyladenine on total RNA and DNA synthesis were next determined in the absence and presence of dCF (Fig. 3). Cordycepin was $\frac{1}{30}$ as potent as xylosyladenine as an inhibitor of total

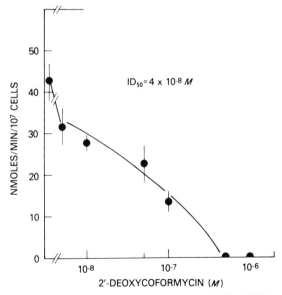

Fig. 2 Inhibition of adenosine deaminase activity by dCF. L1210 cells were incubated for 30 minutes with dCF, and adenosine deaminase was assayed in the 100,000 g supernatant fluid. (From Glazer *et al.*, 1978.)

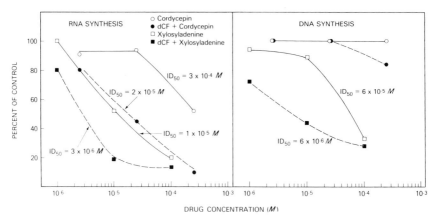

Fig. 3 Effect of dCF on the inhibitory effect of cordycepin and xylosyladenine on total RNA and DNA synthesis. L1210 cells were preincubated with or without dCF for 15–30 minutes followed by a 30-minute incubation with drug. Labeling with [³H]uridine or [³H]thymidine was carried out for 30 minutes (From Glazer *et al.*, 1978; Peale and Glazer, 1978.)

cellular RNA synthesis, but $\frac{1}{15}$ as potent as xylosyladenine in the presence of dCF.

Cordycepin did not significantly inhibit DNA synthesis during short-term incubations even in the presence of dCF. However, xylosyladenine was inhibitory, particularly in the presence of dCF, and the ID_{50} of xylosyladenine for RNA and DNA synthesis only differed by a factor of 2 (Fig. 3).

Detailed studies of the action of cordycepin and xylosyladenine on three species of nRNA were next performed. By this procedure, nuclear rRNA, non-poly(A) heterogeneous RNA (hnRNA), and poly(A) hnRNA are fractionated by the use of differential sodium dodecyl sulfate–phenol extraction and affinity chromatography (Glazer *et al.*, 1978). Cordycepin at 2.5 10^{-5} M significantly inhibited rRNA and poly(A) hnRNA, but not non-poly(A) hnRNA (Fig. 4), whereas xylosyladenine at 5 10^{-5} M inhibited predominantly rRNA and non-poly(A) hnRNA and, to a lesser extent, poly(A) hnRNA (Fig. 5).

That the ineffectiveness of cordycepin on non-poly(A) hnRNA synthesis was an artifact resulting from the rapid deamination of the drug was suggested by dose–response experiments in the presence of dCF (Fig. 6). Only at low concentrations of cordycepin in the absence of dCF was there a lack of inhibition of non-poly (A) hnRNA, whereas little if any differential inhibition was noted in the presence of the adenosine deaminase inhibitor. Similarly, the lesser sensitivity of poly(A) hnRNA to xylosyladenine in comparison to rRNA and non-poly(A) hnRNA was completely eliminated when cells were preincubated with dCF (Fig. 7).

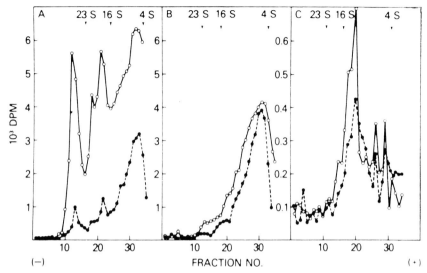

Fig. 4 Agarose gel electrophoresis of nRNA after treatment of L1210 cells with cordycepin. L1210 cells were incubated for 30 minutes with (●) or without (○) 2.5 × 10⁻⁵ M cordycepin. RNA was labeled by an additional 30-minute incubation with [³H]uridine and was fractionated into rRNA(A), non-poly(A) hnRNA (B), and poly (A) hnRNA (C). (From Glazer *et al.*, 1978.)

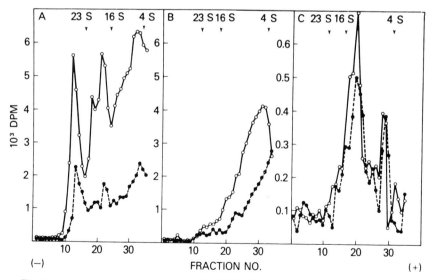

Fig. 5 Agarose gel electrophoresis of nRNA after treatment of L1210 cells with xylosyladenine. L1210 cells were incubated for 30 minutes with (●) or without (○) 5 × 10⁻⁵ M xylosyladenine. RNA was labeled by an additional 30-minute incubation with [³H]uridine and was fractionated into rRNA (A), non-poly (A) hnRNA (B), and poly(A) hnRNA (C). (From Peale and Glazer, 1978.)

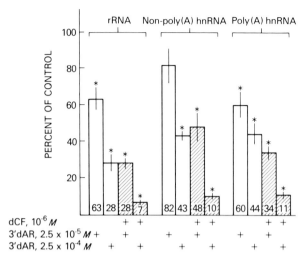

Fig. 6 Dose–response effects of cordycepin (3'-dAR) on nRNA synthesis. L1210 cells were preincubated for 30 minutes with or without 1×10^{-6} M dCF and were further incubated for 30 minutes with cordycepin. RNA was labeled by an additional 30-minute incubation with [^{3}H]uridine and fractionated. Each value is the mean $\pm$ S.E. of six assays. Numbers indicate the percentage of the control value. Asterisks indicate statistically significant differences ($P < 0.01$) versus untreated or dCF-treated controls. (From Glazer *et al.*, 1978.)

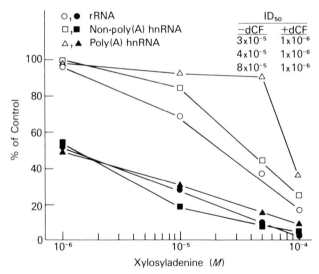

Fig. 7 Dose–response effects of xylosyladenine on nRNA synthesis. L1210 cells were incubated for 15 minutes with (solid symbols) or without (open symbols) 1×10^{-6} M dCF and incubated for 30 minutes with xylosyladenine. RNA was labeled by an additional 30-minute incubation with [^{3}H]uridine. Each value is the mean of five assays. Control values (means $\pm$ S.E., picomoles per A_{260} per 30 minutes) were: rRNA, 660 $\pm$10; non-poly(A) hnRNA, 710 $\pm$40; poly(A) hnRNA, 180 $\pm$20. (From Peale and Glazer, 1978.)

TABLE I

The Effect of dCF on the Inhibitory Effect of Cordycepin and Xylosyladenine on Nuclear Poly(A) Synthesis in L1210 Cells *in Vitro*[a,b]

	Poly(A) synthesis (pmoles/30 minutes per 5 × 10[7] cells)			
Treatment	Without dCF	Percent	With dCF[c]	Percent
Control	0.30	100	0.27	100
Cordycepin				
$2.5 \times 10^{-5}\ M$	0.24	80	0.13	48
$2.5 \times 10^{-4}\ M$	0.12	40	0.08	30
Xylosyladenine				
$1 \times 10^{-5}\ M$	0.30	100	0.13	48
$1 \times 10^{-4}\ M$	0.20	65	0.05	19

[a] From Glazer *et al.* (1978) and Peale and Glazer (1978).

[b] Incubations were carried out as described in Fig. 3 except that [³H] adenosine was used as a precursor.

[c] $1 \times 10^{-6}\ M$.

Examination of the effects of cordycepin and xylosyladenine on nuclear poly(A) synthesis showed that both drugs inhibited polyadenylylation at higher concentrations in the absence of dCF, but that a 10-fold potentiation resulted in the presence of the deaminase inhibitor (Table I). No differences in poly(A) size were produced by cordycepin upon agarose–urea

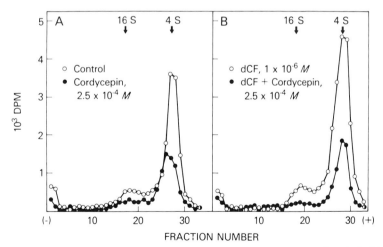

Fig. 8 Effect of cordycepin on poly(A) synthesis. L1210 cells were incubated for 30 minutes with or without $1 \times 10^{-6}\ M$ dCF and were further incubated for 30 minutes with $2.5 \times 10^{-4}\ M$ cordycepin. Poly(A) was labeled by an additional 30-minute incubation with [³H]adenosine. (From Glazer *et al.*, 1978.)

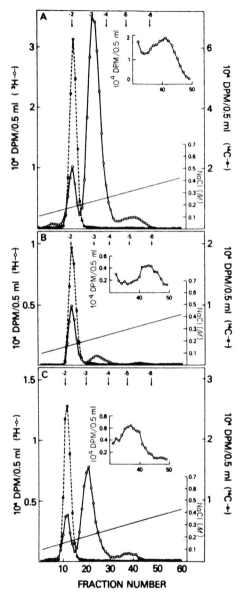

Fig. 9 DEAE Sephadex chromatography of alkaline hydrolyzates of nRNA labeled with [*methyl*-³H]methionine and [¹⁴C]uridine. L1210 cells were incubated in the absence (A) or presence of 5 ×10⁻⁵ M xylosyladenine (B) or 2.5 ×10⁻⁴ M cordycepin (C). Total nRNA was extracted, hydrolyzed, and chromatographed on DEAE Sephadex equilibrated with 7 M urea–20 mM Tris–HCl (pH 7.6). The insets represent the −5.5 oligonucleotide fraction with the scale on the ordinate decreased 10-fold (from Glazer and Peale, 1978a.)

TABLE II

Inhibition by Cordycepin and Xylosyladenine of the Methylation of nRNA in Alkaline Hydrolyzates Following DEAE Sephadex–Urea Chromatography[a,b]

	Fraction −2		Fraction −3	Fraction −5.5
	^{3}H	^{14}C	^{3}H	^{3}H
Control	130.1 ± 16.7 (100)	670.9 ± 130.7 (100)	684.8 ± 86.6 (100)	53.1 ± 5.0 (100)
Cordycepin, 2.5 × 10⁻⁴ M	54.4 ± 4.1 (42)	287.1 ± 49.1 (43)	186.9 ± 18.1 (27)	15.2 ± 1.5 (29)
Xylosyladenine, 5 × 10⁻⁵ M	71.4 ± 1.4 (55)	278.8 ± 59.4 (42)	53.7 ± 4.6 (8)	14.0 ± 1.2 (26)

[a] From Glazer and Peale (1978a).

[b] Total radioactivity represents that coinciding with the peaks at −2, −3, −5.5 charge in Fig. 9. Each value is the mean ± S.E. of three assays and is expressed as total disintegrations per minute (×10⁻³). Percentages are given in parentheses.

gel electrophoresis of poly(A) irrespective of whether or not dCF was present in the medium (Fig. 8).

Since there was previous evidence that cordycepin affected other processes besides transcription, namely, nuclear protein kinase activities and phosphorylation of nonhistone chromosomal proteins (Hirsch and Martelo, 1976; Glazer and Kuo, 1977; Legraverend and Glazer, 1978a,b), experiments were designed to assess if these drugs also affected the post-transcriptional process of methylation of nRNA. DEAE Sephadex–urea chromatography of alkaline hydrolyzates of total nRNA from L1210 cells labeled with [*methyl*-³H]methionine and [¹⁴C]uridine revealed marked inhibition of methylation of the dinucleotide (−3) and oligonucleotide (−5.5) fractions by cordycepin and xylosyladenine (Fig. 9). Equipotent concentrations of the two drugs with respect to inhibition of RNA synthesis reduced methylation in the −3 fraction (representing mainly 2′-O-methylation) by 73 and 92% and methylation in the −5.5 fraction (representing the 5′-terminus or cap) by 70–75% (Table II). Base methylation in the −2 fraction and RNA synthesis were inhibited to equal extents.

Thus the results of these experiments demonstrated that cordycepin and xylosyladenine possessed some similarities in their action on nRNA

TABLE III

Effect of Cordycepin and Xylosyladenine on S-Adenosyl-L-methionine Synthesis in L1210 Cells *in Vitro*[a,b]

Addition	S-Adenosyl-L-methionine synthesis (pmoles/hour per 10⁷ cells)			
	Without dCF	Percent	With dCF[c]	Percent
Control	13.8	100	13.0	100
Cordycepin				
2.5×10^{-5} M	14.8	107	15.9	122
2.5×10^{-4} M	13.1	97	15.9	122
Xylosyladenine				
1×10^{-6} M	12.8	93	10.6	77
5×10^{-6} M	13.7	99	5.8	42
1×10^{-5} M	12.1	88	4.7	34
5×10^{-5} M	9.8	71	2.3	17
5×10^{-4} M	2.9	21	2.1	15
ID₅₀ (M)	1×10^{-4}	—	3×10^{-6}	—

[a] From Glazer and Peale (1979).

[b] S-adenosyl-L-methionine levels were measured as described by Glazer and Peale (1978b). Incubations were carried out as described in Fig. 3, except that [methyl-³H] methionine was used as a precursor and labeling was for 1 hour.

[c] 1×10^{-6} M.

synthesis and the posttranscriptional processes of polyadenylylation and methylation. Further experiments designed to elucidate the mechanism of the inhibition of methylation of nRNA have resulted in the observation of an interesting difference between the two drugs. Xylosyladenine in either the absence or presence of dCF inhibited the synthesis of S-adenosyl-L-methionine at concentrations similar to those that inhibited methylation of nRNA (Table III). Surprisingly, cordycepin was without effect on the synthesis of this methyl donor. Neither drug directly affected nRNA methyl transferase activity *in vitro* (Glazer, unpublished data).

III. Discussion

The results of these studies indicate that the catabolism of cordycepin and xylosyladenine via adenosine deaminase has a differential quantitative effect on the two drugs with respect to inhibition of nRNA synthesis. Inhibition of adenosine deaminase by dCF reduced the ID_{50} of cordycepin for inhibition of total RNA synthesis 15-fold, while the ID_{50} of xylosyladenine was reduced 3-fold. A greater potentiation of cordycepin versus xylosyladenine by dCF was also found for the *in vitro* cytotoxicity of the two drugs in P388 leukemia cells (Adamson *et al.*, 1977), but to a lesser degree for their antitumor activity (Adamson *et al.*, 1977) and inhibition of the phosphorylation of nonhistone chromosomal proteins (Legraverend and Glazer, 1978b). These experiments suggest that the extent of potentiation of xylosyladenine and cordycepin by dCF may be related to their relative degree of utilization as substrates by adenosine deaminase. Indeed, cordycepin is deaminated three times more efficiently than xylosyladenine (Adamson *et al.*, 1977), which explains in part the differential action of dCF.

The first studies of cordycepin documented that this inhibitor had a lesser effect upon hnRNA versus rRNA and poly(A) (Darnell *et al.*, 1971; Kann and Kohn, 1972; Mendecki *et al.*, 1972; Penman *et al.*, 1970; Truman and Frederiksen, 1969). This was confirmed for low concentrations of cordycepin, but not at higher doses or in the presence of dCF where extensive inhibition of all species of nRNA was observed. In this respect, xylosyladenine did not mimic cordycepin in the absence of dCF, since non-poly(A) hnRNA was inhibited to an equal extent as rRNA and, in fact, more than poly(A) hnRNA.

It is now evident that a single site of action cannot be assigned to either adenosine analogue. Several studies have clearly shown that all eukaryotic RNA polymerases and poly(A) polymerase are equally affected by cordycepin 5'-triphosphate (Desrosiers *et al.*, 1976; Horowitz *et al.*, 1976;

Maale *et al.*, 1975; Müller *et al.*, 1977; Neissing, 1975). However, an analogous mode of action for xylosyladenine via its 5′-triphosphate may not be sufficient to explain its inhibitory effects, since it is 30-fold more potent than cordycepin but metabolizes to the 5′-triphosphate at only twice the rate (Klenow, 1963; Ellis and LePage, 1965).

Recently, competitive inhibition by cordycepin and cordycepin 5′-triphosphate of nuclear protein kinases (Glazer and Kuo, 1977; Hirsh and Martelo, 1976), and the phosphorylation of nonhistone chromosomal proteins in isolated nuclei (Legraverend and Glazer, 1978a), were demonstrated. Cordycepin and xylosyladenine were both effective inhibitors of the phosphorylation of nonhistone chromosomal proteins in L1210 cells *in vitro* (Legraverend and Glazer, 1978b). The inhibitory concentrations of cordycepin and xylosyladenine were equivalent to those that inhibited RNA synthesis. Since it is hypothesized that the phosphorylation of nuclear proteins may play a regulatory role in modulating transcription (Stein *et al.*, 1974; Park *et al.*, 1977), it is equally probable that the inhibitory action of cordycepin and xylosyladenine on transcription is mediated in part by their effects on nuclear protein kinases.

It was also ascertained that the multifarious effects of cordycepin and xylosyladenine involved impairment of the methylation of nRNA. 2′-O-Methylation and 5′-cap methylation were particularly sensitive to these drugs. Since these methylated constituents are derived mainly from rRNA (Iwanami and Brown, 1968) and mRNA (Shatkin, 1976), respectively, it is likely that cordycepin and xylosyladenine impair the normal maturation and functioning of these species of RNA.

Acknowledgment

The author expresses his appreciation to Ms. Ann L. Peale for her excellent and diligent technical assistance.

References

Adamson, R. H., Zaharevitz, D. W., and Johns, D. G. (1977). *Pharmacology* **15**, 84.
Adamson, R. H., Chassin, M. M., Chirigos, M. A., and Johns, D. G. (1978). *Curr. Chemother.* p. 1116.
Agarwal, R. P., Spector, T., and Parks, R. E., Jr. (1977). *Biochem. Pharmacol.* **26**, 359.
Darnell, J. E., Philipson, L., Wall, R., and Adesnik, M. (1971). *Science* **174**, 507.
Desrosiers, R. C., Rottman, F. M., Boezi, J. A., and Towle, H. C. (1976). *Nucleic Acids Res.* **3**, 325.
Ellis, and LePage, G. A. (1965). *Mol. Pharmacol.* **1**, 231.
Glazer, R. I. (1975). *Biochim. Biophys. Acta* **418**, 160.

Glazer, R. I. (1978). *Toxicol. Appl. Pharmacol.*

Glazer, R. I., and Kuo, J. F. (1977). *Biochem. Pharmacol.* **26,** 1287.

Glazer, R. I., and Peale, A. L. (1978a). *Biochem. Biophys. Res. Commun.* **81,** 521.

Glazer, R. I., and Peale, A. L. (1978b). *Anal. Biochem.* **91,** 516.

Glazer, R. I., and Peale, A. L. (1979). *Cancer Letters* **6,** 193.

Glazer, R. I., Lott, T. J., and Peale, A. L. (1978). *Cancer Res.* **38,** 2233.

Hirsch, J., and Martelo, O. J. (1976). *Life Sci.* **19,** 85.

Horowitz, B., Goldfinger, B. A., and Marmur, J. (1976). *Arch. Biochem. Biophys.* **172,** 143.

Iwanami, Y., and Brown, G. M. (1968). *Arch. Biochem. Biophys.* **126,** 8.

Johns, D. G., and Adamson, R. H. (1976). *Biochem. Pharmacol.* **25,** 1441.

Kann, H. E., Jr., and Kohn, K. W. (1972). *Mol. Pharmacol.* **8,** 551.

Klenow, (1963). *Biochim. Biophys. Acta* **76,** 347.

Legraverend, M., and Glazer, R. I. (1978a). *Cancer Res.* **38,** 1142.

Legraverend, M., and Glazer, R. I. (1978b). *Mol. Pharmacol.* **14,** 1130.

LePage, G. A., Worth, L. S., and Kimball, A. P. (1976). *Cancer Res.* **37,** 1481.

Maale, G., Stein, G., and Mans, R. (1975). *Nature (London)* **255,** 80.

Mendecki, J., Lee, S. Y., and Brawerman, G. (1972). *Biochemistry* **11,** 792.

Müller, W. E. G., Seiberg, G., Beyer, R., Breter, H. J., Maidhof, A., and Zahn, R. K. (1977). *Cancer Res.* **37,** 3824.

Neissing, J. (1975). *Eur. J. Biochem.* **59,** 127.

Park, W., Jansing, R., Stein, J., and Stein, G. (1977). *Biochemistry* **16,** 3713.

Peale, A. L., and Glazer, R. I. (1978). *Biochem. Pharmacol.* **27,** 2543.

Penman, S., Rosbash, M., and Penman, M. 1970. *Proc. Natl. Acad. Sci. U.S.A.* **67,** 1878.

Rizzo, A. J., Kelly, C., and Webb, T. (1972). *Can. J. Biochem.* **50,** 1010.

Shatkin, A. J. (1976). *Cell* **9,** 645.

Smith and Henderson (1976). *Can. J. Biochem.* **54,** 341.

Stein, G. S., Spelsberg, T. C., and Kleinsmith, L. J. (1974). *Science* **183,** 817.

Truman, J. T., and Frederiksen, S. (1969). *Biochim. Biophys. Acta* **182,** 36.

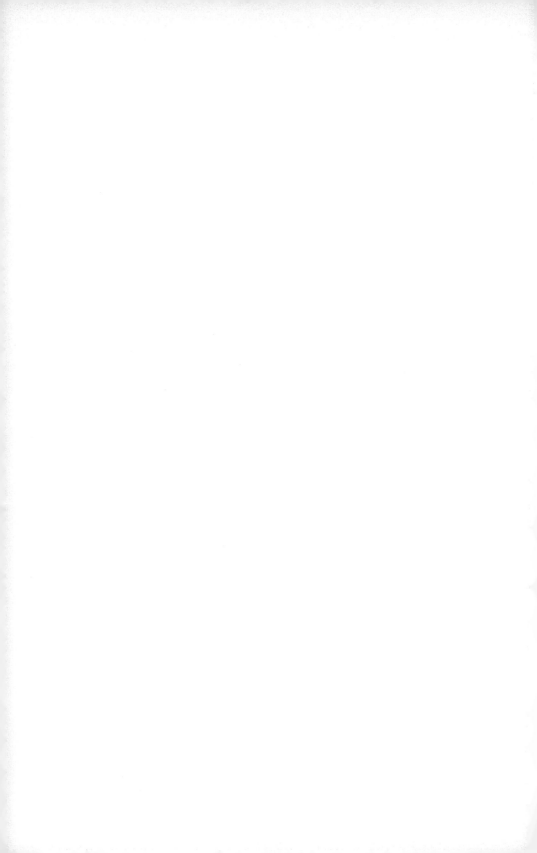

14

Effects of Chemical Mutagens on Chromosomes

T. C. HSU AND WILLIAM AU

1. Introduction

The effects of chemicals on chromosomes have been studied by cytologists for several decades, but only during recent years have activities been increased. The concern over our environment and genetic toxicity has stimulated biologists and biochemists to analyze the effects of environmental mutagens using various test systems at various levels of inquiry. Cytogenetic studies have been considered an integral part of the overall program.

Chromosomes and the mitotic apparatus are complex supramolecules. Analyses of drug effects on these molecules are less precise than those dealing with one type of molecule (e.g., DNA). However, because chromosomes represent the vehicles of genetic material, visualization of damage to chromsomes and division mechanisms contributes as much as the determination of damage to one type of molecule. Actually, studying drug effects on chromosomes has two important aspects: (1) identifying toxic agents and their degree of damage, and (2) interpreting the structure and physiology of chromosomes and the mitotic apparatus by means of drug actions. In this chapter we present a panorama of the various categories of cytogenetic effects induced by environmental chemical mutagens and discuss the differences between chemical mutagens and ionizing radiations and the correlation between chromosome damage and repair mechanisms.

II. Methodology

Cytogenetic effects of mutagens may be roughly classified in two major categories: (1) those that induce chromosome breakage (clastogens), and (2) those that induce disjunctional abnormalities (mitotic poisons). Some compounds may induce both abnormalities. Unfortunately, mitotic poisons have not received as much attention as they deserve, probably because the methodology has not been well established.

It should be borne in mind that chromosome damage in interphase cannot be observed using conventional procedures. The cell must be able to move through the cell cycle and enter the ensuing metaphase (M_1) for cytogenetic observations. This disadvantage creates difficulty in estimating the extent of chromosome damage, because DNA repair (hence chromosome restitution) plays an important role in the expression of damage.

In earlier years, plant materials were almost exclusively used for studies on clastogens. As mammalian cytogenetics has progressed, cells in culture have been employed more extensively because they offer several experimental advantages: (1) They can be propagated quickly in large quantities; (2) they have a relatively short generation time; (3) they have good chromosome characteristics; (4) they can be synchronized; (5) they can be cloned to produce single-cell colonies; and (6) they can be hybridized with other cells. In this discussion, we concentrate on mammalian somatic cells as far as experimental protocol is concerned. It is recognized that responses of cells in culture do not always parallel those of cells *in vivo;* but methodology for *in vivo* studies is still not as sophisticated.

A number of long-term cell lines, as well as short-term human lymphocyte cultures, may be used for studies on the effects of chemicals on chromosomes. The protocol is simple, namely, introducing a concentrated solution of the test compound into culture flasks to a desired final concentration. In most experiments the cells should be in the exponentially growing phase to ensure a plentiful supply of mitotic divisions in the control samples.

Knowledge of the cell cycle of the test cells is essential in such experiments. In Chinese hamster cells, the generation time is usually 12 hours, with a 2-hour G_2, 6 to 7 hour S, 3-hour G_1, and 0.5-hour mitosis. In order to estimate the effects of a given compound on various phases, the harvest times, after introduction of the drug, should be 2 hours (G_2), 5–6 hours (mid-S), and 8–10 hours (G_1). In continuous drug treatments, a 10-hour treatment means that the cell has been exposed to the drug nearly throughout the entire cell cycle. Therefore the observed chromosome damage represents the cumulative effects of the drug on all stages, not just on one phase.

To analyze drug effects on chromosomes in a specific phase it is necessary to use a pulse treatment, e.g., treating the cells for 1 or 2 hours, removing the test compound, and harvesting the cells about 8 hours later. Presumably, the damage represents that inflicted in G_1-phase. With ionizing radiations, this scheme is acceptable; but for chemical mutagens, another factor may complicate the design. Many compounds bind DNA but do not themselves induce DNA breaks. They cause disturbances only when the cells replicate DNA (S-phase). Since cytogeneticists observe chromosome aberrations in mitosis, the damage may be induced in S-phase instead of in G_1. It is possible to differentiate phase-specific damage by the appearance of chromosome aberrations (chromatid breaks versus chromosome breaks), but these are not absolute criteria.

Probably the most reasonable method for determining phase-specific chromosome damage induced by chemical mutagens is to use synchronized cell populations and observe the aberrations in prematurely condensed chromosomes (PCC). We discuss this point in Section III, C.

Many drugs are highly toxic to cells through interference with cellular DNA synthesis, especially at higher concentrations. Under continuous treatment, even 5 or 6 hours may yield practically no mitotic divisions. A few cells, especially those in late S-phase, may escape and enter mitosis. The results from the few mitotic cells in these samples do not reflect the extent of chromosome damage in the majority of cells. A remedy for this defect involves treating cell populations with drugs for a shorter period (2–4 hours) and allowing them to recover in a drug-free medium. Such pulse treatment and recovery experiments are useful in many respects. Agents that cause chromosome stickiness may cause mechanical rupturing of chromatid fibers during first anaphase (A_1), which is expressed as breaks and exchanges in second mitosis (M_2). Without recovering cell populations, a number of phenomena are not noticed.

It is well known that a number of compounds must be metabolically converted before they become carcinogens. Conversely, a mutagen may be metabolically inactivated and become innocuous. In microorganisms and in cell culture test systems, metabolic conversion may not occur. Therefore, in Ames' tests, the liver extract fraction S9 is routinely employed for testing potential mutagens to compare its effect with that of the same compounds without S9 (Ames *et al.*, 1973). Natarajan *et al.* (1976) were the first to observe that two indirectly acting nitrosamines were activated in the presence of liver extract to become potent chromosome-damaging agents. However, very few cytogenetic experiments on mutagen effects have added the liver extract in the protocol.

Table I summarizes the advantages of using S9 in the cytogenetic analyses of mutagens conducted in our laboratory. The liver extract was introduced into the cultures simultaneously with the test agent. Gentian violet proved to be a clastogen (Au *et al.*, 1978a), but S9 almost completely nullified its effects (Au *et al.*, 1978b). The clastogenic potential of some can-

TABLE I
Effect of S9 on the Frequency of Chromosome Breakage

Agent	Dosage	Effect of S9
Biological stains	(μM)	
Azure A	10	Reduction
Gentian violet	10	Inactivation
Toluidine blue	10	Reduction
Anticancer drugs	$(\mu g/ml)$	
Adriamycin	0.1–1.0	Reduction
Actinomycin D	0.1–1.0	Not significant
Bleomycin	1.0–10.0	Not significant[a]
Cyclophosphamide	50–500	Activation
AraC	1.0–10.0	Not significant
Mitomycin C	1.0–10.0	Not significant
Methotrexate	5.0–25.0	No effect
Neocarzinostatin	0.01–1.0	Inactivation
Vincristine	1.0–10.0	No effect
Experimental drugs	$(\mu g/ml)$	
NSC 279836	0.01–0.10	Reduction
NSC 287513	0.01–0.10	Reduction
NSC 299195	0.01–0.10	Reduction

[a] The presence of S9 increased the number of cells with chromosome damage significantly but not the amount of damage per cell.

cer chemotherapeutic agents was found to be enhanced, while that of others was reduced or unchanged (Au *et al.*, 1979). Therefore we strongly recommend that, in clastogen studies, S9 experiments be run concomitantly with and without S9.

A. Chromosome Aberrations

Although the description above contains some general points, it presents principles pertaining especially to analyses of chromosome aberrations. Technically, cell harvest and chromosome preparations follow the conventional procedure: Colcemid arrest of mitoses, hypotonic pretreatment, fixation with a methanol–acetic acid (3:1) mixture, and air-dried preparations stained with Giemsa or orcein. For studies on mitotic poisons, Colcemid and hypotonic solution pretreatments are avoided, since Colcemid is a mitotic poison itself. Bright-field microscopy is used for all observations and photography (for details, see Hsu *et al.*, 1977).

B. Sister Chromatid Exchange

Many cytogenetic laboratories conducting screening tests avoid using chromosome aberrations as criteria for routine work and have recently employed the sister chromatid exchange (SCE) system as a replacement. A brief description of the SCE system is presented below.

Latt (1973) discovered that cells incorporating 5-bromodeoxyuridine (BrdU) into DNA for two cycles exhibited differential fluorescence for the two sister chromatids when the preparations were stained with 33258 Hoechst. One sister chromatid showed bright fluorescence, while the other had dull fluorescence. Along the chromosomes, there may be exchange points between the sister chromatids. Under a given set of experimental conditions, the SCE frequency of a complement is relatively constant (for review of SCE, see Wolff, 1977; Kato, 1977).

An exchange between sister chromatids must involve an exchange of DNA, whatever the mechanism. This notion supported the finding that the frequency of SCE was greatly increased in the cells of patients with Bloom's syndrome, a hereditary defect causing spontaneous chromosome breaks and exchanges (Chaganti *et al.*, 1974). It appeared therefore that SCE could be utilized as a system for estimating mutagen effects. Indeed, Latt (1974), and later other investigators (Perry and Evans, 1975; Carrano *et al.*, 1978), presented evidence that many known mutagens caused a significant increase in SCE.

The test cell culture should receive a sufficient amount of BrdU for two cell cycles. DNA incorporating BrdU in both strands has a staining behavior different from that of native DNA or DNA with only one strand substituted. Either fluorescence microscopy with 33258 Hoechst (Latt, 1973) or Giemsa staining (Perry and Wolff, 1974; Korenberg and Freedlender, 1974) may be used for slide preparations.

C. DNA Repair Synthesis

Since most mutagens induce DNA damage, the extent of damage can be estimated by DNA repair synthesis. Treated cells are labeled with [^{3}H]thymidine, and grain counts over the nuclei in the autoradiographs provide quantitative data (Stich and San, 1970). This method is good as an additional check, but in our opinion it is more time-consuming than direct cytogenetic methods.

III. Cytogenetic Effects of Chemical Mutagens

Chemical agents can cause numerous types of cytogenetic responses in cells, some of which may or may not be detrimental. For example, a number of substances (phytohemagglutinin, pokeweed mitogens, and so on) can induce dedifferentiation of mature lymphocytes in culture. Collectively, they are referred to as mitogens. Many flourochromes bind DNA and can exhibit differential flourescence along metaphase chromosomes under specific optical conditions. These compounds have been effectively utilized to recognize chromosomes and chromosome segments. In this discussion, however, we limit out description to those that produce detrimental effects on chromosomes, and even within this area we can only present a brief summary.

A. Mitotic Poisons

Comparatively, mitotic poisons (agents that cause cell divisional distrubances) have received less attention from workers studying mutagenesis than clastogens (agents that cause chromosome damage). There are several reasons for this disparity. The target structures of mitotic poisons are the mitotic apparatus (spindle, centrioles, and accessory structures). These structures are made of special proteins, not DNA. Strictly speaking, mitotic poisons are not mutagens by definition. However, divisional abnormalities cause a gross chromosomal imbalance, such as aneuploidy, whose effects on cells and on individuals are more devastating than point mutations. In most systems for mutagen testing, agents causing DNA damage (mutagens) are emphasized. Since microorganisms do not employ spindles for cell division, many mitotic poisons are nonmutagens.

Even cytogeneticists pay less attention to mitotic poisons than to clastogens. In clastogen studies, a number of quantitative approaches can be taken to estimate the genetic toxicity of a given agent; but good assay systems have not yet been devised for mitotic poisons. If the mitotic poison completely arrests spindle formation, e.g., colchicine, the mitotic index can be used to give an estimate of its activity. The mitotic index should be directly proportional to the exposure time if a threshold concentration of colchicine (or other mitotic arrestant) is used. However, mitotic poisons do not always arrest metaphase. They may induce abnormal mitoses, such as endoreduplication, multipolar spindles, nondisjunction, and so on. In such cases, other methods for recording should be used.

Probably one can classify mitotic poisons in the following categories.

1. *Mitotic Arrest*

Mitotic arrestants usually block the polymerization of tubulin, the essential protein of microtubules. They do not destroy preformed microtubules. Thus existing metaphases and anaphases are not affected, but cells in prophase or interphase are not able to form a spindle, resulting in arrested metaphase. In this category are numerous types of chemicals, including colchicine, Colcemid, vincristine, rotanone, and others.

In plants meristem tissues treated with colchicine become polyploid. The arrested mitoses eventually enter interphase without anaphase movement. The metaphase chromosomes decondense as if they are in anaphase and telophase (C mitosis), and tetraploid cells result. In animal cells, the fate of arrested cells is not thoroughly understood. In most cases, the chromosomes undergo a similar series of C-mitotic behavior and presumably become polyploid. Perhaps the best illustration can be found in the work of Sawada and Ishidate (1978) on diethylstilbestrol (DES). In several types of cell cultures, DES acts as a mitotic arrestant. Metaphases were accumulated, and after prolonged exposures (24 hours or longer), most mitotic cells were found to be polyploid. When DES was removed after a period of treatment, anaphase occurred. From the data of these investigators, the regeneration of the spindle was considerably faster in the DES-treated series than in the Colcemid-treated series.

Whether arrested cells can regenerate spindles probably depends upon the concentration of the arrestant. If the concentration of the arrestant is barely above the threshold, some cells may be able to regenerate spindles despite the presence of the drug. Stubblefield (1964) observed, from time-lapse cinematographic records, that some Chinese hamster cells treated with Colcemid were able to divide following a period of metaphase block.

In cell cultures, if the mitotic arrestant is removed from the culture medium, most arrested cells regenerate spindles and enter anaphase. However, many of the recovering cells exhibit multipolarity, especially after prolonged periods of arrest. Apparently the ability to regenerating a spindle is not responsible for this anomaly, but the centrioles may be the deciding factor. During the period of arrest, daughter centrioles may become mature and separate from the mother centrioles, thus becoming capable of organizing spindles in addition to the mother centrioles (Stubblefield, 1967). In the *in vivo* condition, most arrestants are excreted or metabolically changed after a period of activity. Thus the *in vivo* situation should be similar to that observed in cell cultures in the recovery experiments.

Another factor to be considered in the analysis of mitotic arrestants is the origin of the test cells. We have known for some time that Syrian hamster cells are highly resistant to colchicine, whereas HeLa cells are extremely susceptible to colchicine. After a moderate period of exposure, HeLa cells fail to regenerate spindles; but HeLa cells are capable of recovery from mitotic arrest caused by nitrous oxide (Rao, 1968).

2. Endoreduplication

Endoreduplication is a special type of polyploid mitotic cell in which sister chromosomes lie side by side. Presumably, a cell undergoes two cycles of DNA replication without an intervening mitosis. Sister chromatids, after the second cycle of replication, are close to each other when the cell finally enters into mitosis. Sister chromosomes arranged in such a way are also known as diplochromosomes.

In cell cultures and in tumor cells *in vivo*, endoreduplicated metaphases are occasionally observed. The frequency of endoreduplication can be increased by a number of chemical agents, e.g., mercaptopyruvate (Jackson and Lindahl-Kiessling, 1963), 6-mercaptopurine (Nasjleti and Spencer, 1966), colchicine (Rizzoni and Palitti, 1973), ethidium bromide (McGill *et al.*, 1974), and a variety of other DNA-intercalating agents, antimetabolites, and antitumor antibiotics (Sutou and Arai, 1975). Most of these agents cause only a slight increase in the frequency of endoreduplication, usually near or below 10%. The most dramatic case was found with Hoechst 33258. When a combined treatment involving Hoechst 33258 and an antitumor antibiotic rubidazone, as many as 70% of metaphases exhibited diplochromosomes in the L strain (Kusyk and Hsu, 1979).

The mechanism for endoreduplication is not known. One of the difficulties in this field of inquiry is the low frequency of endoreduplicated cells that can be induced in cell populations. With the possibility of attaining

70% or more endoreduplication, significant advances will hopefully be made in this direction.

3. Abnormal Spindle Formation

Some chemicals do not prevent the formation of a spindle but cause abnormal spindle formation (multipolarity, nondisjunction, and so on). Probably all anesthetics possess such a property (Sturrock and Nunn, 1975; Grant et al., 1977). The frequency of multipolar spindles can be recorded in anaphase, but it is not feasible to identify unequivocally nondisjunction unless the distribution of chromosomes to the daughter nuclei is highly unequal. Cells with drastically unbalanced chromosome constitutions probably do not survive, but those with less disturbed aneuploidy may. The preponderance of aneuploid individuals in human and some animal populations suggests that nondisjunction in mitotic and meiotic divisions occurs frequently, and conceivably chemical and viral agents play a significant role here.

Because of the mitotic arrest and/or abnormal anaphases induced by mitotic poisons, multinucleation and micronucleation result. However, chromosome breakage can also produce micronucleation, and sticky chromosomes can result in multinucleation. Effective assay methods must be developed to analyze the effects of mitotic poisons, since they comprise an important group of environmental mutagens.

It should be pointed out that aneuploidy formation probably contributes heavily to embryonic mortality. Gropp and associates demonstrated that, in the mouse, monosomics seldom survives beyond 3 days of gestation, whereas trisomics may last much longer during fetal development, depending upon the chromosomes (Gropp, 1975; Gropp et al., 1976). In dominant lethal tests, embryonic wastage is recorded without finding the underlying causes. A certain proportion of the mortality could conceivably be ascribed to chromosome imbalance.

4. Chromosome Decondensation and Stickiness

Arrighi and Hsu (1965) reported that actinomycin D could induce a severe degree of decondensation of metaphase chromosomes. Subsequently, Shafer (1973) discovered that actinomycin D could induce G-band patterns if the cells were incubated with the drug for a few hours. The ability of drugs to induce chromosome banding is not limited to actinomycin D (Hsu et al., 1973; Goodpasture and Arrighi, 1976). Presumably prefixation induction of chromosome banding is related to the failure of proper condensation of specific chromosome regions. This may also be related to the phenomenon of sticky chromosomes.

A number of agents, particularly DNA intercalators, cause a character-istic cytological response, namely, chromosome stickiness. The meta-phase chromosomes are tangled in various degrees such that they cannot be spread even with a hypotonic solution pretreatment. Electron micro-scope observations on sticky chromosomes showed that chromatin fibers of different chromosomes may become entwined with one another (McGill *et al.*, 1974; Pathak *et al.*, 1975).

Because of the fiber entanglement, the chromosomes cannot divide nor-mally during anaphase. In severe cases, anaphase movement is inhibited, and the entire set of chromosomes enters interphase; this is similar to the colchicine effect even though the spindle is present. In less severe cases, tangled chromosomes may move during anaphase, but rupturing of chro-matin fibers may result. In such cases, agents causing sticky chromo-somes may themselves cause no chromosome breakage but may induce chromosome breakage as a secondary effect, i.e., mechanics rupturing of chromatin fibers during cell division. The broken fibers are expressed as breaks or rearrangements in the next cell generation (M_2).

Many DNA intercalators cause chromosome stickiness and/or banding. For example, quinacrine and Hoechst 33258 do not induce chromosome breakage even at relatively high concentrations, but they induce exten-sive chromosome stickiness (Hsu *et al.*, 1977). Our unpublished data show that azure and toluidine blue also belong in this category. During cell division, many chromosome fibers are apparently ruptured, because in M_2 a significantly higher frequency of breakage (mostly of the chromo-some type) is observed. On the other hand, ethidium bromide, which also induces sticky chromosomes, is a clastogen (Hsu and Au, unpublished data).

Hoechst 33258 has another peculiar effect. It induces decondensation specifically in the heterochromatin regions of mouse (*Mus musculus*) chromosomes (Hilwig and Gropp, 1973).

B. Clastogens

Cytogeneticists have been paying more attention to clastogenic effects of chemical mutagens than to any other type of cytogenetic toxicity. Al-though different drugs have different mechanisms of action and the mech-anisms of action of many of them have not been elucidated, all types of chromosome aberrations induced by radiations have been found in drug-treated cells.

When a cell is irradiated, regardless of the phase of the cell cycle, le-sions are induced. The lesions may subsequently be repaired, or may per-sist. The types of aberration in M_1 and the time of cell harvest usually tell in which phase irradiation was performed. For example, chromosome-type aberrations (acentric fragments, rings, dicentrics) indicate that the damage was incurred in G_1 phase, whereas chromatid-type aberrations (chromatid breaks, gaps, exchanges, interstitial deletions, and so on) indicate that the damage was induced in S- and G_2-phases. Once the irradiation stops, generally no new lesions are created; the so-called delayed effect is a rare event. Chemical clastogens, on the other hand, behave differently. Many drugs cause DNA damage, e.g., cross-linking, but do not immediately cause chromosome breakage. Breakage usually occurs when the cell enters S-phase. Cytogenetic analyses of clastogens rely on the recording of chromosome aberrations in metaphase. In such cases, cells treated with a drug in G_1-phase do not express G_1-type aberrations but exhibit S- or G_2-type aberrations. Therefore the situation for chemical clastogens and radiation is considerably different. Furthermore, a persistent effect is common with chemicals, presumably because they continue to react with cellular DNA in one way or another, thereby continuing to create new lesions in the following cell generations (Hsu *et al.*, 1975).

Another major difference between radiation-induced and chemical-induced chromosome aberrations is that many drugs induce a nonrandom distribution of breaks. Incorporation of BrdU causes several highly specific breakpoints in Chinese hamster chromosomes (Hsu and Somers, 1961), while hydroxylamine causes a different set of localized lesions (Somers and Hsu, 1962). The most well-known drug that induces preferential breaks in constitutive heterochromatin areas is mitomycin C (Cohen and Shaw, 1964; Hoehn and Martin, 1973; Hsu, 1975). Actinomycin D preferentially induces damage in nucleolus organizer regions (Pathak *et al.*, 1975). Probably all alkylating agents can induce some degree of nonrandom distribution of chromosome breaks, but no detailed data are available.

C. Prematurely Condensed Chromosomes

Since Johnson and Rao (1970) discovered that an interphase cell could be induced to condense its chromosomes prematurely when such a cell was fused with a mitotic cell, this phenomenon has been employed to study chromosome damage induced by radiation (Waldren and Johnson, 1974; Hittelman and Rao, 1974a) and by chemical mutagens (Hittelman and Rao, 1974b). As mentioned, assessment of cytogenetic damage must rely on the damaged cells moving into M_1 or M_2 for microscopic examination. Severely damaged cells may fail to enter M_1, and those entering M_1 may have lesions repaired. In drug-treated cells, phase determination cannot be critically identified by examining metaphases, because some drugs do not induce lesions in G_1 and others do.

PCCs therefore provide a means for examining the chromosomes of interphase. Hittelman and Rao (1974c) have shown that bleomycin can induce breaks in G_1 chromosomes, whereas the majority of drugs do not until S-phase is reached. The PCC procedure also provides a method for the analysis of repair potential (Hittelman and Rao, 1974c; Sognier *et al.*, 1979). Unfortunately this very useful tool has not been capitalized on by most cytogeneticists, but in future studies of drug effects, PCCs should yield much pertinent information in the field of genetic toxicology.

D. Sister Chromatid Exchange

The method for visualizing SCEs (Latt, 1973) has created an additional tool for studies on mutagen effects. The SCE system of testing mutagens has some advantages over the classic system of scoring chromosome aberrations; namely, SCE recording requires no interpretation, hence is more amenable to routine work by technicians. Another advantage is that, in most cases, induction of SCE requires a lower concentration than that needed to induce chromosome breaks. On the other hand, SCE also has some shortcomings. The experiments require BrdU incorporation for two cell cycles; when the test compound delays the cell cycle time, one must take multiple samples in order to obtain a sample in which SCE is manifested. Moreover, the mechanism for SCE still has not yet been elucidated. Induction of SCE may have a mechanism different from that of chromosome breakage. Some agents that can induce a high frequency of chromosome breakage, e.g., X rays and bleomycin, do not induce a significant increase in SCE. Therefore much work is required in this area of research before SCE can be used as a routine assay procedure for environmental mutagens.

E. Drug Resistance

Several cases of drug resistance showed strong evidence for gene amplification in mammalian systems (Alt *et al.*, 1978). Biedler and Spengler (1976) found that methotrexate-resistant cells contained long chromosome segments (HSRs) stained homogeneously in G-band preparations. Whether HSRs indeed represent amplified genes (in the case of methotrexate resistance, genes determining dihydrofolic reductase) has not yet been verified, but a strong possibility exists that they do.

IV. Discussion

Studies on chemical clastogens have led to a modification of the classic concept of chromosome breakage. Prior to studies on chemical mutagens, cytological data on the effects of external agents on chromosomes were based primarily on experiments involving ionizing radiations. The general conclusion was that the distribution of induced breaks along chromosomes was random. This conclusion led to an important concept, namely, the probability that chromosome breaks occur at precisely the same loci is extremely small. Since many chromosome aberrations (e.g., inversion, translocation, interstitial deletion, and so on) require two breaks each, the probability that the same aberration will occur at precisely the same breakpoints is so small that for practical purpose it can be disregarded. Biologists have utilized this concept in tracing relationships among individuals, populations, races, and species. Since the same inversion or translocation does not recur, it must come from one original aberration. Thus two individuals, regardless of their present location, are considered related if they share a common inversion or translocation. Similarly, in karyological analyses of cell populations *in vitro*, marker chromosomes (abnormal chromosomes with distinctive morphology and, more recently, banding patterns) are considered strain-specific. For example, several investigators have identified four to six marker chromosomes in the HeLa line (Nelson-Rees *et al.*, 1975; Lavappa *et al.* 1976; Heneen, 1976). Any cell line exhibiting HeLa marker chromosomes was considered HeLa contamination because, according to the classic concept, identical chromosome rearrangements cannot recur. This approach is largely correct, but adjustment must be made in view of recent data on cancer chromosomes and drug-induced chromosome damage.

Cytogeneticists have analyzed several types of human neoplasms, employing a number of cases for each type. The most extensively recorded neoplasm has been chronic myelogenous leukemia. The well-known Philadelphia chromosome, a specific anomaly in the overwhelming majority of cases, involved translocation of the long arm of chromosome 22 to the terminal portion of the long arm of chromosome 9 (Rowley, 1973). Since all cases were independent, the specific rearrangement must have occurred hundreds or even thousands of times. Similarly, a specific chromosome anomaly has been found in Burkitt lymphomas (Manolov and Manolova, 1972), retinoblastomas (Orye *et al.*, 1974), and others. Therefore nonrandom aberrations can and do recur, not only once but numerous times.

Nonrandom chromosome breaks located in heterochromatic regions should be particularly common, since some chemical agents, e.g., mitomycin C, can preferentially induce damage in these chromosome segments. Thus when a cell receives multiple breaks in heterochromatic regions, nonrandom translocations can again occur easily and repeatedly. In murine and human karyotypes, constitutive heterochromatins are located in the paracentromeric regions. Breaks occurring in these regions can result in centric fusions and total arm translocations, and some of these may involve the same segments. In the HeLa line, marker chromosome 1 is the product of a total arm translocation between the long arm of chromosome 1 and the long arm of chromosome 3. A chemical with an affinity for heterochromatin can conceivably induce such translocations. Therefore finding a HeLa marker chromosome 1 does not necessarily suggest that the cell line in question is a HeLa contaminant. Indeed, Pathak *et al.* (1979) found such a chromosome in a pleural effusion sample of a patient with breast cancer. Cytological preparations were made directly from the fluids without cell culture. Finding similar marker chromosomes for the identification of cell line contamination, though highly accurate, is not an absolute assurance. On the other hand, it is also a fallacy to claim that, because of the possibility of recurring aberrations, all cell lines are bona fide original lines. Cell line contamination is prevalent in many laboratories, and marker chromosomes are still extremely useful objects for use in throwing suspicion on a cell population unless other facts indicate the opposite.

In the human population, a number of congenital genetic traits have been found to be related to defective DNA repair systems. These syndromes apparently represent different biochemical defects and their cytological expression. The following synopsis briefly presents the cytogenetic observations for these diseases.

Syndrome	Sensitive to:	Significant chromosome damage induced by:
Ataxia telangiectasia	Ionizing radiation	X rays
Faconi's anemia	Cross-linking agents	Mitomycin C
Xeroderma pigmentosum (XP)	Ultraviolet (UV) light	UV light
Bloom's syndrome	Inconclusive	—

San *et al.* (1977) investigated the correlation between induced chromosome damage and repair deficiencies in XP patients. They analyzed fibroblast cultures from four XP patients with different DNA deficiencies in the ability to repair NQO and *N*-acetoxy-2-AAF damage. The amount of chromosome damage induced by these two agents increased corresponding to the decrease in repair ability in these four cell lines. On the other hand, xeroderma cells have been known to be proficient in the repair of DNA damage induced by alkylating agents such as (MNNG). These investigators found no significant difference in chromosome breakage induced by MNNG in XP cells and normal human cells. From these data, it appears that chromosome breakage corresponds well with defects in DNA repair mechanisms.

Interestingly, among the repair-deficient syndromes, only patients with Bloom's syndrome have shown an increased spontaneous rate of SCEs (Chaganti *et al.*, 1974; Latt *et al.*, 1975; Bartram *et al.*, 1976). In XP patients, the deficiency in ability to repair uv-induced damage is reflected in an elevated rate of induced SCEs (Schonwald and Passarge, 1977). Also of interest is the finding that an increased rate of SCE occurred in XP cells exposed to agents believed to be not normally effective, e.g., MMS, MNNG (Cleaver, 1977; Wolff *et al.*, 1977). Thus a great deal remains to be explored with regard to DNA repair defects, chromosome damage, and SCE.

Because of the differences in the mode of action of different chemical agents, analyses of the genetic toxicity of drugs should be considered only at the infant stage. Cytogeneticists must advantageously utilize information obtained by biochemists, molecular biologists, and parmacologists for their own studies on clastogens and mitotic poisons, which may provide a return of information to biochemists. Much more information is expected to surface in the future, especially on mitotic poisons and other aspects of cytogenetic toxicity.

Acknowledgments

These studies were supported in part by research grants ES-01304 from the National Institute of Environmental Health Sciences and ENV 76-82241 from the National Science Foundation.

References

Alt, F. W., Kellems, R. E., Bertino, J. R., and Schimke, R. T. (1978). Selective multiplication of dihydrofolate reductase genes in methotrexate-resistant variants of cultured murine cells. *J. Biol. Chem.* **253,** 1357–1370.

Ames, B. N., Durston, W. E., Yamasaki, E., and Lee, F. D. (1973). Carcinogens are mutagens: A simple test system combining liver homogenates for activation and bacteria for detection. *Proc. Natl. Acad. Sci. U.S.A.* **70,** 2281–2285.

Arrighi, F. E., and Hsu, T. C. (1965). Experimental alteration of metaphase chromosome morphology. *Exp. Cell Res.* **39,** 305–318.

Au, W., Pathak, S., Collie, C. J., and Hsu, T. C. (1978a). Cytogenetic toxicity of gentian violet and crystal violet on mammalian cells *in vitro*. *Mutat. Res.* **58,** 269–276.

Au, W., Butler, M. A., Bloom, S. E., and Matney, T. S. (1978b). Further study of the genetic toxicity of gentian violet. *Mutat. Res.* **66,** 103–112.

Au, W., Johnston, D. A., Collie, C. J., and Hsu, T. C. (1979). Short-term cytogenetic assays of nine cancer chemotherapeutic drugs with metabolic activation. *Cancer Res.* (Submitted for publication).

Bartram, C. R., Koske-Westphal, T., and Passarge, E. (1976). Chromatid exchanges in ataxia telangiectasia, Bloom syndrome, Werner syndrome and xeroderma pigmentosum. *Ann. Hum. Genet.* **40,** 79–86.

Biedler, J. L., and Spengler, B. A. (1976). Metaphase chromosome anomaly: Association with drug resistance and cell-specific products. *Science* **191,** 185–187.

Carrano, A. V., Thompson, L. H., Lindl, P. A., and Minkler, J. L. (1978). Sister chromatid exchange as an indicator of mutagenesis. *Nature (London)* **271,** 551–553.

Chaganti, R. S. K., Schonberg, S., and German, J. (1974). A many fold increase in sister chromatid exchanges in Bloom's syndrome lymphocytes. *Proc. Natl. Acad. Sci. U.S.A.* **71,** 4508–4513.

Cleaver, J. E. (1977). Repair replication and sister chromatid exchanges as indicators of excisable and non-excisable damage in human (xeroderma pigmentosum) cells. *J. Toxicol. Environ. Health* **2,** 1387–1394.

Cohen, M. M., and Shaw, M. W. (1964). Effects of mitomycin C on human chromosomes. *J. Cell Biol.* **23,** 386–395.

Goodpasture, C. E., and Arrighi, F. E. (1976). Effects of food seasonings on the cell cycle and chromosome morphology of mammalian cells *in vitro* with reference to tumeric. *Food Cosmet. Toxicol.* **14,** 9–14.

Grant, C. J., Powell, J. N., and Radford, S. G. (1977). The induction of chromosomal abnormalities by inhalation anaesthetics. *Mutat. Res.* **46,** 177–184.

Gropp, A. (1975). Developmental failure due to monosomy and trisomy. *In* "New Approaches to the Evaluation of Abnormal Development" (D. Neubert and H. J. Merker, eds.), pp. 361–374. Thieme, Stuttgart.

Gropp, A., Putz, B., and Zimmermann, U. (1976). Autosomal monosomy and trisomy causing developmental failure. *Curr. Top. Pathol.* **62,** 177–192.

Heneen, W. K. (1976). HeLa cells and their possible contamination of other cell lines: Karyotype studies. *Hereditas* **82,** 217–248.

Hilwig, I., and Gropp, A. (1973). Decondensation of constitutive heterochromatin in L cell chromosomes by a benzimidazole compound ("33258 Hoechst"). *Exp. Cell Res.* **81,** 474–477.

Hittelman, W. N., and Rao, P. N. (1974a). Premature chromosome condensation. I. Visualization of X-ray-induced chromosome damage in interphase cells. *Mutat. Res.* **23,** 251–258.

Hittelman, W. N., and Rao, P. N. (1974b). Premature chromosome condensation. II. The nature of chromosome gaps produced by alkylating agents and ultraviolet light. *Mutat. Res.* **23,** 259–266.

Hittelman, W. N., and Rao, P. N. (1974c). Bleomycin-induced damage in prematurely condensed chromosomes and its relationship to cell cycle progression in CHO cells. *Cancer Res.* **34,** 3433–3439.

Hoehn, H., and Martin, G. M. (1973). Clonal variants of constitutive heterochromatin of human fibroblasts after recovery from mitomycin treatment. *Chromosoma* **43,** 203–210.

Hsu, T. C. (1975). Chromosome structure. A possible function of constitutive heterochromatin: The bodyguard hypothesis. *Genetics* **79,** 137–150.

Hsu, T. C., and Somers, C. E. (1961). Effect of 5-bromodeoxyuridine on mammalian chromosomes. *Proc. Natl. Acad. Sci. U.S.A.* **47,** 396–403.

Hsu, T. C., Pathak, S., and Shafer, D. A. (1973). Induction of chromosome crossbanding by treating cells with chemical agents before fixation. *Exp. Cell Res.* **79,** 484–487.

Hsu, T. C., Pathak, S., and Kusyk, C. (1975). Continuous induction of chromatid lesions by DNA intercalating compounds. *Mutat. Res.* **33,** 417–420.

Hsu, T. C., Collie, C. J., Lusby, A. F., and Johnston, D. A. (1977). Cytogenetic assays of chemical clastogens using mammalian cells in culture. *Mutat. Res.* **45**, 233–247.

Jackson, J. F., and Lindahl-Kiessling, K. (1963). Polyploidy and endoreduplication in human leukocyte cultures treated with β-mercaptopyruvate. *Science* **141**, 424–425.

Johnson, R. T., and Rao, P. N. (1970). Mammalian cell fusion: Induction of premature chromosome condensation in interphase nuclei. *Nature (London)* **226**, 717–722.

Kato, H. (1977). Spontaneous and induced sister chromatid exchanges as revealed by the BUdR labelling method. *Int. Rev. Cytol.* **49**, 55–97.

Korenberg, J. R., and Freedlender, E. F. (1974). Ciemsa technique for the detection of sister chromatid exchanges. *Chromosoma* **48**, 355–360.

Kusyk, C., and Hsu, T. C. (1979). Induction of high frequencies of endoreduplication in mammalian cell cultures with 33258 Hoechst and rubidazone. *Cytogenet. Cell Genet.*

Latt, S. A. (1973). Microfluorometric detection of deoxyribonucleic acid replication in human metaphase chromosomes. *Proc. Natl. Acad. Sci. U.S.A.* **70**, 3395–3399.

Latt, S. A. (1974). Sister chromatid exchanges, indices of human chromsome damage and repair: Detection by fluorescence and induction by mitomycin C. *Proc. Natl. Acad. Sci. U.S.A.* **71**, 3162–3166.

Latt, S. A., Stetten, G., Juergens, L. A., Buchanan, G. R., and Gerald, P. S. (1975). Induction by alkylating agents of sister chromatid exchanges and chromatid breaks in Fanconi's anemia. *Proc. Natl. Acad. Sci. U.S.A.* **72**, 4066–4070.

Lavappa, K. S., Macy, M. L., and Shannon, J. E. (1976). Examination of ATCC stocks for HeLa marker chromosomes in human cell lines. *Nature (London)* **259**, 211–213.

McGill, M., Pathak, S., and Hsu, T. C. (1974). Effects of ethidium bromide on mitosis and chromosomes: A possible material basis for chromosome stickiness. *Chromosoma* **47**, 157–167.

Manolov, G., and Manolova, Y. (1972). African Burkitt's lymphomas 14qt. *Nature (London)* **237**, 33–34.

Nasjleti, C. E., and Spencer, H. H. (1966). Chromosome damage and polyploidization induced in human peripheral leukocytes *in vivo* and *in vitro* with nitrogen mustard, 6-mercaptopurine, and A-649. *Cancer Res.* **26**, 2437–2443.

Natarajan, A. T., Tates, A. D., Van Buul, P. P. W., Meijers, M., and de Vogel, N. (1976). Cytogenetic effects of mutagens/carcinogens after activation in a microsomal system *in vitro*. I. Induction of chromosome aberrations and sister chromatid exchanges by diethylnitrosamine (DEN) and dimethylnitrosamine (DMN) in CHO cells in the presence of rat liver microsomes. *Mutat. Res.* **37**, 83–90.

Nelson-Rees, W. A., Flandermeyer, R. R., and Hawthorne, P. K. (1975). Distinctive banded marker chromosomes of human tumor cell lines. *Int. J. Cancer* **16**, 74–82.

Orye, E., Delbeke, M. J., and Vandenabeele, B. (1974). Retinoblastoma and long arm deletion of chromosome 13. Attempts to define the deleted segment. *Clin. Genet.* **5**, 457–464.

Pathak, S., McGill, M., and Hsu, T. C. (1975). Actinomycin D effects on mitosis and chromosomes: Sticky chromatids and localized lesions. *Chromosoma* **50**, 79–88.

Pathak, S., Siciliano, M. J., Cailleau, R., Wiseman, C. L., and Hsu, T. C. (1979). A human breast adenocarcinoma with chromosome and isoenzyme markers similar to those of the HeLa line. *J. Natl. Cancer Inst.* (in press).

Perry, P. E., and Evans, H. J. (1975). Cytological detection of mutagen-carcinogen exposure by sister chromatid exchange. *Nature (London)* **258**, 121–125.

Perry, P. E., and Wolff, S. (1974). New Giemsa method for the differential staining of sister chromatids. *Nature (London)* **251**, 156–158.

Rao, P. N. (1968). Mitotic synchrony in mammalian cells treated with nitrous oxide at high pressure. *Science* **160**, 774–776.

Rizzoni, M., and Palitti, F. (1973). Regulatory mechanism of cell division. I. Colchicine-induced endoreduplication. *Exp. Cell Res.* **77**, 450–458.

Rowley, J. D. (1973). A new consistant chromosomal abnormality in chronic myelogenous leukemia identified by quinacrine fluorescence and Giemsa staining. *Nature (London)* **243**, 290–293.

San, R. H. C., Stich, W., and Stich, H. F. (1977). Differential sensitivity of xeroderma pigmentosum cells of different repair capacities towards the chromosome breaking action of carcinogens and mutagens. *Int. J. Cancer* **20**, 181–187.

Sawada, M., and Ishidate, M., Jr. (1978). Colchicine-like effect of diethylstilbestrol (DES) on mammalian cells *in vitro*. *Mutat. Res.* **57**, 175–182.

Schonwald, A. D., and Passarge, E. (1977). UV-light induced sister chromatid exchanges in xeroderma pigmentosum lymphocytes. *Hum. Genet.* **36**, 213–218.

Shafer, D. A. (1973). Banding chromosomes during G_2 with actinomycin D. *Mamm. Chromosomes Newl.* **14**, 16.

Sognier, M. A., Hittelman, W. N., and Rao, P. N. (1979). The effect of DNA repair inhibitors on the induction and repair of bleomycin-induced chromosome damage. *Mutat. Res.* **60**, 61–72.

Somers, C. E., and Hsu, T. C. (1962). Chromosome damage induced by hydroxylamine in mammalian cells. *Proc. Natl. Acad. Sci. U.S.A.* **48**, 937–953.

Stich, H. F., and San, R. H. C. (1970). DNA repair and chromatid anomalies in mammalian cells exposed to 4-nitroquinoline-1-oxide. *Mutat. Res.* **10**, 389–404.

Stubblefield, E. (1964). DNA synthesis and chromosomal morphology of Chinese hamster cells cultured in media containing *N*-deacetyl-*N*-methylcolchicine (Colcemid). *In* "Cytogenetics of Cells in Culture" (R. J. C. Harris, ed.), Symposia of the International Society for Cell Biology, Vol. 3, pp. 223–248. Academic Press, New York.

Stubblefield, E. (1967). Centriole replication in a mammalian cell. *In* "The Proliferation and Spread of Neoplastic Cells", 21st Annual Symposium on Fundamental Cancer Research, pp. 175–193. Williams & Wilkins, Baltimore, Maryland.

Sturrock, J. E., and Nunn, J. F. (1975). Mitosis in mammalian cells during exposure to anesthetics. *Anesthesiology* **43**, 21–33.

Sutou, S., and Arai, Y. (1975). Possible mechanisms of endoreduplication induction. *Exp. Cell Res.* **92**, 15–22.

Waldren, C. A., and Johnson, R. T. (1974). Analysis of interphase chromosome damage by means of premature chromosome condensation after X- and ultraviolet-irradiation. *Proc. Natl. Acad. Sci. U.S.A.* **71**, 1137–1141.

Wolff, S. (1977). Sister chromatid exchange. *Annu. Rev. Genet.* **11**, 183–201.

Wolff, S., Rodin, B., and Cleaver, J. E. (1977). Sister chromatid exchanges induced by mutagenic chemicals in normal and xeroderma pigmentosum cells. *Nature (London)* **265**, 347–349.

The Influence of Nitrosoureas on Chromatin Nucleosomal Structure and Function

MARK E. SMULSON, S. SUDHAKAR, K. D. TEW,
T. R. BUTT, and D. B. JUMP

Initially we were led to the studies outlined below by observations that a number of carcinogenic and cytotoxic agents markedly reduced intracellular levels of NAD (Schein, 1969; Schein and Loftus, 1968). The nonhistone protein poly ADP-ribose polymerase (Fig. 1) is an enzyme tightly associated with eukaryotic chromatin. This enzyme consumes considerable intracellular NAD for the modification of various nuclear proteins. Origi-

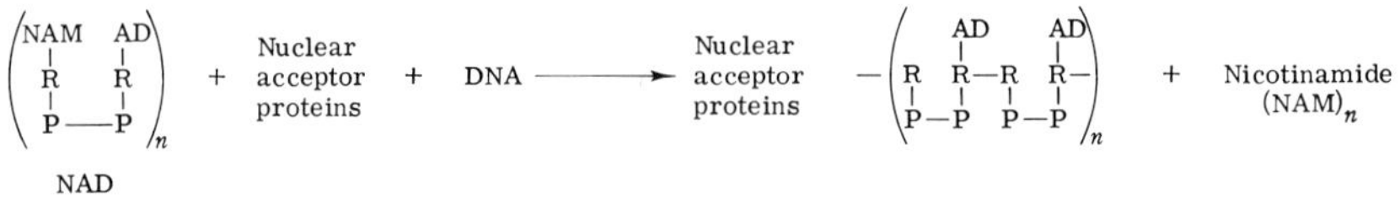

$$\begin{pmatrix} \text{NAM} & \text{AD} \\ | & | \\ R & R \\ | & | \\ P\!-\!\!-\!P \end{pmatrix}_n + \begin{matrix} \text{Nuclear} \\ \text{acceptor} \\ \text{proteins} \end{matrix} + \text{DNA} \longrightarrow \begin{matrix} \text{Nuclear} \\ \text{acceptor} \\ \text{proteins} \end{matrix} - \begin{pmatrix} & \text{AD} & & \text{AD} \\ & | & & | \\ R & R\!-\!R & R\!- \\ | & | & | & | \\ P\!-\!P & P\!-\!P \end{pmatrix}_n + \begin{matrix} \text{Nicotinamide} \\ (\text{NAM})_n \end{matrix}$$

NAD

Fig. 1 The reaction catalyzed by poly ADP-ribose polymerase.

nally we wondered whether these two processes were in some way related to each other in the eukaryotic cell. Poly ADP-ribose polymerase, when purified from chromatin, requires DNA and exogenous nuclear protein acceptors such as histones and nonhistone proteins for activity. Chain lengths of polymer bound to these proteins vary from mono ADP-ribose to oligomers of 20 units or greater. In addition, the polymer has recently been shown to be capable of covalently cross-linking two histone H_1 molecules (Stone *et al.*, 1977). Effective inhibition of the enzyme is achieved by nicotinamide, thymidine, and caffeine. This enzyme has fascinated but frustrated investigators for a number of years. Problems may relate to the biochemical employment of NAD in a nonoxidative fashion and also to the diversity of nuclear reactions with which the enzyme system has been purported to be involved.

Recently our laboratory has been primarily concerned with the precise interaction of this nonhistone protein with the nucleosomal substructure of eukaryotic chromatin (Mullins *et al.*, 1977; Giri *et al.*, 1978a, 1978b; Butt, *et al.* 1978). Although an exact biological function for this nucleoprotein modification has not been determined, the studies presented below suggest that one function might be related to an alteration in chromatin structure at sites of DNA alkylation damage to allow access for DNA repair enzymes (Smulson *et al.*, 1975).

I. Effects of Drugs on Poly ADP Ribosylation

Both methylnitrosourea (MNU) and streptozotocin are reported to cause a reduction in NAD levels in eukaryotic cells. Accordingly, HeLa cells in suspension culture were incubated for 2 hours with each of these drugs, after which nuclei were prepared; lowered cytoplasmic NAD levels were noted under these experimental conditions (Smulson *et al.*, 1975, 1977). The data in Fig. 2 demonstrate the rate of poly ADP-ribose polymerase activity, as measured by the incorporation of radioactive NAD into polymer, in nuclei derived from control and drug-treated cells. A marked activation of enzyme activity was noted, especially in the case of MNU, which chemically is the active cytotoxic moiety of streptozotocin. A similar stimulation of polymerase activity by streptozotocin has

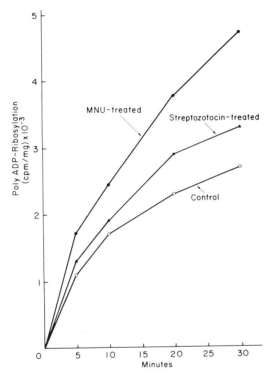

Fig. 2 Effects of *in vivo* incubation of HeLa cells with MNU and streptozotocin for 2 hours. Cell viability was estimated to be essentially 100%. After treatment, cells were centrifuged and washed with a 0.9% NaCl solution and nuclei were isolated. Poly ADP-ribose polymerase activity was determined. ●, Nuclei from MNU-treated cells; ▲, nuclei from streptozotocin-treated cells; ○, nuclei from control cells. Taken from Smulson *et al.* 1977.

been noted by Whish *et al.* (1975) in *Physarum polycephalum*. Based upon these and other data we concluded tentatively that the NAD depression noted with these and other cytotoxic drugs was related in part to enhanced cellular poly ADP ribosylation.

To determine the relationship between the structure and activity of nitrosoureas, a study was made of the effects of methyl and chloroethyl nitrosoureas on nuclear enzyme activity (Table I). A dose–response study was performed on all the nitrosoureas listed in Table I at five different concentrations between 0.1 and 4.0 mM (Sudhakar *et al.*, 1979a). Chloroethyl nitrosoureas had a slight inhibitory effect on enzyme activity at concentrations up to 4 mM. The data in Table I indicate that there was no apparent relationship between the *in vitro* alkylation and carbamoyla-

TABLE I

Comparative Effects of Methyl and Chloroethyl Nitrosoureas on Alkylation, Carbamoylation, NAD Levels, and Poly ADP Ribose Polymerase Specific Activity in Nuclei[a]

Drug[a]	Structure	Carbamoylated [14C]lysine (%)	Alkylating Activity MNU (%)	Alkylating Activity CNU (%)	Effect on cellular NAD levels	Effect on poly ADP-ribose polymerase specific activity (% of control)
Methyl nitrosoureas						
MNU	R'H	48[b]	(100)[b]		Decrease	279
C-1 glucose-substituted MNU		42[b]	40[b]		Decrease	133

Structure:

$$R' = N - C - N - CH_3$$
(with O and N=O on carbonyl/nitroso, H below)

$$R'' = N - C - N - CH_2CH_2Cl$$
(with O and N=O, H below)

	R"H				
Chloroethyl nitrosoureas CNU		100[b]	—	(100)[c]	None	60
Chlorozotocin		4[c]	—	64[c]	None	90
CCNU		94[c]	—	10[c]	None	86

[a] Cells were treated with a 2 mM concentration of the drug, CNU.
[b] From Panasci et al. (1977a).
[c] From Panasci et al. (1977b).

tion activities of the drugs and their effects on poly ADP-ribose polymerase activity. However, it was of significance that, in all cases,
chloroethyl nitrosoureas, which have been reported to have no effect on
intracellular NAD concentrations (Schein, 1969), had a slightly inhibitory
effect on poly ADP-ribose polymerase activity. Methyl nitrosoureas,
which depress NAD levels in cells, stimulated the activity of the enzyme.

II. Biological Effect of Nitrosoureas at the Nucleosomal Level

It became apparent that, before a precise understanding of the relationship between poly ADP ribosylation of nucleoproteins and the cytotoxic
events produced by various drugs could be understood, a better
characterized nuclear subcomponent was required for study. During the
past few years, significant advances have been made in elucidation of the
subunit structure of eukaryotic chromatin. Therefore it seemed of importance to begin a comprehensive study on drug interaction with nonhistone
proteins at the nucleosomal subunit of eukaryotic chromatin.

In brief, chromatin consists of DNA packaged at successive intervals
into small particles, nucleosomes (see Fig. 3). Exactly 140 base pairs of
DNA are located around a globular disk-shaped particle, the nucleosome,
which in turn is composed of an octamer of two asymmetric pairs of the
four histones H3, H4, H2a, and H2b. Although the DNA is located on the
outside of this particle, the amino-terminal regions of the histones are
known to interact with specific locations of the DNA. The region between
nucleosomes has been termed the linker or internucleosomal region and
varies in length from 0 to 60 base pairs of DNA, depending upon the physiological function of the region of chromatin and also upon the specific cell
tissue type. The polynucleosome is in turn thought to be coiled into its
own superstructure within native chromatin.

As shown in Fig. 3, the enzyme micrococcal nuclease is experimentally
used to isolate a variety of subsets of nucleosomes (i.e., monomer, monomer containing linker DNA and H1, dimer, $3N$, $4N$, and so on). This enzyme possesses specificity for the cleavage of internucleosomal DNA.
This property of micrococcal nuclease has been exploited in the experiments described below not only to ascertain the level of chromatin organization at which enhancement of poly ADP-ribose polymerase activity
occurs following drug treatment, but in addition to determine which types
of DNA in chromatin are preferentially modified by alkylation and carbamoylation by nitrosoureas.

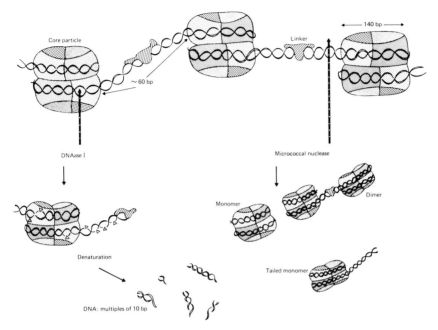

Fig. 3 The polynucleosomal structure of chromatin. Selective digestion by various nucleases.

Nuclei isolated from cells incubated in the presence and absence of MNU were digested with micrococcal nuclease (Fig. 4). Chromatin fragments generated were fractionated on 5–20% linear sucrose gradients. Note that this fractionation procedure separates chromatin into 11 S nucleosomal regions of chromatin (Giri et al., 1978b). Thus, as shown in Fig. 4A, activity was detected only in particles (>1N) containing linker DNA. The activity of this nonhistone protein enzyme was enhanced more than twofold in dimer and higher oligomer subfractions derived from MNU-treated cells as compared to control cells.

Further evidence that the enzyme is bound to internucleosomal DNA is provided by the experiments shown in Fig. 5, where enzymic activity was assayed in individual fractions throughout a mononucleosome region in both control and MNU-prepared chromatin. Significant activity was found only in the faster-sedimenting regions of the gradient where monomers containing internucleosomal linker DNA fragments would be expected to sediment (Giri et al., 1978b). For example, when a purified preparation of nucleosomal dimer was redigested in vitro with micrococcal nuclease to generate mononucleosomes with linkers, the enzyme ac-

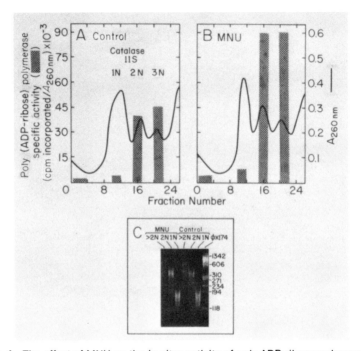

Fig. 4 The effect of MNU on the *in vitro* activity of poly ADP-ribose polymerase assayed at the nucleosomal level. HeLa cells (4×10^7) in 20 ml were incubated in the absence (A) or presence (B) of MNU (7.5 mM) for 1 hour at 37°C. Nuclei were prepared and digested with micrococcal nuclease to isolate nucleosomal subfractions by sucrose gradient centrifugation. The direction of sedimentation is from left to right. Catalase was utilized as an 11 S marker. The optical density was monitored at 260 nm (—). Approximately 0.2 A_{260} units of pooled fractions were assayed for poly ADP-ribose polymerase activity as indicated by the cross-hatched bars. 1N, 2N, and 3N refer to mononucleosomes, dinucleosomes, and trinucleosomes, respectively. DNA was isolated from the pooled fractions corresponding to each peak and analyzed under nondenaturating conditions by 6% polyacrylamide gel electrophoresis. Hae III-digested ϕX174 DNA fragments were used as base pair markers. Taken from Sudhakar, S., Tew, K. D., and Smulson, M. E., 1979a.

tivity previously associated with the dimer was shifted to heavy monomer particles. In addition, direct assays for this enzyme on chromatin gels, which separated particles with and without linker regions, showed definitively that only the former type of particles possessed activity.

In order to assess the potential difference in nucleoprotein acceptors for poly ADP ribosylation, a slightly different protocol has been employed. Nuclei from control and MNU-treated cells were preincubated prior to the preparation of nuclease-treated chromatin with [³H]NAD.

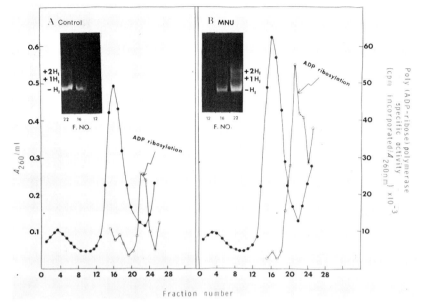

Fig. 5 Distribution of poly ADP-ribose polymerase activity in 11 S mononucleosomes isolated from control and MNU-treated cells. Nuclei (40 A_{260}/ml) isolated from cells incubated in the absence (A) and presence (B) of MNU (2 mM) were digested with micrococcal nuclease (4 U/A_{260}) for 1.5 minutes ($\sim$9% perchloric acid-soluble material). Approximately 5 A_{260} units of nuclease-prepared chromatin was layered on 8–14% linear sucrose gradients and centrifuged for 18 hours at 38 K (4°C) in an SW-40 rotor. The direction of sedimentation is from left to right. Each gradient fraction was assayed for absorbance at 260 nm (●) and poly ADP-ribose polymerase activity (○). Taken from Sudhakar, S., Jump, D., and Smulson, M., 1979.

Following separation of the resultant chromatin fractions by sucrose gradient centrifugation, aliquots corresponding to peak nucleosome fractions were pooled and assessed for acid-insoluble radioactivity, representing poly ADP-ribose (Fig. 6). In contrast to the data in Fig. 4, which indicated negligible enzyme activity in the 11 S mononucleosome chromatin fraction, the results of this experiment showed that, when modification was performed in native chromatin prior to digestion with micrococcal nuclease, considerable amounts of poly ADP-ribose polymer were associated with nucleosomes of all sizes, including mononucleosomes. The data emphasize the fact that the conformation of chromatin, in the native state, allows the nucleosome core histones to be accessible for modification by this enzyme which is internucleosomal in location. The extent of ADP ribosylation of proteins in the subfractions from MNU-treated cells was twice as great as in nucleosomes derived from untreated cells (Fig. 6).

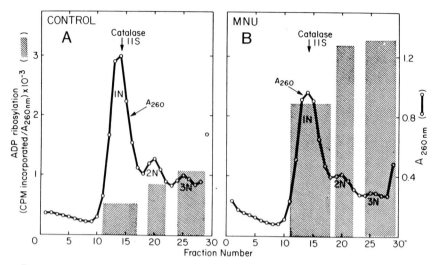

Fig. 6 Incubation of nuclei with [³H]NAD: distribution of ADP ribosylation at the nucleosomal level. HeLa cells (8×10^7) in 40 ml of medium were incubated in the absence (A) and presence (B) of MNU (7.5 mM) for 1 hour after which nuclei were prepared. The nuclei were incubated under conditions optimal for poly ADP-ribose polymerase. The reaction was stopped by the addition of ice-cold isotonic buffer, and the nuclei were collected by centrifugation. Isolation of chromatin by micrococcal nuclease digestion from the *in situ* modified nuclei and its subsequent fractionation were performed as before. Sedimentation is from left to right. Fractions corresponding to each peak were separately pooled and assessed for the presence of acid-insoluble radioactivity representing ADP-ribosylated proteins as indicated by the hatched bars. Taken from Sudhakar, S., Tew, K., and Smulson, M. E., 1979a.

III. Differential ADP Ribosylation of Nuclear Proteins Induced by MNU

Incorporation of [³²P]NAD into chromatin associated with proteins (both histone and nonhistone) from control and MNU-treated nuclei were compared using Triton–acetic acid–urea gels (Fig. 7). The interaction of

Fig. 7 Differential ADP ribosylation caused by MNU treatment revealed by electrophoresis of histones in a Triton–acetic acid–urea gel. Nuclei (4×10^7/ml) from control and MNU-treated cells were incubated with 0.2 µmole [³²P]NAD (20 mCi/µmole) under conditions optimal for poly ADP-ribose polymerase activity for 15 minutes. Nuclear histones were extracted. (A) Coomassie blue stain of the gel and its densitomer scan. Histone proteins were identified by comparison with calf thymus histones. (B) Autoradiograph of the ADP-ribosylated histones from a negative of the photograph shown. (C) Same as in (B), from MNU-treated nuclei. Taken from Sudhakar, S., Tew, K., and Smulson, M. E., 1979a.

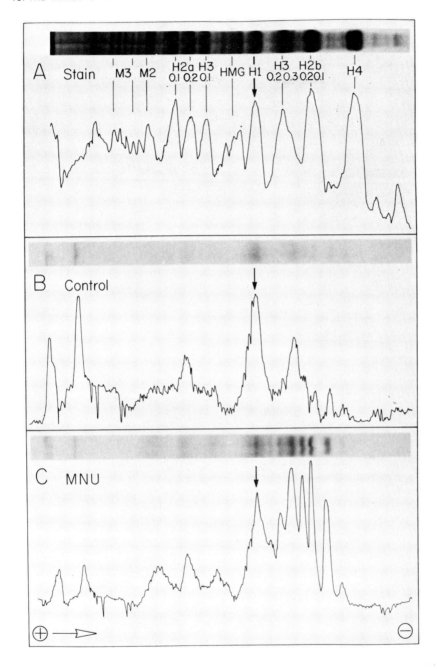

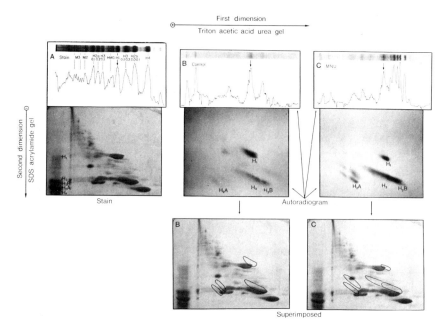

Fig. 8 Two-dimensional gel electrophoretic analysis of poly ADP-ribosylated histones from nuclei derived from cells incubated in the presence or absence of MNU. Nuclei (4 × 10^7/ml) isolated from control and MNU (2 mM)-treated cells were incubated with 0.2 μmole [^{32}P]NAD (20 mCi/μmole) under conditions optimum for poly ADP-ribose polymerase activity. Histones were extracted with 0.4 N H$_2$SO$_4$. An aliquot of the extracted histones was subjected to Triton–acetic acid–urea tube gel electrophoresis in the first dimension, followed by second-dimensional electrophoresis on an SDS acrylamide slab gel, with purified calf thymus histones as standards. After staining (A) with Coomassie blue, the gel was subjected to autoradiography (B and C). Since the electrophoretic patterns of the stained proteins from control and MNU nuclei were identical, only one gel is shown. The photographs and densitometer scans of the negatives refer to the one-dimensional electrophoretic run of an identical sample on a Triton–acetic acid–urea slab gel. The radioactive spots are outlined in the diagrammatic representation (B' and C') of the autoradiograph superimposed on the stained gel. Taken from Sudhakar, S., Tew, K., and Smulson, M. E., 1979a.

MNU with chromatin resulted in an increased and altered pattern of modification of proteins by poly ADP ribosylation (Sudhakar *et al.*, 1979a). MNU did not appear to change the level of ADP ribosylation of histone Hl, the major acceptor in the control. However, there was significantly greater modification of nucleosomal core histones than in untreated cells. Multiple peaks of radioactivity in the region corresponding to H$_2$B (Fig. 7C) indicated that either there were multiple sites of ADP-ribose incorporation into H$_2$B or, more probably, that the ADP-ribose polymer attached to the histone was of variable chain length. The mobilities of the proteins could possibly have been altered as a result of a change in charge and/or hydrophobicity introduced by the various modifications such as MNU carbamoylation and poly ADP ribosylation. Accordingly, the MNU-induced increase in ADP ribosylation of proteins migrating in the Triton–acetic acid–urea gel at a mobility corresponding to the core histones was confirmed by sodium dodecyl sulfate (SDS) gel electrophoresis in a second dimension (Fig. 8).

IV. Modification of Nuclear Proteins by Nitrosoureas

Nitrosoureas exhibit a dual capacity for interacting with nucleic acids and proteins. Thus their differential effects on poly ADP-ribose polymerase activity might be explained by their characteristic interactions with chromatin-bound proteins. It was therefore of importance to identify which proteins were modified by these agents. HeLa cells were treated with [*carbanoyl*-^{14}C]MNU for 1 hour and [*cyclohexyl*-^{14}C]-1-(2-chloroethyl)-3-cyclohexyl-1-nitrosourea (CCNU) for 2 hours at 37°C (Sudhakar *et al.*, 1979b). The data in Fig. 9A indicate that histone H2B, which is present in the nucleosome core, is more accessible for carbamoylation by MNU than H1, present in the internucleosome region of chromatin. The slight but significant modification of H3 and H4, coupled with the above data, indicates that MNU modification could result in a significant alteration of nucleosome structure (see below).

In contrast, negligible carbamoylation of nucleosomal core histones was found following treatment with CCNU (Fig. 9B), a drug we have used in a number of comparative experiments because it does not cause stimulation of poly ADP ribosylation (Sudhakar *et al.*, 1979a). Histone H1 was modified to a minor extent. The nondistone proteins and the histone-like high-mobility group (HMG) proteins, M1 amd M4, appeared to be the primary nuclear protein targets for CCNU carbamoylation. The proteins modified by MNU were analyzed in a second dimension on SDS acrylamide gels (similar to Fig. 8), and the radioautogram pattern when superimposed upon the stained gel confirmed the identity of the carbamoylated histones (data not shown). A major difference found in these studies was that MNU, in contrast to CCNU, caused extensive carbamoylation of histone proteins.

In view of the differential effect (Table I) or chloroethyl versus methyl nitrosourea, on poly ADP-ribose polymerase, a more extensive comparative cellular uptake and chromatin-binding study was carried out with normal and butyrate-pretreated HeLa cells and CCNU and chlorozotocin (Tew *et al.*, 1978). Butyrate was used because of its pronounced influence

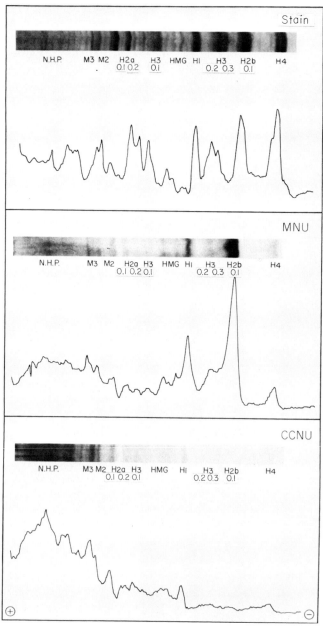

Fig. 9 Modification of nuclear proteins by [*carbonyl*-¹⁴C]MNU and [*cyclohexyl*-¹⁴C]CCNU. HeLa cells (5 × 10⁷) in 1 ml were incubated with 30 μCi of [*carbanoyl*-¹⁴C]MNU (7.9 Ci/mole) and [*cyclohexyl*-¹⁴C]CCNU (8.3 Ci/mole) for 1 and 2 hours, respectively. Nuclei were isolated and proteins extracted with 0.4*N* H₂SO₄ and analyzed on a Triton–acetic acid–urea slab gel. (A) Autoradiograph of MNU-modified histones and densitometer scan. (B) Same as in (A), for CCNU-modified histones. Taken from Sudhakar, S., Tew, K., Smulson, M., 1979b.

on nuclear protein structure (Vidali *et al.*, 1978). These data are presented in Table II. Maximal nuclear incorporation of both drugs occurred at 2 hours. Incorporation of cyclohexyl-labeled CCNU was greater than that of chloroethyl-labeled drugs both at the whole cell and the nuclear level, suggesting that the parent drug underwent partial chemical dissociation in the medium and that there was preferential uptake of the carbamoylating isocyanate moiety. Uptake of the alkylating moiety of chlorozotocin was higher than that of CCNU in both the whole cell (ratio, 1.5) and the nucleus (ratio, 3). The cyclohexyl-labeled CCNU data reflect quantitative protein carbamoylation. In butyrate-treated cells the extent of carbamoylation was increased by a factor of 2.4, the nonhistone fraction accounting for this butyrate-induced increase in drug binding.

Butyrate treatment resulted in an approximate twofold increase in cellular uptake for cyclohexyl-labeled CCNU. This may have resulted from a butyrate-induced effect upon the cell membrane. However, nuclear incor-

TABLE II

A Comparison of Nitrosourea Uptake in Control and Butyrate-Treated Cells[a,b]

	Control (C)	Butyrate (B)	Ratio B/C
[*Cyclohexyl*-1-^{14}C] CCNU			
Whole cells[c]	4.1 ± 0.3	7.2 ± 0.5	1.8
Nuclei[d]	1.1 ± 0.1	2.5 ± 0.6	2.3
Histone and nonhistone[e]	41.4 ± 8	100.1 ± 12	2.4
Chromatin[f]	41.9 ± 6	70.1 ± 8	1.7
[*Ethyl*-2-^{14}C] CCNU			
Whole cells[c]	0.8 ± 0.3	1.03 ± 0.05	1.3
Nuclei[d]	0.1 ± 0.05	0.23 ± 0.06	2.3
Histone and nonhistone[e]	1.6 ± 0.4	2.9 ± 0.6	1.8
Chromatin[f]	6.9 ± 2.9	15.2 ± 3.7	2.2
[*Ethyl*-1-^{14}C] chlorozotocin			
Whole cells[c]	1.2 ± 0.2	1.6 ± 0.2	1.3
Nuclei[d]	0.31 ± 0.1	0.81 ± 0.2	2.6
Histone and nonhistone[e]	0.6 ± 0.2	0.8 ± 0.3	1.3
Chromatin[f]	12.6 ± 2.8	24.0 ± 6.8	1.9

[a] Taken from Tew *et al.* (1978).

[b] Log-phase cells (5.7×10^5) were incubated with 20 μCi radiolabeled drug at a concentration of 30 μM for 2 hours. Butyrate treatment was at 5.0 mM for 24 hours.

[c] Whole cells were washed twice with isotonic saline before counting. Values are expressed as percent of total disintegrations per minute added to the culture.

[d] Nuclei were extracted. Values are expressed as percent of total disintegrations per minute added to culture.

[e] Histone and nonhistone functions were acid-extracted. Values are expressed as picomoles per A_{230}.

[f] Values are expressed as picomoles per A_{260}.

poration was more than doubled by butyrate treatment, and this could not be explained by the increased cellular uptake.

Data for sonically disrupted chromatin gave a ratio of drug incorporation in butyrate-pretreated cells versus control cells similar to that for the other fractions. Chromatin alkylation by chlorozotocin was approximately twice that of CCNU.

V. Sites of Alkylation by Nitrosoureas in Nucleosomal Substructures

The relative accessibility of regions of chromatin substructure for alkylation by carcinogenic agents is of importance in view of the fact that DNA connecting nucleosome core particles is more susceptible *in vitro* to various enzymes such as endonucleases and might, as suggested by our recent data, also be primary sites of drug interaction. Furthermore, we have shown that poly ADP-ribose polymerase is bound to this region of chromatin. Chromatin was labeled *in vivo* with alkyl-labeled MNU and CCNU for 1 and 2 hours, respectively, and subsequently digested with micrococcal nuclease and DNase I (Fig. 10A–E). Treatment of chromatin with the former enzyme (see Fig. 2) initially results in a preferential digestion of internucleosome DNA and subsequent conversion of chromatin into nucleosome monomers. In contrast, treatment of chromatin with DNase I initially results in the digestion of nucleosomal core DNA. It has recently been shown that functionally active regions of chromatin, i.e., replicating and transcriptionally active regions, are also preferentially digested by these nucleases.

The results with MNU (Fig. 10) indicate that, during the entire period of digestion with micrococcal nuclease, the rate of release of radioactivity (methylated products) was greater than the A_{260}. The data suggest that the majority of [*methyl*-^{14}C]MNU molecules reacted with the accessible regions of DNA between nucleosomes. This nonrandom methylation of chromatin by MNU was confirmed by following DNase I digestion (Fig. 10D). A reversal of the digestion pattern with micrococcal nuclease was observed.

In contrast, the release of [*chloroethyl*-^{14}C]CCNU bases, following micrococcal nuclease digestion, was significantly lower than the A_{260} at early time periods (Fig. 10B). However, after 5 minutes, considerable cleavage of 200-base-pair particles was evident, and alkylated bases resulting from CCNU were released late during digestion with the enzyme. In confirmation, alkylated bases were released rapidly when nuclei were digested by DNase I (Fig. 10E). To determine which macromolecules were the pre-

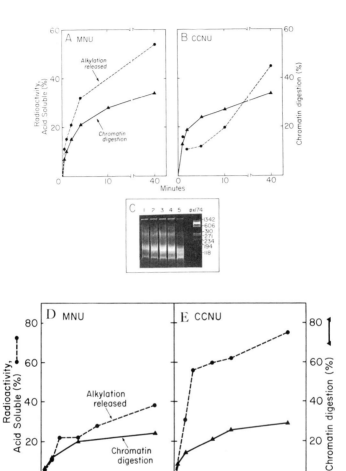

Fig. 10 Distribution of [*methyl*-^{14}C]MNU and [*chloroethyl*-^{14}C]CCNU alkylation within chromatin structure as probed by digestion with micrococcal nuclease and DNase I. HeLa nuclei (4×10^7) in 1 ml of isotonic buffer were incubated with 10μCi [*methyl*-^{14}C]MNU (10.7 Ci/mole) (A and D) for 1 hour, or 10 μCi [*chloroethyl*-^{14}C]CCNU (10.9 Ci/mole) (B and E) for 2 hours. The nuclei were centrifuged at 3000 rpm to remove unincorporated drug, washed once with the isotonic buffer, and resuspended in nuclease digestion buffer; digestions were then performed. The results are expressed as the percentage of total DNA nucleotides (▲) and DNA-bound nitrosourea radioactivity (●). (C) DNA fragments produced my micrococcal nuclease digestion of HeLa nuclei were isolated at each time point and analyzed by 6% polyacrylamide gel electrophoresis. *Hae* III-digested ϕX174 DNA fragments were used as base pair markers. Nuclei were digested with micrococcal nuclease for 1 minute (1), 2 minutes (2), 5 minutes (3), 10 minutes (4), and 40 minutes (5). Taken from Sudhakar, S., Tew, K., Smulson, M., 1979.

dominant alkylated targets of MNU and CCNU, labeled chromatin was subjected to exhaustive digestion by DNase, RNase, and protease. Only DNases were capable of significantly reducing the covalently bound radioactivity. When free DNA, alkylated *in vivo* or *in vitro* and purified from HeLa chromatin, was used instead of nuclei in the nuclease digestion reaction, the rates of release of nucleotides and of the alkylated products were identical.

In a similar type of study (Fig. 11) the nitrosourea chlorozotocin showed digestion kinetics similar to those found above with CCNU. Additional data utilizing these approaches should ultimately aid in our understanding of the repair reactions resulting from differing types of drugs which might preferentially interact with different regions of chromatin.

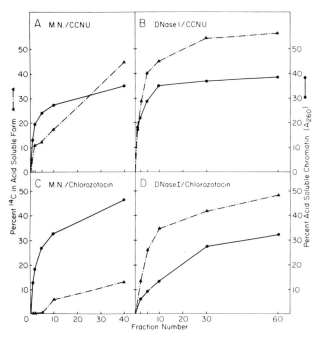

Fig. 11 Limit digest of HeLa cell nuclei treated with 0.3 mM [^{14}C]chlorozotocin or 0.3 mM [*chloroethyl*)-^{14}C]CCNU. (A and C) Micrococcal nuclease (M.N.); (B and D) DNase I. The release of trichloroacetic acid-soluble ^{14}C was monitored (▲) and compared with the digestion of nuclear chromatin (●). The abscissa represents the time in minutes. Taken from Tew, K. D., Sudhakar, S., Schein, P. S., and Smulson, M. E., 1978.

VI. Higher Orders of Chromatin Structure

In native chromatin, polynucleosomes assume a 100-Å solenoidal superstructure. This conformation of chromatin accounts for the interaction of neighboring and distal particles and internucleosomal regions of chromatin with each other. A further degree of condensation of the genome is achieved by such supercoiling. Our knowledge of the structural differences between functionally active (primarily euchromatin) and inactive (presumably heterochromatin) chromatin is limited. Ultimately, drugs, hormone complexes, and mutagens are able to penetrate certain regions of condensed chromatin, yet little is known about the mechanics of these significant events. However, studies with poly ADP ribosylation have in a preliminary fashion increased our understanding of the interaction of drugs with these higher forms of chromatin.

It was observed that the specific activity of poly ADP-ribose polymerase increased progressively in preparations of oligonucleosomes of increasing repeat number (Butt *et al.*, 1978). Activity reached a maximum at 8–10 nucleosomes (Fig. 12). These results led us to perform a detailed kinetic analysis of the digestion by micrococcal nuclease of higher-ordered forms of chromatin (Fig. 13). The data show that two major forms of chromatin can be detected as selective sites of cleavage of chromatin

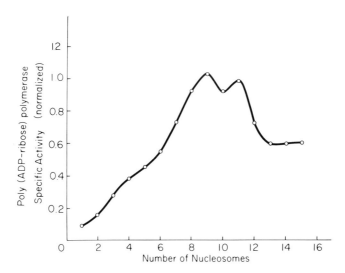

Fig. 12 The relationship between poly ADP-ribose polymerase specific activity and the number of nucleosomes on a chromatin fragment. Taken from Butt, T. R., Brothers, J. F., Giri, C. R., and Smulson, M. E., 1978.

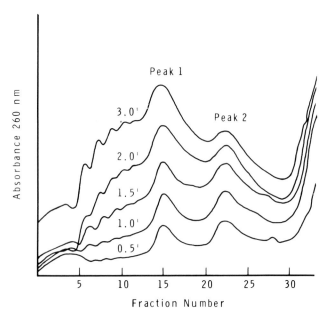

Fig. 13 Higher-order chromatin forms preferentially cleaved by micrococcal nuclease HeLa cell nuclei (1×10^8/ml) were incubated in 1.0 ml of nuclease buffer for 5 minutes at 37°C. Micrococcal nuclease (30 units/10^8 nuclei) was added, and samples were made 1 mM EDTA at times 30 (3×10^8 nuclei), 60 (2×10^8), 90 (2×10^8), 120 (2×10^8), and 180 seconds (1×10^8), respectively. The nuclei were centrifuged and lysed. The supernatant, containing between 4 and 15 A_{260} units was layered on a 12-ml 10–30% linear sucrose gradient containing 0.2 mM EDTA, 1 mM NaPO$_4$, pH 6.8, and 80 mM NaCl and centrifuged in a SW-40 rotor at 40,000 rpm at 4°C for 4.5 hours. Fractions of 0.33 ml were collected and monitored for optical density at A_{259} utilizing an ISCO ultraviolet monitor. The direction of sedimentation is from left to right. Taken from Butt, T. R., Jump, D., and Smulson, M. E., 1979.

by this enzyme (30 seconds). By various criteria, including DNA size determination and native chromatin gel electrophoresis, we have shown that peaks 1 and 2 represent octanucleosomes and 16N polynucleosomes, respectively (Butt *et al.*, 1979). Significantly, it is thought that one complete turn in a 100-Å fiber contains approximately 7–10 nucleosomes. A variety of experimental evidence suggests that perhaps poly ADP-ribose polymerase per se is bound to chromatin at such turns in a chromatin helix. Preliminary data suggest that treatment of HeLa cells with MNU activates poly ADP-ribose in octanucleosomes. A significant increase in single-strand DNA breaks can readily be detected in such large structures.

Experiments are currently underway to ascertain whether various alkylating agents might also (like micrococcal nuclease) attack such regions in chromatin. The data emphasize the significance of an understanding of chromatin sub- and superstructure as a potential aid in the ultimate understanding of drug interactions with nuclear components.

VII. Effects of Methyl Nitrosourea on Chromatin Substructure as Probed by DNase I

Recent advances in understanding the structure of chromatin have revealed that its basic sub-unit nature is stabilized by cooperative interactions between nucleic acids and protein. Chemical modification (i.e., carbamoylation by MNU) of these proteins that participate in the organization of chromatin would be expected to have a significant influence on the structure and function of the nucleus. It has been observed (Fig. 9) that histone H2B and, to a lesser extent, H3 and H4 are the primary targets of the carbonyl moiety of MNU. The digestion of core nucleosomes with trypsin selectively removes several amino acid residues from the amino terminus of each histone, generating a trypsin-resistant nuclear complex (Simpson *et al.*, 1976). We have shown (data not presented) that a significant level of core histone carbamoylation by MNU occurs at the amino-terminal ends of core histones—regions that are capable of interaction with core DNA. To test the effect of this modification on nucleosomes, HeLa cells were incubated with MNU, and 140-base-pair core nucleosomes were isolated (essentially as described by the experimental protocols in Fig. 5B). DNase I generates single-strand cuts in the DNA of nucleosomes (see Fig. 2). Electrophoretic analysis of DNA under denaturing conditions reveals a series of discrete fragments that migrate as multiples of 10-base-pair nucleotides (10–140 base length). The technique described by Simpson and Whitlock (1976) involves phosphorylating the 5'-end of core mononucleosome DNA with polynucleotide kinase and [γ32P]ATP. Analysis of DNase I-generated DNA fragments by electrophoresis followed by radioautography reflects the distance from the 32P-labeled 5'-end where cleavage occurred. DNase I digestion kinetics of 5'-end-32P-labeled nucleosomes with and without the MNU-induced modification are presented in Fig. 14. The rate of DNase I digestion of MNU-modified nucleosomes was two- to three fold more rapid than that of control nucleosomes. A comparison of the relative rates of cleavage at specific sites within the nucleosome between the two samples (Fig. 14) revealed that sites 90, 70, 60, 50, and 40 nucleotides from the 5'-end of nucleosomal DNA became more accessible to DNase I as a result of carbamoylation (Jump *et al.*, 1979). These data suggest that a small molecule, the carbanoyl moiety of MNU, may penetrate the relatively hydrophobic domain of the histone core. Covalent modification in this region would be expected to alter pro-

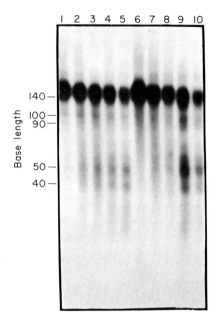

Fig. 14 DNase I digestion of control and carbamoyl-modified nucleosomes. Nucleosomes (0.3 A_{260} units) labeled with ^{32}P at the 5'-end of the DNA (specific activity 1.25×10^6 dpm/A_{260}) at 37°C were digested for the indicated times. The data show a radioautograph of single-stranded DNA fragments generated during DNase I digestion and separated by denaturing polyacrylamide electrophoresis. Columns 1–5 represent DNA fragments of control nucleosomes digested for 0, 1, 2, 4, and 16 minutes, respectively; columns 6–10 represent those from carbamoyl-modified nucleosomes digested for 0, 1, 2, 8, 16 minutes, respectively. Taken from Jump, D., Sudhakar, S. and Smulson, M., 1979.

tein interactions, thus altering the protection of DNA by such proteins. This experimental approach emphasizes the potential of utilizing the technology developed for the analysis of chromatin substructure to determine the precise influence of various classes of drugs within the nucleus.

VIII. Drug-Mediated Fragmentation of DNA May Signal Nuclear Protein Modifications

Two experiments (Figs. 15 and 16) suggest that poly ADP-ribose modification might function in part to alter chromatin structure in response to single-strand breaks induced by cellular interaction with drugs possessing alkylating activity. As indicated above (Fig. 1), poly ADP-ribose polymerase requires DNA for nucleoprotein modification. With the use of a

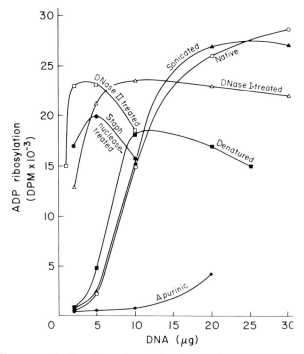

Fig. 15 The concentration dependence of native and fragmented DNA on a partially purified poly ADP-ribose polymerase activity from HeLa cells. The reaction was carried out with an optimal histone concentration (20 μg), and calf thymus DNA was nicked by the respective nucleases to 25% activation in each case. Taken from Smulson et al., 1977.

semipurified polymerase it was found (Fig. 15) that, in the presence of optimal concentrations of histones for the *in vitro* assay, DNA (containing equivalent strand breaks) activated the enzyme at a 10-fold lower concentration than native DNA (Smulson *et al.*, 1977). This observation that the enzyme was stimulated by breaks in DNA was expanded to the cellular situation by the experiment shown in Fig. 16. Cells were incubated in the presence and absence of MNU; significant stimulation of poly ADP-ribose polymerase specific activity resulted from such treatment. DNase I treatment of HeLa nuclei *in vitro* was shown to stimulate poly ADP-ribose polymerase activity, presumably by the generation of single-strand breaks in DNA. However, this nuclease-induced stimulation was not observed in nuclei derived from MNU-treated cells which already possessed considerable DNA fragmentation.

DNase I was found to be stimulatory only to enzyme activity in these cells when they were allowed a 4.5-hour postincubation period to recover from MNU damage. The level of poly ADP-ribose polymerase activity

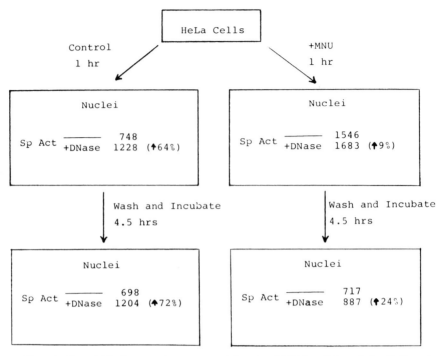

Fig. 16 Poly ADP-ribose polymerase activity after MNU insult to cellular DNA and subsequent recovery. HeLa cells (2×10^8) in 100 ml were incubated at 37°C in the presence or absence of MNU (7.5 mM final concentration) for 1 hour and then washed with sterile 0.9% NaCl solution. Cells (1×10^8) were removed for nuclear isolation, and the remaining cells were suspended at 2×10^6/ml in fresh S-MEM and incubated for an additional 4.5 hours before washing and isolation of nuclei. Poly ADP-ribose polymerase activity was measured in the four nuclear samples for 20 minutes, either in the absence or presence of DNase I (30 μg/500 μl assay). Specific activity (Sp Act) is defined as disintegrations per minute of ADP-ribose incorporated per microgram of protein. Taken from Smulson *et al.*, 1977.

had also returned to basal levels. These data are suggestive that this nucleoprotein modification might be responsive to DNA fragmentation. The resultant increased synthesis of chains of poly ADP-ribose on nuclear proteins in turn might alter chromatin structure (indicated by a number of experiments mentioned above). This alteration could aid in the penetration of various repair enzymes to such regions of chromatin. A similar hypothesis has been suggested for the effects of alkylating agents on nuclear protein phosphorylation drug-resistant and -sensitive tumor cells (Harrap *et al.*, 1975). The same type of chromatin alterations might be required by the cell during normal semiconservative DNA replication.

The experimental approach above illustrates one example of many in which exploitation of a pronounced effect of drugs on the nucleus has helped elucidate the multifaceted interaction of various nucleus-targeted drugs and their influence on macromolecular control reactions within the nucleus.

Acknowledgment

This work was supported by grants CA-13195 and CA-25344 from the National Institutes of Health.

References

Butt, T. R., Brothers, J. B., Giri, G. P., and Smulson, M. E. (1978). *Nucleic Acid Res.* **8,** 2775–2788.
Butt, T. R., Jump, D. B., and Smulson, M. E. (1979). *Proc. Natl. Acad. Sci. U.S.A.* **74,** 1628–1632.
Giri, C. P., West, M. H. P., and Smulson, M. E. (1978a). *Biochemistry* **17,** 3495–3500.
Giri, C. P., West, M. H. P., Ramirez, M. L., and Smulson, M. E. (1978b). *Biochemistry* **17,** 3501–3504.
Gottesfeld, J. M., and Butler, P. J. G. (1977). *Nucleic Acid Res.* **4,** 3155–3172.
Harrap, K. R., Riches, P. G., Gascoigne, E. W., Sellwood, S. M., and Cashman, C. C. (1975). *Proc. Int. Symp. Biol. Characterization Human Tumors, 6th, 1975 Excerpta Med.* Proceedings of the Sixth International Symposium on the Biological Characterisation of Human Tumors, Copenhagen, 1975. Excerpta Medica Foundation, Amsterdam: pp. 106–121.
Hildebrand, C. E., and Walters, R. A. (1976). *Biochem. Biophys. Res. Commun.* **73,** 157–163.
Jump, D. B., Sudhakar, S., and Smulson, M. E. (1979). (Submitted to *Chem. Biol. Interactions.*)
Mullins, D. W., Jr., Giri, C. P., and Smulson, M. *Biochemistry* **16,** 506–513.
Panasci, L. C., Fox, P. A., and Schein, P. S. (1977a). *Cancer Res.* **37,** 3321–3328.
Panasci, L. C., Green, D., Nagourney, R., Fox, P. A., and Schein, P. S. (1977b). *Cancer Res.* **37,** 2615–2617.
Schein, P. S. (1969). *Cancer Res.* **29,** 1226–1232.
Schein, P. S., and Loftus, S. (1968). *Cancer Res.* **28,** 1501–1506.
Simpson, R. T., and Whitlock, J. P., Jr. (1976). *Cell* **9,** 353–374.
Smulson, M. E., Stark, P., Gazzoli, M., and Roberts, J. H. (1975). *Exp. Cell Res.* **90,** 175–182.
Smulson, M. E., Schein, P., Mullins, D. W., Jr., and Sudhakar, S. (1977). *Cancer Res.* **37,** 3006–3012.
Stone, P. R., Lorimer, W. S., and Kidwell, W. R. (1977) *Eur. J. Biochem.* **81,** 9–18.
Sudhakar, S., Tew, K. D., and Smulson, M. E. (1979a) *Cancer Res.* **39,** 1405–1410.
Sudhakar, S., Tew, K. D., and Smulson, M. E. (1979b). *Cancer Res.* **39,** 1411–1417.
Tew, K. D., Sudhakar, S., Schein, P. S., and Smulson, M. E. (1978). *Cancer Res.* **38,** 3371–3378.
Vidali, G., Boffa, L. C., Bradbury, E. M., and Allfrey, V. G. (1978) Proc. Natl. Acad. Sci. U.S., **75,** 2239–2243.
Whish, W. G. D., Daives, M. I., and Shall, S. (1975) *Biochem. Biophys. Res. Commun.* **65,** 722–730.

16

Gene Regulation in Steroid-Responsive Cells

GEORGE E. SWANECK, MING-JER TSAI, and
BERT W. O'MALLEY

I. Essential Features of Hormone-Responsive Cells and Some Major Questions

In a given organism, the genetic information in most of the cells is identical to that of every other cell. The diversity of cell phenotypes—differentiated cells—derives from the fact that each type of cell expresses only a limited amount of its total genetic information and diverse cell types express different parts of their genome. Thus differentiated cells perform distinct functions by synthesizing specific proteins. This differentiation of cell function is the result of a series of coordinated cell divisions which in an orderly progression reach a stage where specific genes are available to be transcribed preferentially in different tissues.

Thus hormone-responsive cells present in an adult organism are the consequence of development (cell multiplication and differentiation) from a single initial cell, which renders cells in which the expression of specific genes is dependent on the interaction of hormones with the genome. Furthermore, in cells responsive to sex steroids, the final steps of differentiation are frequently dependent also on the presence of these hormones (O'Malley and Means, 1974; Yamamoto and Alberts, 1975; Teng and Teng, 1975).

Target cells that are responsive to steroid hormones have receptors, i.e., intracellular binding proteins, that recognize and bind steroids to nuclear acceptor sites. There is a substantial body of evidence that all steroid hormones, including vitamin D, act in the following way: The free steroid diffuses from the extracellular space into the target cell and binds to the receptor protein. This complex is capable of translocation to the nucleus where it binds to chromatin components (Jensen *et al.*, 1974; O'Malley and Means, 1974; Edelman, 1975; Yamamoto and Alberts, 1976). There it triggers biochemical events of which the first measurable response is the accumulation of specific mRNAs (Feigelson *et al.*, 1975; Harris *et al.*, 1975; McKnight *et al.*, 1975; Ringold *et al.*, 1975; Palmiter *et al.*, 1976; Tata, 1976). As a result of this, there is an increase in protein synthesis, which accounts for the physiological effects observed in every steroid-responsive tissue.

The interaction of steroid–receptor complexes with chromatin has led to the assumption that this could be a regulatory step for transcription in a way similar to that observed in bacterial systems, where positive and negative transcriptional elements have been identified as proteins that function by interaction with the genome (Jacob and Monod, 1961; Greenblatt and Schlief, 1971; Dickson *et al.*, 1975; Majors, 1975). On the other hand, the assumptions that the concentration of mRNA is directly proportional to the rate of synthesis, and that the regulation of transcription is the principal step involved in control of the intracellular concentration of mRNA, have substantiated proposals for the role of the steroid–receptor complex as a selective regulator for the transcription of few specific genes. If this were so, a low number of high-affinity binding sites would be enough to account for this regulatory effect. This has not been demonstrated yet, and most observations have shown *in vivo* a high number of binding sites for steroid–receptor complexes in nuclei that exceeds the number of expected regulatory sites and does not allow their localization (Yamamoto and Alberts, 1975, 1976; Williams and Gorski, 1972; Vedeckis *et al.*, 1978).

Thus the appearance of steroid–receptor complexes in the nucleus and the increase in intracellular accumulation of specific mRNAs are two related and successive phenomena, but there is no evidence for a molecular linkage between them. Furthermore, although the primary regulatory event for hormone response is thought to be a modification reaction at the genome, steroid hormones may also affect the rate of synthesis of specific proteins by regulating the different posttranscriptional processes required to transform the information encoded in nuclear RNA transcripts into the final polypeptide gene product (Rosen and O'Malley, 1975).

These are some of the major questions that for one steroid-responsive tissue, the chick oviduct, we have been examining in our laboratory for the past 10 years. Steroid hormones have also different effects at different concentrations, and there are also coordinated effects of diverse steroids in one target tissue where they can either stimulate or inhibit cell functions. It is the purpose of this chapter to present some of the experimental evidence that points to the most efficient level at which estrogen and progesterone regulate the synthesis of specific proteins.

II. Hormonal Regulation of Egg-White Protein Synthesis: Primary and Secondary Induction

The chick oviduct is a very efficient experimental system for study of the reversible induction, by estrogen, of synthesis of the egg-white proteins ovalbumin, conalbumin, ovomucoid, and lysozyme (O'Malley *et al.*, 1969; Chan *et al.*, 1973; Rhoads *et al.*, 1973; Palmiter, 1973; Cox *et al.*, 1974; Palmiter *et al.*, 1976; Hynes *et al.*, 1977; Roop *et al.*, 1978; S. Y. Tsai *et al.*, 1978; McKnight, 1978). Also, specific steroid receptors have been found in this hormone-responsive tissue (Sherman *et al.*, 1970; O'Malley *et al.*, 1971; Smith *et al.*, 1979; Harrison and Toft, 1973). The administration of estrogen to an immature chicken produces (1) cell proliferation and differentiation of the oviduct epithelia, with subsequent development of tubular gland cells, and (2) synthesis of specific egg-white proteins in these tubular gland cells. Primary development is completed after 7–10 days of continuous treatment, and the length of this lag period in absolute terms is a function of the sensitivity of the assay for detection of the proteins.

After withdrawal of the primary estrogen stimulus there is involution of the oviduct and the synthesis of egg-white protein ceases, but the differentiated tubular gland cells persist. The readministration of estrogen after withdrawal (secondary stimulation) induces again the synthesis of egg-white proteins in preexisting gland cells. This secondary response has virtually no lag period, and the rate of protein synthesis is rapidly established, reaching its maximum in 24–40 hours, coupled with enhancement of the growth and differentiation of the oviduct. In a similar fashion, administration of progesterone can stimulate synthesis of the same egg-white proteins in differentiated tubular gland cells.

Ovalbumin is the major component of egg-white proteins, and most of our studies on the chick oviduct have been directed toward determining the molecular mechanisms that mediate the action of estrogen and progesterone in the induction of ovalbumin synthesis. Lately work has been in progress in order to study the induction of ovomucoid. The increase in the synthesis of ovalbumin and ovomucoid observed after primary and secondary inductions is preceded by an increase in the intracellular concentration of specific mRNAs (Chan *et al.*, 1973; Harris *et al.*, 1975; Rhoads *et al.*, 1973; Palmiter, 1973; Cox *et al.*, 1974; Hynes *et al.*, 1977; Roop *et al.*, 1978; S. Y. Tsai, *et al.*, 1978). This effect has allowed us to study the early events of induction after estrogen stimulation, and our results (see below) indicate that, for ovalbumin, the regulatory steps for the estrogen response are associated with a specific increase in the rate of transcription of the ovalbumin gene (Swaneck *et al.*, 1979). We report here the direct measurement, in an isolated nuclei system, of the transcription of structural and intervening sequences of the ovalbumin gene after *in vivo* induction by estrogen.

III. Effects of Estrogen in Gene Expression in the Chick Oviduct

A. The Requirement of Isolating Ovalbumin mRNA

In order to demonstrate that the increase in the rate of ovalbumin synthesis was due to an increase in the amount of specific mRNA ($mRNA_{ov}$), our earlier studies were directed toward isolating and purifying this messenger. Subsequently it was used for the synthesis of complementary DNA (cDNA) which could serve as a hybridization probe for the quantitation of $mRNA_{ov}$ in oviducts under estrogen stimulation. The procedures used were designed for the isolation and selective purification of the poly(A) RNA (putative mRNA) from total nucleic acid extracts of hen oviducts, and the presence of pure mRNA$_{ov}$ was assayed for its ability to direct the specific synthesis of ovalbumin in a wheat germ cell-free translation assay. This yielded polypeptides that (1) were specifically immunoprecipitated with ovalbumin antiserum, (2) migrated as a single peak in sodium dodecyl sulfate (SDS) polyacrylamide gel electrophoresis in correspondence to an ovalbumin standard, and (3) were free of rRNA (Rosenfeld *et al.*, 1972; Rosen *et al.*, 1975).

The molecular weight of mRNA$_{ov}$ was estimated by sucrose gradient centrifugation and sedimentation velocity determination, and its molecular size was ascertained by electron microscopy under denaturing conditions. A molecular weight of 650,000 was thus obtained, and this value corresponded to a polyribonucleotide chain of 1890 residues, which is 600 nucleotides longer than the nucleotide sequence required to code for the 387 amino acids present in the ovalbumin protein. The poly(A) region constituent of the mRNA$_{ov}$ was heterogeneous in size, and the adenosine number ranged from 20 to 140 residues (Woo *et al.*, 1975).

The complete sequence of chicken ovalbumin mRNA has been determined on a full-length duplex DNA copy of the mRNA$_{ov}$ cloned in the *Escherichia coli* plasmid pMB9 (McReynolds *et al.*, 1977, 1978), and it has been found to be 1859 residues long, excluding the poly(A) region and its cap terminus. It has a leader sequence of 64 noncoding nucleotides at the beginning of the 5'-end, and the 1158 coding nucleotides are separated from the poly(A) region by 637 nucleotides. Studies of the secondary structure of mRNA$_{ov}$ have shown that it has extensive base pairing between neighboring sequences, similar in proportion to that found in rRNAs and tRNA but with fewer GC-rich stems and with AU pairs in short regions (Van *et al.*, 1977). These unique features raise the possibility that the conformation that derives from this secondary structure may be important for certain posttranscriptional events in the cytoplasm.

B. Induction and Synthesis of mRNA$_{ov}$ *in Vivo*

After the purification of mRNA$_{ov}$, a complementary DNA (cDNA$_{ov}$) was synthesized *in vitro* using RNA-dependent DNA polymerase from avian myeloblastosis virus. This cDNA$_{ov}$ was then employed in DNA excess hybridization assays to determine the effects of estrogen on the concentration of mRNA$_{ov}$ extracted from the chick oviduct (Harris *et al.*, 1975). The concentration of mRNA$_{ov}$ per tubular gland cell was measured in immature chicks during primary stimulation, after hormone withdrawal, and again following secondary stimulation with estrogen. The initial stimulation of the immature tissue resulted in growth of the oviduct, differentiation of epithelial cells to tubular glands, and a corresponding increase in the concentration of $mRNA_{ov}$ in the tubular gland cell from essentially zero before estrogen administration to ~48,000 molecules per cell after 18 days of estrogen treatment (Table I). Withdrawal of estrogen from the chick for 12 days was followed by a decrease in the cellular $mRNA_{ov}$ concentration to an almost undetectable level. Readministration of a single dose of estrogen (secondary stimulation) to these chicks resulted in a rapid increase in the concentration of $mRNA_{ov}$ that was significant within 60 minutes and by 30 hours had reached 17,000 molecules per tubular gland cell.

These data indicated that estrogen increased the cellular concentration of $mRNA_{ov}$ molecules in the oviduct of unstimulated and withdrawn chickens. With the use of the previous data, a half-life for $mRNA_{ov}$ of approximately 24–40 hours was calculated for stimulated oviducts. But it has been shown that this half-life varies according to the hormonal state of the chick and decreases from the reported value to 2–3 hours in the withdrawn animal (Cox, 1977). In this context, estrogen not only increases the concentration of $mRNA_{ov}$, but its presence is also required for the prevention of RNA degradation at a posttranscriptional (nuclear or cytoplasmic) level of regulation. It was therefore important to measure the *de novo* synthesis of $mRNA_{ov}$ after estrogen administration. If direct RNA-labeling studies show that ovalbumin mRNA sequences are newly synthesized, then it could be concluded that, for the most part, the level of regulation of $mRNA_{ov}$ concentration is at the transcriptional step.

TABLE I

Effect of Estrogen Administration on the Intracellular Concentration of $mRNA_{ov}$ in the Chick Oviduct[a]

Hormonal state[b]	Tubular gland cells (% of total)	Number of molecules of $mRNA_{ov}$ per tubular gland cell
Unstimulated		
After 4 days	34	20,000
After 9 days	50	44,000
After 18 days	85	52,000
Withdrawn[c]	15	0–10
After 1 hour	15	50
After 4 hours	15	2,300
After 8 hours	20	5,100
After 29 hours	25	17,000

[a] From Harris et al. (1975).
[b] DES (2.5 mg) was injected daily into immature chicks.
[c] After 2 weeks of daily injection with DES, hormonal treatment was discontinued for 12 days and then a single dose of DES (2.5 mg) was injected.

IV. Synthesis of mRNA$_{ov}$ in Isolated Oviduct Nuclei after *in Vivo* Induction by Estrogen

A. Characteristics of the *in Vitro* Synthesis of mRNA$_{ov}$

In an attempt to define the mechanisms of the estrogen-induced accumulation of mRNA$_{ov}$ we measured the rate of transcription of the chicken ovalbumin gene *in vitro* after *in vivo* induction by estrogen. We have studied the optimal conditions for the synthesis of radiolabeled RNA by nuclei isolated from different tissues of estrogen-treated chicks and from oviducts in different hormonal states. The conditions for the isolation of nuclei and for the synthesis of radiolabeled RNA have been established according to the previous work of several authors (Marzluff *et al.*, 1973; Tsai *et al.*, 1975; Ernest *et al.*, 1976; Weber *et al.*, 1977).

Table II summarizes the results obtained when nuclei from stimulated oviducts were incubated in the presence of [^{3}H]UTP. The direct measurement of the incorporation of radioactive nucleotides into trichloroacetic acid-precipitable material, which represents *de novo* synthesized RNA, reached a plateau in about 15 minutes in the isolated nuclei reaction mixture at 37°C. The incorporation was rapid during the first 5 minutes, and the addition of a 100-fold excess of nonlabeled UTP to the reaction mixture after 10 minutes showed no decrease in this value for the following 60 minutes, indicating that there was no major degradation of the newly synthesized [^{3}H]RNA. The time course of the [^{3}H]RNA synthesis was linear for about 60 minutes when the incubation was performed at 25°C.

In nuclei isolated from diethylstilbestrol (DES)-stimulated oviducts (Table II) 45–52% of the total [^{3}H]RNA synthesis was sensitive to concentrations of α-amanitin (0.5 μg/ml) that inhibit transcription by polymerase II (Weinman and Roeder, 1974; Weil and Blatti, 1975). In the presence of concentrations of α-amanitin (100 μg/ml) that inhibit polymerases II and III, about 20–38% of the activity remained, indicating that polymerase I also was active under the conditions employed. In order to rule out the possibility of RNA-dependent [^{3}H]RNA synthesis, actinomycin D (40 μg/ml) was added in the reaction mixture, and RNA synthesis was inhibited by 95%.

B. Quantitation of Nascent Hormone-Induced [^{3}H]mRNA$_{ov}$ Sequences

The concentration of [^{3}H]mRNA$_{ov}$ in the radiolabeled RNA synthesized by nuclei from oviducts under different states of estrogen stimulation and from nontarget tissues was determined by hybridizing the total

TABLE II

Effect of Temperature and of Various Inhibitors of RNA Polymerases on [³H] RNA Synthesis in Nuclei Isolated from Hormone-Stimulated Oviducts[a]

	[³H]UMP incorporated (pmoles/μg DNA)		
Conditions	5 minutes	10 minutes	15 minutes
At 37°C	0.15	0.18	0.20
α-Amanitin, 0.5 μg/ml	0.08	0.09	0.09
α-Amanitin, 100 μg/ml	0.03	0.04	0.08
1 mM UTP after 10 minutes	0.15	0.18	0.19
Actinomycin D, 40 μg/ml	0.008	0.009	0.012
At 25°C	0.04	0.09	0.14
Actinomycin D (40 μg/ml)	0.002	0.004	0.008

[a] Nuclei were purified from oviducts by homogenization in 10 volumes of 0.5 M sucrose, 50 mM Tris, 20 mM KCL, 5 mM MgCl$_2$ (TKM) buffer in a Tissuemizer blender at 70 V for 1 minute. The homogenate was filtered through cheesecloth and organza, layered over a cushion of 0.88 M sucrose–TKM, and centrifuged at 2000 g for 10 minutes. The pellet was resuspended in 2 ml of 0.88 M sucrose and homogenized in 30 ml of 2.1 M sucrose–TKM, filtered through organza, and centrifuged through a 2.1 M sucrose–TKM cushion at 12,000 g for 90 minutes. The nuclear pellets were finally suspended in 25% glycerol, 5 mM MgCl$_2$, 5 mM dithiotreithol (DTT), 0.1 mM EDTA, 50 mM Tris, pH 7.8. Nuclei from chick liver and spleen were isolated by the same method. Nuclei prepared this way were free of cytoplasmic debris, and were round or oval-shaped with one or two nucleoli as observed by light microscopy. The in vitro [³H]RNA synthesis of 0.8–2.2×10^8 nuclei/ml was tested in duplicate in 5-ml reaction mixtures that contained 0.8 mM ATP, GTP, and CTP, 0.014 mM [³H]UTP (specific activity, 45.4 Ci/mmole), 3 mM MgCl$_2$, 1.5 mM MnCl$_2$, 3 mM DTT, 0.5 mM EDTA, 100 mM KCl, 12.5% glycerol, 50 mM Tris–HCl, pH 7.8. At the end of the [³H]RNA synthesis incubation, 100-μl aliquots were taken in duplicate for measuring the incorporation of ³H into RNA by precipitation with cold 10% trichloracetic acid, 50 mM pyrophosphate.

[³H]RNA to filters containing cloned ovalbumin cDNA (pOV230), according to techniques previously reported (Jacquet et al., 1977; Roop et al., 1978) and as shown in Table III. Cloned pOV230 DNA contains a full-length ovalbumin DNA insert (1847 nucleotides) except for 12 nucleotides at the 5′-end (McReynolds et al., 1977, 1978). Table III shows the concentration of mRNA$_{ov}$ sequences present in the total [³H]RNA. Oviduct nuclei from chickens stimulated chronically with DES synthesized mRNA$_{ov}$ sequences at a concentration of 0.2–0.3% of the total [³H]RNA, while no detectable mRNA$_{ov}$ sequences were found in [³H]RNA synthesized in spleen and liver nuclei. This tissue-specific response represents a preferential synthesis in the sense that it corresponds to at least a significant 50 to 100-fold increase over the random transcription of the total chick genome. Also shown in Table III, the lack of mRNA$_{ov}$ synthesis in isolated

TABLE III

Specificity of In Vitro Nuclear [³H]mRNA Synthesis from Different Tissues [a]

Sources of [³H]RNA	Total [³H]RNA synthesis (pmoles UMP/mg DNA)	Input of [³H]RNA to hybridize (cpm × 10⁻⁶)	[³H]RNA hybridized (cpm)	[³²P]cRNA_ov recovery (%)	Specific hybridizable sequences (cpm)	mRNA_ov in total RNA (%)
Oviduct, DES [b]	186	1.02	437	18.6	2350	0.238
		2.92	971	14.7	6950	0.238
Spleen, DES [b]	78	3.0	—	18.9	—	<0.001 [d]
Liver, DES [b]	110	0.6	—	16.9	—	<0.001 [d]
Oviduct, withdrawn after 3 days [c]	130	1.1	—	17.1	—	<0.001 [d]
Oviduct, withdrawn after 14 days [c]	71	0.9	—	15.0	—	<0.001 [d]
Oviduct, DES plus 40 µg/ml Actinomycin D [b]	12	1.1	468	18.2	2576	0.234
Oviduct, DES plus 0.5 µg/ml α-amanitin [b]	83	1.6	—	18.3	—	<0.001 [d]
Oviduct DES, pOV230 filters saturated with mRNA_ov [b]	186	3.0	—	—	—	<0.001 [d]

[a] The concentration of [³H]mRNA_ov in the transcripts was determined by hybridizing the total [³H]RNA to filters containing cloned ovalbumin DNA pOV230. The hybridization reaction started with the addition of these filters to the [³H]RNA suspended in 50% formamide, and incubation proceeded for 16 hours at 42°C; filters were then removed, rinsed, and treated with pancreatic RNase, and the radioactivity was measured. In parallel vials, nonradiolabeled mRNA_ov was added to the reaction as a competitor, and the radioactivity present in these filters was subtracted from the total [³H]RNA hybridized to pOV230. With this technique the amount of newly synthesized [³H]mRNA_ov was measured. As an internal standard, ³²P-labeled complementary RNA_ov transcribed from ovalbumin cDNA was used in order to correct for the efficiency of hybridization and loss of hybridizable sequences during the washing and RNase treatment step. Tsai et al (1978) have described these procedures in detail.

[b] Chickens were implanted with DES pellets weekly.

[c] Chickens were injected daily with 2.5 mg of DES in 0.25 ml of sesame oil.

[d] mRNA_ov sequences cannot be measured at a concentration less than 0.001% in our assay.

nuclei from oviducts after withdrawal from hormonal treatment confirms the importance of estrogen in maintaining the synthesis of mRNA$_{ov}$. Total [^{3}H]RNA and [^{3}H]mRNA$_{ov}$ synthesis was inhibited about 96% when actinomycin D (40 μg/ml) was present in the reaction mixture. This inhibition appeared to be random in that the total mass of newly synthesized [^{3}H]RNA was greatly decreased (Table III), but there was no preferential inhibition of [^{3}H]mRNA$_{ov}$ sequences, since their concentration remained unaltered in the presence of actinomycin D (Table III). These results are consistent with the idea that the synthesis of mRNA$_{ov}$ sequences is a DNA-dependent process. The fact that the hybridizable [^{3}H]RNA can be competed by an excess of unlabeled mRNA$_{ov}$ indicated that these transcripts were indeed mRNA$_{ov}$ sequences (Table III), and inhibition of the synthesis of mRNA$_{ov}$ by α-amanitin at low concentrations substantiated that they were transcribed by RNA polymerase II. The values for the mRNA$_{ov}$ sequences synthesized by nuclei *in vitro* shown here are higher than the corresponding values obtained in previous reports using chromatin. This could be explained by the presence of endogenous nuclear RNA polymerases and the preservation of nuclear structure that possibly constitutes a condition for an *in vitro* system where specific genes can be transcribed more efficiently (Stallcup *et al.*, 1978).

The direct measurement of [^{3}H]mRNA$_{ov}$ sequences by the filter hybridization technique implies the detection of only *de novo* synthesized RNA. Nevertheless, it is likely that the large majority of the RNA synthesis is due to the completion of chains initiated *in vivo* prior to the *in vitro* incubation and thus reflects the transcriptional activity present in the intact animal and its own hormonal milieu. Table III also shows that the filter hybridization technique is highly specific, and its reproducibility and validity were evident when a close range of values for mRNA$_{ov}$ sequences was obtained at different input levels of [^{3}H]RNA synthesized in nuclei from stimulated chicks. To validate the transcription in nuclei we have assayed whether the correct strand of DNA is transcribed *in vitro*. pOV230 filters were presaturated with mRNA$_{ov}$ before the hybridization was carried out, and in this condition only the anticoding DNA sequences were free to hybridize. In Table III the results show that the [^{3}H]RNA did not hybridize, thus indicating that the nascent nuclear transcripts corresponded to the coding strand.

Next we examined the effects of hormone withdrawal on expression of the ovalbumin gene in oviduct nuclei. The decrease was rapid and appeared to be exponential (Fig. 1A). After 60 hours there was no detectable mRNA$_{ov}$ in the transcripts, while the total [^{3}H]RNA synthesis in nuclei was not altered greatly. This preferential loss of expression of the ovalbumin gene after 60 hours of hormone withdrawal was readily reversible

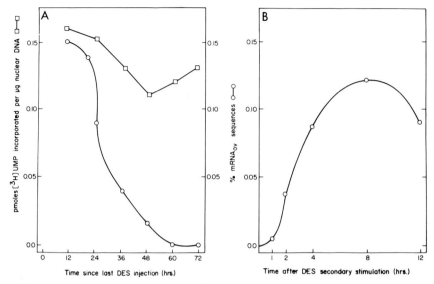

Fig. 1   Time course of decrease in mRNA$_{ov}$ synthesis by nuclei from chick oviducts after withdrawal from DES treatment (A) and of recovery of mRNA$_{ov}$ synthesis after readministration of 2.5 mg of DES (B). □, Total [³H]RNA synthesis; ○, [³H]mRNA$_{ov}$ synthesis.

within 1–2 hours after readministration of a single injection (secondary stimulation) of estrogen (Fig. 1B). There was an acute increase in the synthesis of mRNA$_{ov}$ sequences that reached a peak by 8 hours. When a second injection was given after 12 hours of secondary stimulation, the synthesis of mRNA$_{ov}$ increased to values approaching those of oviduct nuclei prepared from chicks chronically treated with DES. Similarly, when chicks were withdrawn from hormone for periods of 72 or 86 hours, induction of mRNA$_{ov}$ synthesis in isolated nuclei was observed but the maximal levels of induction were suppressed (Swaneck *et al.*, 1979).

These results support the hypothesis that estrogen induces the accumulation of mRNA$_{ov}$ primarily by increasing its rate of transcription. If another mechanism, such as inhibition of its rate of degradation, were responsible for changes in the level of mRNA$_{ov}$, one would expect the rate of transcription of the ovalbumin gene in isolated nuclei to be less dependent on the hormonal state of the chick. However, since we detect no synthesis (Table III) and little mRNA$_{ov}$ mass (see below) in withdrawn chicks, ovalbumin sequences would have to be degraded at the rate of their synthesis in order to account for the lack of any *de novo* synthesized ovalbumin transcripts in nuclei derived from the withdrawn oviduct. Thus, while pretranslational stabilization of mRNA$_{ov}$ is probably involved in the overall regulation of the level of mRNA$_{ov}$ by estrogen, its role appears to be secondary to that of gene transcription.

In further support of transcriptional regulation is the observation that the kinetics of induction of synthesis of mRNA$_{ov}$ sequences in isolated nuclei by estrogen resembled the accumulation of mRNA$_{ov}$ *in vivo* (Harris *et al.*, 1975; Roop *et al.*, 1978). Significant increases occurred under both conditions after 1–2 hours of secondary estrogen stimulation and continued to increase for at least 8 hours.

V. *In Vitro* Transcription of the Natural Ovalbumin Gene

Recently it has been shown that the structural sequences of the ovalbumin gene are interrupted by multiple regions of nonstructural intervening sequences (Fig. 2) at least three times the length of the structural regions (Breathnach *et al.*, 1977; Dugaiczyk *et al.*, 1978). Similar findings have been reported for the globin gene, and in addition the 15 S precursor of globin mRNA has been shown to contain both structural and intervening sequences of the globin gene (Jeffreys and Flavell, 1977; Tilghman *et al.*, 1978). Similarly, transcripts of both types of ovalbumin sequences accumulated *in vivo* in oviduct nuclei after stimulation with estrogen (Table IV). In addition, we have demonstrated the existence of high-molecular-weight species of ovalbumin RNA in nuclear extracts of oviducts stimulated chronically with estrogen. Since these molecules contain sequences complementary to intervening as well as to structural sequences of the ovalbumin gene, it is likely that these RNAs are precursors of mature mRNA$_{ov}$ (Roop *et al.*, 1978; Swaneck *et al.*, 1979).

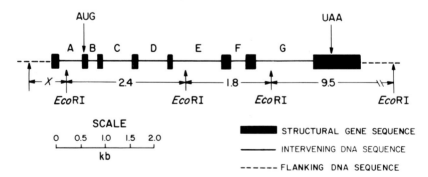

Fig. 2 Molecular organization of the natural ovalbumin gene resulting from *EcoR* I digestion. The structural sequences are separated by intervening sequences (A–G). This organization derives from a more detailed restriction analysis of cloned DNA fragments and from data of electron microscopy of R-loop hybrids between DNA and mRNA$_{ov}$ (Dugaiczyk *et al.*, 1978, Lai *et al.*, 1978).

TABLE IV

In Vivo **Accumulation of Transcripts of Structural and Intervening Sequences of the Ovalbumin Gene in Oviduct Nuclei**[a]

| | Number of molecules per tubular gland cell nucleus[b] | | |
| | Structural sequences | Intervening sequences | |
Hormonal state	pOV230	2.4	1.8
Stimulated	3075	233	286
Withdrawn from DES			
After 14 days	2	1	1
Restimulated with DES			
After 2 hours	6	2	3
After 4 hours	71	—	15
After 8 hours	440	25	33

[a] Nuclear RNA was isolated as described by Roop *et al.* (1978).

[b] Concentration of $mRNA_{ov}$ sequences in total nuclear RNA was measured by hybridization of excess RNA to [^{3}H]DNA probes corresponding to structural and intervening sequences (2.4 and 1.8 kb).

The presence of transcripts of intervening sequences from the chicken ovalbumin gene in nuclear RNA indicated that RNA polymerases were able to transcribe selectively *in vivo* the entire gene. The ability of isolated nuclei to perform this preferential synthesis has also been examined, and in order to define the mechanism of steroid hormone-induced accumulation of $mRNA_{ov}$ we have studied the rate of transcription of the ovalbumin gene *in vitro* and the size of ovalbumin gene transcripts *in vivo*. We have measured the *in vitro* nuclear transcription of intervening sequences of the ovalbumin gene by hybridizing total nuclear [^{3}H]RNA to filters containing cloned ovalbumin DNA restriction fragments pOV2.4 DNA and pOV1.8 DNA which represent most of the intervening sequences in the ovalbumin gene (Lai *et al.*, 1978; Breathnach *et al.*, 1977; Roop *et al.*, 1978). The results (Table V) showed that 0.17–0.18% of the total [^{3}H]RNA from chronically stimulated oviduct nuclei corresponded to intervening sequences. Since about 20% of pOV1.8 and pOV2.4 DNA sequences are structural sequences (Lai *et al.*, 1978), $mRNA_{ov}$ (7 μg) was included in this experiment to compete out any structural sequence hybridization.

The kinetics of induction of transcripts of intervening sequences were next examined in the [^{3}H]RNA synthesized by nuclei from oviducts restimulated with estrogen after 60 hours of hormone withdrawal. These results (Table V) indicated that the synthesis of intervening transcripts was detectable after 1 hour of DES treatment and increased five- to six-fold

TABLE V

In Vitro **Transcription of Ovalbumin Gene Structural and Intervening Sequences by Oviduct Nuclei**[a]

Hormonal state	[³H]RNA hybridized to filters (%)		
	pOV230	pOV2.4	pOV1.8
DES daily	0.23	0.18	0.17
Withdrawn from DES after 60 hours	<0.001	<0.001	<0.001
After 1 hour DES	0.010	0.005	0.004
After 2 hours DES	0.031	0.010	0.008
After 4 hours DES	0.060	0.026	0.025

[a] [³H]RNA ($1-5 \times 10^6$ cpm) synthesized in nuclei from oviducts of stimulated, withdrawn, and secondarily stimulated chicks was incubated with filters containing pOV230 DNA, pOV2.4 DNA, or pOV1.8 DNA and the appropriate [³²P]RNA internal standard (2000 cpm) in the presence and absence of competitor RNA (7.5 μg of mRNA$_{ov}$ or 9 μg of either RNA 2.4 or RNA 1.8) was also present in duplicate vials. Conditions were the same as described for Table II. Values represent the percent of hybridized [³H]RNA that could be specifically competed out by the unlabeled RNA.

within 4 hours, in parallel with increased transcription of structural sequences. Nevertheless, the maximum level of intervening sequence transcripts never equals that of structural transcripts. Although this result may reflect a faster turnover rate for the intervening sequence RNA, *in vitro* labeling conditions and hybridization conditions may be also suboptimal for quantitating intervening sequence transcripts.

All the studies described above indicated that the transcription of the ovalbumin gene *in vitro*, after *in vivo* induction, proceeded to an equivalent extent as observed in the *in vivo* studies. Furthermore, our data indicated that ovalbumin mRNA synthesis was a process that (1) was estrogen-responsive, (2) was preferentially lost after estrogen withdrawal, (3) was dependent on the coding strand template, and (4) was effected by RNA polymerase II. It was then necessary to study the site of termination of the *in vitro* transcription, as we have observed that *in vivo* transcription terminates near the end of the 3'-terminus of the structural sequences. In order to study the approximate site of termination, *in vitro* transcripts were hybridized to filters containing the restriction fragment pOV9.5 DNA and, as shown in Table VI, the hybirdization values indicated that the transcript was complementary to this fragment. When the hybridization assay was done in the presence of competitor OV9.5 RNA (unlabeled transcripts of the OV9.5 fragment), the hybridized radioactivity was reduced to background level. Further details of the termination site were provided by competition with the unlabeled transcripts of the restriction fragments 2.7, 3.4, 1.7, and 1.8 kb generated after *Hind* III digestion of the 9.5-kb

TABLE VI

Hybridization of [³H]RNA Synthesized in
Nuclei Isolated from Oviduct to pOV9.5 DNA[a,b]

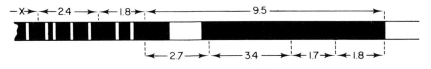

Competitor	[³H]RNA hybridized (cpm)
—	1050
RNA, 9.5	125
RNA, 2.7	250
RNA, 3.4	885
RNA, 1.7 + 1.8	975

[a] From Roop *et al.* (1979).

[b] White areas correspond to structural sequences of the natural ovalbumin gene. After digestion by *EcoR* I, three major fragments were generated: 2.4, 1.8, and 9.5 kb. Further digestion of the 9.5-kb fragment by *Hind* III produces four different fragments of 2.7, 3.4, 1.7, and 1.8 kb. Results show the radioactivity (cpm) hybridized to filters containing pOV9.5 DNA (see text).

fragment (Fig. 2). The competition with unlabeled RNA 2.7 (Table VI) established that the *in vitro* transcript contained sequences complementary to that DNA region, while the other transcripts (RNA 3.4, 1.7, and 1.8 kb) did not compete, indicating that *in vitro* termination of transcription occurred at a region in the DNA correspondingly located, by restriction enzyme analysis, in the 2.7-kb fragment. This is strong evidence that the 3'-end of most of the *in vitro* transcripts is similar to that of the mRNA$_{ov}$ isolated from nuclei (Roop *et al.*, 1979).

VI. Hormone-Induced Accumulation of Putative mRNA$_{ov}$ Precursors

Electrophoresis of oviduct nuclear RNA from chicks stimulated chronically with DES have revealed the existence of multiple species (labeled a–f in Fig. 3) of high-molecular-weight ovalbumin sequence-containing RNA (Fig. 3A). The mRNA$_{ov}$ band represents mature (18 S) mRNA$_{ov}$. Species of RNA larger than mRNA$_{ov}$ are not found in oviduct cytoplasm and are not aggregates of mRNA$_{ov}$. Since these molecules contain sequences complementary to intervening as well as to structural sequences of the ovalbumin gene, it is likely that they are precursors of mRNA$_{ov}$.

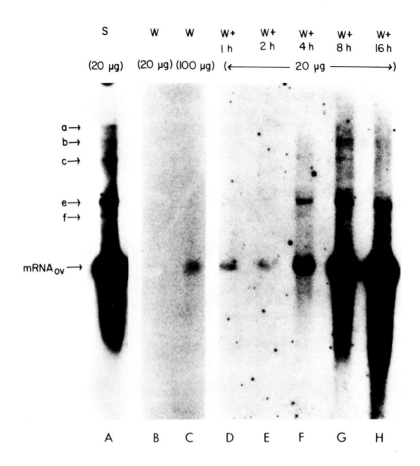

Fig. 3 Induction of high-molecular-weight ovalbumin RNA by secondary estrogen stimulation. Oviduct nuclear RNA, isolated from chicks subjected to the indicated hormonal treatments, was electrophoresed (40 V, 16 hours) on 1.5% agarose gels containing 10 mM methylmercury hydroxide. The RNA was transferred to DBM paper (12 × 14 cm) and hybridized with the [^{32}P]-labeled pOV230 probe (2 × 10^7 cpm, 2.5 × 10^8 cpm). Species of ovalbumin RNA larger than mRNA$_{ov}$ where labeled a, b, c, e, f. Bands d and g, which are minor species, were not detected in this figure. (A), Oviduct nuclear RNA (20 μg) from chicks chronically stimulated with DES. (B), Oviduct nuclear RNA (20 μg) from chicks stimulated with DES and then withdrawn from hormone for 14 days. (C), Same as lane (B), except 100 μg. Lane (D) oviduct nuclear RNA (20 μg) from chicks withdrawn for 14 days and restimulated with DES for 1 hour. (E) Same as (D), except restimulation period was 2 hours. (F) Same as (D), except restimulation period was 4 hours. (G) Same as (D), except restimulation period was 8 hours. (H) Same as (D), except restimulation period was 16 hours.

Evidence for this hypothesis has been presented elsewhere (Roop *et al.*, 1978; Nordstrom *et al.*, 1979).

From 20 μg of nuclear RNA isolated from chicks that had been withdrawn from estrogen for 14 days, neither high-molecular-weight ovalbumin RNA nor mature $mRNA_{ov}$ was detected (Fig. 3, lane B). However, a slight amount of $mRNA_{ov}$ was detected when 100 μg of withdrawn nuclear RNA was assayed (Fig. 3C). Since no high-molecular-weight ovalbumin RNA was observed in this experiment (Fig. 3C), these data indicate that the low amount of mature $mRNA_{ov}$ in withdrawn oviduct nuclei is not due to a block in RNA processing which would have permitted the accumulation of high-molecular-weight species of ovalbumin RNA (Swaneck *et al.*, 1979).

After 1 hour of secondary estrogen stimulation, a band of $mRNA_{ov}$ was detected (Fig. 3D). After 2 hours, an additional band of high-molecular-weight ovalbumin RNA (band e) was also faintly detected (Fig. 3E); after 4 hours significant increases in the concentration of mature $mRNA_{ov}$ and high-molecular-weight forms were apparent (Fig. 3F), and after 8 hours all major species of high-molecular-weight were detected (Fig. 3G). By 16 hours of secondary stimulation, the concentration of the high-molecular-weight ovalbumin RNA species, particularly the largest ones, began to decline. In contrast, that of mature $mRNA_{ov}$ continued to increase.

The kinetics of accumulation of nuclear species of ovalbumin RNA larger than mature $mRNA_{ov}$ (Fig. 3) closely mimic those observed previously for nuclear RNA transcripts corresponding to the intervening sequences of the ovalbumin gene (Table IV). The concentrations of high-molecular-weight ovalbumin RNA and intervening sequence transcripts both remain low for 2 hours, increase sharply at 4 hours, reach a maximum at 8 hours, and then appear to decline. These results support the hypothesis that RNA sequences corresponding to the intervening sequences of the ovalbumin gene are present in oviduct nuclei mainly in the form of RNA molecules higher in molecular weight than mature $mRNA_{ov}$.

At all times after secondary estrogen stimulation, the concentration of mature $mRNA_{ov}$ was greater than that of the high-molecular-weight forms of ovalbumin RNA and, at short times after injection, less than detectable amounts of the high-molecular-weight forms were observed. After short periods of restimulation, however, the accumulation of small amounts of precursors divided among multiple species may be difficult to detect relative to that of $mRNA_{ov}$, which is a discrete species. In addition, rapid processing activity already present in withdrawn oviduct nuclei or very rapidly activated by estrogen may lead to the preferential accumulation of mature $mRNA_{ov}$. Thus more detailed and more sensitive studies are required to assess accurately the precursor–product relationships of the ovalbumin RNA molecules.

VII. Summary

De novo synthesis of RNA sequences corresponding to intervening as well as to structural sequences of the ovalbumin gene have been detected in isolated oviduct nuclei. Their presence in the nuclear transcripts and their time course of induction support the hypothesis that structural and intervening sequences are transcribed from the natural ovalbumin gene in response to steroid hormones. These results are in agreement with our previous demonstration of high-molecular-weight species of ovalbumin RNA in nuclei that contain structural as well as intervening RNA sequences and are thus likely precursors of mature cytoplasmic $mRNA_{ov}$ (Roop *et al.*, 1978; Swaneck *et al.*, 1979).

Analysis of the size of *in vivo* nuclear RNA by denaturing gel electrophoresis revealed that withdrawal of hormone depleted the level of high-molecular-weight ovalbumin RNA as well as that of mature $mRNA_{ov}$ and that readministration of estrogen induced the accumulation of both species. These results are consistent also with transcriptional regulation of the ovalbumin gene. In addition, they rule out the possibility that the rapid accumulation of mature $mRNA_{ov}$ after secondary stimulation results from the processing of ovalbumin RNA precursors that might have been stored in the withdrawn oviduct.

The results presented here indicate that it is possible to assay the *in vitro* nuclear synthesis of hormone-inducible specific mRNA and that modulation of the preferential expression of the ovalbumin gene *in vivo* is maintained in isolated oviduct nuclei. With the use of isolated nuclei it will be possible to quantify the rate of synthesis of other mRNAs induced by estrogen and progesterone. This approach is feasible, since the highly organized, complex structure necessary for the selective expression of inducible genes appears to be preserved in nuclei where transcription continues to proceed faithfully under the *in vitro* labeling conditions described.

Our efforts to elucidate the mechanism of action of sex steroids in the chick oviduct have led us to a better understanding of the organization of the eukaryotic gene. We have used sex steroid hormones in order to study the regulation of gene expression, i.e., the synthesis of specific proteins, and of the many possible regulatory steps for the induction of ovalbumin by estrogen in the chick oviduct; and we have presented evidence that regulation occurs primarily at the level of transcription.

At present, we do not know in precise detail how estrogen induces the preferential transcription of the ovalbumin gene *in vivo*. While new experimental approaches must be developed to understand fully the regulation of gene expression in eukaryotes, we are aware that many of the assumptions regarding regulatory steps have been derived from prokaryotic systems. In these organisms DNA is the primary genetic material expressed through an intermediate, mRNA, which directs protein synthesis. However, the structure and function of the genetic apparatus of eukaryotic cells is quite different from that of bacteria; the complex nuclear architecture, the presence of intervening sequences in genes, the existence of chromosomal proteins, the transcription and processing of precursors mRNAs, the posttranscriptional modifications of RNA, and so on, constitute some of the differences indicating that the mechanisms that regulate gene expression may also be significantly different.

The cells of eukaryotes appear to have more complex mechanisms to process genetic information for the development of differentiated tissues and the expression of specific genes. It is conceivable that the regulation of gene expression has evolved as a more efficient process and selective agents such as hormones have been achieved. In this respect, steroid–receptor complexes most certainly play an important role in the control of differentiation and regulation of gene expression in eukaryotic cells.

References

Breathnach, R., Mandel, J. L., and Chambon, P. (1977). *Nature (London)* **270**, 314–319.

Chan, L., Means, A. R., and O'Malley, B. W. (1973). *Proc. Natl. Acad. Sci. U.S.A.* **70**, 1870–1874.

Cox, F. R. (1977). *Biochemistry* **16**, 3433–3443.

Cox, R. G., Haines, M. E., and Emtage, J. S. (1974). *Eur. J. Biochem.* **47**, 225–236.

Dickson, R., Abelson, J., Barnes, W., and Reznikoff, W. (1975). *Science* **187**, 27–30.

Dugaiczyk, A., Woo, S. L. C., Lai, E. C., Mace, M. L., McReynolds, L. A., and O'Malley, B. W. (1978). *Nature (London)* **274**, 328–333.

Edelman, I. S. (1975). *J. Steroid Biochem.* **6**, 147–153.

Ernest, M. J., Schutz, G., and Feigelson, P. (1976). *Biochemistry* **15**, 824–829.

Feigelson, P., Beato, M., Colman, P., Kalimi, M., Killewich, L., and Schutz, G. (1975). *Recent Prog. Horm. Res.* **31**, 213–249.

Greenblatt, J., and Schlief, R. (1971). *Nature (London), New Biol.* **273**, 166–169.

Harris, S. E., Rosen, J. M., Means, A. R., and O'Malley, B. W. (1975). *Biochemistry* **14**, 2072–2081.

Harrison, R. W., and Toft, D. O. (1973). *Biochem. Biophys. Res. Commun.* **55**, 857–863.

Hynes, N. E., Grover, B., Sippel, A. E., Nguyen-Hu, M. C., and Schutz, G. (1977). *Cell* **11**, 923–932.

Jacob, F., and Monod, F. (1961). *J. Mol. Biol.* **3**, 318–356.

Jacquet, M., Levy, S. T., Robert, B., and Gros, G. (1977). *Gene* **1**, 373–383.

Jeffreys, A. J., and Flavell, R. A. (1977). *Cell* **12**, 429–436.

Jensen, E. V., Mohla, S., Gorell, T. A., and DeSombre, E. R. (1974). *Vitam. Horm. (N.Y.)* **32**, 89–127.

Lai, E. C., Woo, S. L. C., Dugaiczyk, A., Catterall, J. F., and O'Malley, B. W. (1978). *Proc. Natl. Acad. Sci. U.S.A.* **75**, 2205–2209.

McKnight, G. S. (1978). *Cell* **14**, 403–413.

McKnight, G. S., Pennequin, P., and Schimke, R. T. (1975). *J. Biol. Chem.* **250**, 8105–8112.

McReynolds, L. A., Catterall, J., and O'Malley, B. W. (1977). *Gene* **2**, 217–230.

McReynolds, L. A., O'Malley, B. W., Nisbet, A. D., Fothergill, J. E., Givol, D., Fields, S., Robertson, M., and Brownlee, G. G. (1978). *Nature (London)* **273**, 723–728.

Majors, J. (1975). *Nature (London)* **256**, 672–675.

Marzluff, W. F., Murphy, E. C., and Huang, R. C. C. (1973). *Biochemistry* **12**, 3440–3446.

Nordstrom, J. L., Roop, D. R., Tsai, M.-J., and O'Malley, B. W. (1979). *Nature (London)* 328–331.

O'Malley, B. W., and Means, A. R. (1974). *Science* **183**, 160–164.

O'Malley, B. W., McGuire, W. L., Kohler, P. O., and Korenman, S. G. (1969). *Recent Prog. Horm. Res.* **25**, 105–160.

O'Malley, B. W.,

Palmiter, R. D. (1973). *J. Biol. Chem.* **248**, 8260–8270.

Palmiter, R. D., Moore, P. B., Mulvihill, E. R., and Emtage, S. (1976). *Cell* **8**, 557–566.

Rhoads, R. E., McKnight, G. S., and Schimke, R. T. (1973). *J. Biol. Chem.* **248**, 2031–2039.

Ringold, G. M., Yamamoto, K. R., Tomkins, G. M., Bishop, J. M., and Varmus, H. E. (1975). *Cell* **6**, 299.

Roop, D. R., Nordstrom, J. L., Tsai, S. Y., Tsai, M.-J., and O'Malley, B. W. (1978). *Cell* **15**, 671–685.

Roop, D. R., Tsai, S. Y., Tsai, M.-J., Stumph, W. E. and O'Malley, B. W. (1979). (Submitted).

Rosen, J. M., and O'Malley, B. W. (1975). *In* "Biochemical Action of Hromones" (G. Litwack, ed.), Vol. 3, p. 271. Academic Press, New York.

Rosen, J. M., Woo, S. L. C., Holder, J. W., Means, A. R., and O'Malley, B. W. (1975). *Biochemistry* **14**, 69.

Rosenfeld, G. C., Comstock, J. P., Means, A. R., and O'Malley, B. W. (1972). *Biochem. Biophys. Res. Commun.* **47**, 387.

Sherman, M. R., Corvol, P., and O'Malley, B. W. (1970). *J. Biol. Chem.* **245**, 6085–6090.

Smith, R. G., Clarke, S. G., Zalta, E., and Taylor, R. N. (1979). *J. Steroid Biochem.* **10**, 31–35.

Stallcup, M. R., Ring, J., and Yamamoto, K. R. (1978). *Biochemistry* **17**, 1515–1521.

Swaneck, G. E., Nordstrom, J. L., Kruezaler, F., Tsai, M.-J., and O'Malley, B. W. (1979). *Proc. Natl. Acad. Sci. U.S.A.* **76**, 1049–1053.

Tata, J. R. (1976). *Cell* **9**, 1.

Teng, C. S., and Teng, C. T. (1975). *Biochem. J.* **150**, 191.

Tilghman, S. M., Curtis, P. J., Tiemeier, D. C., Leder, P., and Weissman, C. (1978). *Proc. Natl. Acad. Sci. U.S.A.* **75**, 1309–1313.

Tsai, M.-J., Schwartz, R. J., Tsai, S. Y., and O'Malley, B. W. (1975) *J. Biol. Chem.* **250**, 5165–5174.

Tsai, M.-J., Tsai, S. Y., Chang, C. W., and O'Malley, B. W. (1978). *Biochem. Biophys. Acta* **521**, 689–707.

Tsai, S. Y., Roop, D. R., Tsai, M.-J., Stein, J. P., Means, A. R., and O'Malley, B. W. (1978). *Biochemistry* **17**, 5773–5780.

Van, N. T., Monahan, J. J., Woo, S. L. C., Means, A. R., and O'Malley, B. W. (1977). *Biochemistry* **16**, 4090–4100.

Vedeckis, W. V., Schrader, W. T., and O'Malley, B. W. (1978). *In* "Biochemical Actions of Hormones" (G. Litwack, ed.), Vol. 5, p. 321. Academic Press, New York.

Weber, J., Jelinek, W., and Darnell, J. E., Jr. (1977). *Cell* **10**, 611–616.

Weil, P. A., and Blatti, S. P. (1975). *Biochemistry* **14**, 1636–1642.

Weinman, R., and Roeder, R. G. (1974). *Proc. Natl. Acad. Sci. U.S.A.* **71,** 1790–1794.
Williams, D., and Gorski, J. (1972). *Proc. Natl. Acad. Sci. U.S.A.* **69,** 3464–3469.
Woo, S. L. C., Rosen, J. M., Liarakos, C., Robberson, D. L., Choi, Y. C., Buxch, H., Means, A. R., and O'Malley, B. W. (1975). *J. Biol. Chem.* **250,** 7027–7039.
Yamamoto, K. R., and Alberts, B. M. (1975). *Cell* **4,** 301–308.
Yamamoto, K. R., and Alberts, B. M. (1976). *Annu. Rev. Biochem.* **45,** 721–748.

17

Biochemical and Morphological Changes Stimulated by the Nuclear Binding of the Estrogen Receptor

JAMES H. CLARK, SHIRLEY A. McCORMACK,
HELEN PADYKULA, BARRY MARKAVERICH, AND
JAMES W. HARDIN

I. Introduction

Estrogens are steroid hormones produced by the ovary, which control sexual growth and development in the female and thus are physiological substances of major importance. Yet it has been recognized for many years that estrogenic stimulation provides an environment conducive to the development of neoplasia (Hertz, 1974). Therefore estrogens have the distinction of being not only significant physiological hormones but also pharmacological compounds of considerable importance. In order to discuss these properties of estrogens it is necessary to present a general picture of their mechanism of action.

At physiological temperatures estrogen (E) readily enters all cells (Fig. 1). In hormone-sensitive cells it is retained by binding to soluble macromolecules in the cytoplasm. These macromolecules are called cytosol receptors (R_c) and, while their exact nature *in vivo* is not known, they appear to be large proteins probably made up of two or more subunits. The binding reaction is specific for estrogens and results in the formation of receptor–estrogen complexes ($R_c E$) which undergo translocation to nuclear sites ($R_n E$). The translocation process depletes the cytosol of R_c sites, and these are subsequently replenished by the mechanisms dis-

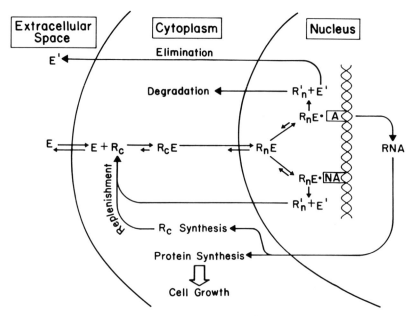

Fig. 1 A generalized model for the interaction of estrogens with target cells. See text for details.

cussed below. Nuclear binding of the $R_n E$ complexes can be classified as to either acceptor (A) or nonacceptor sites (NA). Acceptor sites are generally visualized as specific complexes of chromosomal proteins, probably nonhistone proteins, which the $R_n E$ complex recognizes and binds to with a very high affinity. Nonacceptor sites are considered to be secondary sites on chromatin where the $R_n E$ complex can bind with a lower affinity. Although these nonacceptor sites have a lower binding affinity for the complex, they are present in such large numbers that they constitute a major component of the chromatin-binding mechanism. These binding interactions between the $R_n E$ complex and nonacceptor sites may serve to maximize the number of $R_n E$ complexes that can be accumulated and thus maximize the chance that binding of complexes to specific acceptor sites will occur.

The binding of $R_n E$ complexes to acceptor sites is thought to make gene sites available for transcription by RNA polymerase, which subsequently results in elevated cellular RNA and protein synthesis. These synthetic events may be very restricted, such that the hormone appears to stimulate only a few cellular functions. This is the case with aldosterone which enhances sodium transport in kidney tubules but does not have a general metabolic or growth effect on renal cells. In contrast, hormones that cause growth, such as estrogens and androgens, stimulate many cellular events which ultimately lead to hypertrophy and hyperplasia of specific target tissues. (For reviews of these concepts, see Jensen and DeSombre, 1972; O'Malley and Means, 1974; Gorski and Gannon, 1976; Clark *et al.*, 1977a.)

One of the events stimulated by nuclear binding of $R_n E$ complexes is the replenishment of R_c sites. This may occur by synthesis of new receptor molecules or reutilization of the same receptor sites ($R_n l$) through a recycling mechanism. Receptor molecules may also undergo degradation; however, little is known about these processes. Elimination of the steroid from the cell is probably accomplished by metabolic conversion of the steroid to a metabolite which has a lower affinity for the receptor, hence diffuses out of the cell (S^1). These various possibilities are illustrated in Fig. 1.

In order to study these interactions of steroids with their receptors it has been necessary to differentiate between occupied receptor ($R_c E$ or $R_n E$) and unoccupied receptors (R_c). This can be accomplished by the use of ^3H-labeled steroid exchange assays as developed in our laboratory (Anderson *et al.*, 1972a). This method is based on the temperature dependence of the rate of estrogen receptor–hormone complex dissociation. At a temperature of 0–4°C, $R_c S$ and $R_n E$ sites dissociate very slowly with a dissociation half-time of 20–30 hours, while R_c sites readily bind [^3H]estradiol. However, at elevated temperatures, previously occupied receptor sites readily dissociate and rebind [³H]estradiol. These conditions make it possible to exchange unlabeled hormone occupying the receptor site for a labeled hormone molecule which can then be measured. The binding of [³H]estradiol to nonreceptor sites is accounted for by competitive inhibition of binding of estradiol to the receptor sites by excess nonlabeled estrogen. This exchange method has been used for the measurement of several steroid hormone receptors and provides a technique for the evaluation of occupied receptor sites under *in vivo* physiological conditions. We have used this method to examine the relationship between nuclear binding of the receptor–estradiol complex and the stimulation of growth processes in the rat uterus (Anderson *et al.*, 1972a, 1973, 1975; Clark *et al.*, 1972).

II. Nuclear Binding of the Estrogen Receptor and Uterine Growth

Estrogen agonists and antagonists vary in their ability to stimulate uterotropic responses. Some produce cellular hypertrophy and hyperplasia (true growth), while others act as partial agonists or antagonists and fail to produce true growth. We have used these differential responses to various estrogens in an attempt to define the obligatory responses that produce true uterine growth.

A single injection of estradiol into a female rat stimulates a number of biochemical and metabolic events in the uterus. Among these are glucose oxidation, amino acid and nucleotide uptake, water imbibition, histamine mobilization, eosinophil accumulation, and stimulation of nuclear RNA polymerase activities (Clark *et al.*, 1978a). These activities are increased within the first 6 hours after hormone administration and are normally termed early uterotrophic events. Late events, such as DNA synthesis, sustained stimulation of RNA polymerase activities, and cellular hypertrophy and hyperplasia occur between 12 and 36 hours after estradiol treatment (Clark *et al.*, 1978b). All these responses can be stimulated maximally by a single injection of a low dose of estradiol (0.2 μg/100 μg body weight). This level of hormone causes nuclear accumulation and retention of approximately 10–20% of the total number of uterine R_c sites (~1000–2000 sites per cell) (Anderson *et al.*, 1972b, 1973, 1975; Clark and Peck, 1976). The retention or occupancy of nuclear sites by this number of complexes for six or more hours appears to be a requirement for stimulation of all the above-mentioned later uterotrophic events (Fig. 2).

The importance of long-term nuclear occupancy by receptor–estrogen

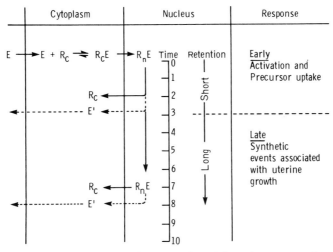

Fig. 2 Relationship between nuclear retention of the estrogen receptor and uterotropic response. E, Estrogen; R_c, cytoplasmic receptor; R_cE, cytoplasmic receptor–estrogen complex; R_nE, nuclear receptor–estrogen complex; E', metabolized estrogen.

complexes has been shown by using short-acting estrogens such as estriol and dimethylstilbestrol (Anderson *et al.*, 1972b, 1973, 1975; Lan and Katzenellenbogen, 1976; Clark *et al.*, 1977b; Capony and Rochefort, 1977). These hormones do not stimulate significant uterine growth after a single injection; however, they stimulate all early uterotropic events (Anderson *et al.*, 1972b). This failure to stimulate true uterine growth is correlated with a rapid loss of receptor–estriol complexes from nuclear sites, which may be due to the rapid clearance and/or dissociation of estriol from receptor sites. It is also possible that receptor–estriol complexes do not bind as tightly to nuclear sites, hence are lost more rapidly. If the receptor is kept continually occupied by either serial injection of estriol or by estriol implants, true uterine growth occurs (Anderson *et al.*, 1975; Clark *et al.*, 1977c). These results are summarized in Table I and Fig. 3.

Estriol has been classified as an estradiol antagonist, and it clearly is when the two hormones are administered as a single injection. However, when the two hormones are implanted, no antagonism is detected. This apparent paradox is resolved by considering the fact that following an injection both complexes are in competition for nuclear binding sites and, since the receptor–estriol complex dissociates before it can fully stimulate uterotropic responses, the net effect of receptor–estradiol complexes is reduced. When the two hormones are implanted, receptor–estriol and receptor–estradiol complexes occupy nuclear retention sites equally

TABLE I
Effects of Estradiol and Estriol on Early and Late Uterotropic Responses

Response	Comparison of estradiol (E_2) and estriol (E_3)
Initial nuclear accumulation of receptor–hormone complex	$E_2 = E_3$
Long-term retention of receptor–hormone complex by the nucleus after an injection	E_2, longer than 6 hours E_3, shorter than 6 hours
Early uterotropic events: RNA polymerase I and II activity, template activity, histamine mobilization, water imbibition	$E_2 = E_3$
Late uterotropic events: sustained and elevated RNA polymerase I and II activity, sustained RNA polymerase initiation sites, RNA and DNA synthesis, cellular growth	$E_2 \gg E_3$
True uterine growth after paraffin implant of hormone	$E_2 = E_3$
Receptor occupancy in the nucleus after paraffin implant of hormone	$E_2 = E_2$

well, therefore late uterotrophic events are maximally stimulated, resulting in no antagonism.

The ability of short-acting estrogens to stimulate all early uterotrophic events while failing to cause significant uterine growth after a single injection indicates that nuclear accumulation of the estrogen receptor and stimulation of early events do not cause a cascade of events culminating in growth. Merely turning on RNA and protein synthesis is not sufficient to cause uterine hypertrophy and hyperplasia. Instead, a sustained input via long-term nuclear retention is an obligatory requirement for true growth.

In contrast to the short nuclear residency of the receptor–estriol complex, Nafoxidine and other triphenylethylene derivatives cause nuclear retention of the receptor for long periods of time (Clark *et al.*, 1973, 1974). These results are compared with those obtained with estradiol and estriol in Fig. 3. Long-term retention of the R_nN complex correlates with the extended stimulation of true uterine growth by Nafoxidine. This stimulation is equal in magnitude to that occurring after a single injection of estradiol and superior to that of estradiol in duration of growth stimulation. Thus the R_nN complex undergoes long-term nuclear retention which is correlated with sustained uterotropic stimulation. In the immature rat this phenomenon of prolonged nuclear retention and the attendant uterotropic stimulation can last for weeks (Clark *et al.*, 1973, 1974).

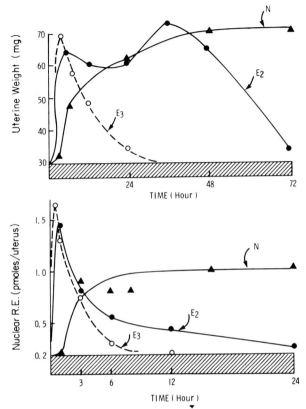

Fig. 3 Uterotropic response and nuclear binding of the estrogen receptor. Immature rats were injected with estradiol (E_2, ●), estriol (E_3, ○), or Nafoxidine (N, ▲), and the uterine wet weight (upper panel) and quantity of nuclear estrogen receptor were measured (lower panel).

III. Nuclear Binding of the Estrogen Receptor and the Control of Transcriptional Events in the Uterus

A. RNA Polymerase Activity

As pointed out above, estrogens stimulate many early uterotropic responses; however, the most important of these probably involve the augmentation of RNA synthesis. It is well known that estrogen administration to either immature or ovariectomized animals increases RNA synthesis in the uterus (for reviews, see Mueller *et al.*, 1958; Hamilton, 1968; O'Malley and Means, 1974; Katzenellenbogen and Gorski, 1975; Segal *et al.*, 1977). Gorski (1964) and Noteboom and Gorski (1965) demonstrated that estradiol stimulated RNA polymerase activity within 60 minutes after treatment. Quantitative changes in RNA synthesis are most marked in rRNA and are measurable within 4–6 hours following hormone administration (Hamilton, 1968; Hamilton et al., 1965, 1968a,b; Billing et al., 1968). Elevated levels of specific mRNA are assumed to occur and have been studied indirectly through the use of RNA synthesis inhibitors (DeAngelo and Gorski, 1970; Keran and Barker, 1976). Several groups have reported an early increase in very high-molecular-weight RNA (DNA-like) and have suggested that the marked increase in total RNA that follows may be dependent on this early appearance of mRNA (Knowler and Smellie, 1971; Luck and Hamilton, 1972; Borthwick and Smellie, 1975). Complementary to these results on high-molecular-weight RNA, estrogen treatment also results in an early increase in endogenous nuclear RNA polymerase II activity. This initial surge of polymerase II activity is followed at later times (2–4 hours) by an increase in the activity of RNA polymerase I and a second rise in RNA polymerase II activity (Glasser et al., 1972; Borthwick and Smellie, 1975). Similar observations have been made in the chick oviduct system by Spelsberg and Cox (1976). These findings suggest that RNA polymerase activity could be used as one end point for the detection of important differences between receptor binding and uterotrophic stimulation by estradiol, estriol, and Nafoxidine. Therefore we have examined the RNA polymerase response profiles induced by these compounds and compared them to their ability to cause long-term retention of the $R_n E$ complex by the nucleus (Hardin et al., 1976).

A single injection of estradiol, estriol, or Nafoxidine causes a transient rise in endogenous nuclear RNA polymerase II activity, which reaches a peak within 1 hour after hormone treatment (Fig. 4). The greatest response at this time is elicited by estradiol and estriol, each of which causes a significant increase in enzymic activity as early as 30 minutes after hormone treatment. Nafoxidine has little, if any, effect at this very early time and evokes less response at 1 hour than the other two compounds. This decreased response is correlated with the slower rate of nuclear accumulation of the receptor–Nafoxidine complex.

The activity of polymerase II declines dramatically by 2 hours after injection in all three groups. This decline is followed by a second elevation in activity in estradiol-treated animals, which reaches a maximum by 4 hours (Fig. 4). The early elevation of polymerase II activity in Nafoxidine-treated animals is followed by a second larger increase which occurs between 12 and 24 hours after the injection. A second elevation in enzyme activity was not observed in estriol-treated animals; rather the activity of polymerase II remained low between 4 and 24 hours.

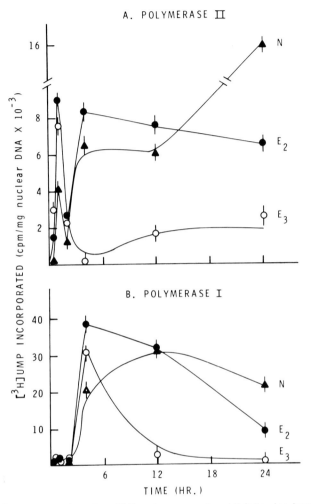

Fig. 4 Time course of nuclear RNA polymerases I and II following hormone injections. Animals were injected with 1 μg estradiol (E_2, ●), 1 μg estriol (E_3, ○), or 50 μg Nafoxidine (N, ▲). At the indicated times, uteri were removed, nuclei isolated, and endogenous RNA polymerase activities determined.

Following the early transient increase in uterine nuclear RNA polymerase II activity, an increase in RNA polymerase I activity occurred in all treatment groups by 4 hours (Fig. 4). Estriol caused a transient rise in this activity, which was characterized by a regression phase between 4 and 12 hours. Estradiol treatment resulted in a marked elevation in RNA polymerase I activity by 4 hours. This rise was followed by a slow decline in activity; however, values remained significantly above those of the control at 24 hours. Nafoxidine treatment resulted in a similar elevation of endogeneous RNA polymerase I activity by 4 hours, which was maintained at levels as high or higher than those induced by estradiol.

The correlations made earlier in this chapter between nuclear retention of the receptor and estrogenic potency are also apparent in these polymerase experiments. The greatest increase in early polymerase II activity occurred in response to estradiol and estriol, the compounds that caused the most rapid accumulation of receptor by the nucleus. On the other hand, Nafoxidine, which accumulated more slowly as R_nN, produced a peak of polymerase II activity which was approximately 50% less than that produced by either estradiol or estriol at early times after hormone administration. The second elevation of polymerase II activity, which was observed by 4 hours in estradiol- and Nafoxidine-, but not in estriol-treated animals, may be dependent upon long-term retention of the receptor by the nucleus. The failure of estriol to stimulate this second rise in activity may be one of the factors involved in the inability of this estrogen to stimulate true uterine growth.

The elevation of polymerase I activity stimulated by all three compounds was maintained for much longer periods of time by treatment with estradiol or Nafoxidine. The rapid decline in polymerase I activity in the estriol-treated animals may result from the short-term residency of the receptor–estriol complex in the nucleus. These data demonstrate that the secondary rise in polymerase II activity, as well as the duration and magnitude of the increase in polymerase I activity, temporally correlate with the nuclear retention of receptor–estrogen complexes.

The early (30 minutes) estrogen-dependent rise in uterine endogenous nuclear RNA polymerase II activity was first measured directly by Glasser et al. (1972) in the mature ovariectomized rat and subsequently confirmed in the immature rat (Hardin et al., 1976) and immature rabbit (Borthwick and Smellie, 1975). It has been suggested that this early stimulation of putative mRNA synthesis (Knowler and Smellie, 1971; Glasser et al., 1972; Borthwick and Smellie, 1975) may be involved in the synthesis of uterine proteins involved in later increases in both polymerase activities. A similar suggestion was made by Raynaud-Jammet et al. (1972) and Baulieu et al. (1972a,b), who found an RNA product which was sensitive to α-amanitin that appeared to be necessary for estrogen-induced RNA polymerase I activity. A similar cascade mechanism has been proposed by DeAngelo and Gorski (1970) for the estrogen-induced protein (IP). Baulieu et al. (1972b) have suggested that IP plays a key intermediary role in the mechanism of action of estrogen, hence is a primary event in a cascade reaction which ultimately culminates in uterine growth.

Our results do not support such a mechanism; instead they indicate that the action of estrogen on RNA synthesis is more complex and difficult to interpret than simply relating an early increase in RNA polymerase II activity to the synthesis of a product that later modulates increases in the activities of both polymerases. Thus an injection of estriol into immature rats, which evokes as great an increase in polymerase II activity at 30–60 minutes as estradiol (Fig. 4), fails to produce the secondary increase in polymerase II activity. The failure of estriol to continue to stimulate RNA synthesis is reflected in both the disappearance of the receptor–estriol complex from the nucleus and the failure of the hormone to stimulate true uterine growth.

Nafoxidine, in comparison, causes only a small early increase in polymerase II activity but produces a substantial and sustained increase in polymerase I and a large secondary stimulation in polymerase II activity as well as true uterine growth. The elevated activity of RNA polymerase II in Nafoxidine- treated animals may mean that many genes are "turned on" and remain in the "on" position. This seems even more likely when one considers the large number of R_nN complexes present in the nucleus. Approximately 10,000 R_nN complexes remain in the nucleus for long periods of time. This quantity exceeds the number of R_nE complexes required to maximize uterine growth by a factor of at least 5 and leads to the speculation that R_nN complexes bind to secondary and tertiary nuclear sites involved in the control of RNA synthesis. If this is the case, these binding interactions might lead to the stimulation of many uterine genes that would not normally be turned on and thus could account for the marked elevation in RNA polymerase II activity. This anomalous nuclear binding behavior may also be linked to the antiestrogenicity of these compounds. One can imagine that either inappropriate genes are turned on or they are activated in an incorrect temporal sequence. The activation of such "right" and "wrong" genes might result ultimately in the inhibition of growth. This is particularly relevant when one considers that estrogens act in concert with other hormones to produce the biochemical changes that occur during the estrous cycle of the rat. These changes involve both synthetic and degradative enzymic activities and account for the fluctuations in uterine size and morphology during the cycle. Thus the uterus is programmed for both anabolic and catabolic events, and any compound that alters the proper sequence of these events could result in the anomalous growth state observed with Nafoxidine.

In summary, the stimulation of true uterine growth is not characteristic of every estrogen when it is administered by injection. Of the varied multiple effects that characterize the biological action of each estrogen only certain correlated sets of events stimulate true uterine growth. It is of prime importance that the estrogen receptor be retained in the nucleus for some critical period in order to effect true uterine growth. Nuclear retention of the receptor correlates with a secondary increase in and sustained activation of RNA polymerase II activity and a sustained elevation in RNA polymerase I activity. These effects on RNA polymerases I and II appear necessary for true uterine growth.

B. RNA Polymerase Initiation Sites on Uterine Chromatin

The changes in RNA polymerase activity discussed above do not appear to be due to an increase in the number of polymerase molecules (Courvalin *et al.*, 1976; Weil *et al.*, 1977). Rather these changes may result from either alterations in chromatin template activity or increases in factor(s) which directly modulate RNA polymerase activity. Among the first demonstrations that estrogens exert an effect on uterine biochemistry at the level of transcription was the observation that estrogen induced changes in chromatin template activity (Barker and Warren, 1966; Hamilton, 1968; Church and McCarthy, 1970; Glasser *et al.*, 1972). However, because of the complexity of the transcription process, these studies provide little information as to which components of the chromatin are altered or which steps in transcription are affected by the hormone.

Procedures for prokaryotic systems have been recently adapted for measuring the specific initiation of RNA chains on eukaryotic chromatin *in vitro* (Tsai *et al.*, 1975). These techniques take advantage of the specific inhibition, by the antibiotic rifampicin, of bacterial RNA polymerase not bound in a highly stable preinitiation complex (Chamberlin, 1974). When a mixture of chromatin and bacterial RNA polymerase is challenged with a mixture of ribonucleoside triphosphates and rifampicin, only those RNA polymerase molecules bound at true initiation sites are capable of synthesizing an RNA chain, while the other polymerase molecules are irreversibly inactivated by rifampicin. Each RNA polymerase molecule bound at an initiation site is capable of synthesizing one RNA chain. This facilitates accurate measurement of the number of RNA chains initiated on a given quantity of chromatin DNA and consequently the number of RNA initiation sites. We have used this technique to examine the effect of various hormones on R_nE complexes and the promotion of RNA polymerase initiation sites.

Figure 5A illustrates typical titration curves of rat uterine chromatin incubated with increasing amounts of *Escherichia coli* RNA polymerase in the presence of rifampicin and heparin. The latter two components are included to inhibit RNA chain reinitiation and RNase activity, respectively (Tsai *et al.*, 1975). Several points are evident from this plot. The amount

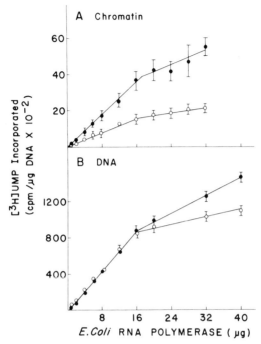

Fig. 5 Titration of rat uterine chromatin DNA with increasing concentrations of *E. coli* RNA polymerase. Animals were injected with either 2.5 µg of estradiol (●) or saline (○) 24 hours prior to sacrifice. (A) Chromatin was isolated, and RNA synthesis was measured in the presence of rifampicin and heparin using 1.5 µg of chromatin DNA as template. (B) The DNA present in the chromatin used in (A) was isolated, and 0.5 µg of the isolated DNA was used in titration assays.

of RNA being synthesized increases linearly with increasing enzyme concentration until a transition point is reached. Tsai *et al.* (1975) have shown that the coordinates of this transition point can be used to calculate the number of high-affinity binding sites for RNA polymerase as well as the number of RNA chains initiated.

The data presented in Fig. 5A also demonstrate that treatment of immature rats with estradiol 24 hours prior to the preparation of chromatin significantly increases the number of rifampicin-resistant RNA chains initiated. Chromatin isolated from both control and estradiol-treated animals saturates at 16 µg of RNA polymerase; however, chromatin from estradiol-treated animals allows the initiation of more than twice as many RNA chains, as reflected by the increased incorporation of [³H]UMP into RNA. These results indicate that estradiol treatment results in a marked increase in the number of RNA chain initiation sites on chromatin. These results agree with previous reports on template activity in the uterus and support the concept that estrogens act, at least partially, at the level of chromatin transcription.

The increased incorporation of [³H]UMP into RNA using chromatin from estradiol-treated animals as compared to controls could be caused by either an increased number of RNA chains initiated or an increased length of the RNA synthesized. This dichotomy results from the nature of the assay in which only RNA polymerase molecules bound to chromatin in a stable preinitiation complex are able to synthesize RNA. The number-average chain length of the RNA synthesized in all portions of this study ranged from 340 to 515 nucleotides. This variation in size was not sufficient to account for any of the treatment effects we observed in the rifampicin assay. In fact, most of the RNA preparations fell into a more narrow size range (390–470 nucleotides). These findings indicate that estradiol-induced increases in [³H]UMP incorporation into RNA were the result of increased numbers of specific RNA chain initiations rather than increased length of the RNA synthesized as suggested by Barry and Gorski (1971).

The role of chromatin structure in steroid-induced RNA synthesis in target tissues was also examined. One approach to this problem is illustrated in Fig. 5B. DNA isolated from the chromatin used as template in Fig. 5A was employed in titration assays in the presence of rifampicin and heparin. Both estradiol and control DNAs had essentially the same transistion point. This is in sharp contrast to the results obtained when chromatin was used as a template (Fig. 5A). Purified DNAs are much more efficient templates for RNA synthesis than chromatin. These data indicate that the structure of chromatin plays an important role in the expression of steroid hormone effects on RNA synthesis.

We have previously discussed the correlation that exists between the patterns of endogenous nuclear RNA polymerase activities and the retention of estrogen–receptor complexes in nuclei of the immature rat uterus (Hardin *et al.*, 1976). All classes of estrogenic compounds we have examined resulted in altered RNA polymerase activities. Only the estrogen–receptor complexes retained in nuclei for periods greater than 6 hours produced a secondary rise in RNA polymerase II activity and the sustained elevation in RNA polymerase I activity required for true uterine growth. When we examined the effects of estradiol, estriol, and Nafoxidine on the number of RNA initiation sites on uterine chromatin, a similar general pattern was observed. As shown in Fig. 6, estradiol treatment gradually elevates the number of initiation sites to very high levels by 12 hours, and this is followed by a slow decline in the number of sites. In contrast, estriol causes a slight elevation in the number of initiation sites, which di-

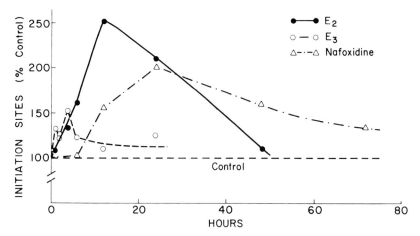

Fig. 6 Time course of chromatin sites capable of initiating RNA synthesis following hormone injections. Immature rats were injected with saline, estradiol (E_2), estriol (E_3), or Nafoxidine and sacrificed at the indicated times. Uteri were removed, and chromatin isolated and used in titration assays as described in Fig. 5. Control levels represent 42,000 initiation sites/pg DNA.

minishes with time. These observations mirror the effect that estradiol and estriol have on long-term retention of the receptor in the nucleus. Likewise, long-term retention of the receptor induced by Nafoxidine is correlated with a high level of sustained numbers of initiation sites for up to 72 hours after treatment. As can be seen in Fig. 6, the number of initiation sites declines by 48 hours in estradiol-treated animals. This is expected, since estradiol does not cause retention of the receptor for as long a period as Nafoxidine (see Fig. 3).

The marked elevations in RNA polymerase II activity observed within 60 minutes after estradiol, estriol, or Nafoxidine (Fig. 4) do not correlate well with the barely detectable increases in initiation site numbers at this time (Fig. 6). Since the amount of polymerase remains constant during this period, it seems likely that factors other than template availability are operating to bring about this elevation in enzyme activity. The secondary rise in RNA polymerase II and the primary elevation in RNA polymerase I activity that are stimulated by estradiol and Nafoxidine, but not by estriol, are correlated with increases in the number of initiation sites. Thus the later increases in both RNA polymerase activity and polymerase initiation sites are stimulated by hormones that cause long-term retention of the receptor in the nucleus. In addition, these increases in initiation sites closely correlate with the conversion of nuclear receptor–hormone complexes to a form that is resistant to $0.4 M$ KCl extraction (Clark and Peck,

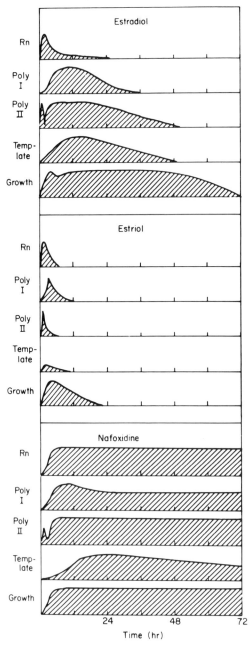

Fig. 7 Summary of the effects of estradiol, estriol, and Nafoxidine on uterotropic responses. Each parameter was measured as a function of time after a single injection of hormone in saline or aqueous solution. Rn, Nucleus-bound receptor; Poly I, RNA polymerase I activity; Poly II, RNA polymerase II activity.

1976; Clark *et al.*, 1977c). Such forms of the receptor molecule may be associated with acceptor sites on chromatin, which results in their long-term retention in the nucleus of target cells.

All the data discussed above are summarized and compared to nuclear retention of the estrogen receptor and uterine growth in Fig. 7. From these data it can be concluded that the duration of nuclear retention is highly correlated with sustained uterotropic responses. This extended period of occupancy may allow a search for nuclear acceptor sites and/or a processing of receptor–hormone complexes, which results not only in the stimulation of RNA and DNA synthesis but also in inactivation of the receptor–hormone complex. Buller and O'Malley (1976) and Palmiter *et al.* (1976) have suggested that receptor–steroid complexes bind to nuclear sites and move along the chromatin in search of specific acceptor sites. This nuclear search function may well be a component of the total picture of nuclear retention; however, interaction of the receptor–hormone complex and acceptor sites could also be a pseudoirreversible phenomenon. Receptor–hormone complexes may undergo conformational changes when they bind to acceptor sites that do not permit ready dissociation of the complex or the hormone from the complex. In order for dissociation of the R_nE complex to take place, processing factors may be required that recognize the complex and bring about changes in the receptor and/or hormone that result in dissociation of the complex from chromatin. This processing may be an important step in the replenishment of cytoplasmic receptors. Occupancy of nuclear acceptor sites by such a pseudoirreversible mechanism may be responsible for the sustained stimulation of RNA polymerase I and II activities and the elevation of RNA polymerase initiation sites that appears to be required for true uterine growth.

IV. Triphenylethylene Derivatives and Estrogen Antagonism

Triphenylethylene derivatives, such as Nafoxidine, are classified as estrogen antagonists. This is paradoxical in light of the data presented above which demonstrate that Nafoxidine causes long-term nuclear retention of the estrogen receptor (Clark *et al.*, 1973, 1974; Capony and Rochefort, 1975; Katzenellenbogen and Ferguson, 1975), stimulation of RNA polymerase activity, and true uterine growth (Hardin *et al.*, 1976). It has been proposed by others that the mechanism of action of triphenylethylene derivatives resides in their ability to compete with estrogens for cytoplasmic receptors, thereby reducing the number of receptor–estrogen complexes in the cytoplasm of estrogen target tissues (Jensen *et al.*, 1966; Terenius,

1971; Rochefort et al., 1972). With subsequent translocation to nuclear sites considered the primary event in the mechanism of estrogen action, this reduction in receptor–estradiol complexes would lead to decreased physiological responses. Implicit in this hypothesis is that the receptor–antagonist complex should have an intrinsic biological activity lower than that of the receptor–estradiol complex. That is, the ability of the receptor –antagonist complex to stimulate estrogenic responses should be less than that of the receptor–estradiol complex.

A. Effects of Triphenylethylene Derivatives on Uterine Growth

Based on the above assumptions, one would predict that estrogen antagonism should be observed following a single injection of estrogen and the antagonists; however, as shown in Fig. 8, this is not the case. Immature rats, 21–22 days old, were injected with 2.5 μg estradiol, 100 μg Nafoxidine, or a combination of the two compounds, and uterine dry weights were determined 24 or 48 hours later. The increases in uterine dry weight following a single injection of estradiol, Nafoxidine, or estradiol plus Nafoxidine were identical 24 hours after the injection. By 48 hours, treatment with Nafoxidine or estradiol plus Nafoxidine was superior to that obtained with estradiol alone in the stimulation of uterine growth (Fig. 8). Therefore, following a single injection of estradiol plus Nafoxidine, there is no antagonism; indeed, Nafoxidine clearly acts as an estrogen. This is also true for CI-628 and clomiphene (Clark et al., 1973; Capony and Ro-

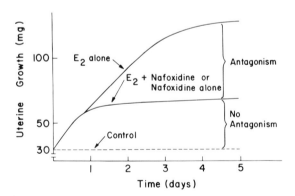

Fig. 8 Effect of daily injections of estradiol (E_2), Nafoxidine, or a combination of the two hormones on uterine growth. Immature rats were injected daily with 1.0 μg of estradiol, 50 μg of Nafoxidine, or a combination of the two hormones. Uterine weight was determined 24 hours after each injection.

chefort, 1975; Emmens, 1970). However, the antagonistic properties of Nafoxidine can be observed when the compounds are administered at 24-hour intervals and the uterine weights determined at 48 hours (Fig. 8). Serial injections of Nafoxidine (three to eight in number) at 24-hour intervals have been used routinely by many investigators to study antagonism, and it is well established that estrogen antagonism can be observed under these conditions (Emmens, 1970; Lerner, 1964). The routine application of this protocol has resulted in the failure to recognize the significance of the agonist properties of these compounds after a single injection. We have used much lower doses of these compounds with similar results; that is, doses of 1–10 μg display both agonistic and antagonistic properties depending on the injection scheme.

Triphenylethylene derivatives could act as estrogen antagonists by stimulating cellular hypertrophy, thereby increasing uterine weight, but fail to stimulate uterine hyperplasia. In such a case the number of cells capable of responding to subsequent estrogen treatment would be reduced, and this reduction would result in diminished uterotropic re-

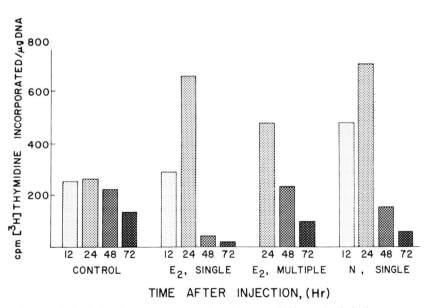

Fig. 9 Effect of either estradiol or Nafoxidine on DNA synthesis in immature rat uteri. Immature rats were injected with saline, a single injection of 1.0 μg of estradiol (E$_2$) at 24-hour intervals, or a single injection of 50 μg of Nafoxidine. Uteri were removed at the indicated times, placed in 2.0 ml of Eagle's HeLa medium containing 25 μCi of [^{3}H]thymidine, and incubated at 37°C for 1 hour. The level of [^{3}H]thymidine incorporated into DNA was determined.

sponses when compared to estrogen treatment alone. This does not appear to be the case, since both estradiol and Nafoxidine increase DNA content by 48 hours (Clark *et al.*, 1974), and no differences are apparent in the capacity of these compounds to elicit uterine hyperplasia or [^{3}H]thymidine incorporation (Fig. 9).

B. Effects of Triphenylethylene Derivatives on Cytoplasmic Replenishment and Nuclear Retention of Estrogen Receptors

We have proposed that triphenylethylene derivatives antagonize estrogen-induced uterine growth as a result of their failure to stimulate replenishment of the cytoplasmic estrogen receptor (Clark *et al.*, 1973, 1974). As previously described, Nafoxidine causes accumulation and long-term retention of the R_n–ligand complex; however, this retention is not accompanied by the usual replenishment of the cytoplasmic receptor (R_c), as is the case after estradiol treatment (Fig. 10). This failure to cause R_c replenishment has been observed by many investigators (Capony and Rochefort, 1975; Katzenellenbogen and Ferguson, 1975; Katzenellenbogen *et al.*, 1977; Ruh and Baudendistel, 1977), and we have suggested that it may render the uterus insensitive to subsequent injection of estrogen and therefore antagonism can be observed. These mechanisms can be visualized according to the following model. Receptor–estrogen complexes and receptor–antagonist complexes stimulate cellular hypertrophy and hyperplasia. Thus uterine growth is observed in both cases after a single injection of the compound. However, the receptor–antagonist complex fails to cause the replenishment of R_c by 24 hours. When the animal receives a second injection of estrogen at this time, the uterus in nonresponsive in animals that received the antagonist and highly responsive in estrogen-treated animals. Therefore the uterus continues to grow in the estrogen-treated rat and remains unstimulated in the antagonist-treated animal. Although this reasoning appears logical, it fails to offer a complete explanation. One must explain how antagonism is expressed when large quantities of estrogen receptor are being retained for long periods of time in the nucleus. This should cause continued stimulation of uterine growth; instead, Nafoxidine, either as a single dose or as multiple injections, causes the uterus to double in size and to remain at this level for long periods of time (Fig. 8). In contrast, serial injection of estradiol causes continued stimulation of uterine growth which produces a uterus five times as large as that in the control.

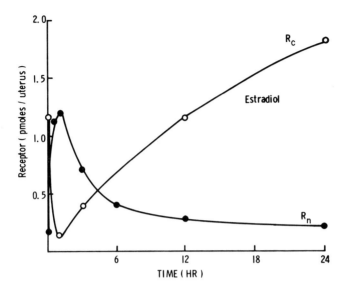

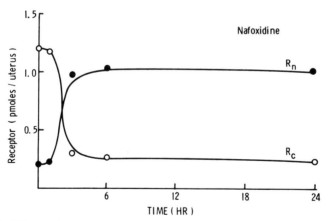

Fig. 10 Effects of estradiol and Nafoxidine on nuclear retention and cytoplasmic replenishment of the estrogen receptor. Immature rats were injected with estradiol (2.5 μg) or Nafoxidine (50 μg), and the quantities of estrogen receptor in the nuclear (R_n, o) and cytoplasmic fractions (R_c, o) were determined by the [^{3}H]estradiol exchange assay.

C. Triphenylethylene Derivatives and Differential Cell Stimulation

As discussed above, daily injections of estradiol, Nafoxidine, or the two compounds together cause the uterus to grow; however, it becomes much larger in animals that receive estradiol alone (Fig. 8). This difference is primarily due to the differential effect of Nafoxidine on the growth of the epithelial layer of the endometrium. From Fig. 11 it is clear that Nafoxidine has stimulated the hypertrophy of epithelial cells to a greater extent than estradiol, while estradiol has stimulated hypertrophy and hyperplasia of the stromal and myometrial layers to a much greater degree than Nafoxidine. Therefore it appears that Nafoxidine and other compounds like it, such as Clomid and CI-628, can act as estrogen agonists in one cell type and estrogen antagonists in others. Nafoxidine causes nuclear binding of receptor in all tissue layers of the uterus, therefore differential cellular binding does not explain this phenomenon. However, we have not examined nuclear retention in these different cell types, hence differential long-term retention could occur. The explanation probably depends on the competence or mode by which a given cell type reacts to the binding of Nafoxidine by the receptor. Regardless of the explanation, the implications of differential cell stimulation are far-reaching. It is possible that nonsteroidal estrogen antagonists react in this fashion in the brain, pituitary, ovary, and other estrogen target organs. If so, this may explain the often observed, but poorly explained, estrogenic and antiestrogenic responses reported by others. Triphenylethylene derivatives have long been recognized as compounds that can either block or stimulate ovulation (Holtkamp *et al.*, 1960). This has been thought to be due to their ability at certain dose levels to block the negative feedback effect of estrogens and thus result in gonadotropin secretion. Instead, at the appropriate dose levels these drugs may act as estrogens having a positive feedback effect on gonadotropin secretion. At other doses, antiestrogenic effects may be noted. It is also possible that these compounds affect the pituitary cells in a fashion that differs from their effect on brain cells. Ross *et al.* (1973) have reported negative (antiestrogenic) effects of CI-628 on ovulation and positive (estrogenic) effects on sexual behavior. Harman *et al.* (1975) have noted that CI-628 blocks estrogen-induced follicular growth but does not increase estrogen-dependent atresia. Nafoxidine has also been shown to inhibit the growth of mammary tumors; however, it never reduces the size of the tumor to that seen in the ovariectomized control animals (Gallez *et al.*, 1973). All the above observations may result from differential cell stimulation by nonsteroidal estrogen antagonists. Therefore any interpretation of the action of these compounds

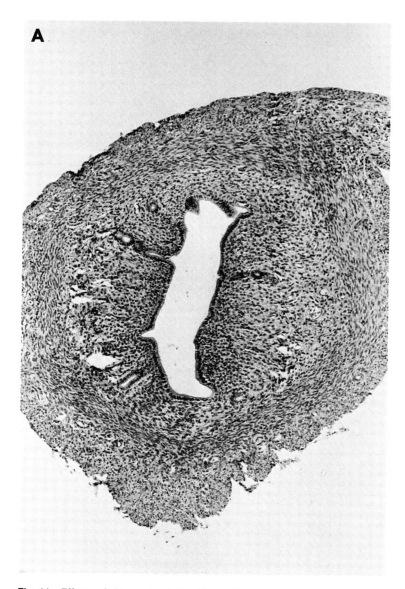

Fig. 11 Effects of either estradiol or Nafoxidine treatment on the morphology of the immature rat uterus. Immature rats were injected at 24-hour intervals for a total of three injections with saline, estradiol (2.5 µg), Nafoxidine (50 µg), or a combination of estradiol and Nafoxidine (2.5 µg plus 50 µg). Twenty-four hours after the last injection, the animals were sacrificed and the uteri removed and fixed for morphological examination. (A) Cross section of uterus from a saline-treated animal.

(Continued)

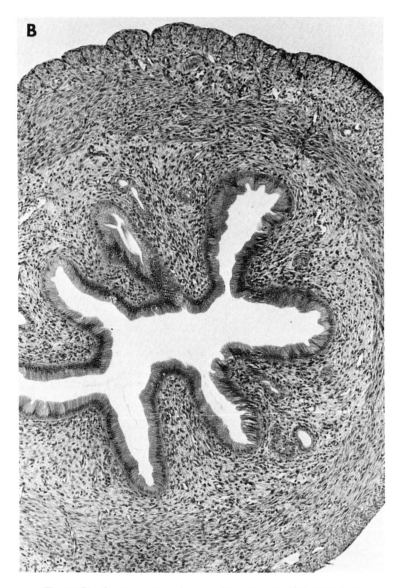

Fig. 11(B) Cross section of uterus from an estradiol-treated rat.

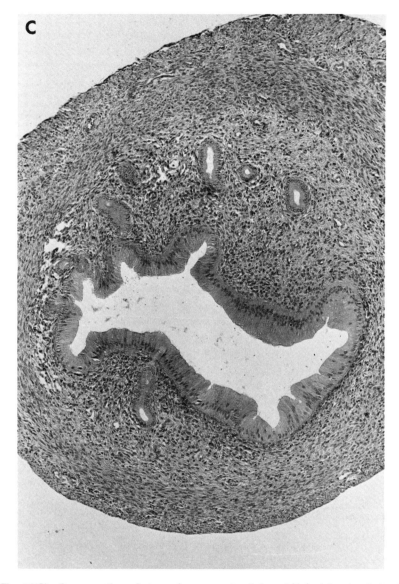

Fig. 11(C)   Cross section of uterus from an estradiol- and Nafoxidine-treated rat.
(Continued)

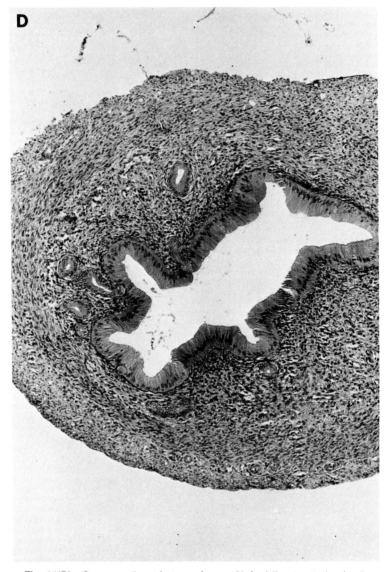

Fig. 11(D)   Cross section of uterus from a Nafoxidine-treated animal.

based solely on their antiestrogenic qualities may lead to invalid conclusions.

V. Hyperestrogenization by Triphenylethylene Derivatives and Reproductive Tract Abnormalities

Chronic exposure to estrogen produces preneoplastic and neoplastic changes in the vagina, uterus, pituitary, and mammary gland (Hertz, 1974). Triphenylethylene derivatives produce effects similar to those of chronic estrogen exposure when given as a single dose in immature rats. We first showed this by administering a single dose of Nafoxidine to 21 to 22-day-old castrated rats and observing uterine weights and receptor levels 7 and 19 days later (Clark *et al.*, 1973). These results demonstrate that a single injection of Nafoxidine can act as a very long-acting estrogen, presumably by continuous occupancy and nuclear retention of the estrogen receptor. This observation led to an attempt to masculinize female neonatal rats using triphenylethylene derivatives (Clark and McCormack, 1977). The rationale for these experiments was based on the concept that androgens masculinize the hypothalamus via conversion to estrogens (Gorski, 1963; Reddy *et al.*, 1974). Since triphenylethylene derivatives have no androgen activity and appear to act only as estrogens, administration of triphenylethylene derivatives to the neonate should cause masculinization.

Nafoxidine or Clomid was administered to neonatal rats at various dose levels on days 1, 5, 10, and 21 of life. During the first and second week after injection, the uteri of these rats showed extensive epithelial stimulation (McCormack and Clark, 1979). Uteri from control rats had a low cuboidal epithelium, and no estrogenic stimulation was observed. This extensive uterotropic stimulation by Nafoxidine or Clomid was accompanied by elevated levels of nuclear estrogen receptor and depletion of cytoplasmic receptor. These results agree with previous studies employing 21 to 22-day-old rats. Vaginal opening occurred in 86% of the rats injected with $100\mu g$ of Nafoxidine or 500 μg of Clomid between days 21 and 34. Vaginal opening occurred in control rats between days 35 and 50. Vaginal smears of treated rats did not show normal cyclic changes; rather a high incidence of estrus smears was noted. Therefore these animals were probably acyclic and in a state that outwardly resembled persistent estrus. These responses are typical of masculinized female rats; however, further analysis demonstrated a much more complicated syndrome. When these animals were autopsied between 60 and 100 days of age, they were found to have a complicated array of abnormalities of the reproductive tract. These included atrophic ovaries with accompaning atrophic uteri in some animals, while others showed cystic ovaries and enlarged uteri.

An examination of the histology of uterine tissue revealed various stages of uterine hyperplasia and squamous metaplasia. Tumors of the uterus were also observed in rats that had received Clomid or Nafoxidine. Although such tumors were observed in only a few animals, it should be noted that no animals older than 100 days were used in this study. The incidence of uterine tumors would probably increase considerably with age. Other abnormalities included hypertrophied and hyperplastic oviducts; ovarian, oviductal, and uterine inflammation accompanied by pyometra; liquid-filled periovarian sacs with small atrophic ovaries; and hylus cell tumors of the ovary. Control animals that received oil injections did not manifest any reproductive tract abnormalities and were cyclic. The types and frequency of abnormalities varied widely among the various treatment groups. The high dose of either Clomid (500 μg) or Nafoxidine (100 μg) produced some form of abnormality in 80–100% of the animals. Intermediate and lower doses have not been completely evaluated at present; however, it is anticipated from preliminary results that 10–15% of the animals will be adversely affected. Uterine metaplasia and infertility accompanied by polycystic degeneration of the ovary have been described by others (Gellert *et al.*, 1977; Fels, 1976). Lobl and Maenza (1975) have observed extensive squamous metaplasia in uteri of androgenized female rats. The relationship between the latter observation and our findings is not clear at the present time.

The variation in the kinds of abnormalities probably relates to both the dose of the compound and the age at which it is administered. The ability of the reproductive organs to respond to estrogenic compounds depends in part on the presence of estrogen receptors. Since the concentration of these receptors is known to increase with time in the neonatal rat (Clark and Gorski, 1969), the effectiveness of the compounds, as well as their mode of action, may vary with time.

Although the possibility of indirect effects of Nafoxidine and Clomid have not been ruled out, it seems likely that these drugs act directly on the various target tissues. Both drugs cause nuclear accumulation and long-term retention of the nuclear receptor complex, as well as extensive stimulation of the uterine epithelium in 5 to 10-day-old rats. Since activation of the hypothalamic–pituitary–gonadal axis is not likely at this time, it seems probable that the triphenylethylene derivatives act in a direct fashion on the affected organs and tissues.

The effects observed with triphenylethylene derivatives may be analogous to the hyperestrogenism observed by many investigators (see Section IV, A). As discussed earlier, continuous exposure of the neonatal mouse to high levels of estrogen will result in neoplastic development of the reproductive tract. Since a single injection of Nafoxidine or Clomid causes continuous occupancy of the estrogen receptor, these drugs mimic the effects of daily injections or implants of other estrogens. Although this is a reasonable suggestion, certain qualifications should be noted relating to peculiar properties of these compounds. As discussed above, both drugs extensively stimulate the epithelial cells of the uterus while having little or no stimulatory effect on stromal or myometrial components. This of course is not true for other estrogens. Therefore this hyperestrogenization of the epithelium may place the triphenylethylene derivatives in a separate category with respect to carcinogenic potential. This point is discussed in more detail below.

Another property that makes triphenylethylene derivatives different from ordinary estrogens is their failure to promote cytoplasmic replenishment of the estrogen receptor. Although it is tempting to equate the hyperestrogenization following exposure to triphenylethylene derivatives with that produced by continuous exposure to estradiol or DES, sufficient differences exist to warrant caution.

VI. Hyperestrogenism and Nuclear Body Formation

As discussed above, a single injection of either Nafoxidine or estradiol into immature rats stimulates endogenous nuclear RNA polymerase activities. The extent and the degree of stimulation correlates with the nuclear retention of the estrogen receptor. When estradiol is implanted, the estrogen receptor is continuously occupied and can be found in the nuclear fraction of the rat uterus (Clark et al., 1978b). This produces effects on RNA polymerase activity similar to those shown in Fig. 7 for a single Nafoxidine injection. Therefore implants of estradiol mimic the effects of a single injection of Nafoxidine on estrogen receptor retention by the nuclei and effects on RNA polymerase activity. A single injection of estradiol has a significant effect on these functions but gradually loses its estrogenic effect by 72 hours after an injection.

To relate these biochemical observations to morphological changes that occur in the normal immature rat uterus in response to Nafoxidine and estradiol, samples of uteri were prepared for light and electron microscopy, and the ultrastructure of uterine luminal epithelial cells was examined. The height of these cells was greatly increased over that of control cells by either Nafoxidine treatment or estradiol implant. The height of luminal epithelial cells 72 hours after a single injection of estradiol was not significantly different from that of controls. This probably represents a regressed state which follows hypertrophy and hyperplasia 24–48 hours after a single injection of estradiol. At the ultrastructural level, the hypertrophied cells resulting from Nafoxidine treatment or an estradiol implant possess an abundance of free polysomes and rough cisternal endoplasmic recticulum, as well as enlarged Golgi systems. These features are indicative of stimulated cytoplasmic protein synthesis. Thus a single injection of Nafoxidine or an estradiol implant causes extensive cellular hypertrophy of the immature rat uterus characterized by long-term nuclear retention of the estrogen receptor and prolonged stimulation of endogenous nuclear RNA polymerase activities. This very active state of uterine epithelial cells appears to be one manifestation of the hyperestrogenized uterus.

In addition to the above observations, several types of nuclear bodies were observed in the nuclei of luminal epithelial cells in tissue from animals either treated with Nafoxidine or implanted with estradiol. An example of one of these nuclear bodies is shown in Fig. 12. Nuclear bodies were quantitated in cells judged to be sectioned in the longitudinal plane. Electron microscope counts were made on ultrathin sections of nuclei, which are referred to as nuclear profiles. The number of nuclei that contained nuclear bodies was similar in control and estradiol-injected animals, 22 and 19%, respectively. The value observed in estradiol-injected animals probably reflects the regressed state of the epithelium 72 hours after the injection. The percent of nuclei that contained nuclear bodies was significantly elevated in animals that had been implanted with estradiol (37%) or injected with Nafoxidine (53%). In addition, 38% of the profiles in Nafoxidine-treated animals contained multiple nuclear bodies, as compared to 28% of the positive profiles in estradiol-implanted animals and only 5% in control animals. No cases of multiple nuclear bodies were seen 72 hours after a single estradiol injection.

Four distinct morphological classes of nuclear bodies were observed during the course of this study. These included singlets with a filamentous capsule and a less dense core (size range, 280–305 nm), nuclear bodies which contained granules in the core (size range, 700–1000 nm), doublets with double cores, and granular bodies with large electron-opaque inclusions. The latter three classes were never observed in control tissues but only in nuclei from luminal epithelium of hormone-treated animals.

These nuclear bodies closely resemble proteinaceous nuclear bodies previously described cytochemically by Bouteille et al. (1967) and Dupay-Coin et al. (1972), who showed that the nuclear bodies in their studies consisted of a filamentous protein capsule and a core that probably contained either RNA or DNA. Recently, LeGoascogne and Baulieu (1977) have described identical nuclear bodies in the immature rat uterus

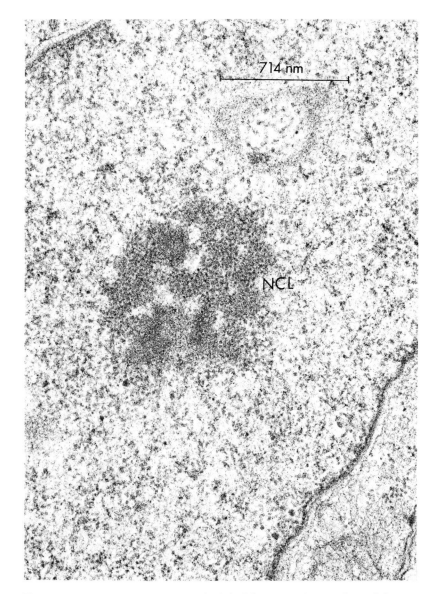

Fig. 12 Nuclear body and nucleolus in Nafoxidine-treated rat uterine cell. Immature rats 22–24 days old were injected with a single dose of 50 μg of Nafoxidine. The animals were sacrificed at 72 hours, and the uteri removed for fixation. A complex nuclear body is shown above the nucleolus (NCL). × 63,000.

and have suggested that they are composed of chromatin. Such bodies have often been identified in neoplastic cells (Krishan *et al.*, 1967).

Two interesting observations concerning nuclear bodies arise from this study. First, the number and complexity of nuclear bodies is increased in a hyperestrogenized animal; second, nuclear bodies appear to be present predominantly in luminal epithelial cells. The latter point probably relates to the fact that Nafoxidine preferentially stimulates growth of luminal epithelial cells while having little effect on the growth of myometrial and stromal cells (see Fig. 11).

The composition and function of nuclear bodies in the hyperestrogenized uterus is not known, though they are visible manifestations of hyperestrogenization. Their presence and complexity is closely related to the transcriptional activity of the uterus; i.e., nuclei of quiescent cells have fewer and morphologically simple nuclear bodies, while nuclei of hyperactive cells contain many bodies of varying complexity. Increased transcriptional activity and the appearance of nuclear bodies are correlated with long-term retention of the estrogen receptor in uterine nuclei. Thus nuclear bodies may represent organelles involved in elevated transcriptional activity or may be by-products of such activity. The relationship between the stimulation of these nuclear bodies by Nafoxidine and the cause of the reproductive tract abnormalities discussed previously is unknown, though it is known that many neoplastic cells contain nuclear bodies (Bouteille *et al.*, 1967; Krishan *et al.*, 1967; Dupay-Coin *et al.*, 1972). Since we have shown that nuclear body formation is promoted by compounds that induce reproductive tract abnormalities and neoplasia, the study of nuclear bodies as precursors of the neoplastic state should be pursued in the future.

VII. Classification and Pharmacology of Estrogen Agonists and Antagonists

Based on the work discussed above we have proposed that estrogen agonists and antagonists be classified as shown in Table II (Clark *et al.*, 1977b). Estriol is a short-acting estrogen, hence acts as a partial agonist or antagonist when injected; however, when it is implanted, it acts as an agonist with no antagonistic properties (Figs. 3 and 6). Estriol has been classified in the past as a weak or impeded estrogen (Hisaw, 1959; Huggins and Jensen, 1955; Wotiz *et al.*, 1968). These terms imply that estriol is less effective under all circumstances. Since this is not the case, the classification of estriol as a short-acting estrogen provides a functional definition that applies in all cases. In this scheme, dimethylstilbestrol, me-

TABLE II

Classification of Estrogen Agonists and Antagonists[a]

Class subclass	Short-acting	Long-acting	
		Intermediate	Extended
Examples	Estriol, dimethyl-stilbestrol, 16-oxoestradiol	Estradiol, diethyl-stilbestrol	Triphenylethyl-ene derivatives, i.e., Nafoxidine, Clomid
Pharmacological characteristics	Partial agonist or antagonists	Agonists when injected	Agonists in some cell types and antagonists in others when injected
Nuclear retention of estrogen receptor	1–4 hours	1–24 hours	24–72 hours or longer
Replenishment of cytoplasmic receptor	12–24 hours	12–24 hours	Greater than 48–72 hours
RNA polymerase I activity	Initial increase but not sustained	Initial increase for >12 hours	Initial increase followed by sustained ac-tivity for >24–48 hours
RNA polymerase II activity	Early increase not followed by secondary rise	Early increase fol-lowed by a sus-tained second-ary rise	Early increase fol-lowed by a sus-tained second-ary rise
RNA polymerase initiation site	Slight increase followed by a rapid decline	Large increase by 12 hours, de-clines to con-trol by 48 hours	Large increase by 12–24 hours, which is sus-tained for >72 hours
Cellular hyper-trophy and hyperplasia	Insignificant	Significant in all tissue layers	Significant in epi-thelium, insig-nificant in other tissue layers

[a] This classification is based on data derived from a single injection in saline or aqueous vehicle to immature rats.

sobutoestrol, and 16-oxoestradiol are similar to estriol and thus may be classified together (Martin, 1969; Terenius, 1971; Rochefort et al., 1972). These compounds have in common the ability to stimulate early uterotropic responses as shown in Table I; however, they fail to influence significantly the long-term responses that promote uterine growth when given as an injection.

The long-acting estrogens are divided into two classes, A and B, according to their retention times in the body. Subclass A includes estradiol and DES because both these hormones are fully agonistic, with no antagonistic properties, and have similar nuclear retention times and biological potencies (Ruh and Baudendistel, 1977). Triphenylethylene derivatives, such as Clomid, Nafoxidine, and CI-628, are placed in a separate subclass, B, because of their ability to cause a sustained nuclear retention of the estrogen receptor and a failure to effect rapid replenishment of the cytoplasmic receptor (see Fig. 10). In addition, these compounds have the capacity to act as long-acting agonists in the epithelium of the uterus, while behaving as long-acting antagonists in other uterine tissues. Therefore triphenylethylene derivatives are distinctly different from steroidal estrogens.

The above classification focuses attention on the complex nature of estrogen agonists and antagonists and relates their functional activity to the retention of the receptor by the nucleus of target cells and their capacity to stimulate various uterotropic responses. Formerly, estriol and similar steroids were designated weak or impeded estrogens, while triphenylethylene derivatives such as Nafoxidine were called estrogen antagonists. Obviously this older classification applies only under certain circumstances and does not present a valid or complete picture of the activity of these compounds.

The establishment of estriol as an estrogen agonist when it is present under steady-state conditions has important implications with respect to certain hypotheses on the role of estriol in physiology and pathology. Estriol is present at high levels in the blood during pregnancy in the human (Hobkirk and Nilsen, 1962) and is the major estrogen present during the menstrual cycle (Goebelsmann et al., 1969). Therefore estriol is likely to be a major contributor to the total estrogen state of the human. Its role in this capacity needs reappraisal in light of the present results.

A protective role has been ascribed to estriol in breast cancer. This suggestion is based on the observation that oriental women, who have a high estriol/(estradiol +estrone) ratio in the blood, also have a low incidence of breast cancer (Jensen et al., 1966; Goebelsmann et al., 1969; Lemon et al., 1971; Cole and MacMahon, 1969). This hypothesis was formulated on the assumption that estriol was a weak estrogen under all circumstances and that during each menstrual cycle estriol acts to reduce the "carcinogenic potential'' of the more potent estradiol. Our results indicate that this theory is suspect and, in light of recent evidence showing that estriol and estradiol are of equal potential in facilitating the onset of mammary tumors in mice (Rudali *et al.*, 1975), we suggest that the estriol theory of mammary cancer protection is untenable.

Although it has long been recognized that the triphenyethylene derivatives possess inherent estrogenicity (Lerner, 1964), these compounds were generally considered to be estrogen antagonists and most experimental results obtained with them were interpreted according to this reasoning. The demonstration that triphenylethylene derivatives should be classified as long-acting estrogens with both agonistic and antagonistic properties results in the reconsideration of previously proposed explanations of the mechanism by which they alter estrogen-stimulated responses.

The long-acting effects of triphenylethylene derivatives and their ability to cause differential cell stimulation has obvious implications for the use of these drugs in humans. Clomid has been widely used for the past 15 years to induce ovulation in anovulatory women. Treatment consists of 50–100 mg of Clomid taken orally for 5 days. If the initial trial fails and no signs of pregnancy are present, the treatment is resumed the following month, ~40 days later. This treatment regimen is often continued for many months, hence the exposure of a woman to Clomid can be extensive. Under these circumstances, Clomid may stimulate some cell types while acting as an antagonist in others. The eventual effects of such stimulation may remain unknown for many years. Just recently we have demonstrated that Clomid administration on day 5 of pregnancy in the rat results in the development of neoplasia in the offspring (McCormack and Clark, 1979). This effect probably originates from the early and intense estrogenic stimulation of developing fetal tissues and demonstrates again the extreme potency of these compounds. The possibility exists that Clomid and other triphenylethylene derivatives could cause hyperestrogenization of certain cell types in humans, hence great caution should be exercised when these drugs are used in humans.

Acknowledgments

This work was supported by grants HDO8436 and CA 20605 from

References

Anderson, J. N., Clark, J. H., and Peck, E. J., Jr. (1972a). *Biochem. J.* 561–567.
Anderson, J. N., Clark, J. H., and Peck, E. J., Jr. (1972b). *Biochem. Biophys. Res. Commun.* **48,** 1460–1468.

Anderson, J. N., Peck, E. J., Jr., and Clark, J. H. (1973). *Endocrinology* **92**, 1488–1495.

Anderson, J. N., Peck, E. J., Jr., and Clark, J. H. (1975). *Endocrinology* **96**(1), 160–167.

Barker, K. L., and Warren, J. C. (1966). *Proc. Natl. Acad. Sci. U.S.A.* **56**, 1298–1302.

Barry, J., and Gorski, J. (1971). *Biochemistry* **10**, 2384–2390.

Baulieu, E. E., Alberga, A., Raynaud-Jammet, C., and Wira, C. R. (1972a). *Nature (London), New Biol.* **236**, 236–239.

Baulieu, E. E., Wira, C. R., Milgrom, E., and Raynaud-Jammet, C. (1972b). *Karolinska Symp. Res. Methods Reprod. Endocrinol. 5th* pp. 396–419.

Billing, R. J., Barbiroli, B., and Smellie, R. M. S. (1968). *Biochem. J.* **109**, 705–706.

Borthwick, N. M., and Smellie, R. M. S. (1975). *Biochem. J.* **147**, 91–101.

Bouteille, M., Kalifat, S. R., and Delarue, (1967). *J. Ultrastruct. Res.* **19**, 474–486.

Buller, R. E., and O'Malley, B. W. (1976). *Biochem. Pharmacol.* **25**, 1–12.

Capony, F., and Rochefort, H. (1975). *Mol. Cell. Endocrinol.* **3**(3), 233–251.

Capony, F., and Rochefort, H. (1977). *Mol. Cell. Endocrinol.* **8**, 47–64.

Chamberlin, M. J. (1974). *Annu. Rev. Biochem.* **43**, 721–775.

Church, R. B., and McCarthy, B. J. (1970). *Biochim. Biophys. Acta* **199**, 103–114.

Clark, J. H., and Gorski, J. (1969). *Biochim. Biophys. Acta* **192**, 508–515.

Clark, J. H., and McCormack, S. A. (1977). *Science* **197**, 164–165.

Clark, J. H., and Peck, E. J., Jr. (1976). *Nature (London)* **260**, 635–637.

Clark, J. H., Anderson, J., and Peck, E. J., Jr. (1972). *Science* **176**, 528.

Clark, J. H., Anderson, J. N., and Peck, E. J., Jr. (1973). *Steroids* **22**, 707–718.

Clark, J. H., Anderson, J. N., and Peck, E. J., Jr. (1974). *Nature (London)* **251**, 446–448.

Clark, J. H., Hardin, J. W., Padykula, H. A., and Cardasis, C. A. (1978b). *Proc. Natl. Acad. Sci* **75**, 2781–2784.

Clark, J. H., Peck, E. J., Jr., and Glasser, S. R. (1977a). *In* "Reproduction in Domestic Animals" (H. H. Cole and P. T. Cupps, eds.), 3rd Ed., pp. 143–174. Academic Press, New York.

Clark, J. H., Hseuh, and Peck, E. J., Jr. (1977b). *Ann. N.Y. Acad. Sci.* **286**, 161–179.

Clark, J. H., Paszko, Z., and Peck, E. J., Jr. (1977c). *Endocrinology* **100**, 91–96.

Clark, J. H., Peck, E. J., Jr., Hardin, J. W., and Eriksson, H. (1978). *In* "Receptors and Hormone Action" (B. W. O'Malley and L. Birnbaumer, eds.), Vol. 2, pp. 1–31. Academic Press, New York.

Cole, P., and MacMahon, B. (1969). *Lancet* **i**, 604–606.

Courvalin, J. C., Bouton, M. M., Baulieu, E. E., Nuret, P., and Chambon, P. (1976). *J. Biol. Chem.* **251**, 4843–4849.

DeAngelo, A. B., and Gorski, J. (1970). *Proc. Natl. Acad. Sci. U.S.A.* **66**, 693–700.

Dupay-Coin, A. M., Kalifat, S. R., and Bouteille, M. (1972). *J. Ultrastruct. Res.* **38**, 174–183.

Emmens, C. W. (1970). *Annu. Rev. Pharmacol.* **4**, 237–254.

Fels, E. (1976). *Arch. Gynaekol.* **221**, 103–118.

Gallez, G., Heuson, J. C., and Waelbroeck, C. (1973). *Eur. J. Cancer* **9**, 699–700.

Gellert, R. J., Lewis, J., and Petra, P. H. (1977). *Endocrinology* **100**(2), 520–528.

Glasser, S. R., Chytil, F., and Spelsberg, T. C. (1972). *Biochem. J.* **130**, 947–957.

Goebelsmann, U., Midgley, A. R., Jr., and Jaffe, R. B. (1969). *J. Clin. Endocrinol.* **29**, 1222–1230.

Gorski, J. (1964). *J. Biol. Chem.* **239**, 889–892.

Gorski, J., and Gannon, F. (1976). *Annu. Rev. Physiol.* **38**, 425–450.

Gorski, R. (1963). *Am. J. Physiol.* **205**, 842–844.

Hamilton, T. H. (1968). *Science* **161**, 649–660.

Hamilton, T. H., Widnell, C. C., and Tata, J. R. (1965). *Biochim. Biophys. Acta* **108**, 168–172.

Hamilton, T. H., Widnell, C. C., and Tata, J. R. (1968a). *J. Biol. Chem.* **243**, 408–417.

Hamilton, T. H., Teng, C. S., and Means, A. R. (1968b). *Proc. Natl. Acad. Sci. U.S.A.* **59**, 1265–1272.

Hardin, J. W., Clark, J. H., Glasser, S. R., and Peck, E. J., Jr. (1976). *Biochemistry* **15**, 1370–1374.

Harman, S. M., Louvet, J.-P., and Ross, G. T. (1975). *Endocrinology* **96**, 1145–1152.

Hertz, R. (1974). *Cancer (Philadelphia)* **38**, 534–540.

Hisaw, F. L., Jr. (1959). *Endocrinology* **64**, 276–289.

Hobkirk, R., and Nilsen, M. (1962). *J. Clin. Endocrinol. Metab.* **22**, 134–141.

Holtkamp, D. E., Greslin, J. G., Root, C. A., and Lerner, L. J. (1960). *Proc. Soc. Exp. Biol. Med.* **105**, 197–198.

Huggins, C., and Jensen, E. V. (1955). *J. Exp. Med.* **102**, 335–346.

Jensen, E. V., and DeSombre, E. R. (1972). *Annu. Rev. Biochem.* **41**, 203–230.

Jensen, E. V., Jacobson, H. I., Flesher, J. W., Saha, N. N., Gupta, G., Smith, S., Colucci, V., Shiplacoff, D., Neumann, H. G., DeSombre, E. R., and Jungblut, P. W. (1966). *In* "Steroid Dynamics" (G. Pincus, T. Nakao, and J. F. Tait, eds.), pp. 133–157. Academic Press, New York.

Katzenellenbogen, B. S., and Ferguson, E. R. (1975). *Endocrinology* **97**, 1–12.

Katzenellenbogen, B. S., and Gorski, J. (1975). *In* "Biochemical Actions of Hormones" (G. Litwack, ed.), pp. 187–243. Academic Press, New York.

Katzenellenbogen, B. S., Ferguson, E. R., and Lan, N. C. (1977). *Endocrinology* **100**, 1252–1259.

Keran, E. E., and Barker, K. L. (1976). *Endocrinology* **99**, 1386–1397.

Knowler, J. T., and Smellie, R. M. S. (1971). *Biochem. J.* **125**, 605–614.

Krishan, A., Uzman, B. G., and Hedley-Whyte, E. T. (1967). *J. Ultrastruct. Res.* **19**, 563–672.

Lan, N. C., and Katzenellenbogen, B. S. (1976). *Endocrinology* **98**(1), 220–227.

LeGoascogne, C., and Baulieu, E. E. (1977). *Biol. Cell:* **30**, 195–206.

Lemon, H. M., Miller, D. M., and Foley, J. F. (1971). *Natl. Cancer Inst., Monogr.* **34**, 77–83.

Lerner, L. J. (1964). *Recent Prog. Horm. Res.* **20**, 435–490.

Lobl, R. T., and Maenza, R. M. (1975). *Biol. Reprod.* **13**, 255–264.

Luck, D., and Hamilton, T. H. (1972). *Proc. Natl. Acad. Sci. U.S.A.* **69**, 157–161.

MacCormack, S. A., and Clark, J. H. (1979). (Submitted).

Martin, L. (1969). *Steroids* **13**, 1–10.

Mueller, G. C., Herranen, A. M., and Jervell, K. (1958). *Recent Prog. Horm. Res.* **14**, 95–139.

Noteboom, W. D., and Gorski, J. (1965). *Arch. Biochem. Biophys.* **111**, 559–568.

O'Malley, B. W., and Means, A. R. (1974). *Science* **183**, 610–620.

Palmiter, R. D., Moore, P. B., and Mulvihill, E. R. (1976). *Cell* **8**, 557–572.

Raynaud-Jammet, C., Cattelli, M. G., and Baulieu, E. E. (1972). *FEBS Lett.* **22**, 93–96.

Reddy, V., Naftolin, F., and Ryan, K. (1974). *Endocrinology* **94**, 117–124.

Rochefort, H., Lignon, F., and Capony, F. (1972). *Gynecol. Invest.* **3**(1), 43–62.

Ross, J. W., Shryne, J., Gorski, R. A., and Marshall, J. R. (1973). *Endocrinology* **92**, 1079–1083.

Rudali, G., Apiou, F., and Muel, B. (1975). *Eur. J. Cancer* **11**, 39–41.

Ruh, T. S., and Baudendistel, L. J. (1977). *Endocrinology* **100**(2), 420–426.

Segal, S. J., Scher, W., and Koide, S. S. (1977). *In* "Biology of the Uterus" (R. M. Wynn, ed.), pp. 139–202. Plenum, New York.

Spelsberg, T. C., and Cox, R. F. (1976). *Biochim. Biophys. Acta* **435**, 376–390.

Terenius, L. (1971). *Eur. J. Cancer* **7**, 57–64.

Tsai, M.-J., Schwartz, R. J., Tsai, S. G., and O'Malley, B. W. (1975). *J. Biol. Chem.* **250,** 5165–5174.

Weil, P. A., Sidikaro, J., Stancel, G. M., and Blatti, S. P. (1977). *J. Biol. Chem.* **252,** 1092–1098.

Wotiz, H. H., Shane, J. A., Vigersky, R., and Brecher, P. I. (1968). *In* "Prognostic Factors in Breast Cancer" (A.P.M. Forrest and B. Kunkler, eds.), pp. 368–376. Livingstone, Edinburgh.

18

Testosterone Effects on the Prostatic Nucleus

KHALIL AHMED, MICHAEL J. WILSON,
SAID A. GOUELI, and MARY E. NORVITCH

I. Introduction

This chapter deals primarily with the testosterone effects on prostatic nuclear phosphoprotein metabolism investigated in the authors' laboratory. We have also included studies concerning factors such as polyamines, which may influence the level of phosphorylation of nonhistone proteins (NHPs) in cell nuclei in general.

The dependence of male accessory sex glands on the constant availability of androgen for their development and activity is now well recognized (Price and Williams-Ashman, 1961; Mann, 1964; Williams-Ashman and Shimazaki, 1967). The prostate gland in mammalian species is a target organ for testosterone, and in this regard rat ventral prostate has been extensively used as an experimental model for carrying out studies on the mechanism of androgen action (see, e.g., Huggins, 1945; Price and Williams-Ashman, 1961; Mann, 1964; Williams-Ashman et al., 1964; Liao and Fang, 1969; Williams-Ashman and Reddi, 1971; King and Mainwaring, 1974; Mainwaring, 1977; Ahmed and Wilson, 1978; Ahmed et al., 1979a). As documented in these reviews, androgen withdrawal from adult animals results in a large number of biochemical and morphological changes in rat ventral prostate epithelium. The alterations in biochemical activities proceed at varying rates since most, if not all, of them are influenced by in vivo changes in androgen levels. Some of the more rapid changes (i.e., within 12 hours) include a decline in nuclear androgen receptor, RNA synthesis, and nuclear protein phosphorylation, whereas among the more slowly declining activities (i.e., at about 3–5 days postorchiectomy) are a generalized reduction in protein synthesis including that of certain enzymes, a decline in respiratory activity, a decrease in polyamine levels, and a cessation of secretory activity. Morphological changes are equally pronounced within a few days and may become evident within 24 hours, e.g., the electron microscope changes in certain subcellular components (Price and Williams-Ashman, 1961). The gland undergoes rapid involution with a decline in intracellular membranes and ribosomes; the nuclei become small and pyknotic. Within a week or so the regression of the gland is very pronounced. Institution of androgen administration to castrated adult rats leads to orderly temporal alterations in various biosynthetic activities. Among the earliest changes are an increase in RNA polymerase activity (Williams-Ashman et al., 1964; Liao et al., 1965; Mainwaring et al., 1971), a transient fall in total ATP level (Ritter, 1966; Coffey et al., 1968), an enhancement in the binding of methionyl-tRNA$_f$ to a cytoplasmic factor (Liang et al., 1977), and an increased phosphorylation of nuclear NHPs (Ahmed and Wilson, 1978). These are followed by dramatic increases in protein synthesis and other macromolecular synthetic activities (see, e.g., Liao and Fang, 1969; Williams-Ashman and Reddi, 1971; King and Mainwaring, 1974). DNA synthesis and activity of enzymes engaged in this function undergo a very substantial (though transitory) elevation between 2 and 5 days after androgen administration (Kosto et al., 1967; Coffey et al., 1968; Williams-Ashman et al., 1975).

II. Model of Androgen Action

Since, as mentioned above, one of the earliest effects of testosterone treatment in the male accessory sex glands is the stimulation of DNA-dependent RNA polymerase followed by increased incorporation of amino acids into proteins by polyribosomes (Liao and Williams-Ashman, 1962; Hancock *et al.*, 1962; Williams-Ashman *et al.*, 1964; Kochakian, 1965; Fujii and Villee, 1969; Liao and Fang, 1969; Mainwaring *et al.*, 1971; King and Mainwaring, 1974; Mainwaring, 1977), current investigations of the mechanism of action of androgen in male accessory glands (as well as of other sex hormones in their target organs) have put major emphasis on the control of transcription by these hormones (O'Malley and Means, 1974; Mainwaring *et al.*, 1974a,b; Harris *et al.*, 1975; McKnight *et al.*, 1975; Woo and O'Malley, 1976).

The discovery by Jensen and Jacobson (1962) that estrogen was preferentially retained by its target organs led the way to the search for receptor(s) for sex steroids in these tissues. Testosterone enters the target cell where it is converted to 5α-dihydrotestosterone (Farnsworth and Brown, 1963; Shimazaki *et al.*, 1965) by the action of an NADPH-dependent 5α-reductase and may be the active metabolite *in vivo* (Bruchovsky and Wilson, 1968a,b; Anderson and Liao, 1968; Wilson and Gloyna, 1970). Nuclear retention of 5α-dihydrotestosterone in prostatic tissue has been demonstrated following an injection of [³H]testosterone (see, e.g., Liao and Fang, 1969; Wilson and Gloyna, 1970; King and Mainwaring, 1974). The mode of appearance of 5α-dihydrotestosterone in the nucleus is a consequence of its interaction in the cytosol with receptor protein(s) which exist with sedimentation coefficients ranging from 3 to 11 S (Fang *et al.*, 1969; Mainwaring and Peterken, 1971). This interaction promotes steroid entry into the nucleus by an energy-dependent process; in the absence of cytosol receptor protein, no steroid is retained in the nucleus (Liao *et al.*, 1974; Mainwaring, 1977). The receptor complex can be extracted from the nucleus with 0.4 M KCl, and in this case it appears to have sedimentation coefficient values of 3.0–4.5 S (Liao *et al.*, 1974; 1975; Mainwaring, 1977). The relationship between cytosol and the nuclear receptor is not clear at the present time. A more detailed discussion of this topic has been given previously (see, e.g., Ahmed and Wilson, 1978; see also reviews cited above).

The next step in this scheme is the binding of the 5α-dihydrotestosterone–receptor complex to specific acceptor sites in the chromatin. The precise nature of these sites remains unresolved at the present time. Although DNA may have some acceptor function in relation to the steroid–receptor complex, specificity is achieved most likely by association of the complex with chromatin proteins. Current observations suggest that

NHPs in the chromatin provide sites for specific interaction with the steroid–receptor complex (see, e.g., King and Gordon, 1972; Lebeau *et al.*, 1973; Davies and Griffiths, 1973a,b; Spelsberg, 1974; Liao *et al.*, 1974, 1975; Chan and O'Malley, 1976; Mainwaring, 1975, 1977; Klyzsejko-Stefanowicz *et al.*, 1976; Nyberg and Wang, 1976; Ahmed and Wilson, 1978). The precise nature of the events following this association with the chromatin, resulting in the synthesis of new RNA species, remains unknown and is currently the subject of intense investigation.

III. Control of Transcription

From the foregoing, it is clear that control of transcriptional activity may be fundamental to the mechanism of androgen action in the prostate. Hence it is important to identify the factors involved in the regulation of transcription and their modulation by testosterone. A large number of recent investigations have suggested that chromosomal proteins play a regulatory role in the control of transcription. NHPs and their derivatives (such as by phosphorylation) appear to be excellent candidates as positive regulatory agents for such a function (for reviews, see Busch *et al.*, 1963; Langan, 1967; Stellwagen and Cole, 1969; MacGillivray *et al.*, 1972; Allfrey, 1974; Baserga, 1974; Kleinsmith, 1974; Ahmed, 1975; Ahmed and Wilson, 1978). The phosphorylation of chromatin proteins appears to be mediated by protein phosphokinase activities endogenous to the nucleus (Ahmed and Ishida, 1971; Takeda *et al.*, 1971; Teng *et al.*, 1971; Ruddon and Anderson, 1972; Ishida and Ahmed, 1974; Kish and Kleinsmith, 1974; Ahmed, 1975; Ahmed and Davis, 1975; Keller *et al.*, 1975; Blat *et al.*, 1976). It is therefore reasonable to assume that the control of chromosomal NHP synthesis and phosphorylation may be germane to androgen action on the prostate. Besides their function in the control of transcription in the nucleus, prostatic chromatin NHPs (as mentioned earlier) may be involved as acceptors in the nuclear binding of the 5α-dihydrotestosterone–receptor complex; in this context it is noteworthy that the phosphorylation of chromatin NHPs may stimulate such acceptor functions (Klyzsejko-Stefanowicz *et al.*, 1976).

IV. Prostatic Nuclear Phosphoproteins

A systematic investigation of the effects of testosterone on prostatic nuclear phosphoprotein metabolism was originally undertaken by us (Ahmed, 1970, 1971; Ahmed and Ishida, 1971). We observed that purified nuclei from rat ventral prostate rapidly incorporated ^{32}P (from [γ-^{32}P]ATP). When incubated under appropriate reaction conditions, the steady state of labeling of nuclear phosphoproteins was achieved within about 6–8 minutes using prostatic nuclei as well as nuclei from other tissues, e.g., submandibular gland and liver (Ahmed, 1971, 1974; Ahmed and Ishida, 1971; Ishida and Ahmed, 1973). Separation of ^{32}P-labeled nuclear phosphoproteins into nonhistone and histone phosphoprotein fractions showed that a preponderant amount of radioactivity was incorporated into the nonhistone fraction. Orchiectomy of rats resulted in a rapid decline in the ability of nuclei to incorporate ^{32}P *in vitro* (from [γ-^{32}P]ATP), so that at 4–5 days postcastration the rates of phosphorylation reactions were reduced by over 80% (Table I). Androgen treatment of castrated rats prevented these alterations. Liver nuclear phosphoprotein phosphorylation *in vitro* was uninfluenced by either of these *in vivo* androgenic manipulations, suggesting a target tissue effect of testosterone on prostatic nuclear phosphoprotein phosphorylation. In order to determine whether or not the phosphorylation of nuclear proteins was related to gene action in the prostate in response to testosterone, we investigated the early effect of a single injection of testosterone into castrated rats. Rats, castrated 5 days previously, were given a single injection of testosterone and killed 30 or 60 minutes later. Nuclei were isolated from pooled prostatic tissue and *in vitro* incorporation of ^{32}P from [γ-^{32}P]ATP was examined in various nuclear phosphoprotein fractions. As shown in Table I, the rate of phosphorylation of total nuclear phosphoproteins was increased by about 50%. On fractionation it was observed that the increase in histone phosphoprotein radioactivity was not significant, whereas that in the nonhistone phosphoprotein fraction was very marked (about 80%). This observation, taken together with the original work of Kleinsmith *et al.* (1966), further implicated NHP phosphorylation in the control of gene action. It may be noted that the androgen effects on nuclear protein phosphorylation described above were not reproduced by the addition of testosterone or 5α-dihydrotestosterone to the reaction media. Rather, the aforementioned experiments and other similar studies from our laboratory (Ishida and Ahmed, 1973; Ahmed, 1974, 1975) demonstrated that *in vivo* manipulations that altered genome activity produced changes in nuclear phosphoprotein metabolism, which were apparent *in vitro* in a cell-free system. ^{32}P incorporation into nuclear phosphoproteins *in vivo* and the effects of androgen thereon have also been reported and corroborate the above observations (Schauder *et al.*, 1974; Kadohama and Anderson, 1976, 1977). Kadohama and Anderson (1976, 1977) also reported that the distribution of phosphorylated proteins and newly synthesized proteins was dissimilar. Thus the synthesis of nuclear NHPs and their postsynthe-

TABLE I

The Effect of Castration and Testosterone Treatment on the Initial Rates of ^{32}P Incorporation into Nuclear Phosphoproteins[a,b]

	^{32}P incorporation (nmoles/mg protein/hour[c])		
Source	Total phospho-proteins	Nonhistone phospho-proteins	Histone phospho-proteins
Ventral prostate			
Normal	25.6 ± 0.5	55	6
Castrated controls[d]	6.2 ± 0.7	9.9 ± 2.2	2.8 ± 1.0
Castrated, single injection of testosterone at 30 minutes[e]	9.5 ± 0.4	17.8 ± 3.5	3.5 ± 0.8
Castrated, maintained with daily testosterone injections[f]	24.9 ± 0.4	55	6
Liver			
Normal	58.6 ± 0.8	—	—
Castrated controls[g]	54.4 ± 0.2	—	—
Castrated, maintained with daily testosterone injections[h]	53.8 ± 2.4	—	—

[a] From Ahmed (1971) and Ahmed and Ishida (1971).

[b] Rats used in these experiments were orchiectomized for 112–137 hours.

[c] The phosphorylation reactions were carried out for 1 minute in medium consisting of 5 mM MgCl$_2$, 115 mM NaCl, 30 mM Tris–HCl, pH 7.5, and 3 mM [γ-^{32}P]ATP. Time course experiments demonstrated that the incorporation of radioactivity into nuclear phosphoproteins was measured within the linear range for nuclei from rats of differing androgenic status.

[d] Castrated control rats received 0.2 ml sesame oil 30 minutes prior to sacrifice. The values for orchiectomized rats receiving a daily treatment with 0.2 ml sesame oil were not significantly different from those shown here for rats receiving a single injection of oil.

[e] These rats received a single injection of testosterone propionate (2 mg in 0.20 ml sesame oil) 30 minutes prior to sacrifice.

[f] Testosterone-maintained, castrated animals received a daily subcutaneous dose of 1 mg testosterone propionate in 0.2 ml sesame oil.

[g] Castrated rats received a daily treatment of 0.2 ml sesarne oil.

[h] Castrated rats were treated as described in footnote e.

tic modification by phosphorylation may not be temporally related, so that the phosphorylation is independent of synthesis (for review, see Ahmed and Wilson, 1978). Androgen-stimulated synthesis of nuclear NHPs has been studied by several investigators (Chung and Coffey, 1971a,b; Anderson *et al.*, 1973). It may also be noted that an early increase in phosphorylation of nuclear NHPs in response to genome activation has now been described in many experimental systems (see, e.g., Jungmann and Kranias, 1977; Stein *et al.*, 1974; Ahmed and Wilson, 1978).

V. Prostatic Nuclear Protein Kinase and Phosphatase Reactions

A. Kinases

1. *Introduction*

As summarized later, several explanations may account for the aforementioned effect of testosterone on nuclear phosphoprotein phosphorylation (see Section V,D). As a first step, we decided to examine the androgen control of enzyme activities engaged in these reactions by utilizing both endogenous and exogenous substrates. The use of the latter would be particularly warranted if there were marked changes in the content of endogenous phosphoprotein substrates. Thus we have explored protein kinase reactions associated with purified chromatin, a NHP fraction derived from chromatin, purified nucleoli compared with extranucleolar material, and separated enzymes as sources of protein kinase activity. As exogenous sources of protein substrates we have utilized lysine-rich histone (as a basic protein substrate) and partially dephosphorylated phosvitin (dephosphophosvitin) as a model acidic protein substrate (Ahmed *et al.*, 1975).

In addition, we have also examined androgen effects on prostatic nuclear protein phosphatase activities, again utilizing basic phosphoprotein and acidic phosphoprotein substrates.

2. *Subnuclear Localization of Protein Kinases*

The results summarized in Table II show the subnuclear localization of protein kinases and their properties for achieving optimal reaction conditions. The activities shown in the nucleolar, extranucleolar, and chromatin fractions show distinct features which indicate a multiplicity of these activities. The properties of nucleolus- and chromatin-associated activities are in general similar; this is expected, since chromatin preparations must include the nucleolar components. The similarities and differences in these fractions are particularly underscored by the similarities and differences in the apparent K_m values for ATP and for protein substrates. Kinase activities toward lysine-rich histone as substrate were only a small fraction of those toward dephosphophosvitin as substrate, which is in accord with the results obtained for the phosphorylation of nuclear proteins

TABLE II

Comparison of the Enzymic Properties of Histone Kinase and Acidic Phosphoprotein Kinase Associated with Nucleolar, Extranucleolar, and Chromatin Subfractions from Rat Ventral Prostate Nuclei[a,b]

Property	Nucleolus		Extranucleolus	Chromatin	
	LRH	DPV	DPV	LRH	DPV
pH optima	8.0–8.2	7.1	7.4, 8.4	8.0–8.2	7.0–7.4, 7.89
Mg²⁺, optimal (mM)	8	5–8	3–6	6	5
Mn²⁺, substitution (% compared to optimal Mg²⁺)	30	60	40[c]	30	40
NaCl, optimal (mM)	120	160	160	80	200
Dithiothreitol (% stimulation)	67	58	—	37	64
K_m values for ATP (mM)	0.02	0.02, 0.05, 1.05	0.05, 0.24	0.01	0.04, 0.41
K_m values for protein substrate (mg/ml)	2	0.03, 0.06, 1.9	0.06, 0.44, 1.9	0.9	0.3
Effect of orchiectomy (% decrease in activity at 24 hours)	2	42	26	8	53

[a] From Wilson and Ahmed (1975, 1976b, 1977) and Ahmed and Wilson (1975).

[b] Histone kinase and acidic phosphoprotein kinase activities associated with nucleolar, extranucleolar, and chromatin fractions were determined as described in the legends for Fig. 1 and Fig. 2 using lysine-rich histones (LRH) and dephosphophosvitin (DPV) as substrates.

[c] The activity in the presence of 0.5 mM Mn²⁺ (compared with Mg²⁺) was 40% but was only 15% at 5 mM Mn²⁺.

TABLE III

Protein Phosphokinase Activities of Euchromatin and Heterochromatin Fractions of Chromatin from Rat Ventral Prostate[a,b]

	Protein phosphokinase activity[c]			
Enzyme source	DPV substrate[d]	LRH substrate[d]	DPV substrate[e]	LRH substrate[e]
Total chromatin	148.9	3.7	310.0	7.8
Heterochromatin	44.0	0.1	70.0	0.5
Euchromatin	326.8	4.8	1660.0	24.3

[a] Norvitch, Wilson, and Ahmed (unpublished data).

[b] Euchromatin and heterochromatin fractions were prepared from rat ventral prostate chromatin by the procedure of Marushige and Bonner (1971).

[c] Protein phosphokinase activities were assayed as described in the legend for Fig. 1.

[d] Activity expressed as nanomoles of ^{32}P per milligram of protein per hour.

[e] Activity expressed as nanomoles of ^{32}P per milligram of DNA per hour.

and chromatin. It is also noteworthy that Mg^{2+} (compared with other divalent cations), a certain ionic strength in the reaction, and the presence of sulfhydryl-protective agents (e.g., dithiothreitol) are necessary for optimal reaction conditions. The characteristics of a NHP-associated protein kinase activity are similar to those of chromatin. The activity tends to be unstable in the reaction which is prevented by the addition of albumin (Ahmed *et al.*, 1978; Ahmed and Wilson, 1978). Compared with the extranucleolar material, the chromatin- and nucleolus-associated kinase activity toward dephosphophosvitin shows a rapid decrease at 24 hours following orchiectomy. The loss of kinase activity in the NHP fraction from chromatin was similar to that of chromatin-associated kinase activity (Ahmed *et al.*, unpublished data). A more detailed account of the properties of these kinase reactions has been given previously (Ahmed and Wilson, 1978). The presence of distinct kinase activity in chromatin (see, e.g., Allfrey, 1974; Kleinsmith, 1974) and the nucleolus (Olson *et al.*, 1978) has been shown in other cell nuclei. An interesting feature of chromatin-associated protein kinases is that they are predominantly localized in the euchromatin fraction (Table III). Similar observations were made by Keller *et al.* (1975) with chick oviduct chromatin in which the euchromatin fraction contained a high template activity as well as acidic protein kinase activity. It may be recalled that euchromatin is the active portion of chromatin engaged in RNA synthesis (see, e.g., Stellwagen and Cole, 1969).

3. Androgen Control of Prostatic Nucleus-Associated Protein Kinases

a. Effects of Orchiectomy and Androgen Treatment

i. Chromatin-Associated Protein Kinases Orchiectomy of adult male rats results in a remarkably rapid decline in chromatin-associated protein kinase activities using exogenous substrates (Fig. 1). Thus kinase activity using dephosphophosvitin as substrate was reduced by 30% at 9 hours, and 50% at 18 hours postorchiectomy, compared with the results for normal controls. Longer postcastration periods resulted in a continuous decline in this kinase activity, so that by 120 hours it was present in minimal amounts. In contrast, the activity toward a basic protein substrate (lysine-rich histone) initially did not decrease as rapidly; it was reduced by only about 10% at 18 hours, and about 30% at 48 hours, postorchiectomy. Nuclear RNA polymerase also declined rapidly after orchiectomy of adult rats; its activity was shown to be reduced by about 27% at 12 hours and 50% at 24 hours postcastration, as compared with normal controls (Liao

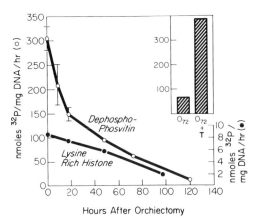

Hours After Orchiectomy

Fig. 1 The effect of orchiectomy on chromatin-associated protein phosphokinase activities toward acidic and basic protein substrates. The acidic phosphoprotein activity was measured using partially dephosphorylated phosvitin (DPV) as a model acidic protein substrate. The reaction medium contained 5 mM $MgCl_2$, 200 mM NaCl, 1 mM dithiothreitol, 30 mM Tris–HCl, pH 7.4 at 37°C, 3 mM [γ-^{32}P]ATP 3000 dpm/nmole ATP), and 2 mg/ml of DPV. The histone kinase activity was assayed using lysine-rich histone as substrate (3 mg/ml) in a medium containing 6 mM $MgCl_2$, 80 mM NaCl, 1 mM dithiothreitol, 30 mM Tris–HCl, final pH 8.1 at 37°C, and 0.1 mM [γ-^{32}P]ATP (10^5 dpm/nmole ATP). The effect of androgen maintenance of castrated rats on acidic phosphoprotein kinase activity was ascertained (see inset). Orchiectomized animals were injected subcutaneously with testosterone propionate (1 mg/100 gm body weight) in 0.2 ml sesame oil (0_{72} + T) or 0.2 ml sesame oil alone (0_{72}) daily for 3 days. (From Ahmed and Wilson, 1975; Wilson and Ahmed, 1977; reproduced with permission.)

and Fang, 1969). Thus chromatin-associated kinases that are active toward an acidic phosphoprotein substrate appear to be as sensitive (or even more so) as the RNA polymerase with regard to the androgenic status of the animal. (Acidic phosphoprotein substrate denotes dephospho-phosvitin as substrate, as opposed to histones which are basic phosphoprotein substrates.) The effects of castration on kinase activities are fully prevented by the administration of androgen to castrated rats. Indeed, under these circumstances (i.e., daily administration of androgen for 72 hours) kinase activities are even somewhat higher than those for normal controls. The mechanism of the aforementioned early decline in chromatin-associated kinases is not clear at present and must await purification of these enzymes. However, it should be noted that these results were the same when expressed per unit of chromatin protein or DNA, and that, at the early times (9 and 18 hours postorchiectomy) when significant reduction in kinase activity was apparent, there was not a significant decrease in the protein/DNA ratio in chromatin preparations (Table IV).

ii. Nucleolus-Associated Protein Kinases It is well-known that the nucleolus is the site of rRNA synthesis and subsequent maturation of ribosomal particles (Busch and Smetana, 1970). In view of the fact that stimulation of nucleolar RNA polymerase activity and RNA synthesis are marked early responses to androgen in rat ventral prostate (Liao and Fang, 1969; Mainwaring *et al.*, 1971), and the presence of certain nonhis-

TABLE IV

Effect of Orchiectomy on the Chemical Composition of Rat Ventral Prostate Chromatin and Its Associated Acidic Phosphoprotein Phosphokinase Activity[a]

Hours after orchiectomy	Decline (%)[b]	
	Protein kinase activity toward DPV[c]	Protein/DNA
9	30	4
18	50	5
48	70	17
96	80	25

[a] From Ahmed and Wilson (1975).

[b] The values for protein phosphokinase activity toward DPV and the ratio of protein to DNA are expressed in terms of percent reduction compared with intact controls.

[c] The conditions for the determination of chromatin-associated protein kinase activity toward DPV are given in the legend for Fig. 1.

tone phosphoproteins in the nucleolus (Olson *et al.*, 1975), it was of particular interest to examine specifically the effects of androgen on nucleolus-associated kinase activities. As observed in the case of chromatin-associated kinases, nucleolus-associated kinase activities toward lysine-rich histone and acidic phosphoprotein substrates showed differential responses to androgen deprivation; e.g., at 24 hours postorchiectomy there was little change in the former but a significant reduction in the latter (Fig. 2). These changes were prevented by androgen administration to castrated animals. It was also noted that the protein kinase activity in the extranucleolar fraction was relatively less sensitive to the androgenic status of the animal. It seems likely that the decline in activity in the extranu-

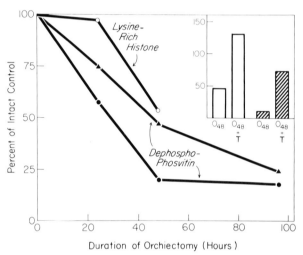

Fig. 2 Effects of orchiectomy on acidic phosphoprotein kinase and histone kinase activities of nucleolar (● and ○) and extranucleolar (▲) fractions of rat ventral prostate nuclei. The acidic phosphoprotein kinase activity of nucleoli was measured using DPV (6 mg/ml) as the protein acceptor substrate in a medium containing 6 mM $MgCl_2$, 160 mM NaCl, 1 mM dithiothreitol, 3 mM [γ-^{32}P]ATP (3000 dpm/nmole ATP), and 30 mM imidazole–HCl, final pH 7.1 at 37°C. The kinase activity in the extranucleolar fraction was ascertained in the same manner as that of the nucleolus, except that the buffer was 30 mM Tris–HCl, pH 7.4 at 37°C. The histone phosphokinase activity of the nucleoli was determined with lysine-rich histone (4 mg/ml) as substrate in a reaction mixture containing 8 mM $MgCl_2$, 120 mM NaCl, 1 mM dithiothreitol, 1 mM [γ-^{32}P]ATP (10^4 dpm/nmole ATP), and 30 mM Tris–HCl, final pH 8.1 at 37°C. The maintenance of castrated rats by daily treatment with testosterone propionate was performed as described for Fig. 1, and the effect on nucleolar protein kinase activity is given in the inset: O_{48}, 48-hour orchiectomized, oil-treated controls; O_{48} +T, 48-hour orchiectomized, testosterone-treated; open bars, activity with lysine-rich histones as substrate; hatched bars, activity with DPV as substrate. (From Wilson and Ahmed, 1976b, 1977; reproduced with permission.)

cleolar fraction was actually a reflection of the presence of a fraction of chromatin (which contains androgen-sensitive kinase activities) and that presumably the activity in the nucleoplasm may be relatively insensitive to androgen withdrawal. A more definitive answer to this will be forthcoming from the current studies on purification of these enzymes in the authors' laboratory.

b. Effects of Antiandrogens

We have already demonstrated that the protein kinase activities associated with the prostatic nucleus are influenced by androgen in a target tissue-specific manner. Androgen withdrawal from, or administration to, castrated rats is without influence on the kinases associated with rat liver. One may therefore conclude that androgen effects on prostatic nuclear kinases (and the phosphorylation of nuclear protein) are mediated via the androgen–receptor system. Another criterion for establishing the specificity of such a mode of action (i.e., the androgen–receptor system) is to demonstrate an effect of antiandrogens on the androgen-sensitive activities in target tissues. For this purpose, compounds that interfere with formation of the hormone–receptor complex and/or its movement into the nucleus may be utilized (Fig. 3). Cyproterone acetate, a steroidal antiandrogen (Neumann, 1977), and flutamide, a nonsteroidal antiandrogen (Neri and Monahan, 1972), have been shown to antagonize the manifestations of androgen-mediated response, including RNA and DNA synthesis in target glands (Fang et al., 1969; Fang and Liao, 1969; Grigorescu and Villee, 1973; Peets et al., 1974; Liao et al., 1974; Sufrin and Coffey, 1976; Mainwaring, 1977). The effects of antiandrogens are thus analogous to those produced by androgen withdrawal via orchiectomy and are taken as evidence for the participation of a 5α-dihydrotestosterone receptor in the

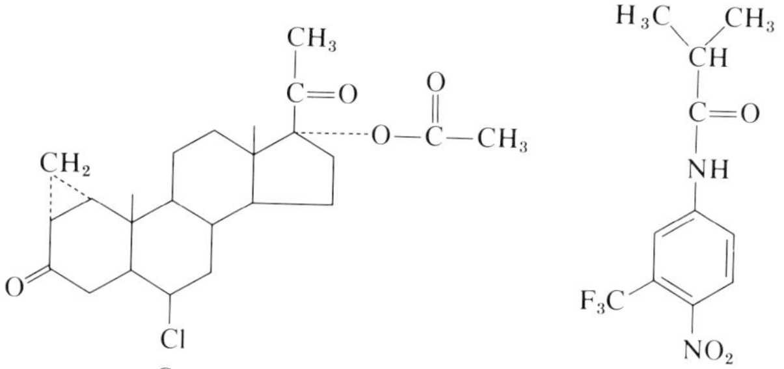

Fig. 3 Structure of cyproterone acetate and flutamide.

testosterone-mediated events. Since prostatic nuclear protein kinase
reactions are profoundly influenced by the androgenic status of the host,
we examined the effects of the above antiandrogens on these reactions.

Intact adult male rats (315–335 gm) were treated daily with a subcutaneous dose of flutamide or cyproterone acetate (each at 10 mg dissolved
in sesame oil) over a period of 48 hours. At the end of this period prostatic
chromatin was prepared, and its associated protein kinase activities
toward acidic phosphoprotein substrate (dephosphophosvitin) and
lysine-rich histone were examined. Both these antiandrogens caused a decline of 33–36% in the activity of the kinase reaction toward dephosphophosvitin. As was observed in the case of orchiectomy, the influence on
histone kinase was less marked than that on acidic protein kinase (Ahmed

TABLE V

**The Effect of Competition of Antiandrogens and Testosterone in 48-Hour
Castrated Rats on the Phosphorylation of Endogenous Prostatic Chromatin
Proteins and Chromatin-Associated Protein Phosphokinase Activity toward
DPV**[a,b]

| Testosterone propionate | Antiandrogen | Percent of testosterone-treated controls[c] | |
		Endogenous protein	DPV
0.01 mg/100 gm	Oil only	100	100
Oil only	Oil only	46	36
0.01 mg/100 gm	Flutamide, 10-fold	65	86
0.01 mg/100 gm	Flutamide, 100-fold	41	55
0.01 mg/100 gm	Cyproterone acetate, 10-fold	70	79
0.01 mg/100 gm	Cyproterone acetate, 100-fold	45	73

[a] From Wilson, Davis, and Ahmed (unpublished data).

[b] Animals were castrated and injected at two independent subcutaneous sites
with testosterone propionate and antiandrogen, both of which were suspended
in sesame oil. The testosterone-treated castrated control animals received hormone and oil; the castrate controls were injected with sesame oil at both sites.
The antiandrogens cyproterone acetate and flutamide were administered in two
doses; one at a 10-fold and the other at a 100-fold higher concentration than the
testosterone propionate dose on a molar basis. Injections of oil, hormone, or
antiandrogen were given immediately upon castration, at 24 hours, and finally
at 48 hours just prior to sacrifice.

[c] Phosphorylation of endogenous chromatin proteins was measured using a reaction mixture containing 30 mM Tris–HCl, pH 7.6 at 37°C, 5 mM, MgCl$_2$, 1 mM
dithiothreitol, 0.1 mM[γ-^{32}P]ATP (specific radioactivity 30,000 dpm/nmole), 30 mM
NaCl, and approximately 50 μg of prostatic chromatin protein. The time of reaction
was 1 minute. Protein kinase activity toward DPV was assayed as described in
the legend for Fig. 1.

and Wilson, 1977; Wilson *et al.*, unpublished data). A clearer demonstration of antiandrogen effects on prostatic chromatin-associated protein kinase toward dephosphophosvitin, as well as endogenous chromatin proteins, was demonstrated by administering antiandrogens simultaneously with a suitable dose of testosterone upon castration of rats (daily treatment for 48 hours). It was established that 10 μg of testosterone propionate administered daily maintained the size of the prostate gland in castrated adult rats, as well as chromatin-associated protein kinase activities. The administration of flutamide or cyproterone acetate at a dose 10 or 100 times that of testosterone gave a dose-dependent reduction in protein kinase reactions involving both endogenous chromatin phosphoproteins and dephosphophosvitin as substrates. The 100-fold dose of antiandrogens administered along with testosterone at 10 μg/100 gm body weight essentially countered the androgen-mediated stimulation of the phosphorylation of endogenous chromatin proteins (Table V). These experiments lend further credence to our view that these enzymes are under the control of events mediated via the 5α-dihydrotestosterone–receptor complex system.

B. Prostatic Nucleus-Associated Phosphatases

Since phosphoprotein metabolism would be regulated not only by protein kinase reactions but also by protein phosphatase reactions, we examined the phosphatase activities associated with the prostatic cell nucleus. Three such activities were detected: (1) nuclear alkaline phosphatase using *p*-nitrophenyl phosphate as substrate, (2) histone phosphatase active toward ^{32}P-labeled lysine-rich histone; and (3) acidic phosphoprotein phosphatase (which designates the activity toward phosvitin used as a model acidic phosphoprotein substrate) active toward [^{32}P]phosvitin. The general properties of these phosphatases are shown in Table VI.

1. *Alkaline Phosphatase*

In these studies nuclei were purified further so that their outer membrane was removed by treatment with 0.5% Triton X-100 (Wilson and Ahmed, 1976a). This treatment removed an acid phosphatase activity from the nucleus. The alkaline phosphatase, bound to the nucleus, had a broad substrate specificity: *p*-nitrophenyl phosphate >phosphothreonine >β-glycerophosphate >phosphoserine. No activity was detected toward glucose 1-phosphate or glucose 6-phosphate. It was denatured by heat or urea treatment and was inhibited by P_i, L-phenylalanine, homoarginine, and EDTA. The EDTA-inhibited enzyme was most effectively regenerated by Zn^{2+} and somewhat less so by Ca^{2+} and Mg^{2+}. The phospha-

TABLE VI

A Comparison of the Properties of Phosphatases Associated with the Nucleus of Rat Ventral Prostate[a]

Property	Acidic phosphoprotein phosphatase[b]	Histone phosphatase[c]	Alkaline phosphatase[d]
Substrate	[^{32}P]phosvitin	^{32}P-labeled lysine-rich histone	p-Nitrophenyl phosphate
pH optimum	6.7	7.1	9.5–10.3
EDTA, 1 mM (% activity)	23	90	2
2-Mercaptoethanol, 3 mM (% activity)	99	140	10
NaCl, 0.2 M (% activity)	52	57	96
Inhibitors (% activity)			
NaF, 10 mM	37	36	96
Ammonium molybdate, 1 mM	81	64	—
ATP, 1 mM	34	18	—
Effect of orchiectomy (% intact controls at 48 hours)	69	81	232

[a] From Wilson and Ahmed (1976a,c, 1978) and Wilson *et al.* (1978). Sonicates of Triton X-100-washed nuclei were used as the source of enzyme.

[b] Acidic phosphoprotein phosphatase activity was assayed by measuring the release of ^{32}P$_i$ from [^{32}P]phosvitin. The reaction medium included 1 mM MgCl$_2$, 32 mM imidazole–HCl (final reaction pH 6.7 at 37°C), and 0.8 mg of [^{32}P]phosvitin in a final volume of 0.25 ml.

[c] The histone phosphatase activity was determined by the release of ^{32}P$_i$ from ^{32}P-labeled lysine-rich histone and was assayed in a final volume of 0.25 ml containing 3 mM 2-mercaptoethanol, 48 mM Tris–HCl (final reaction pH 7.1 at 37°C), and 125–200 μg ^{32}P-labeled lysine-rich histone.

[d] The alkaline phosphatase activity was determined by the p-nitrophenol split from p-nitrophenyl phosphate. The reaction medium included 3 mM p-nitrophenyl phosphate and 50 mM sodium carbonate–bicarbonate buffer (final reaction pH 9.68 at 37°C).

tase was uninfluenced by the ionic concentration in the reaction (tested by adding up to 300 mM NaCl). Sulfhydryl-reducing agents (dithiothreitol, 2-mercaptoethanol) were potent inhibitors of the enzyme, suggesting the importance of disulfide linkages for the activity of this enzyme. The properties of this enzyme that distinguish it from other total cellular alkaline phosphatases in the prostate are: (1) Its nuclear localization distinguishes it from other phosphatases predominantly in basal and luminal plasma membrane (Stafford *et al.*, 1949); (2) strong inhibition by L-phenylalanine; and (3) opposing androgen effect; i.e., its activity increases upon castration concomitant with declining prostatic function (see later). This phosphatase may function as a protein phosphatase or an ATPase, however, these are only speculations at the present time. A more detailed discussion of this topic has been given previously (Ahmed and Wilson, 1978).

2. Histone and Acidic Phosphoprotein Phosphatases

Prostatic nuclear protein phosphatase activities toward phosphohistone and acidic phosphoprotein substrates appear to have distinct characteristics despite certain similarities (Table VI). Their pH optima are not remarkably different, and increased ionic strength appears to reduce both these activities. However, unlike acidic phosphoprotein phosphatases, histone phosphatase does not show a divalent cation requirement. This feature distinguishes nuclear-associated histone phosphatase from some cytosol enzymes which are activated by Mn^{2+} (Maeno and Greengard, 1972; Albin and Newburgh, 1975) and stimulated by increased ionic strength (Meisler and Langan, 1969; Ullman and Perlman, 1975). However, the characteristics of nuclear histone phosphatase (Wilson and Ahmed, 1978; Ahmed and Wilson, 1978) are similar to those described for a nucleolar phosphatase active toward nucleolar sulfuric acid-soluble proteins (Olson and Guetzow, 1976).

A number of features distinguish acidic phosphoprotein phosphatase (Wilson *et al.*, 1978; Ahmed and Wilson, 1979) from the aforementioned histone phosphatase. These include the requirement for divalent cations (primarily Mg^{2+}) for maximal activity and its insensitivity to sulfhydryl-protective agents such as dithiothreitol and 2-mercaptoethanol.

Recent preliminary studies on the purification of these two types of nuclear phosphatases have further indicated the distinct nature of these enzymes. A 0.35 M NaCl extract containing over 60% of the nucleus-associated protein phosphatase activities was subjected to DEAE-Sephadex column chromatography. This separated the histone phosphatase activity in a distinct peak which was only slightly active toward acidic phosphoprotein substrate. However, the phosphatase(s) active toward acidic phosphoprotein substrate eluted from the DEAE-Sephadex column in about two peaks which showed a minimal overlap with that of the histone phosphatase (Wilson *et al.*, unpublished data).

3. Effects of Orchiectomy and Antiandrogens

The effects of orchiectomy and antiandrogen treatment of intact animals on the various aforementioned nucleus-associated phosphatases are shown in Table VII. As shown, there was only a small decrease (20–30%) at 48 hours postorchiectomy toward the basic and acidic phosphoprotein substrates. This decrease was apparent when the data were expressed per unit of DNA but not when expressed per unit of nuclear protein. This suggests that the reduction in phosphatases per unit of DNA reflected the de-

TABLE VII

The Effects of Castration, Testosterone Maintenance of Castrated Animals, and Antiandrogen Treatment of Intact Animals on Phosphatase Activities Associated with the Nucleus of Rat Ventral Prostate[a]

Treatment	Acidic phosphoprotein phosphatase (nmoles ^{32}P/mg DNA/hour)[b]	Histone phosphatase (nmoles ^{32}P/mg DNA/hour)[b]	Alkaline phosphatase (nmoles p-nitrophenol/mg DNA/hour)[b]
Intact	1039 (100)	24.1 (100)	1348 (100)
Castration[c]			
24 hours	—	23.6 (98)	2568 (190)
48 hours	717 (69)	19.6 (81)	3138 (232)
96 hours	724 (70)	15.3 (63)	—
48 hours plus oil[c]	630 (61)	19.7 (82)	2960 (220)
48 hours plus testosterone[c]	1380 (133)	28.6 (119)	1742 (129)
Antiandrogen, 2-day treatment[d]			
Flutamide, 5 mg/day	948 (91)	21.0 (87)	2116 (157)
Cyproterone acetate, 5 mg/day	834 (80)	22.4 (93)	2938 (218)

[a] From Wilson and Ahmed (1976a,c, 1978), Ahmed and Wilson (1977), and Wilson et al. (1978).

[b] Acidic phosphoprotein phosphatase, histone phosphatase, and alkaline phosphatase activities were determined as described in the footnotes to Table VI. Data in parentheses represent percent of intact controls.

[c] Orchiectomized rats were maintained with testosterone propionate (see legend for Fig. 1) or oil alone with injections given upon orchiectomy and then 24 hours later.

[d] Antiandrogens (5 mg/day) were injected subcutaneously in sesame oil at the beginning of treatment and 24 hours later. The animals were sacrificed 24 hours after the last treatment.

cline in the protein/DNA ratio in the nucleus. Treatment of normal rats for 2 days with 5 mg/day of flutamide or cyproterone acetate yielded the same result for these phosphatases.

Alkaline phosphatase activity, on the other hand, showed a marked increase on castration, reaching a maximal level of activity at 48 hours postorchiectomy. Similar results were obtained in response to antiandrogen treatments.

In all the above cases, the effects of orchiectomy were prevented by androgen treatment of the animals.

C. Developmental Changes in Prostatic Chromatin

At the time of sexual maturation (puberty), the accessory sex glands undergo dramatic morphological and biochemical changes. As discussed earlier, these developments, once stabilized at adulthood, are strictly maintained by the constant availability of sex hormones. It seems logical that chromatin controls in the prostate would be modified at the onset of puberty through adulthood. We therefore initiated a study of prostatic chromatin composition and phosphoprotein metabolism in rats at age 21 days through puberty (Norvitch *et al.*, 1978).

The average body weight of rats at 28 days of age is 70 gm and increases to 335 gm by 90 days, i.e., adulthood. The average weight of the prostate also gradually increases from 30 mg at age 28 days to about 300 mg in 90-day-old rats.

The chromatin from 28-day-old rat ventral prostate was used as the starting point to determine changes in the chromatin-associated protein phosphokinase reactions in later periods of life and those due to androgenic stimulation of immature animals. [The circulating androgen levels in rats at this age are low, but just at the point of beginning to rise (Lee *et al.*, 1975; Gupta *et al.*, 1975).] Protein kinase activity toward exogenous lysine-rich histone increased by about 110% from 28 days to 48 days of age and then declined by 55% from 48 to 90 days of age (adult animals) (Fig. 4). Protein kinase activity toward dephosphophosvitin changed in a similar manner, but the increase at 48 days was smaller (about 45%). In contrast, no change in the *in vitro* phosphorylation of endogenous chromatin proteins was observed between 28 and 48 days of age, although it increased by 47% in adult animals (Norvitch *et al.*, 1978). This finding of the presence of high protein kinase activities toward the exogenous phosphoprotein substrates compared with that toward endogenous chromatin proteins at 48 days of age suggests that, at this age period, chromatin is deficient in the levels of endogenous chromosomal acceptor phosphoproteins despite the presence of protein kinase activities in it. These experiments

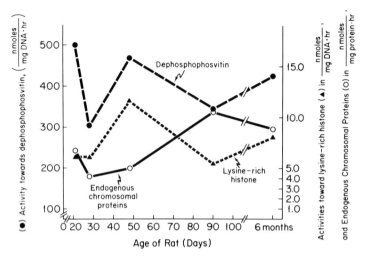

Fig. 4 The effect of age during sexual maturation into adulthood on prostatic chromatin-associated protein phosphokinase activities and phosphorylation of endogenous chromatin proteins. Protein phosphokinase activities toward DPV (●) and lysine-rich histone (▲) were measured as described in the legend for Fig. 1. The phosphorylation of endogenous chromatin proteins (○) was determined as described in footnote *b* of Table V. (From Norvitch *et al.,* 1978; Norvitch, Wilson, and Ahmed, unpublished data.)

suggest that, in response to androgen, prostatic chromatin-associated protein kinases increase prior to the maximal appearance of phosphoprotein substrates endogenous to the chromatin.

D. Summary

In the foregoing we have shown that nucleus-associated protein kinase reactions of rat ventral prostate show multiplicity by virtue of discrete localization as well as distinct varying androgen sensitivity. In particular, nucleolus- and chromatin-associated protein kinase reactions involving acidic protein substrates (rather than histones) are greatly influenced by the androgenic status of the animals. The temporal relationship of the androgen dependence of chromatin-associated (and nucleolar) protein kinase reactions in relation to other androgen-dependent activities in the prostate is shown in Fig. 5. It is clear that the decline in protein kinase is as marked as that in RNA polymerase activity following androgen withdrawal; the fall in these activities in turn appears to be a consequence of the very rapid diminution in the nuclear receptor levels. On the other hand, the changes in nucleus-associated protein phosphatase activities appear to go hand in hand with the changes in wet weight of the tissue.

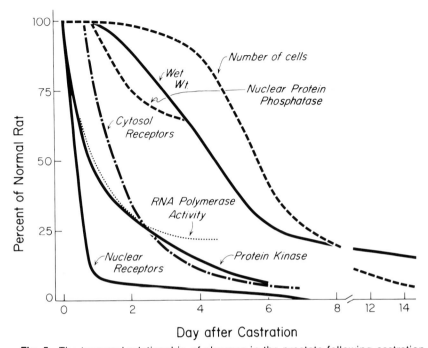

Fig. 5 The temporal relationship of changes in the prostate following castration. (Data adapted from Liao and Fang, 1969; Lesser and Bruchovsky, 1974; Ahmed and Wilson, 1975; vanDoorn *et al.*, 1976; Wilson and Ahmed, 1978; Wilson *et al.*, 1978.)

Studies from the authors' laboratory discussed above lend strong support to the view that nuclear NHP phosphorylation reactions are primarily modulated by endogenous nuclear kinases rather than by the translocation of cytosol cyclic AMP (cAMP)-dependent kinase. Similar conclusions were arrived at by others working with different tissues (Kamiyama *et al.*, 1972; Keller *et al.*, 1975, 1976). The prostatic cytosol cAMP-dependent protein kinase is relatively insensitive to androgen administration or withdrawal (Reddi *et al.*, 1971; Fuller *et al.*, 1978). Also, it seems unlikely that cAMP-mediated events are involved in the initial response of prostatic cells to androgenic stimulation; a detailed discussion of this subject has been given elsewhere (Ahmed, 1975; Mainwaring, 1977; Ahmed and Wilson, 1978).

The variety of evidence presented in the foregoing strongly suggests that control of prostatic chromatin-associated and nucleolar protein kinases is mediated via the androgen–receptor complex systems. Hence regulation of nuclear phosphoprotein phopshorylation may be germane to androgen action on the prostate. The enhanced capacity of androgen–receptor complex binding by prostatic chromatin due to phosphorylation of the latter is analogous to these considerations. A number of reviews have discussed the possible role of nonhistone phosphoproteins in the control of gene action (references cited earlier). Therefore a study of the possible mechanisms underlying the enhancement of nuclear phosphoprotein phosphorylation reactions in experimental models of cell growth is of fundamental importance. We have enumerated some of the possibilities that may be considered in attempts to decipher the androgen control of prostatic nuclear protein kinase reactions (Fig. 6). This outline scheme, which by no means covers all the possibilities, suggests some of the ways that may result in augmentation of nuclear protein kinase activities. Nuclear phosphoproteins and/or protein kinases may activate RNA polymerase reactions by several modes. Among the suggested possibilities are that specific phosphoproteins may combine with the polymerase in order to activate it. Alternately, phosphoproteins may bind at specific sites on

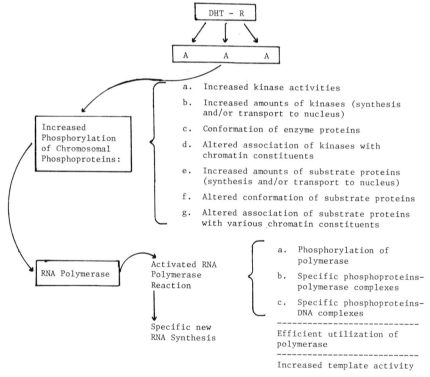

Fig. 6 A schematic representation of androgen-mediated chromatin controls in the prostate. The factors listed in the brackets on the right are presented to give possible explanations for the events listed on the left.

DNA, producing a conformational change in DNA (by the removal of histones or by a direct effect), resulting in a more efficient utilization of RNA polymerase (Allfrey, 1974; Kleinsmith, 1974; Ahmed and Wilson, 1978). An equally plausible possibility is that some chromatin or nucleolar protein kinases may be involved in phosphorylating RNA polymerase itself, which may be a mechanism to control its activity. A number of studies have recently suggested the possibility of such a control (Martelo and Hirsch, 1974; Dahmus, 1976; Jungmann and Kranias, 1977).

VI. Polyamines and Nuclear Protein Kinase Reactions

A. Introduction

Various nucleus-associated protein kinase reactions described so far have shown the requirement for a certain level of monovalent salts (e.g., NaCl, KCl) in the reaction for maximal rates. This hints at the possibility that an optimal concentration of monovalent salt in the reaction may influence the phosphorylation reaction by promoting a suitable conformation of substrate and/or enzyme for proper interaction. However, a simple ionic strength effect due to salts does not necessarily account for the observed effects on phosphorylation reactions. For example, Imai *et al.* (1975) observed that polyamines stimulated the phosphorylation of endogenous chromatin protein of hog liver. Analogous to these considerations was the report that histone and polylysine stimulated the phosphorylation of chromatin-associated NHPs, a result most likely due to effects of these molecules on the conformation of the acidic protein substrate (Kaplowitz *et al.*, 1971).

In view of the androgen dependence of prostatic nuclear protein kinase reactions, and considering that adult rat ventral prostate and its secretions contain relatively high levels of spermine and spermidine and that polyamine synthesis in this organ is strictly controlled by androgenic hormones (Williams-Ashman *et al.*, 1969; Pegg *et al.*, 1970), we decided to undertake a systematic investigation of effects of polyamines on various prostatic nucleus-associated protein kinase reactions (Ahmed *et al.*, 1976, 1978). It may be recalled that aliphatic polyamines (spermine, spermidine, and putrescine) are present in substantial concentrations in all nucleated cells. Their concentrations and those of their biosynthetic enzymes are markedly elevated in concert with induced growth of many tissues; these changes usually precede or are concomitant with increases in RNA, DNA, and protein contents in the cell (for reviews, see Williams-Ashman *et al.*, 1969, 1976; Stevens, 1970; Cohen, 1971; Bachrach, 1973; Raina and Jänne, 1975; Tabor and Tabor, 1976).

B. Protein Kinase Reactions Involving Exogenous Phosphoprotein Substrates

Chromatin- and NHP-associated protein kinase reactions toward de-phosphophosvitin as substrate, assayed under optimal ionic conditions (Ahmed *et al.*, 1978), were not influenced by the addition of 1–2 mM spermine or spermidine to the reaction (Table VIII). However, in the presence of suboptimal NaCl in the reaction (i.e., about 10 mM NaCl or less) very significant stimulations of these reactions were noted. Since polyamines are cationic compounds, corresponding controls containing equivalent amounts of NaCl to compensate for the increase in ionic strength owing to the presence of spermine or spermidine were included in the reaction (Hirschman *et al.*, 1967). Thus, at 4.5 and 8 mM NaCl (compared with no added NaCl), the increase in chromatin-associated protein kinase activity toward dephosphophosvitin was only 8 and 15%, respectively. The stimulation by 2 mM spermine of this reaction was 133% compared to only 31% by 16 mM NaCl, which provided an increment in total ionic strength equivalent to that given by 2 mM spermine. The effects of polyamines on NHP-associated protein kinase activity toward dephosphophosvitin are also recorded in Table VIII and were the same as those observed with chromatin as the source of enzyme activity. Casein as a substrate gave about 40% of activity compared with dephosphophosvitin, however, the effects of spermine were similar in both these cases (Goueli *et al.*, unpublished data). It is noteworthy that the rates of chromatin and NHP-associated protein kinase reactions produced by 1–2 mM spermine were essentially similar to those obtained under optimal experimental conditions.

In other experiments, polyamine stimulation of these kinase reactions was demonstrated to require an optimal Mg^{2+} concentration in the reaction, and that polyamines did not substitute for Mg^{2+} (Ahmed *et al.*, 1978). Further, the ionic charge of the amino compound alone did not seem to be responsible for the effects observed with spermine or spermidine, since the even more highly ionized polyamine analogue methylglyoxal bis(guanylhydrazone) [also a specific inhibitor of putrescine-activated S-adenosylmethionine decarboxylase (Williams-Ashman and Schenone, 1972)] did not stimulate the protein kinase reaction (Ahmed *et al.*, 1978).

Table VIII also shows that chromatin and NHP-associated protein kinase reactions toward lysine-rich histone were uninfluenced by spermine or spermidine under the various experimental conditions. This hinted at the possibility that polyamine effects on nuclear protein kinase reactions toward dephosphophosvitin were stimulated by an influence of the polyamine on the conformation of the acidic protein substrate rather than on the enzyme per se. To test this hypothesis, we investigated the effect of

N,N-dimethylation of dephosphophosvitin substrate with respect to spermine stimulation of chromatin-associated protein kinase reactions. N,N-Dimethylation of protein substrates alters their activity (as a result of altered conformation) toward proteolytic enzymes (Lin *et al.*, 1969). The results presented in Table IX show that, although N,N-dimethylation of dephosphophosvitin markedly reduced its activity as a substrate (which was not due to a change in the apparent K_m) but also altered the relative stimulation by spermine. These observations are in agreement with the above hypothesis concerning polyamine effects on protein substrate in the nuclear protein kinase reaction toward acidic protein substrate.

C. Protein Kinase Reactions Involving Endogenous Chromatin Phosphoprotein Substrates

The result in Fig. 7 shows that the phosphorylation of endogenous chromatin-associated proteins requires a relatively small ionic concentration (NaCl) in the medium for maximal rates of ^{32}P incorporation from [γ-

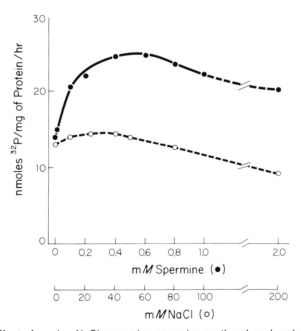

Fig. 7 Effect of varying NaCl or varying spermine on the phosphorylation of chromatin phosphoproteins. The phosphorylation of endogenous chromatin proteins was performed as described in the footnotes to Table V, except the concentrations of NaCl and spermine were as indicated. (From Ahmed *et al.*, 1978; Ahmed, Goueli, and Wilson, unpublished data.)

TABLE VIII

Effects of Spermine, Spermidine, and NaCl on Prostatic Chromatin- and NHP-Associated Protein Kinase Reactions toward Dephosphophosvitin and Lysine-Rich Histone as Substrates[a]

| NaCl[e] (mM) | Polyamine (mM) | | Protein kinase activity associated with:[b] | | | |
| | Spermine | Spermidine | Chromatin (nmoles ^{32}P/hour/mg DNA)[c] | | NHPs (nmoles ^{32}P/hour/mg protein)[d] | |
			DPV substrate	LRH substrate	DPV substrate	LRH substrate
—	—	—	130	5.0	—	—
4.5	—	—	140	—	—	—
8.0	—	—	150	6.2	407	7.6
16.0	—	—	170	—	476	8.3
80	—	—	—	6.9	—	—
160	—	—	321	—	827	—
200	—	—	215	—	—	—
—	1.0	—	303	6.0	810	7.8
—	2.0	—	193	6.0	855	8.1
—	—	1.0	211	—	642	—
—	—	2.0		—	763	—

160	1.0	—	—	—	873	—
160	—	1.0	—	—	887	—
200	1.0	—	324	—	—	—
200	—	1.0	300	—	—	—

[a] From Ahmed et al. (1976, 1978).

[b] The reactions were initiated by the addition of chromatin (equivalent to 10 µg of DNA) or NHPs (5 µg of protein) and continued for 10 minutes.

[c] Chromatin-associated protein kinase activity was assayed as described in the legend for Fig. 1, except for the variation in NaCl concentrations and the inclusion of polyamines as indicated in the table.

[d] The assay of NHP-associated protein kinase activity toward DPV was carried out in medium containing 4 mM $MgCl_2$, 1 mM dithiothreitol, 3 mM $[\gamma\text{-}^{32}P]ATP$ (specific radioactivity of 3000 dpm/nmole), 30 mM Tris–HCl, pH 7.45 at 37°C, albumin (100 µg/ml), and saturating amounts of DPV. NaCl and polyamines were included in the reaction mixture as indicated. The NHP-associated protein kinase activity toward lysine-rich histone was determined in reaction medium consisting of lysine-rich histone (3 mg/ml), 4 mM $MgCl_2$, 0.1 mM $[\gamma\text{-}^{32}P]ATP$ (specific radioactivity 60,000 dpm/nmole), 1 mM dithiothreitol, 30 mM Tris–HCl, pH 7.45 at 37°C, and albumin (100 µg/ml). NaCl and polyamines were added to the reaction media as indicated. In these kinase assays some 8 mM NaCl was contributed to the reactions because of its presence in the NHP preparations.

[e] Assays containing 4.5–16 mM NaCl provided control ionic-strength values corresponding to various concentrations of polyamines; 160 mM, 200 mM, and 80 mM NaCl are optimal salt requirements for NHP-associated kinase activity toward DPV, chromatin-associated kinase activity toward DPV, and chromatin-and NHP-associated kinase activity toward lysine-rich histones, respectively.

TABLE IX

Effect of Methylation of Dephosphophosvitin Substrate with Respect to Spermine Stimulation of Chromatin-Associated Protein Kinase[a]

Addition	Protein kinase (nmoles ^{32}P/hour/mg DNA)[b]		Inhibition of protein kinase owing to methylation (%)
	DPV substrate	Methylated[c] DPV substrate	
None	110	21	81
8.0 mM NaCl	139 (26)	28 (33)	80
1.0 mM spermine	181 (65)	57 (170)	68
200 mM NaCl	231 (110)	46 (119)	80

[a] From Ahmed *et al.* (1978).

[b] Protein phosphokinase assays were performed as described in the legend for Fig. 1, except for the concentrations of NaCl and spermine which were as indicated. Percentages are shown in parentheses.

[c] Methylated dephosphophosvitin was prepared by chemical *N,N*-dimethylation by adapting the procedure of Lin *et al.* (1969) as described in Ahmed *et al.* (1978).

^{32}P]ATP. Thus the increase in the reaction rate due to 24–30 mM NaCl, which appears to be optimal, is only about 10%; at higher NaCl concentrations an inhibition of ^{32}P incorporation is observed. Also shown in Fig. 7 is the effect of varying concentrations of spermine on the phosphorylation of chromatin-associated phosphoproteins. It is clear that near-maximal rates of reaction are achieved by spermine at a concentration of about 5×10^{-4} M. Compared with the effect of varying NaCl, the reaction rates were remarkably stimulated in the presence of various concentrations of spermine. The effect of 1 mM spermine on the incorporation of ^{32}P into chromatin proteins over a time course when compared with 0, 8, or 30 mM NaCl-containing reaction media clearly showed not only that spermine enhanced by at least 60%, the initial rate of this phosphorylation reaction but also that the stimulation was apparent even when the trans-phosphorylation had plateaued in the controls (e.g., at 30 minutes), so that in the presence of 1 mM spermine it was 48% greater than that with various NaCl-containing controls (Ahmed *et al.*, 1978).

The effect of spermine on endogenous chromosomal protein phosphorylation is apparent even in the presence of optimal or even higher concentrations of NaCl (which are by themselves inhibitory, as shown in Fig. 7). This result, shown in Table X, stands in contrast with the aforementioned studies with dephosphophosvitin as substrate, in which the stimulation by polyamines was elicited only at suboptimal salt concentrations. Finally, it is shown in Fig. 8 that 1 mM spermine (compared with no NaCl)

TABLE X

Effect of Spermine in the Presence of Varying Amounts of NaCl on the Incorporation of ^{32}P from $[\gamma\text{-}^{32}P]$ATP into Endogenous Phosphoproteins of Rat Ventral Prostate Chromatin[a]

NaCl (mM)	Spermine (1 mM)	^{32}P Incorporated into chromatin phosphoproteins (nmoles/mg protein/hour)[b]	Percent change
—	—	8.76	—
—	+	13.26	+51
30	—	8.64	—
30	+	12.36	+43
50	—	8.40	—
50	+	11.64	+39
100	—	7.38	—
100	+	9.36	+27

[a] Adapted from Ahmed et al. (1978).

[b] The rate of phosphorylation of endogenous chromatin proteins was determined as described in the footnotes to Table V, except that NaCl and spermine were present as indicated.

did not cause a generalized enhancement of the phosphorylation of non-histone chromatin-associated proteins as judged by the electrophoretic pattern of these proteins. Rather, it is clear that the phosphorylation of the different proteins is stimulated to different extents. Again, this would be expected if these stimulatory effects of spermine were mediated via alterations in the conformation of the various substrates.

D. Summary

The aforementioned stimulatory effects of polyamines are not restricted only to prostatic nuclear protein kinase reactions, since similar observations were made with chromatin preparations from other tissues such as liver (Imai et al., 1975; Ahmed et al., 1978), salivary gland (Ahmed et al., unpublished data), and human benign hypertrophic prostate (Ahmed et al., unpublished data). Similar results are also obtained when chromatin from 96-hour castrated rats is examined with respect to spermine effects; however, the results do not indicate that androgen effects on prostatic protein kinases are mediated via polyamines (see Ahmed et al., 1978, for discussion of this point). Murray et al. (1976) and Mäenpää (1977) have reported stimulation of cAMP-independent cytosol

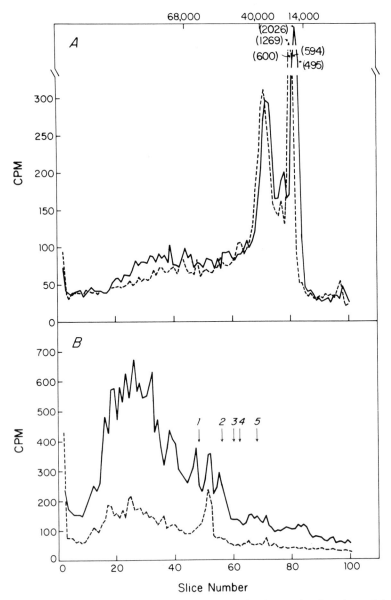

Fig. 8 The electrophoretic separation of prostatic chromatin phosphoproteins on polyacrylamide gels. (A) SDS–urea gel-electrophoresed nonhistone phosphoproteins which had been phosphorylated in the presence (—) or absence (-----) of 1 m*M* spermine. (B) Acid–urea gel-electrophoresed sulfuric acid-soluble phosphoproteins which had been phosphorylated in the presence (—) or absence (-----) of 1 m*M* spermine. The phosphorylation of chromosomal proteins was carried out as described in Table V

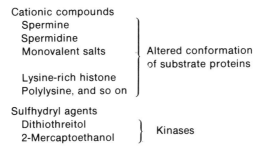

Cationic compounds
  Spermine
  Spermidine
  Monovalent salts   Altered conformation
                       of substrate proteins
  Lysine-rich histone
  Polylysine, and so on

Sulfhydryl agents
  Dithiothreitol
  2-Mercaptoethanol   Kinases

Fig. 9 Factors that may be involved in controlling nuclear NHP phosphorylation reactions. Possible sites of action are indicated on the right-hand side.

kinases by polyamines with casein and phosvitin as substrates. However, the soluble cAMP-dependent kinase that phosphorylates histones and other basic proteins was uninfluenced by spermine and spermidine. Thus, based on these observations and the foregoing results presented by us, it seems that polyamine stimulation pertains primarily to protein kinase reactions involving acidic (or nonbasic) protein substrates.

From the foregoing, it is possible to summarize some of the factors that may be required for the optimal phosphorylation of nuclear phosphoproteins mediated by nuclear-associated protein kinases (Fig. 9). The presence of sulfhydryl-protective agents (Ahmed, 1975; Ahmed and Davis, 1975; Ahmed and Wilson, 1978) has been shown to stimulate the various protein kinase reactions, presumably by an effect on the enzyme activity. Kaplowitz *et al.* (1971) showed that histone and polylysine may influence the levels of phosphorylation of NHPs. Similar observations have been made by us with prostate NHPs (Ahmed *et al.*, unpublished data). Our demonstration of the markedly increased extent of phosphorylation of chromosomal NHPs due to low concentrations of spermine, even in the presence of relatively high salt concentrations, suggests that these compounds may act as effective biological cations (even more so than mono-

---

without NaCl in the reaction medium and a reaction time of 20 minutes. The ATP concentration in the reaction was 25.8 μM with a specific radioactivity of 2×10^6 dpm/nmole. A duplicate incubation was carried out as described above but included 1 mM spermine. The reaction was stopped by adding 1 N H$_2$SO$_4$ to a final concentration of 0.2 N, and the sulfuric acid-soluble proteins were extracted (Bonner *et al.*, 1968) and electrophoresed on acid–urea polyacrylamide gels (10% acrylamide) (Panyim and Chalkley, 1969). The remaining proteins were extracted from the sulfuric acid-insoluble material with 0.4 M guanidine–HCl and 6.0 M urea by the method of Levy *et al.* (1972) and electrophoresed on 7.5% polyacrylamide gels containing 0.1% SDS and 4 M urea (MacGillivray *et al.*, 1972). (From Ahmed *et al.*, 1978; Ahmed, Davis, Goueli, and Wilson, 1979b.)

valent salts) in these protein kinase reactions, and that this effect is mediated via an influence on the conformation of the protein substrate. These conclusions are, however, speculative at the present time.

Acknowledgments

The original investigations were supported in part by research grant CA-15062 from the National Cancer Institute, Department of Health, Education, and Welfare, and by the U. S. Veterans Administration Medical Research Fund.

References

Ahmed, K. (1970). *Pharmacologist* **12**, 229.
Ahmed, K. (1971). *Biochim. Biophys. Acta* **243**, 38–40.
Ahmed, K. (1974). *Res. Commun. Chem. Pathol. Pharmacol.* **9**, 771–774.
Ahmed, K. (1975). *In* "Molecular Mechanisms of Gonadal Hormone Action" (J. A. Thomas and R. L. Singhal, eds.), Advances in Sex Hormone Research, Vol. 1, pp. 129–165. Univ. Park Press, Baltimore, Maryland.
Ahmed, K., and Davis, A. T. (1975). *In* "Normal and Abnormal Growth of the Prostate" (M. Goland, ed.), pp. 317–327. Thomas, Springfield, Illinois.
Ahmed, K., and Ishida, H. (1971). *Mol. Pharmacol.* **7**, 323–327.
Ahmed, K., and Wilson, M. J. (1975). *J. Biol. Chem.* **250**, 2370–2375.
Ahmed, K., and Wilson, M. J. (1977). *Endocrinology* **100**, 81A.
Ahmed, K., and Wilson, M. J. (1978). *In* "The Cell Nucleus" (H. Busch, ed.), Vol 6, Part C. pp. 409–459. Academic Press, New York.
Ahmed, K., Wilson, M. J., and Davis, A. T. (1975). *Biochim. Biophys. Acta* **377**, 80–83.
Ahmed, K., Wilson, M. J., and Williams-Ashman, H. G. (1976). *Pharmacologist* **18**, 744.
Ahmed, K., Wilson, M. J., Goueli, S. A., and Williams-Ashman, H. G. (1978). *Biochem. J.* **176**, 739–750.
Ahmed, K., Wilson, M. J., Goueli, S. A., and Steer, R. C. (1979a). *In* "Accessory Glands of the Male Reproductive Tract" (E. S. E. Hafez and E. Spring-Mills, eds.), Perspectives of Human Reproduction, Vol. 6. pp. 69–108 Ann Arbor Sci. Publ., Ann Arbor, Michigan.
Ahmed, K., Davis, A. T., Goueli, S. A., and Wilson, M. J. (1979b). *Proc. Int. Congr. Biochem., 11th, Toronto,* pp. 53.
Albin, E. E., and Newburgh, R. W. (1975). *Biochim. Biophys. Acta* **337**, 381–388.
Allfrey, V. G. (1974). *In* "Acidic Proteins of the Nucleus" (I. L. Cameron and J. R. Jeter, Jr., eds.), pp. 1–27. Academic Press, New York.
Anderson, K. M., and Liao, S. (1968). *Nature (London)* **219**, 277–279.
Anderson, K. M., Slavik, M., Evans, A. K., and Couch, R. M. (1973). *Exp. Cell Res.* **77**, 143–158.
Bachrach, U. (1973). "Function of Naturally Occurring Polyamines." Academic Press, New York.
Baserga, R. C. (1974). *Life Sci.* **15**, 1057–1071.
Blat, C., DeMorales, M. M., and Harel, L. (1976). *Exp. Cell Res.* **98**, 104–110.
Bonner, J., Chalkley, G. R., Dahmus, M., Fambrough, D., Fujimura, F., Huang, R.-C. C., Huberman, J., Jensen, R., Marushige, K., Ohlenbusch, H., Olivera, B., and Widholm,

J. (1968). *In* "Nucleic Acids" (L. Grossman and K. Moldave, eds.), Methods in Enzymology, Vol. 12, pp. 3–65. Academic Press, New York.

Bruchovsky, N., and Wilson, J. D. (1968a). *J. Biol. Chem.* **243,** 2012–2021.

Bruchovsky, N., and Wilson, J. D. (1968b). *J. Biol. Chem.* **243,** 5953–5960.

Busch, H., and Smetana, K. (1970). "The Nucleolus." Academic Press, New York.

Busch, H., Steele, W. J., Hnilica, L. S., Taylor, C. W., and Movioglu, H. (1963). *J. Cell. Comp. Physiol.* **62,** 95–110.

Chan, L., and O'Malley, B. W. (1976). *New Engl. J. Med.* **294,** 1322–1328, 1372–1381, 1430–1437.

Chung, L. W. K., and Coffey, D. S. (1971a). *Biochim. Biophys. Acta* **247,** 570–583.

Chung, L. W. K., and Coffey, D. S. (1971b). *Biochim. Biophys. Acta* **247,** 584–596.

Coffey, D. S., Shimazaki, J., and Williams-Ashman, H. G. (1968). *Mol. Pharmacol.* **124,** 184–198.

Cohen, S. S. (1971). "Introduction to the Polyamines." Prentice-Hall, Englewood Cliffs, New Jersey.

Dahmus, M. E. (1976). *Biochemistry* **15,** 1821–1829.

Davies, P., and Griffiths, K. (1973a). *Biochem. Biophys. Res. Commun.* **53,** 373–382.

Davies, P., and Griffiths, K. (1973b). *Biochem. J.* **136,** 611–622.

Fang, S., and Liao, S. (1969). *Mol. Pharmacol.* **5,** 428–431.

Fang, S., Anderson, K. M., and Liao, S. (1969). *J. Biol. Chem.* **244,** 6584–6595.

Farnsworth, W. E., and Brown, J. R. (1963). *Natl. Cancer Inst., Monogr.* **12,** 323–325.

Fujii, T., and Villee, C. A. (1969). *Proc. Natl. Acad. Sci. U.S.A.* **62,** 836–843.

Fuller, D. J. M., Byus, C. V., and Russell, D. H. (1978). *Proc. Natl. Acad. Sci. U.S.A.* **75,** 223–227.

Grigorescu, A., and Villee, C. A. (1973). *Biochim. Biophys. Acta* **319,** 165–173.

Gupta, D., Rager, K., Zarzycki, J., and Eichner, M. (1975). *J. Endocrinol.* **66,** 183–193.

Hancock, R. L., Zelis, R. F., Shaw, M., and Williams-Ashman, H. G. (1962). *Biochim. Biophys. Acta* **55,** 257–260.

Harris, S. E., Rosen, J. M., Means, A. R., and O'Malley, B. W. (1975). *Biochemistry* **14,** 2072–2081.

Hirschman, S. Z., Leng, M., and Felsenfeld, G. (1967). *Biopolymers* **5,** 227–233.

Huggins, C. (1945). *Physiol. Rev.* **25,** 281–295.

Imai, H., Shimoyama, M., Yamamoto, S., Tanigawa, Y., and Ueda, I. (1975). *Biochem. Biophys. Res. Commun.* **66,** 856–862.

Ishida, H., and Ahmed, K. (1973). *Exp. Cell Res.* **78,** 31–40.

Ishida, H., and Ahmed, K. (1974). *Exp. Cell Res.* **84,** 127–136.

Jensen, E. V., and Jacobson, H. I. (1962). *Recent Prog. Horm. Res.* **18,** 387–414.

Jungmann, R. A., and Kranias, E. G. (1977). *Int. J. Biochem.* **8,** 819–830.

Kadohama, N., and Anderson, K. M. (1976). *Exp. Cell Res.* **99,** 135–145.

Kadohama, N., and Anderson, K. M. (1977). *Can. J. Biochem.* **55,** 513–520.

Kamiyama, M., Dastugue, B., Defer, N., and Kruh, J. (1972). *Biochim. Biophys. Acta* **277,** 576–583.

Kaplowitz, P. B., Platz, R. D., and Kleinsmith, L. J. (1971). *Biochim. Biophys. Acta* **229,** 739–748.

Keller, R. K., Socher, S. H., Krall, J. F., Chandra, T., and O'Malley, B. W. (1975). *Biochem. Biophys. Res. Commun.* **66,** 453–459.

Keller, R. K., Chandra, T., Schrader, W. T., and O'Malley, B. W. (1976). *Biochemistry* **15,** 1958–1967.

King, R. J. B., and Gordon, J. (1972). *Nature (London)* **240,** 185–187.

King, R. J. B., and Mainwaring, W. I. P. (1974). "Steroid-Cell Interaction." Univ. Park Press, Baltimore, Maryland.

Kish, V. M., and Kleinsmith, L. J. (1974). *J. Biol. Chem.* **249**, 750–760.

Kleinsmith, L. J. (1974). *In* "Acidic Proteins of the Nucleus" (I. L. Cameron and J. R. Jeter, Jr., eds.), pp. 103–135. Academic Press, New York.

Kleinsmith, L. J., Allfrey, V. G., and Mirsky, A. E. (1966). *Science* **154**, 780–781.

Klyzsejko-Stefanowicz, L., Chiu, J. F., Tsai, Y. H., and Hnilica, L. S. (1976). *Proc. Natl. Acad. Sci. U.S.A.* **73**, 1954–1958.

Kochakian, C. D. (1965). *In* "Mechanisms of Hormone Action" (P. Karlson, ed.), pp. 192–242. Thieme, Stuttgart.

Kosto, B., Calvin, H. I., and Williams-Ashman, H. G. (1967). *Adv. Enzyme Regul.* **5**, 25–37.

Langan, T. A. (1967). *In* "Regulation of Nucleic Acid and Protein Biosynthesis" (V. V. Konigsberger and L. Bosch, eds.), pp. 233–242. Elsevier, Amsterdam.

Lebeau, M. C., Masson, N., and Baulieu, E. E. (1973). *Eur. J. Biochem.* **36**, 294–300.

Lee, V. W. K., DeKretser, D. M., Hudson, B., and Wang, C. (1975). *J. Reprod. Fertil.* **42**, 121–126.

Lesser, B., and Bruchovsky, N. (1974). *Biochem. J.* **142**, 429–434.

Levy, S., Simpson, R. T., and Sober, H. A. (1972). *Biochemistry* **11**, 1547–1554.

Liang, T., Castaneda, E., and Liao, S. (1977). *J. Biol. Chem.* **252**, 5692–5700.

Liao, S., and Fang, S. (1969). *Vitam. Horm. (N.Y.)* **27**, 17–90.

Liao, S., and Williams-Ashman, H. G. (1962). *Proc. Natl. Acad. Sci. U.S.A.* **48**, 1956–1964.

Liao, S., Leininger, K. R., Sagher, D., and Barton, R. W. (1965). *Endocrinology* **77**, 763–765.

Liao, S., Howell, D. K., and Chang, T.-M. (1974). *Endocrinology* **94**, 1205–1209.

Liao, S., Tymoczko, J. L., Castaneda, E., and Liang, T. (1975). *Vitam. Hormon. (N.Y.)* **33**, 297–317.

Lin, Y., Means, G. E., and Feeney, R. E. (1969). *J. Biol. Chem.* **244**, 789–793.

MacGillivray, A. J., Paul, J., and Threfall, G. (1972). *Adv. Cancer Res.* **15**, 93–162.

McKnight, G. S., Pennequin, P., and Schimke, R. T. (1975). *J. Biol. Chem.* **250**, 8105–8110.

Mäenpää, P. H. (1977). *Biochim. Biophys. Acta* **498**, 294–305.

Maeno, H., and Greengard, P. (1972). *J. Biol. Chem.* **247**, 3269–3277.

Mainwaring, W. I. P. (1975). *Vitam. Horm. (N.Y.)* **33**, 223–244.

Mainwaring, W. I. P. (1977). "The Mechanism of Action of Androgens." Springer-Verlag, Berlin and New York.

Mainwaring, W. I. P., and Peterken, B. M. (1971). *Biochem. J.* **125**, 285–295.

Mainwaring, W. I. P., Mangan, F. R., and Peterken, B. M. (1971). *Biochem. J.* **123**, 619–628.

Mainwaring, W. I. P., Mangan, F. R., Irving, R. A., and Jones, D. A. (1974a). *Biochem. J.* **144**, 413–426.

Mainwaring, W. I. P., Wilce, P. A., and Smith, A. E. (1974b). *Biochem J.* **137**, 513–524.

Mann, T. J. (1964). "The Biochemistry of Semen and the Male Reproductive Tract." Methuen, London.

Martelo, O. J., and Hirsch, J. (1974). *Biochem. Biophys. Res. Commun.* **58**, 1008–1015.

Marushige, K., and Bonner, J. (1971). *Proc. Natl. Acad. Sci. U.S.A.* **62**, 2941–2944.

Meisler, M. H., and Langan, T. H. (1969). *J. Biol. Chem.* **244**, 4961–4968.

Murray, A. W., Froscio, M., and Rogers, A. (1976). *Biochem. Biophys. Res. Commun.* **71**, 1175–1181.

Neri, R., and Monahan, M. (1972). *Invest. Urol.* **10**, 123–130.

Neumann, F. (1977). *Horm. Metab. Res.* **9**, 1–13.

Norvitch, M. E., Wilson, M. J., and Ahmed, K. (1978). *Proc. Int. Conf. Differ. 3rd, Minneapolis* pp. 31.

Nyberg, L. M., and Wang, T. Y. (1976). *J. Steroid Biochem.* **7**, 267–273.

Olson, M. O. J., and Guetzow, K. (1976). *Biochem. Biophys. Res. Commun.* **70**, 717–722.

Olson, M. O. J., Ezrailson, E. G., Guetzow, K., and Busch, H. (1975). *J. Mol. Biol.* **97**, 611–619.

Olson, M. O. J., Hatchett, S., Allan, R., Hawkins, T. C., and Busch, H. (1978). *Cancer Res.* **38**, 3421–3426.

O'Malley, B. W., and Means, A. R. (1974). *Science* **183**, 610–620.

Panyim, S., and Chalkley, R. (1969). *Arch. Biochem. Biophys.* **130**, 337–346.

Peets, E. A., Henson, M. F., and Neri, R. (1974). *Endocrinology* **94**, 532–540.

Pegg, A. E., Lockwood, D. H., and Williams-Ashman, H. G. (1970). *Biochem. J.* **117**, 17–31.

Price, D., and Williams-Ashman, H. G. (1961). *In* "Sex and Internal Secretions" (W. C. Young, ed.), pp. 366–488. Williams & Wilkins, Baltimore, Maryland.

Raina, A., and Jänne, J. (1975). *Med. Biol.* **53**, 121–147.

Reddi, A. H., Ewing, L. L., and Williams-Ashman, H. G. (1971). *Biochem. J.* **122**, 333–345.

Ritter, C. (1966). *Mol. Pharmacol.* **2**, 125–133.

Ruddon, R. W., and Anderson, S. L. (1972). *Biochem. Biophys. Res. Commun.* **46**, 1499–1508.

Schauder, P., Starman, B. J., and Williams, R. H. (1974). *Proc. Soc. Exp. Biol. Med.* **145**, 331–333.

Shimazaki, J., Kurihara, H., Ito, Y., and Shida, K. (1965). *Gunma J. Med. Sci.* **14**, 313–325.

Spelsberg, T. C. (1974). *In* "Acidic Proteins of the Nucleus" (I. L. Cameron and J. R. Jeter, Jr., eds.), pp. 248–296. Academic Press, New York.

Stafford, R. O., Rubinstein, I. N., and Meyer, R. K. (1949). *Proc. Soc. Exp. Biol. Med.* **71**, 353–357.

Stein, G., Spelsberg, T. C., and Kleinsmith, L. J. (1974). *Science* **183**, 817–824.

Stellwagen, R. H., and Cole, R. D. (1969). *Annu. Rev. Biochem.* **38**, 951–990.

Stevens, L. (1970). *Biol. Rev. Cambridge Philos. Soc.* **45**, 1–27.

Sufrin, G., and Coffey, D. S. (1976). *Invest. Urol.* **13**, 429–434.

Tabor, C. W., and Tabor, H. (1976). *Annu. Rev. Biochem.* **45**, 285–306.

Takeda, M., Yamamura, H., and Oga, Y. (1971). *Biochem Biophys. Res. Commun.* **42**, 103–110.

Teng, C. S., Teng, C. T., and Allfrey, V. G. (1971). *J. Biol. Chem.* **246**, 3597–3609.

Ullman, B., and Perlman, R. L. (1975). *Biochim. Biophys. Acta* **403**, 393–411.

vanDoorn, E., Craven, S., and Bruchovsky, N. (1976) *Biochem. J.* **160**, 11–21.

Williams-Ashman, H. G., and Reddi, A. H. (1971). *Annu. Rev. Physiol.* **33**, 31–82.

Williams-Ashman, H. G., and Schenone, A. (1972). *Biochem. Biophys. Res. Commun.* **46**, 288–295.

Williams-Ashman, H. G., and Shimazaki, J. (1967). *In* "Endogenous Factors Influencing Host–Tumor Balance" (R. W. Wissler, T. L. Dao, and S. Wool, Jr., eds), pp. 31–41. Univ. of Chicago Press, Chicago, Illinois.

Williams-Ashman, H. G., Liao, S., Hancock, R. L., Jurkowitz, L., and Silverman, D. A. (1964). *Recent Prog. Horm. Res.* **20**, 247–292.

Williams-Ashman, H. G., Pegg, A. E., and Lockwood, D. H. (1969). *Adv. Enzyme Regul.* **7**, 291–323.

Williams-Ashman, H. G., Tadolini, B., Wilson, J., and Corti, A. (1975). *Vitam. Horm.* *(N.Y.)* **33**, 39–60.

Williams-Ashman, H. G., Corti, A., and Tadolini, B. (1976). *Ital. J. Biochem.* **25**, 1–32.

Wilson, J. D., and Gloyna, R. E. (1970). *Recent Prog. Horm. Res.* **2**, 309–336.

Wilson, M. J., and Ahmed, K. (1975). *Exp. Cell Res.* **93**, 261–266.

Wilson, M. J., and Ahmed, K. (1976a). *Biochim. Biophys. Acta* **429**, 439–447.

Wilson, M. J., and Ahmed, K. (1976b). *Endocrine Res. Commun.* **3**, 63–69.

Wilson, M. J., and Ahmed, K. (1976c). *Endocrinology* **98**, 75A.

Wilson, M. J., and Ahmed, K. (1977). *Exp. Cell Res.* **106**, 151–157.

Wilson, M. J., and Ahmed, K. (1978). *Exp. Cell Res.* **117**, 71–78.

Wilson, M. J., Ahmed, K., and Fischbach, T. J. (1978). *Biochim. Biophys. Acta* **542**, 12–20.

Woo, S. L. C., and O'Malley, B. W. (1976). *Life Sci.* **17**, 1039–1048.

19

Drug Effects on the Cell Cycle

SAM C. BARRANCO

I. Introduction

The cell cycle was described originally by Howard and Pelc (1953) and is composed of four major compartments—mitosis (M), a pre-DNA synthesis phase (G_1), a DNA synthesis phase (S), and a post-DNA synthesis phase (G_2). Cells in an exponential growth state have rather fixed time parameters for each of these phases. Under a variety of conditions cell populations may cease dividing or divide very slowly and conceptually can be described as having entered either an extended G_1 or G_2 period or as comprising a compartment of noncycling cells (G_0) which may reenter the cycle on demand (Fig. 1).

Mammalian cells respond to treatment with physical and chemical agents as a function of their position in the cell cycle. In the last few years a concept or model of the cell cycle has emerged in which a highly inte-

The Cell Cycle

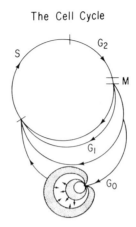

Fig. 1 An idealized view of the mammalian cell cycle.

grated control mechanism is considered to be a series of biochemical events which, when ordered in a specific sequence, move the cell toward division. Factors having a direct or indirect influence on the cell's response are controlled both qualitatively and quantitatively by the specific biochemical events being carried out in the cell at the time of treatment. This view of cell cycle-modulated response to any agent then leads to the inevitable conclusion that, in order to understand the mechanism of action of a perturbing agent, we will have to know a great deal more about specific normal events occurring during the cell cycle.

Puck and Marcus (1956) developed the now classical quantitative method for determining the effect of radiation on single mammalian cells *in vitro*. The criterion of survival is based on the ability of a cell to divide at least five to six times when plated into an appropriate growth medium. The method (Fig. 2) is straightforward, is adaptable to most mammalian cell lines, and yields precise kinetic data on the killing efficiency of radiation and chemicals.

The question of cell cycle-dependent or non-cell cycle-dependent response was answered when Terasima and Tolmach (1961) reported on the effects of X rays on the survival of HeLa cells irradiated in different phases of the cell cycle. In terms of survival the most sensitive phases were M, G_2, and late G_1, while the most resistant phases were early G_1 and S. The patterns of response have shown some differences, but the phenomenon has been observed in every cell line tested (Frindel and Tubiana, 1971). The obvious conclusion has been that the radiation response of mammalian cells is cell cycle phase-dependent. Furthermore, it appears that M-phase cells are universally the most sensitive and at least some S-phase cells are the most resistant.

PLATING TECHNIQUE

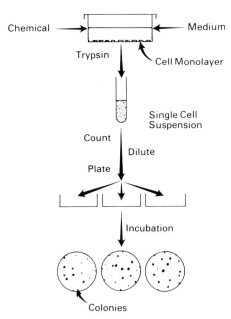

Fig. 2 Treatment and plating scheme used in survival curve determinations *in vitro*.

Similar experiments with mouse L cells were conducted by Walker and Helleiner (1963) using nitrogen mustards and sulfur mustard. They showed that the survival response for these chemicals was cell cycle-dependent. In this case S-phase cells were the most sensitive, while G_1 and G_2 were more resistant. Since this first, original report in 1963, the major types of chemicals used as mutagens and chemotherapy agents have been investigated in a wide variety of mammalian cells ranging from rodent to human (Hoffman and Poet, 1973).

The purpose of this chapter is to discuss the effects of a variety of drugs on survival and cell kinetics and to demonstrate how knowledge of these factors might be used to manipulate the cell cycle of human tumors in an effort to optimize treatment schedules.

II. Drug Effects on Dividing and Nondividing Cells

The effects of Ara-C on the survival of Chinese hamster ovary (CHO) cells treated *in vitro* are shown in Fig. 3. The cells were treated either during exponential growth or during a nondividing or plateau phase. The re-

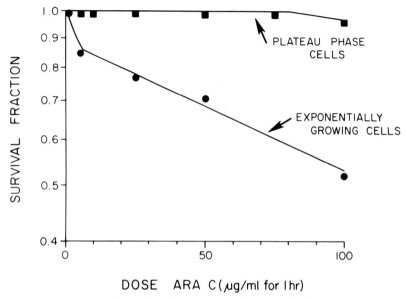

Fig. 3 The effects of Ara-C on the survival of exponentially growing or plateau-phase CHO cells. (Barranco, et al., 1974).

sults show that this drug is effective only against dividing cells, whereas nondividing cells are totally resistant through doses of 75 μg/ml (for 1 hour). Even at the 100 μg/ml does, plateau cell survival is still greater than 95% (Barranco and Novak, 1974). The antitumor activity of Ara-C is attributed to its ability to inhibit DNA synthesis after being phosphorylated by cytidine kinase to Ara-CTP (Chu and Fischer, 1966; Kessel *et al.*, 1967). This inhibition may result from a direct effect on DNA polymerase (Furth, & Cohen, 1968), with ensuing cell lethality caused by unbalanced growth (Atkinson and Stacey, 1968). Since there are few if any cells replicating DNA during the plateau phase (or in G_0 *in vivo*), no Ara-C effect would be expected.

Contrary to the Ara-C results, plateau-phase CHO cells are almost two times more sensitive than dividing cells to 1,2:5,6-dianhydrogalactitol (galactitol). Galactitol has been shown to inhibit DNA, RNA, and protein synthesis and produces cross-linking in DNA (Hidvégi *et al.*, 1967). We showed (Barranco and Flournoy, 1977) that the survival curves of galactitol-treated cells were characterized as having shoulder regions up to 12.5 μg/ml doses in both dividing and nondividing populations, followed by exponential decreases in survival at higher drug concentrations (Fig. 4). The *n*-values, the intercepts obtained by extrapolation of the exponential portion of the survival curve to 0 dose, were 8 and 20 for dividing and nondi-

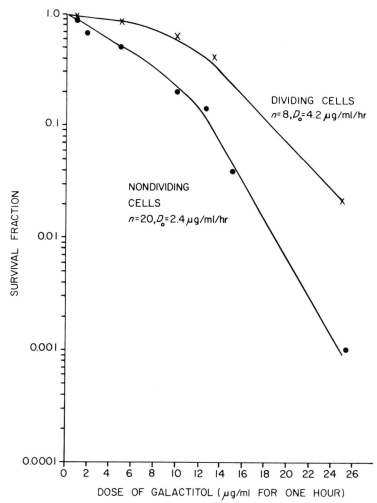

Fig. 4 The survival responses of dividing or plateau-phase CHO cells to galactitol. (Barranco, et al., 1977).

viding cells, respectively. The D_0 was 4.2 μg/ml per hour for dividing cells and 2.4 μg/ml per hour for nondividing cells, making the nondividing cells almost two times more sensitive to the drug (relative to the D_0 values) and 22 times more sensitive at the 25 μg/ml dose points (0.02 survival fraction in dividing cells versus 0.0009 survival fraction in plateau cells).

The apparent high efficiency of this anticancer drug in killing nondividing cells *in vitro* does not necessarily mean that G_0 tumor cells *in vivo* will exhibit a similar response, although hematopoietic stem cells (thought to reside in a G_0 compartment) have been shown to be sensitive (Fuzy *et al.*, 1975). In animal tumor models the size of the G_0 population increases as the tumor grows larger and as the distance between cells and capillaries increases (Tannock, 1968). This is generally taken to mean that less oxygen and nutrients can reach these G_0 cells; therefore anticancer drugs may also have difficulty in reaching these G_0 areas within the tumor. However, Hahn *et al.* (1973) showed that the G_0 cells in an EMT6 tumor *in vivo* were

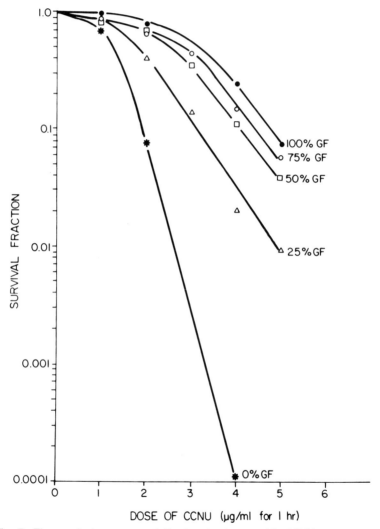

Fig. 5 The survival responses following treatment with CCNU observed as the growth fraction (GF) decreases. (Barranco et al., 1979).

more sensitive to bleomycin than the dividing cells, thus confirming *in vitro* bleomycin findings (Barranco *et al.*, 1973c). Hageman *et al.* (1973) also demonstrated greater *in vivo* G_0 tumor sensitivity to 1,3-bis(2-chloroethyl)-1-nitrosourea (BCNU), another anticancer drug shown to be more effective against nondividing cells *in vitro* (Barranco *et al.*, 1973c; Hahn *et al.*, 1974).

An example of how the sensitivity of a population changes as more cells enter the nondividing state is shown in Fig. 5. Known numbers of dividing and nondividing CHO cells were mixed together and then treated immediately with 1-(2-chloroethyl)-3-cyclohexyl-1-nitrosourea (CCNU). It can be seen in Fig. 5 that the sensitivity of the population increased as the fraction of cells in the growth fraction decreased (Barranco *et al.*, 1979). Hence there is a possibility that considerable killing in a G_0 tumor population *in vivo* may be observed following treatment with drugs shown to kill both dividing and nondividing cells.

III. Cell Cycle Phase-Related Drug Effects

A. Survival

As discussed earlier, the response to drug treatment depends somewhat on the biochemical events occurring in a particular cell at the time of treatment (Kim and Kim, 1972). Thus it may be assumed that cells would respond differently if treated in various phases of the cell cycle. In Fig. 6, the survival responses of cells treated with 5 μg adriamycin/ml for 1 hour are shown to vary with the stage of the cell cycle. From these data it can be seen that cells in M-, late G_1-, and early to mid-S-phases were about equally sensitive. The most resistant cells were found in early G_1- and late S-phases, and the difference in survival among these groups of cells at this dose level was a factor of about 20.

B. Cell Progression Kinetics

Each chemical, based on its mode of action may block cells at specific positions in the cell cycle. Thus a chemical that inhibits DNA synthesis either prevents cells from initiating DNA replication so that they remain in late G_1-phase or reduces the rate of replication so that they remain in S-phase. Therefore, once a chemical is applied to an *in vitro* or *in vivo* cell population, the kinetics of cellular progression will be altered and impose on the remaining viable population a completely changed pattern of response. From this fact, it follows that the action of a second agent must be

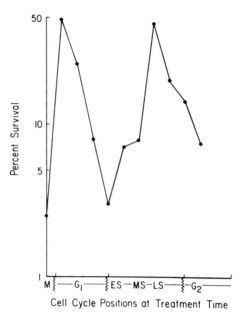

Fig. 6 Cell cycle phase sensitivity to adriamycin of cells treated in various phases of the cell cycle. (Barranco et al., 1973a).

influenced in some way by the first, the action of a third agent influenced by a summation of the first and second, and so on.

In Fig. 7, the kinetics effects of a relatively new anticancer agent, diglycoaldehyde (DGA), are shown. This drug is an inhibitor of ribonucleotide reductase (Cory *et al.*, 1976) and has been shown to *kill cells most effectively in S-phase,* while cells in G_0, M, G_1, and G_2 are relatively resistant (Bhuyan and Fraser, 1974; Barranco *et al.*, 1978).

Mitotic cells treated with 500 μg/ml DGA progressed at control rates into G_1-phase. It can be seen in Fig. 7A that the mitotic index decreased from 93% to almost 0% within 1.5 hours in both the treated and control populations, indicating normal progression into G_1-phase.

Cells treated for 1 hour (see arrows in Fig. 7B) during early G_1-phase were delayed for approximately 2 hours but then progressed at a slightly reduced rate into S-phase. The labeling index (LI) was essentially 0% at 0–2 hours after plating mitotic cells, indicating that the cells were in G_1 at the time of treatment. As the G_1 cells in the control populations progressed into S phase, the LI increased. The ruse in the LI of the treated population was delayed until the fourth hour and then increased at a rate slower than that for the controls, thus demonstrating the DGA effect on G_1 progression kinetics.

The LI in the control S-phase populations in Fig. 7C rose to 92% by the

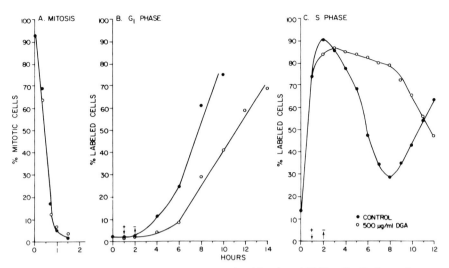

Fig. 7 The effects of DGA on cell progression kinetics of CHO cells. ●, Control population; ○, treated population. (Barranco et al., 1978).

second hour after the end of synchrony and decreased when the majority of cells began progressing out of S-phase and into G_2. The LI decreased to 30% by the eighth hour and rose again as some cells reentered the subsequent S-phase. Cells treated for 1 hour in early S-phase with 500 μg/ml DGA were delayed almost 5 hours longer in S-phase before progression into G_2 (Fig. 7C). At doses below 500 μg/ml, there were no effects on cell progression from G_1 to S, or from S to G_2-phase of the cell cycle. A dose-dependent effect of DGA on G_2 progression into M was also observed.

It is important to note here that the inhibition of progression of cells from G_1-phase into S-phase (the most sensitive phase for this drug's lethal effects) puts self-limiting restrictions on the effectiveness of DGA as an anticancer agent. The data suggest that multiple single exposures (perhaps separated by one cell cycle time) might be the most useful treatment regimen, since this schedule might allow repopulation of the sensitive S-phase between exposures.

Presented in Fig. 8 is a selected group of agents showing where they block cells at different positions in the cell cycle. The group headed by amethopterin consists of chemicals that inhibit DNA synthesis. They prevent cells from entering S-phase and reduce the progression of cells from S-phase. The majority of agents thus far analyzed fall into this category, although they may act at other positions as well. An example of the latter is actinomycin D. Three chemicals, listed in Fig. 8, were chosen as examples of agents that are rather specific in the block they produce. They were (1) the alkaloid represented by Colcemid, which inhibits completion

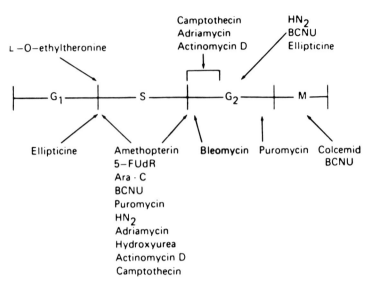

Fig. 8 Blockage of cell cycle traverse by chemical agents.

of mitosis, (2) bleomycin, which inhibits completion of G_2, and (3) L-O-ethyltheronine, which inhibits the initiation of DNA synthesis. BCNU is an example of a chemical that affects progression of cells in all phases of the cell cycle.

The position of blockage may or may not have any relationship to the killing effectiveness of a chemical. The alkaloids colchicine, vinblastine, and vincristine are very effective specific inhibitors of mitosis in all mammalian cells. However, it has been reported (Mauro and Madoc-Jones, 1970) that in HeLa cells these alkaloids are most effective in killing S-phase cells. A relationship exists for bleomycin in which the block is in G_2 and the phases most sensitive to killing are M and G_2 (Barranco and Humphrey, 1971). Hydroxyurea serves as an example illustrating a very close relationship between blockage and cell killing efficiency. Hydroxyurea kills cells specifically in S-phase, blocks cells in S-phase, and prevents cells in G_1-phase from entering into S-phase. Cells arrested in G_1 are not killed unless they remained blocked for a time approximately equal to one cell cycle time (Sinclair, 1967).

IV. Use of Drug-Induced Kinetics Effects to Manipulate Human Tumor Kinetics

Because of a better knowledge of drug effects on the cell cycle obtained through experiments such as those described in this chapter, and because of the recent development of instruments that allow rapid cell cycle analysis, it may now be possible to manipulate a patient's tumor kinetics in a way that would optimize treatment scheduling. For example, most large solid tumors contain only small fractions of cells in the growth fraction (Tannock, 1968). The cell cycle-active anticancer drugs, specific for dividing cells, are usually only minimally effective. Likewise, the effectiveness of cell cycle phase-specific anticancer drugs will be determined by the "size" of a particularly sensitive population in the cell cycle. A tumor with only 8–10% of its cells in S-phase will not be very sensitive to S-phase agents such as hydroxyurea and Ara-C. However, if the fraction of cells in S-phase could be *enriched*, the tumor might become more sensitive to S-phase-specific anticancer drugs. Such enrichment may be achieved through the use of drug treatments that induce partial synchronization in the cell population. Although the synchrony obtained from such drug treatments may not be perfect, the resulting enrichment may be of significant value in scheduling multiple drug and radiation combination therapy.

We have employed such techniques, using bleomycin to produce partially synchronized cell populations in human melanomas *in vivo* (Barranco *et al.*, 1973b), and have used changes in the patient's own tumor kinetics to direct the timing of the second drug treatment. Bleomycin has been shown to block cells near the $S-G_2$ boundary *in vitro* (Fig. 8); and the blockage is reversible, depending on the dose given. After a 4-day synchronizing treatment by infusion with bleomycin, tumor cells blocked at the $S-G_2$ boundary progressed through the cell cycle in a partially synchronized manner, reaching the next S-phase 1–3 days later.

The enrichment or synchrony was measured in our studies with the use of a flow microfluorometry (FMF) system. Such a system employs the use of a laser beam to exite a fluorescent dye in the DNA of the cells. The amount of fluorescent light emitted is related to the amount of DNA in the cells, and therefore the fraction of cells in G_1, S, and G_2 and M phases can be quantitated. Generally the method used is as follows. Tumor biopsies obtained before bleomycin infusion (baseline kinetics) and at various times after bleomycin are dissociated into single cells by pepsin treatment (Zante *et al.*, 1976; Barranco *et al.*, 1979b). The DNA in the cells is stained with a fluorescent dye, propidium iodide (Crissman and Steinkamp, 1973; Krishan, 1975). The cell sample is then introduced into a rapid sheath flow system in which each cell interacts with the laser beam. The emitted fluorescent light characteristic of each cell is processed in a 128 multichannel analyzer, and the resulting histograms display increasing fluorescence (DNA) on the x axis and the number of cells having a specific fluorescence on the y axis.

FMF histograms obtained from a human malignant melanoma are

shown in Fig. 9. Tumor cells with a G_1 quantity of DNA exhibit a peak in channel 30. G_2 cells that have already replicated their DNA have two times more DNA than G_1 cells and peak in channels 59–60. The mathematical analysis of the baseline histogram (Fig. 9A) obtained for a melanoma nodule prior to the start of the bleomycin infusion showed that the frac-

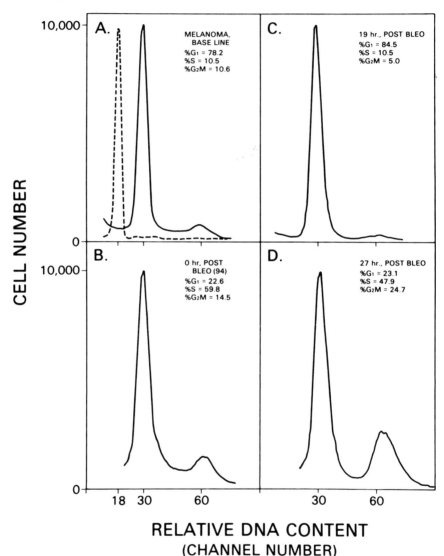

Fig. 9 FMF DNA histograms of human malignant melanoma showing changes in cell kinetics parameters following treatment with bleomycin.

tion of cells in G_1 or G_0 was 78.2%, in S-phase 10.5%, and in G_2M 10.6%. The dashed line is a histogram of the patient's lymphocytes obtained from peripheral blood and isolated by a Hypaque-Ficoll gradient. The fact that its G_1 peak is to the left of the G_1 of the tumor indicates that the tumor is hyperdiploid. Figure 9B shows that at the end of the ninety-fourth hour of bleomycin infusion (25 units/24 hours) the fraction of cells in S and G_2M phases of the cell cycle had risen to 59.8 and 14.5%, respectively, suggesting that the kinetics blockage had occurred at the $S-G_2$ boundary. Nineteen hours later (Fig. 9C) the fraction of cells in S-phase had dropped to 10.5% and G_2M to 5%, indicating that the bleomycin block was reversible. By the twenty-seventh hour (Fig. 9D) the G_1 fraction had decreased from 84.5 to 23.1%, while 47.9% of the cells had moved into S-phase, with an extremely large fraction (24.7%) returning to the G_2M compartment. This represented an almost 5-fold increase in the fraction of cells in S phase and about a 2.5 fold increase in G_2M.

Figure 10A indicates that the baseline measurements for a carcinoma of the cervix were: G_1, 49.1%; S, 40.5%; and G_2M, 10.4%. Another fraction of cells in the tumor preparation peaked at channel 23, and that coincided with the peak for the patient's peripheral blood lymphocytes (dashed line). (The pathology examination of this biopsy sample indicated lymphocyte and macrophage infiltration.) At the end of a 60-hour infusion with bleomycin (25 units/24 hours), the fraction of cells in S-phase had increased to 59.2%. Twelve hours later (Fig. 10C) the fraction of cells in S-phase had droped to 42.6% and the fraction in G_2M had increased to 26.1%, indicating the progression of this partially synchronized population through the cell cycle. The fraction of cells in S-phase ultimately increased to 64.6% by the thirty-fifth hour after bleomycin infusion—a factor 1.6 times greater than that present in the baseline biopsy (Fig. 10A).

Although the changes in kinetics seen in the FMF histograms suggest that bleomycin induces a reversible partial synchronization in human tumors, we cannot be sure at this time whether these synchronized cells were truly alive or whether they had been killed by the bleomycin and were doomed to die after dividing once or twice. We also do not know whether any of the synchrony observed was the result of recruitment from G_0. These and other questions can be answered only after studying a large group of patients. The significance of studies such as those described in this chapter is that the patient's own tumor kinetics help to direct the optimal timing of a second drug or radiation treatment.

A better knowledge of perturbed and unperturbed kinetics within a specific tumor is now possible because of the development of rapid and accurate instrumentation and techniques. This, coupled with a more thorough understanding of drug-induced cell cycle effects, and with the use of

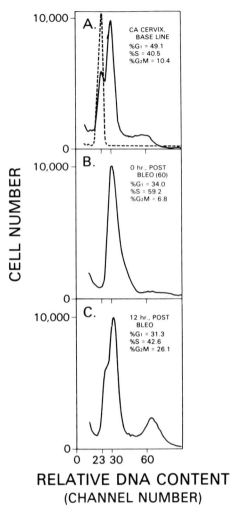

Fig. 10 FMF DNA histograms of human carcinoma of the cervix showing changes in cell kinetics parameters following treatment with bleomycin.

mathematical modeling and computer simulation methods, makes it important at this time to expand such studies in humans.

Acknowledgment

These studies were supported by grant DHEW 1P01 CA 23114-01 from the National Institutes of Health.

References

Atkinson, C., and Stacey, K. A. (1968). *Biochim. Biophys. Acta* **166**, 705–707.

Barranco, S. C., and Flournoy, D. R. (1977). *J. Natl. Cancer Inst.* **58**, 657–663.

Barranco, S. C., and Humphrey, R. M. (1971). *Cancer Res.* **31**, 1218–1223.

Barranco, S. C., and Novak, J. K. (1974). *Cancer Res.* **34**, 1616–1618.

Barranco, S. C., Gerner, E. W., Buck, K. H., and Humphrey, R. M. (1973a). *Cancer Res.* **33**, 11–16.

Barranco, S. C., Luce, J. K., Romsdahl, M. M., and Humphrey, R. M. (1973b). *Cancer Res.* **33**, 882–887.

Barranco, S. C., Novak, J. K., and Humphrey, R. M. (1973c). *Cancer Res.* **33**, 691–694.

Barranco, S. C., Bolton, W. E., and Novak, J. K. (1979). *Cell Tissue Kinet.* **12**, 11–16.

Barranco, S. C., Fluornoy, D. R., Bolton, W. E., and Oka, M. S. (1978). *J. Natl. Cancer Inst.* **61**, 1307–1310.

Bhuyan, B. K., and Fraser, T. J. (1974). *Cancer Chemother. Rep.* **58**, 149–155.

Chu, M. Y., and Fischer, G. A. (1966). *Biochem. Pharmacol.* **15**, 1417–1428.

Cory, J. G., Mansell, M. M., and Whitford, T. W., Jr. (1976). *Cancer Res.* **36**, 3166–3170.

Crissman, H. A., and Steinkamp, J. A. (1973). *J. Cell Biol.* **59**, 766–771.

Frindel, E., and Tubiana, M. (1971). *In* "The Cell Cycle and Cancer" (R. Baserga, ed.), Vol. 1, pp. 391–447. Dekker, New York.

Furth, J. J., and Cohen, S. S. (1968). *Cancer Res.* **28**, 2061–2067.

Fuzy, M., Lelieveld, P., and Van Putten, L. M. (1975). *Eur. J. Cancer* **11**, 169–173.

Hageman, R. F., Schenken, L. L., and Lesher, S. (1973). *J. Natl. Cancer Inst.* **50**, 467–474.

Hahn, G. M., Ray, G. R., and Gordon, L. F. (1973). *J. Natl. Cancer Inst.* **50**, 529–533.

Hahn, G. M., Gordon, L. F., and Kurkjian, S. D. (1974). *Cancer Res.* **24**, 2373–2377.

Hidvégi, E. J., Lonai, P., and Holland, J. (1967). *Biochem. Pharmacol.* **16**, 2143–2153.

Hoffman, J., and Poet, J. (1973). *In* "Drugs and the Cell Cycle" (A. M. Zimmerman, G. M. Padilla, and I. L. Cameron, eds.), pp. 219–247. Academic Press, New York.

Howard, A., and Pelc, S. R. (1953). *Heredity* **6**, 261–273.

Kessel, D., Hall, T. C., and Woodinsky, I. (1967). *Science* **156**, 1240–1241.

Kim, S. H., and Kim, J. H. (1972). *Cancer Res.* **32**, 323–325.

Krishan, A. (1975). *J. Cell Biol.* **66**, 188–193.

Mauro, F., and Madoc-Jones, H. (1970). *Cancer Res.* **30**, 1397–1408.

Puck, T. T., and Marcus, P. I. (1956). *J Exp. Med.* **103**, 653–666.

Sinclair, W. K. (1967). *Cancer Res.* **27**, 297–308.

Tannock, I. F. (1968). *Br. J. Cancer* **22**, 258–273.

Terasima, T., and Tolmach, L. J. (1961). *Nature (London)* **190**, 1210–1211.

Walker, I. G., and Helleiner, G. W. (1963). *Cancer Res.* **23**, 734–738.

Zante, J., Schumann, J., Barologie, B., Göhde, W., and Büchner, J. (1976). *In* "Pulse Cytophotometry" (W. Göhde, J. Schumann, and J. Büchner, eds.), pp. 97–106. European Press, Ghent.

Discussion

Z. DARZYNKIEWICZ

In reference to the point previously raised, regarding the presence of G_0 or quiescent cells in cell populations, I would like to mention some of our recent observations on this subject. Three independent flow cytometric techniques to distinguish quiescent from cycling cells have been developed recently in our laboratory (Darzynkiewicz et al., 1975, 1976, 1977, 1978; Traganos et al., 1977). Applying these techniques to a variety of cell systems, including normal and neoplastic cells, we observed certain general features characteristic of the transition from the cycling phase to quiescence (or cell differentiation), and vice versa. Namely, in populations of normal cells the transition occurs predominantly at the 2c (G_0–G_1) DNA level (Darzynkiewicz et al., 1975, 1976, 1977, 1978; Traganos et al., 1977), whereas in neoplastic systems the transition may occur at all levels, i.e., at G_1, S, and G_2 (Kurland et al., 1978; Traganos et al., 1979). In other words, neoplastic cells may be blocked in the cycle not only at G_1-phase but also at G_2- and S-phases.

As an illustration of this point Fig. 1 can be compared with Figs. 2 and 3.

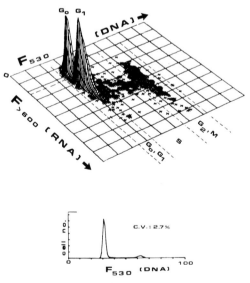

Fig. 1

Figure 1 represents populations of quiescent and cycling normal lymphocytes. The cells are displayed in the form of a two-parameter frequency histogram. The height of the peaks or ridges in these histograms is proportional to cell number, while their position with respect to the ordinates is a relative measure of cellular DNA and RNA, stained ortho- and metachromatically, respectively, with the fluorescent dye acridine orange (Darzynkiewicz *et al.*, 1975, 1976, 1977; Traganos *et al.*, 1977). Based on DNA content cells may be subclassified into G_0/G_1-, S-, and G_2/M-phases. RNA content distinguishes quiescent (G_0) cells from cycling ones; in most of the cell systems studied noncycling cells have been found to have a lower RNA content than cycling cells (Darzynkiewicz *et al.*, 1975, 1976, 1978; Kurland *et al.*, 1978; Traganos *et al.*, 1977, 1979). Note that quiescent cells have the same DNA content as G_1 cells. Thus, in lymphocytes, as well as in other normal cells, transition from the quiescent to the cycling phase occurs at the 2c DNA level.

Figure 2 illustrates a murine erythroleukemic cell population. In these two-parameter scattergrams, cells are represented by individual points whose distance from the abscissa and the ordinate reflects the relative values of DNA and RNA, respectively. On the right there is a control cell population from exponentially growing cultures. The G_1 cells are located in the main cluster; there are also numerous S and G_2/M cells. The left scattergram represents cells that are fully differentiated and noncycling, from cultures incubated with dimethyl sulfoxide (DMSO) for 6 days (Tra-

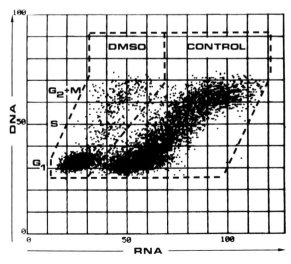

Fig. 2

ganos *et al.*, 1979). At that time, DMSO induced not only erythroid differentiation of these cells but also completely stopped their progression
through the cell cycle. In this quiescent population, though the cells are
preferentially blocked in G_1, there are still a large number of cells with
DNA values characteristic of S and G_2/M. These low-RNA S-phase
cells do not synthesize DNA, and G_2 cells do not enter mitosis. Thus they
represent a genuine, noncycling, differentiated cell population blocked in
S and G_2.

BL -CML: Effect of DVA

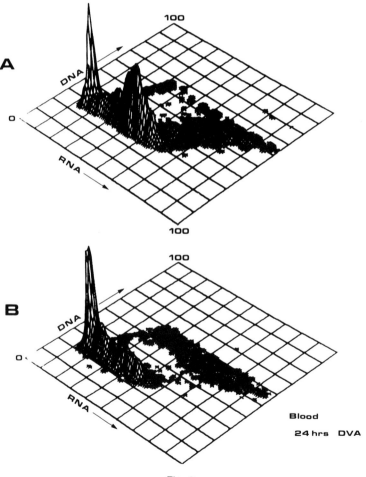

Fig. 3

Figure 3 shows histograms of blast cells from the blood of a patient with chronic myeloid leukemia in blastic crisis. Figure 3A represents cells obtained prior to any treatment and indicates the presence of two cell subpopulations, one with a low RNA content and the other one with a high RNA content. Note that in both subpopulations there are cells with a G_1 DNA content (two highest peaks) as well as cells with an S and G_2/M DNA content. Based on a number of control studies, we presume that the subpopulation with low RNA represents noncycling cells blocked in G_1-, S-, and G_2-phases, while cycling cells are represented by a high-RNA subpopulation.

Figure 3B shows cells from the same patient but 24 hours after treatment with the vinblastine analogue desacetylvinblastine amide sulfate, i.e., with a drug expected to block cells in mitosis. The treatment perturbed only the high-RNA subpopulation. In this subpopulation there is an accumulation of cells with doubled DNA content (G_2/M locus), most likely mitotic cells, and a proportional decrease in the number of G_1 and S cells. In contrast, the noncycling cells represented by the low-RNA supopulation are not affected. After the treatment they still show a prominent G_1 peak and also display a similar number of S and G_2/M cells as prior to treatment. It appears therefore that in this *in vivo* situation the noncycling subpopulation arrested in G_1-, S-, and G_2-phases is not sensitive to the drug treatment. This example perhaps best illustrates the problem raised concerning the lack of sensitivity of quiescent cells to cell cycle-specific drugs.

References

Darzynkiewicz, Z., Traganos, F., Sharpless, T., and Melamed, M. R. (1975). *Exp. Cell Res.* **95**, 143–153.

Darzynkiewicz, Z., Traganos, F., Sharpless, T., and Melamed, M. R. (1976). *Proc. Natl. Acad. Sci. USA* **73**, 2881–2884.

Darzynkiewicz, Z., Traganos, F., Sharpless, T., and Melamed, M. R. (1977). *Cancer Res.* **37**, 4635–4640.

Darzynkiewicz, Z., Andreeff, M., Traganos, F., Sharpless, T., and Melamed, M. R. (1978). *Exp. Cell Res.* **115**, 31–35.

Kurland, J., Traganos, F., Darzynkiewicz, Z., and Moore, M. (1978). *Cell. Immunol.* **36**, 318–330.

Traganos, F., Darzynkiewicz, Z., Sharpless, T., and Melamed, M. R. (1977). *J. Histochem. Cytochem.* **25**, 46–56.

Traganos, F., Darzynkiewicz, Z., Sharpless, T., and Melamed, M. R. (1979). *J. Histochem. Cytochem.* **27**, 382–389.

20

G$_2$ Arrest Induced by Anticancer Drugs

POTU N. RAO

I. Introduction

The life cycle of mammalian cells, either normal or malignant, usually consists of a pre-DNA synthesis (G$_1$) period, a period of DNA synthesis (S), a post-DNA synthesis (G$_2$) period, and mitosis. Soon after cell division, the daughter cells may either stop in G$_1$-phase for prolonged periods of time or prepared for another round of cell division. Once the cell is triggered to proceed through the cell cycle, biochemical events necessary for the initiation of DNA synthesis are set in motion. One of the most important aspects of the G_1-period is the synthesis and gradual accumulation of the inducers of DNA synthesis (Rao *et al.*, 1977). The cell enters S-phase when the concentration of these inducers reaches a critical level. As the cell proceeds through DNA synthesis, biosynthetic activities related to entry of the cell into mitosis, which reach a peak at the G_2–mitosis transition, are also initiated. While the G_1-period is important for preparing the cell to replicate its DNA, the G_2-period serves the purpose of preparing the cell for the equal distribution of genetic material between the daughter nuclei through mitosis. The earliest event associated with cell division is the gradual and progressive condensation of chromatin, which is initiated as soon as DNA synthesis is completed. It is generally accepted that transformation of the diffused chromatin into highly condensed chromosomes during mitosis is brought about by the synthesis or activation of one or more factors as cells traverse through G_2. Continued protein synthesis is known to be essential for cells to complete the G_2-period and enter mitosis (Taylor, 1963; Kishimoto and Lieberman, 1964; Tobey *et al.*, 1966). In Chinese hamster cells, it has been shown that protein synthesis is required up to 60 minutes prior to the initiation of mitosis.

Knowledge of cell cycle events is helpful in designing and synthesizing more effective anticancer drugs. A variety of anticancer agents block the progression of tumor cells at different points in the cell cycle. The majority of these compounds are antimetabolites that interfere with DNA synthesis. They include arabinosylcytosine, 5-fluorouracil, 6-mercaptopurine, 6-thioguanine, and methotrexate. Anthracycline compounds, e.g., adriamycin, actinomycin D, daunorubicin, and mithramycin, intercalate into DNA and block RNA synthesis. Certain antibiotics, bleomycin and neocarzinostatin in particular, are very effective in causing DNA strand breaks. Another important and most effective group of anticancer drugs are alkylating agents, for example, nitrosoureas. Nitrosoureas, which cause DNA–DNA and DNA–protein cross-links, usually block cells in the G_2 period. Ionizing radiations that cause DNA damage are also known to induce G_2 arrest. This chapter examines the nature of the G_2 block induced by a variety of agents including certain anticancer drugs.

II. Reversible G_2 Arrest

Naturally synchronous or experimentally synchronized cell populations are ideal for the delineation of various biochemical events taking place at different points in the mammalian cell cycle. There are a variety of methods for synchronizing mammalian cells in various phases of the cell cycle. For example, cells can be synchronized (1) in mitosis by Colcemid or N_2O (Rao, 1968) or by selective detachment (Terasima and Tolmach, 1963), (2) in G_1-phase by the reversal of any one of the above-mentioned mitotic blocks or by deprivation of certain amino acids, i.e., leucine (Everhart and Prescott, 1972) and isoleucine (Tobey and Ley, 1971), and (3) in S-phase by the use of amethopterin (Rueckert and Mueller, 1960), hydroxyurea (Tobey and Crissman, 1972), or an excess dose of thymidine (TdR) (Rao and Engelberg, 1966). Only recently, a new method has been found to block mammalian cells reversibly in G_2-phase.

The substitution for phenylalanine by its analogue p-fluorophenylalanine (FPA) in the medium was reported to block the progression of a random population of HeLa cells from G_2 to mitosis (Wheatley and Inglis, 1977). Removal of FPA from the medium by washing the cells and resuspending them in regular medium with elevated levels of phenylalanine resulted in resumption of the progression of G_2 cells into mitosis, but without any evidence of synchrony (Wheatley and Henderson, 1975). However, by exposing a synchronized S-phase population of HeLa cells to FPA (0.5 mM) it was possible to block most of the cells in G_2 in a reversible manner (Sunkara *et al.*, 1978).

A. Effect of FPA on Synchronized S-Phase HeLa Cells

In these experiments (Sunkara *et al.*, 1978), HeLa cells were synchronized in S-phase by the excess Tdr double-block method (Rao and Engelberg, 1966) and plated in a number of 60-mm culture dishes at 2×10^6 cells per dish. At various times after reversal of the second TdR block, the medium was replaced with medium containing FPA (0.5 mM) instead of phenylalanine. Colcemid (0.05 μg/ml) was also added to determine the percentage of cells that were able to reach mitosis in the presence of FPA. These cells were incubated for 16 hours to allow the completion of DNA synthesis. At the end of this period the cells were pulsed with [³H]TdR (1.0 μCi/ml; specific activity, 6.7 Ci/mM) for 15 minutes and trypsinized; part of the sample was used to determine the labeling index after autoradiography. The cells in the remaining sample were fused with synchronized mitotic HeLa cells using ultraviolet-inactivated Sendai virus for cell cycle analysis by the prematurely condensed chromosome (PCC) method as described by Rao *et al.* (1977).

These experiments showed that the time of addition of FPA to the medium after reversal of the TdR block had a profound effect on the ability of the cells to complete DNA synthesis (Table I). Addition of FPA within 2 hours after reversal of the block prevented most of the cells from completing S-phase, as revealed by the high labeling index at the end of the FPA treatment. However, when FPA was added 4 hours after reversal (mid-S), most of the cells were able to complete DNA synthesis but were blocked in G_2. This was further confirmed by the PCC method; 93% of the PCCs scored exhibited G_2 morphology, while the remaining were in S-sphase. The longer the interval between reversal of the second TdR block and the addition of FPA, the greater the fraction of cells able to complete DNA synthesis and proceed to mitosis. These results suggest that maximum G_2 synchrony could be obtained by adding FPA 4 hours after reversal of the TdR block. The addition of FPA earlier than 4 hours would prevent completion of S-phase in most of the cells (Table I). These data indicate that the substitution of phenylalanine by its analogue, FPA, in cellular proteins impairs their activity, and as a result cells fail to progress through the cell cycle. However, if FPA is added to cells in mid- to late S-phase, they can complete DNA synthesis but are blocked in G_2-phase.

B. Reversibility of G_2 Block Induced by FPA

Removal of FPA by washing and incubating the cells in the presence or absence of an excess dose of phenylalanine (1 mM) allowed the cells to progress from G_2 to mitosis in a fairly synchronous manner (Fig. 1). However, in the presence of excess phenylalanine, the cells entered mitosis a little faster than those in regular medium. It appears that the phenylalanine present in the regular medium (0.2 mM) is enough to reverse the effects of FPA, since an excess amount of this amino acid (1 mM) made little difference in the rate of progression of these cells from G_2 to mitosis.

TABLE I

Effect of the Time of Addition of FPA after the Reversal of a TdR Block on the Progression of S-Phase HeLa Cells through the Cell Cycle[a,b]

Medium[c]	Hours after reversal of TdR block FPA (0.5 mM) was added	Labeling index	Mitotic index	G_2 PCCs (%)
Regular	—	—	94.0	—
Phe⁻	—	—	92.0	—
Phe⁻	0	80.2	9.0	19.5
Phe⁻	2	76.5	14.0	23.5
Phe⁻	4	7.0	10.0	93.0
Phe⁻	6	4.0	65.5	96.0

[a] From Sunkara et al. (1978).
[b] Determinations of labeling index, mitotic index, and percent G_2 PCC were performed on cultures incubated for 16 hours with Colcemid and with or without FPA.
[c] Phe⁻, Phenylalanine-deficient.

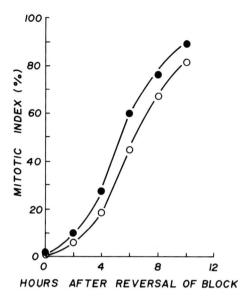

Fig. 1 The kinetics of mitotic accumulation in HeLa cells following the reversal of a FPA-induced G_2 block. Colcemid (0.05 μg/ml) was added immediately after reversal of the FPA block. ○, Cells plated in regular medium; ●, cells plated in MEM containing 1 mM of phenylalanine. (From Sunkara et al., 1978).

Although the FPA treatment blocked most of the cells in G_2, the rate of entry into mitosis following removal of the drug suggests that the cells are not blocked at a single point in G_2 phase (Fig. 1). This is in agreement with the observations of Wheatley and Henderson (1975), who could not detect any measurable degree of synchrony in the G_2-mitosis transition of a random population following reversal of a FPA block. Even though the degree of synchrony, with regard to the progression of cells from G_2 to mitosis, in FPA-blocked cells is about the same as that achieved by the TdR double-block method, the advantage of the present method lies in the fact that we are able to arrest most of the cells in G_2 phase and that this G_2 block is quickly and completely reversible. The reversal appears to be due to the synthesis of new proteins following the replacement of FPA with phenylalanine in the medium.

III. Anticancer Agents That Induce G₂ Arrest

Many cancer chemotherapeutic agents currently in clinical use, as well as X-irradiation, arrest cells preferentially in G_2-phase of the cell cycle. These include adriamycin, neocarzinostatin (NCS), the polypeptide complex of m-[di(2-chloroethyl)amino]-L-phenylalanine (peptichemio), 4'-de-methylepipodophyllotoxin   9-(4,6-O-2-thenylidene-β-D-glucopyranoside) (VM-26), and nitrosourea compounds.

A. Adriamycin

Adriamycin, which intercalates into DNA, is one of the most potent anticancer agents of the anthracycline antibiotics. Exposure of synchronous human lymphoma cells to adriamycin induced a concentration- and exposure time-dependent accumulation of cells in G_2-phase (Barlogie et al., 1976). Similar results were obtained with human lymphoblasts in vitro (Krishan et al., 1975), human acute myelogenous leukemia, and Ehrlich ascites tumor cells (Gohde et al., 1974). Barlogie et al. (1976) observed some reversibility of this G_2 block after 1- and 3-hour incubations with 0.5 μg/ml of adriamycin, whereas higher concentrations and longer exposure times produced an irreversible arrest of 70–90% of the cells in G_2-phase.

B. Neocarzinostatin

NCS is an acidic antitumor protein, with a molecular weight of 11,000 isolated from a culture of Streptomyces carzinostaticus (Ishida et al., 1965; Tsuruo et al., 1971; Tatsumi et al., 1974; Meienhoffer et al., 1972). NCS, at lower concentrations, inhibits DNA synthesis and mitosis in HeLa cells (Kumagai et al., 1966; Homma et al., 1970) but induces degradation of DNA at higher concentrations (>20 μg/ml) by causing DNA strand breaks (Ohtsuki and Ishida, 1975). Further studies by Ebina et al. (1975), using random and synchronized populations of HeLa S3 cells, revealed that the first mode of action of NCS was the inhibition of DNA synthesis, the second being the block in G_2 phase. It appears that the G_2 block is not dependent upon the inhibition of DNA synthesis by the antibiotic.

C. Peptichemio

Peptichemio, which is closely related to L-phenylalanine mustard, is an alkylating agent. Exposure of cultured human lymphoma cells to peptichemio results in a prolongation of S- and G_2-phases, and the increase in G_2 period is very dramatic. The induction of a G_2 block is dependent on the position of the cell in the cell cycle at the time of treatment (Barlogie et al., 1977). A pulse treatment of early G_1- and early S-phase cells with peptichemio (5 μg/ml for 1 hour) blocked these cells in the subsequent G_2 period, whereas late S and G_2 cells underwent one cell division without significant delay and were arrested in G$_2$-phase before the second mitosis after treatment.

D. VM-26

VM-26 is a semisynthetic derivative of podophyllotoxin, which is obtained from the root of *Podophyllum* spp. Podophyllotoxin and its other derivatives cause metaphase arrest, whereas VM-26 has been reported by Misra and Roberts (1975) to block CCRF-CEM cells in G$_2$ phase of the cell cycle. These authors found that the inhibition of incorporation of precursors into DNA, RNA, and protein was delayed, and probably secondarily to the arrest of cells in G$_2$ phase. These results were further confirmed by Krishan *et al.* (1975), who studied the DNA content by flow microfluorometric analysis of human lymphoid cells exposed to cytostatic concentrations (0.01 μg/ml) of VM-26 for 24 hours. A majority (40–60%) of the treated cells had a G$_2$ amount of DNA, but no cells were arrested in mitosis. However, higher concentrations (0.1 μg/ml) of VM-26 inhibited cell cycle traverse and, after 24 hours of exposure, most of the population was arrested in S-phase. The cytostatic effects of VM-26 have been found to be irreversible (Krishan *et al.*, 1975).

E. X-Irradiation

Exposure to small doses of X rays is known to cause a dose-dependent, reversible G$_2$ lag in mammalian cells (Puck, 1963). Recently, Bedford and Mitchell (1977) reported that S3 HeLa cells could be arrested in G$_2$ either by exposing cells continuously (37°C) for 30 hours to a dose of 37 rads or by administering an X-ray dose of 1000 rads over a very short period of time to a population synchronized in late S-phase. This G$_2$ block is probably irreversible.

Do all these agents arrest cells at a single point or at different points in the G$_2$-period? Tobey (1975) tried to answer this question by measuring the increase in cell number of exponentially growing cultures of Chinese hamster ovary (CHO) cells at different times before and after addition of drug to the culture medium. He determined the time that cells continued to divide at the exponential rate after the addition of each drug or various concentrations of the same drug. The terminal point of action in the G$_2$-period was found to be 60 minutes before mitosis for neocarzinostatin irrespective of drug concentration. Similarly, Tobey (1975) determined the terminal point of action for various drugs that cause accumulation of cells in G$_2$ (Fig. 2). These data indicate that different agents stop cells at different stages in G$_2$.

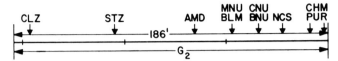

Fig. 2 Drug-specific arrest of progression at different stages within the G_2-phase of the cell cycle in asynchronous cultures of CHO cells. The terminal point of action was determined for the following agents: CLZ, chlorozotocin; STZ, streptozotocin; AMD, actinomycin D; MNU, 1-*trans*-(2-chloroethyl)-3-(4-methylcyclohexyl)-1-nitrosourea; BLM, bleomycin; CNU, CCNU; BNU, BCNU; NCS, neocarzinostatin; CHM, cyclohexi-mide; PUR, puromycin. The drug solutions were prepared immediately before use. The terminal point of action for each agent was determined in multiple cultures using 20 to 80-fold concentration ranges for each drug. (From Tobey, 1975).

IV. The Cause of G_2 Arrest

Even though the mode of action of these various anticancer drugs is different, the drugs have one thing in common: They induce G_2 arrest. What is the nature of this G_2 block? Is it the result of metabolic deficiency or damage to the genetic material? To answer this question, we applied the PCC method. In this study (Rao and Rao, 1976), CHO cells in exponential growth were treated with one of the drugs for 1 hour, washed free of drug, and incubated in regular medium for 30 hours. At the end of this period, the treated cells were pulse labeled with [^{3}H]TdR for 15 minutes and then fused with mitotic HeLa cells using uv-inactivated Sendai virus. The frequency of PCC in the treated cells in G_1-, S-, and G_2-phases were scored for each drug. The drugs studied included VM-26, NCS, and three alkylating agents, 1,3-bis(2-chloroethyl)-1-nitrosourea (BCNU), 1-(2-chloroethyl)-3-cyclohexyl-1-nitrosourea (CCNU), and cis-4-({[2-chloroethyl)-nitrosoamino]carbonyl}amino)cyclohexane carboxylic acid (cis acid). The data indicate a significant increase in the G_2 fraction with all the treatments (Table II).

A. Correlation between G_2 Accumulation and Chromosome Damage

In almost every case, the G_2 PCC of the treated cells exhibited extensive chromosome damage (Fig. 3). For each drug treatment the frequency of extensively damaged G_2 PCC correlated with the extent of G_2 accumulation (Fig. 4). The linear relationship between these two parameters clearly suggests that extensive chromosome damage contributes to the arrest of cells in G_2.

What does this correlation between chromosome damage and G_2 arrest indicate? The necessity for protein synthesis until about 60 minutes

TABLE II

Effect of Drugs on the Cell Cycle Traverse: Percent of Cells in Various Phases of the Cell Cycle at 30 Hours after Treatment[a]

Treatment	Dose (μg/ml)	Mitotic index (%)[b]	Frequency (%)		
			G$_1$	S	G$_2$
Control	No drug	34.0	43.0	46.0	12.0
VM-26	1	14.7	43.0	21.5	35.5
BCNU	50	0.6	43.0	20.0	37.0
CCNU	50	0.3	6.6	30.9	62.5
Cis acid	50	9.8	11.5	17.5	71.0
NCS	1	7.0	28.0	34.0	39.0

[a] From Rao and Rao (1976).

[b] These data represent the extent of mitotic accumulation (in the presence of Colcemid) between 30 and 38 hours after a 1-hour drug treatment.

before the initiation of mitosis in order for G$_2$ cells to enter mitosis is well documented (Tobey *et al.*, 1966). On the basis of this and other evidence, we suggest that exposure of cells to X rays or other clastogenic agents, such as the anticancer drugs included in this study, may result in the loss or modification of a gene or genes necessary for the synthesis of specific proteins required for the initiation of chromosome condensation and mitosis. The higher the incidence of chromosome damage, the greater the possibility of a loss or modification of gene(s) regulating the flow of cells from G$_2$ to mitosis.

B. G$_2$-Phase-Specific Proteins

To test whether specific proteins are involved in the G$_2$–mitosis transition, we compared the total cellular proteins of G$_2$-synchronized, G$_2$-arrested, and S-phase HeLa cells by two-dimensional polyacrylamide gel electrophoresis (Al-Bader *et al.*, 1978). Cells were synchronized by the excess TdR double-block method (Rao and Engelberg, 1966). Cells in S- and G$_2$-phases were obtained by harvesting at 1 and 7 hours, respectively, after reversal of the second TdR block. To induce G$_2$ arrest, synchronized S-phase cells were exposed to cis acid (75 μg/ml) for 60 minutes, the drug was removed, and the cells were incubated in drug-free medium for 16 hours; at the end, 90% of cells were blocked in G$_2$.

Whole cells were frozen immediately after collection, lyophilized, and stored at $-20°C$ until use. Total cellular proteins from G$_2$-arrested and G$_2$-synchronized cells were separated by sodium dodecyl sulfate (SDS) polyacrylamide slab gels. Long slab gels (26 cm long) were used to facilitate separation of the protein bands. A few protein bands in the molecular

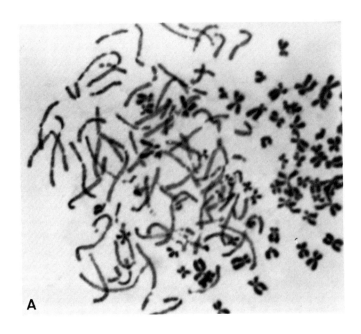

A

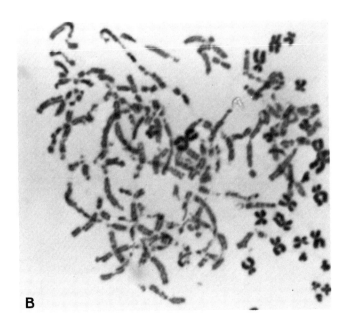

B

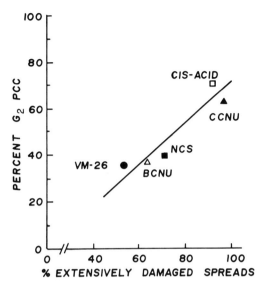

Fig. 4 Relationship between G_2 accumulation and chromosome damage. (From Rao and Rao, 1976.)

weight range of $4–5 \times 10^4$ were missing from the G_2-arrested cells (Fig. 5). Since these protein bands might represent more than one protein fraction of the same molecular weight, high-resolution two-dimensional gel electrophoresis (O'Farrell, 1975) was used. This technique allowed the complex protein patterns to be separated, first, according to their isoelectric point, and second, according to their molecular weight. Protein spots in different regions of the gel were circled in clusters for easier comparison and recognition of the missing spots. The number of protein spots present in each of the 14 clusters in the three different cell populations is shown in Table III. The number of spots in each cluster varied depending on the cell cycle phase. A significant number of proteins present in clusters G, J, K, and M of both G_2-synchronized and G_2-arrested cells were absent in S-phase cells. They are probably specific for the G_2-phase. A major difference between G_2-arrested and G_2-synchronized cells could be seen in cluster E. At least nine protein spots present in G_2-synchronized

---

Fig. 3 Prematurely condensed chromosomes (PCC) of HeLa cells synchronized in G_2-phase (A) and HeLa cells arrested in G_2 phase due to cis acid treatment (B). Extensive chromosome damage such as breaks and exchanges can be seen in these G_2 PCC of drug-treated cells. The highly condensed and darkly stained chromosomes to the right of the PCC spreads are from the mitotic HeLa cells.

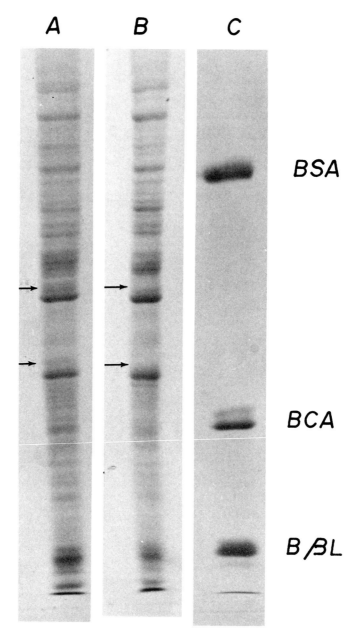

Fig. 5 One-dimensional polyacrylamide gradient (7.5–15.0%) gel of total cellular proteins of HeLa cells. (A) G₂-synchronized. (B) G₂-arrested cells. (C) Molecular-weight markers. BSA, Bovine serum albumin; BCA, bovine carbonic anhydrase; BβL, bovine β-lactoglobulin. Protein bands missing in G₂-arrested cells are indicated by arrows. (From Al-Bader *et al.*, 1978.)

TABLE III

Comparison of the Protein Profiles of S-phase, G$_2$-synchronized, and G$_2$-arrested HeLa Cells[a]

Cluster	Number of protein spots			Major difference in number of spots between:		
	S-phase	G$_2$-arrested	G$_2$-synchronized	G$_2$-synchronized and S-phase	G$_2$-arrested and S-phase	G$_2$-synchronized and G$_2$-arrested
A	12	12	13	—	—	—
B	14	10	14	—	—	—
C	12	9	10			
D	12	7	9			
E	6	6	15	9	0	9
F	10	8	11			
G	4	10	11	7	6	1
H	12	11	11			
I	9	7	9			
J	4	10	10	6	6	0
K	11	18	18	7	7	0
L	7	7	7			
M	3	9	9	6	6	0
N	4	4	6			
Total	120	128	153	35	25	10

[a] From Al-Bader et al. (1978).

cells were missing in S-phase and G_2-arrested cells. These proteins are probably required for the G_2–mitosis transition.

These experiments clearly demonstrated a correlation between the absence of certain proteins and the inability of the drug-treated cells to enter mitosis. However, when these proteins were supplied to the G_2-arrested cells by fusing them with G_2-synchronized cells, the treated cells were able to enter mitosis in synchrony with the untreated nucleus (Fig. 6). The mono-, bi, and trinucleate cells of the unlabeled (G_2-arrested) parent failed to enter mitosis. In about 50% of the "hybrid" binucleate cells carrying a labeled and an unlabeled nucleus, the unlabeled nucleus entered mitosis in synchrony with the labeled nucleus. In other words, a normal G_2 cell, upon fusion with a G_2-arrested cell, supplies the necessary factors so that both nuclei can enter mitosis synchronously.

If these agents cause damage to DNA, why are the cells not blocked in

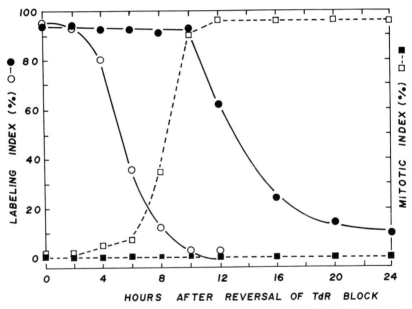

Fig. 6 Effect of cis acid treatment on the cell cycle progression of S-phase cells. HeLa cells were synchronized in S-phase by the excess TdR double-block method. Immediately after the reversal of the second TdR block, the cells were exposed to cis acid (75 μg/ml) for 1 hour. After removal of the drug, Colcemid (0.5 μg/ml) was added to the cultures and samples taken at regular intervals. The cell samples were pulse-labeled with ^{3}H[TdR] for 30 minutes and processed for autoradiography. The labeling index and mitotic accumulation are plotted as a function of time. Labeling index: ○, untreated control; ●, cis acid-treated cultures. Mitotic index: □, untreated control; ■, cis-acid-treated cultures. (From Al-Bader and Rao, unpublished data.)

other stages of the cell cycle? The damaging effects of alkylation of DNA become manifest during the first round of DNA replication after treatment. At this time, DNA strand breaks and realignment occur that would ultimately result in chromatid or chromosome breaks, deletions, fragments, and exchanges. At the dose of cis acid required to induce G_2 arrest, the integrity of the cellular genome was practically destroyed and its cloning ability was reduced to almost zero. This could result in the inactivation or alteration of some genes, which in turn could lead to the failure of protein synthesis. Since the damage occurs in S-phase, the synthesis of RNA and protein necessary for the transition of cells from G_2 to mitosis is affected. If these proteins are not made, the cells are not able to enter mitosis. However, supplying the missing proteins to the G_2-arrested cells by cell fusion with normal G_2 cells enabled the former to enter mitosis in synchrony with the latter.

V. Summary

The objective of this chapter has been to examine the cause of G_2 arrest induced by a variety of agents in mammalian cells. Reversible G_2 arrest in HeLa cells can be induced by substituting FPA for phenylalanine in the medium when the cells are in the middle to late part of S-phase. Replacing FPA-containing medium with regular culture medium, which contains 0.2 mM of phenylalanine, is adequate to reverse the G_2 block and allow the cells to enter mitosis. However, the G_2 block induced by most of the anticancer drugs is irreversible. Examination of the PCC of G_2-arrested HeLa or CHO cells revealed extensive chromosome damage. Studies with a variety of anticancer drugs revealed a positive correlation between their ability to induce chromosome damage and the frequency of G_2 arrest. Polyacrylamide gel electrophoretic examination of total cellular proteins indicated that certain protein bands in the range of $4-5 \times 10^4$ daltons, present in the G_2-synchronized and mitotic cells, were absent in G_2-arrested cells. Supplying the missing proteins to the G_2-arrested cells by fusing them with normal G_2 cells enabled them to enter mitosis.

On the basis of these data, we suggest the following working hypothesis. Specific proteins are synthesized during the G_2 period that are essential for the G_2–mitosis transition. Exposure of cells to clastogenic agents, such as anticancer drugs, leads to chromosome damage and consequently results in the inactivation or modification of certain genes that regulate the flow of cells from one phase of the cell cycle to the next. Since the damage to the genome is manifest during the first round of DNA replication after exposure to an alkylating agent, the gene(s) regulating the progress of cells through the G_2 period are affected. If these genes are inactivated or modified, the factors necessary for the initiation of mitosis are not synthesized, hence the cells are arrested in G_2.

References

Al-Bader, A. A., Orengo, A., and Rao, P. N. (1978). *Proc. Natl. Acad. Sci. U.S.A.* **75,** 6064.

Barlogie, B., Drewinko, B., Johnston, D. A., and Freireich, E. J. (1976). *Cancer Res.* **36,** 1975.

Barlogie, B., Drewinko, B., Gohde, W., and Bodey, G. P. (1977). *Cancer Res.* **37,** 2583.

Beford, J. S., and Mitchell, J. B. (1977). *Radiation Res.* **70,** 641.

Ebina, T., Ohtsuki, K., Seto, M., and Ishida, N. (1975). *Eur. J. Cancer* **11,** 155.

Everhart, L. P., and Prescott, D. M. (1972). *Exp. Cell Res.* **75,** 170.

Gohde, W., Schumann, J., Buchner, T., and Barlogie, B. (1974). *In* "Ergebnisse der Adriamycin-Therapie. Adriamycin-Symposium" (M. Ghione, J. Fetzer, and H. Maier, eds.), pp. 14–23. Springer-Verlag, Berlin and New York.

Homma, M., Koide, T., Saito-Koide, T., Kamo, I., Seto, M., Kumagai, K., and Ishida, N. (1970). *Proc. Int. Congr. Chemother, 6th,* Tokyo **2,** 410.

Ishida, N., Miyazaki, K., Kumagi, K., and Rikimaru, M. (1965). *J. Antibiot., Ser. A* **18,** 68.

Kishimoto, S., and Lieberman, I. (1964). *Exp. Cell Res.* **40,** 12.

Krishan, A., Paika, K., and Frei, E., III (1975). *J. Cell Biol.* **66,** 521.

Kumagai, K., Ono, Y., Nishikawa, T., and Ishida, N. (1966). *J. Antibiot., Ser. A* **19,** 69.

Meienhoffer, J., Maeda, H., Glaster, C. B., Czombos, J., and Kuromizu, K. (1972). *Science* **178,** 865.

Misra, N. C., and Roberts, D. (1975). *Cancer Res.* **35,** 99.

O'Farrell, P. H. (1975). *J. Biol. Chem.* **250,** 407.

Ohtsuki, K., and Ishida, N. (1975). *J. Antibiot.* (Tokyo) **28,** 143.

Puck, T. T., and Steffan, J. (1963). *Biophys. J.* **3,** 379.

Rao, A. P., and Rao, P. N. (1976). *J. Natl. Cancer Inst.* **57,** 1139.

Rao, P. N. (1968). *Science* **160,** 774.

Rao, P. N., and Engelberg, J. (1966). *In* "Cell Synchrony: Studies in Biosynthetic Regulation" (I. L. Cameron and G. M. Padilla, eds.), pp. 332–352. Academic Press, New York.

Rao, P. N., Wilson, B. A., and Puck, T. T. (1977). *J. Cell. Physiol.* **91,** 131.

Rueckert, R. R., and Mueller, G. C. (1960). *Cancer Res.* **20,** 1584.

Sunkara, P. S., Chakraborthy, B., and Rao, P. N. (1978). Unpublished data.

Tatsumi, K., Nakamura, T., and Wakisaka, G. (1974). *Gann* **65,** 459.

Taylor, E. W. (1963). *J. Cell Biol.* **19,** 1.

Terasima, T., and Tolmach, L. J. (1963). *Exp. Cell Res.* **30,** 344.

Tobey, R. A. (1975). *Nature (London)* **254,** 245.

Tobey, R. A., and Crissman, H. A. (1972). *Exp. Cell Res.* **75,** 466.

Tobey, R. A., and Ley, K. D. (1971). *Cancer Res.* **31,** 46.

Tobey, R. A., Petersen, D. F., Anderson, E. C., and Puck, T. T. (1966). *Biophys. J.* **6,** 567.

Tsuruo, T., Satoh, H., and Ukita, T. (1971). *J. Antibiot.* **24,** 423.

Wheatley, D. N., and Henderson, J. Y. (1975). *Exp. Cell Res.* **92,** 211.

Wheatley, D. N., and Inglis, M. S. (1977). *Exp. Cell Res.* **107,** 191.

21

Perspectives on the Research of New Anticancer Agents

A. DI MARCO

I. Introduction

The empirical approach to the pharmacological therapy of cancer is certainly the most ancient; South American and African Sciamani employed plant extracts for antitumor therapy long before western science acknowledged an imbalance in the regulation of cellular proliferative activity as the starting point of cancer. Some of these plant extracts have been recently reconsidered as sources of powerful antitumor agents, e.g., maytansine (Kupchan, 1976), which can be added to the list of drugs, such as colchicine and the *Vinca* alkaloids, of similar origin. Dependent from the observation of the leucopenic effect, was the introduction in cancer chemotherapy of nitrogen mustard (Gilman and Philips, 1946; Goodman *et al.*, 1946) later developed to the modern alkylating agents.

II. Discussion

The origin of powerful antitumor drugs, such as 5-fluorouracil and methotrexate, may be traced to the theory of the competition of synthetic substances with natural substracts, or coenzymes with essential biochemical functions (Fildes, 1940; Wood, 1940). The antibacterial drug sulfanilamide selectively kills bacterial cells and spares mammalian cells, since the biosynthetic pathway sensitive to the inhibition is not present in the latter. This is unfortunately not true of antitumor agents, because of the presence of identical pathways of nucleic acid synthesis from small precursors in normal and cancer cells. When actinomycin was discovered by Waksman and Woodruff (1940) and its antitumor effect recognized, many felt that this empirical approach (so fruitful in antibacterial therapy) could lead to agents active in cancer therapy. It was soon realized that this substance interfered with cellular activity in a very peculiar manner, binding to DNA and inhibiting its ability to function as a template in the transcription of genetic information.

Many other microbial products were subsequently isolated, and a few, such as mitomycin, bleomycins, and anthracyclines, were recognized to have clinical usefulness. Their antiproliferative effect is generally understood to be based on damage to DNA or, as regards anthracyclines, impairment in its template activity in replication and transcription (Di Marco, 1967, 1978; Di Marco et al., 1975). A selective effect on the genetic material could arise from preferential binding of the antibiotic to a specific base sequence or as a consequence of a peculiar feature in the structure of the chromatin.

Actinomycin D has been observed to bind preferentially to guanine-containing sequences (purine–pyrimidine) | (purine–pyrimidine), whereas an increased number of binding sites for adriamycin has been recognized in the alternating copolymer poly (dA-dT) | poly (dA-dT) (Phillips et al., 1978). The latter finding is consistent with inactivation of the template properties of DNA polymerase I from *Escherichi coli* and DNA polymerase from rat liver. A high frequency of these base pairs in repetitive sequences with regulatory functions could help explain the preferential inhibition of some polymerase systems, such as MSV polymerase (Zunino et al., 1974).

In the *in vivo* situation, however, nuclear proteins influence considerably the interaction of intercalating agents with the native chromatin structure. According to the intercalation model (Pigram et al., 1972), daunorubicin lies in the large groove of DNA and should therefore compete with the terminal amino groups of lysine in the H_4 histone (Lovie et al., 1974). Since neutralization of the negative charge of DNA phosphate radicals by the cationic amino group reduces the electrical repulsion between the two DNA strands, the intercalator may cause local denaturation of DNA by this mechanism. In agreement with the observed reduction in affinity and in the number of chromatin-binding sites (Table I) (Zunino et al., 1978) of adriamycin, if compared to DNA, it is possible that histones, and most likely nonhistone nuclear proteins (NHNP), control a specific binding to DNA sequences with a regulatory function.

A question that arose soon after the discovery of antimicrobial antibi-

TABLE I

Interaction of Adriamycin with DNA and Chromatin

Parameter	DNA–adriamycin	Chromatin–adriamycin
$K_{app.}$	17.5×10^6	$5.9 \pm 0.8 \times 10^6$
n	0.230	0.137 ± 0.001

otics was: What is their function in the producing organism? It appears now that some of them, e.g., gramicidin (and tyrocidins), may have a specific regulatory function as inhibitors of transcription initiation during the transition from vegetative growth to sporulation (Paulus and Sarkar, 1976). The mechanism of action consists of inhibition of formation of the binary complex between RNA polymerase and DNA and an increase in its dissociation rate. A similar mechanism appears to operate in the inhibiting effect of actinomycin D on transcription in the producing organism (Yoshida *et al.*, 1966).

The recognized ability of the oligopeptide distamycin to form complexes with DNA by the interaction of amide groups with AT base pairs (Gursky *et al.*, 1976) may be taken as a model for specific DNA–protein interactions similar to the interaction of lac and lambda repressors with their specific operators. Since the specificity of the interaction appears to be determined by the nature of the side chains of the peptide backbone, polypeptides active in regulation should have an high degree of complexity.

Could these antibiotics have a specific effect on the regulation of gene expression in eukaryotic cells? It is amazing that actinomycin D, when administered to cultured cells in very low doses, has a paradoxical enhancing effect on RNA synthesis. As suggested by Tomkins *et al.* (1972), this may be due to the inhibitory effect of the antibiotic on the transcription of regulatory DNA sequences. In the Britten and Davidson model (Britten and Davidson, 1969), regulatory RNA molecules or their translation products, coded for by integrator genes, presumably interact with receptor DNA sequences contiguous to each producer gene in a battery of functionally related genes. Since the inhibition of transcription of the regulatory gene by actinomycin D causes enhancement of total RNA synthesis, it could be deduced that the physiological function of integrator RNA, or the corresponding protein, is to repress the transcription of a series of integrator genes (Fig. 1).

Since the effect on regulatory gene activity is observed at a lower concentration than in the case of structural genes, the drug appears to have an higher affinity for the chromatin structure of regulatory genes.

Low doses of adriamycin (1 ng/ml) enhance thymidine incorporation in growing (or conditioned) MEF (Fig. 2); this effect may be the conse-

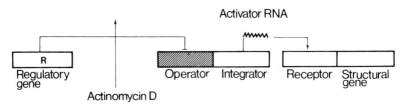

Fig. 1 Supposed effect of actinomycin D on the regulation of gene expression.

quence of early stimulation of RNA synthesis in the same cells and therefore of derepression of a regulatory gene.

There is evidence that a similar negative control is present in regulation of the cell cycle; it was observed, in fact, that the number of mitotic figures in epidermal cells after wounding was reduced by translation inhibitors but increased by actinomycin D (Gelfant and Candelas, 1972). The antibiotic effect would consist of inhibiting the synthesis of a regulatory RNA coding for a specific repressor (chalone) of the transition between G_2 and M. Negative control of cellular replication mediated by chalones appears to regulate the transition between G_0- and G_1- or S-phases in most tissues (Honck, 1976).

It has been suggested (Attallah and Honck, 1976) that the glycoprotein with chalone activity has two active sites: one specific for the cell membrane and the other nonspecifically stimulating the activity of adenyl cyclase. A consequence of binding of the chalone to the cell surface would therefore be an increase in the concentration of the nucleotide 3′,5′-cyclic adenosine monophosphate (cAMP) over the critical concentration.

This negative regulation at certain critical stages in cell replication ap-

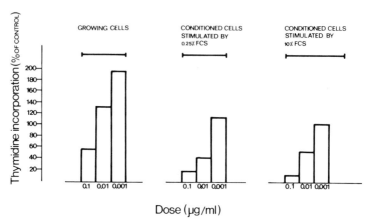

Fig. 2 Activity of adriamycin on thymidine incorporation in MEF.

pears to overlap a positive regulation; initiation of RNA or protein synthesis in G_1 is required, in fact, to permit the cells to enter S-phase. Nuclear transplantation and cellular fusion experiments suggest, furthermore, that the initiation of DNA synthesis in the many replicons of eukaryotic chromosomes is under the positive control of cytoplasmic factors (Lewin, 1976). Since coordinated gene expression is certainly preprogrammed at the genetic level, it may be supposed that the influence of cytoplasmic or external factors on the flow of information from the genome is due to the specific interaction of proteins with certain genes. The ability of proteins to interact specifically with small molecules could be the bridge between external information and the genome. The coordinated expression of functionally related genes in eukaryotic cells may be achieved by the interaction of more copies of regulatory proteins with the regulatory sequences adjacent to each functional gene.

The hypothesis of the role played by NHNPs in regulation is supported by observations made on reconstituted chromatin. Kostraba and Wang (1972) demonstrated, by RNA–DNA hybridization experiments, the presence of RNA species similar to those synthesized from Walker tumor when (NHCPs) were used to activate the *in vitro* transcription of rat liver chromatin. Conversely, RNA species similar to those synthesized from rat liver chromatin were demonstrated when NHCPs from normal rat liver were used to activate the *in vitro* transcription of Walker tumor chromatin, which suggests that NHCPs are at least partially responsible for the transcriptional differences between rat liver and Walker tumor (Stein *et al.*, 1978).

The sensory structure originally proposed by Davidson and Britten might result, in its simpler form, from a sensory protein located at the cell membrane or in the cytoplasm (receptor) and able to interact specifically with hormones or inducers (Fig. 3). This scheme is consistent with the known pattern of nuclear activation by estrogens following interaction with the specific cytoplasmic (4 S) receptor, its consequent modification to the 5 S form, nuclear transport, and interaction with the chromatin receptor. Whereas the molecular basis of the transcriptional effect of steroid hormones is still not well understood, more is known about the chain of biochemical events following interactions with the cell membrane of polypeptide hormones, which are transduced to the level of the regulation of metabolic activities by the second messenger, cAMP. The metabolic role of this nucleotide may be deduced also from studies on the mechanism of action of anthracyclines.

The inhibiting effect of adriamycin on MEF is highest when the drug is administered during the first few hours after serum addition (Fig. 4) (Supino *et al.*, 1977), when DNA synthesis has not yet begun.

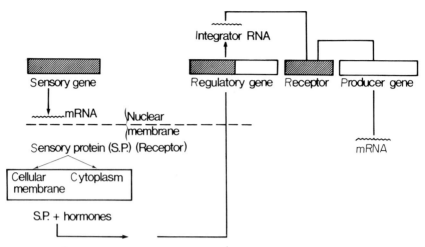

Fig. 3 Interaction of sensory proteins with regulatory genes.

It appears likely therefore that the antibiotic interferes with an early event, occurring shortly after serum addition, that is required for the cells to enter the S-phase.

It is well known that enhanced RNA and protein synthesis are caused by the addition of fresh serum to conditioned cultures, and it is therefore easy to observe an early inhibition in total RNA synthesis in MEF cultures stimulated by serum and immediately treated with adriamycin (Fig. 5).

The question arises, however, of possible drug interference with an earlier process triggered by the growth factors present in fetal serum. To answer this question we have measured the effect of the addition of serum on the level of cAMP in MEF conditioned cultures. As shown in Fig. 6

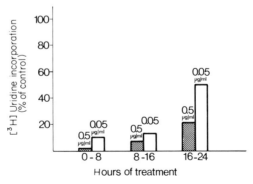

Fig. 4 Effect of adriamycin on DNA synthesis in serum-stimulated MEF.

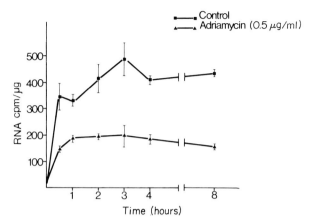

Fig. 5 Effect of adriamycin on RNA synthesis in serum-stimulated MEF.

(Supino and Di Marco, 1978), the addition of serum causes a rapid increase in the cAMP level which afterward returns to lower values. Adriamycin at the cytotoxic concentration (10^{-6} or 10^{-7} M) has a pronounced
inhibitory effect on this early peak of cAMP synthesis.

It has been postulated (Kuo and Greengard, 1969) that the known effects of this nucleotide on transcription and transcriptionally controlled
enzyme induction are mediated through activation of cellular cAMP-dependent protein kinases (PKs). Genetic analysis supports this contention;
Insel et al. (1975) in fact showed that in mutant 849 lymphoma cells,
which lack cAMP-dependent PK, and their wild type, which possess this
enzyme, only the wild-type cells responded to cAMP by induction of
phosphodiesterase. Costa et al. (1975, 1976) established a close temporal
correlation between the elevation of cAMP in the adrenal medulla, activation of cAMP-dependent PK, nuclear translocation of the C-unit, activation of RNA synthesis (total RNA and RNA), and transsynaptic induction

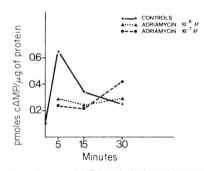

Fig. 6 Effect of adriamycin on cAMP levels induced by serum in MEF cultures.

of tyrosine hydroxylase. Jungmann and Kranias (1977) have recently proposed that cAMP-dependent PK from the cytoplasm achieves phosphorylation of nuclear proteins after translocation of the dissociated catalytic and regulatory unit to chromatin acceptor sites.

The precise mechanism of the modulating effect of phosphorylation on gene expression is still unclear and may involve increased availability for the transcription of specific sites of DNA, or a more direct effect on RNA polymerases through covalent phosphorylative modification of the enzyme subunits. This change may be brought by cAMP-dependent as well as cAMP-independent kinases. The latter type of enzyme is localized in the nucleus and maintains a constant specific activity throughout the cell cycle, in contrast to cytoplasmic cAMP-dependent PK which shows activation and synthesis throughout the transition from G_1 to S (Costa et al., 1977). The increase in activity and the synthesis of cAMP-dependent PK during the G_1–S transition suggests that phosphorylation of some proteins is required for cells to enter S-phase. This appears to be in contrast to the negative regulatory effect of cAMP on the cellular activity of cultures approaching confluence (Fig. 7) (Perdue and Raizada, 1976). This paradoxical effect may be understood by assuming that cAMP below a certain concentration is required for enzyme induction, while over this critical concentration it exerts an direct inhibitory effect on many enzymes by allosteric modifications or by enzyme phosphorylation as reported for PK (Rion, 1978). This may explain the inhibitory effect observed at confluence on cAMP PD and Na^+, K^+-ATPase.

It has been recently proposed (Hadden et al., 1972; Rudland et al., 1974) that most cellular activities are regulated by the balance of cAMP and cGMP. Coffey et al. (1977) have shown, in fact, that the capacity of mitogens to stimulate DNA synthesis in human lymphocytes is correlated with the capacity to increase the cGMP concentration and that the participation of Ca^{2+} is essential to mediate the mitogenic effect (Hadden et al., 1975). The messenger activity of cGMP has been related to the increase in synthesis, phosphorylation, and DNA binding of NHNPs (Johnson et al., 1974a,b), to the synthesis of DNA-dependent RNA polymerases I and III, and to RNA synthesis (Goldberg et al., 1976; Hadden et al., 1976; John-

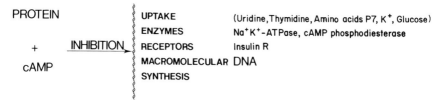

Fig. 7 Effect of cAMP on cellular activity in confluent cultures.

son and Hadden, 1975). It is known that many hormones (such as acetyl-choline, α-adrenergic agonists, histamine, serotonin, prostaglandin F, estrogens, oxytocin, and insulin) increase the level of cGMP in sensitive cells. Regulation of the proliferative activity in some tissues could therefore be achieved by a multikey system of interaction of chemical mediators (hormones, chalones) with receptors at the cell surface or periphery. This first stage of interaction could be transduced by the activity of the key enzymes, adenyl cyclase and guanyl cyclase, and cAMP or cGMP association with specific proteins, with effects at the nuclear level.

It is a widely expressed view that neoplastic growth is due to the loss of a regulatory mechanism of gene expression; this may result from an impairment in one or more of the different steps in which cyclic nucleotides are involved. A decrease in adenyl cyclase activity is considered a consistent change in virus-transformed cells (Pastan and Johnson, 1976). Furthermore, a different response to environmental influences may be present; in highly differentiated Morris hepatoma the enhancing effect of glucagon on cAMP synthesis is of the same order of magnitude as that of adult rat liver, but on the least differentiated hepatoma it is like the effect on fetal neonatal rat liver (Butcher *et al.*, 1972). Knowledge of these physiological mechanisms is essential not only for a clear understanding of important adverse effects on differentiated tissues but also for a more sophisticated approach to therapy.

Regulatory mechanisms, which are essential for a correct specialized function, may be dispensed with in tumor cells. This, however, does not necessarily mean that neoplastic cells have lost all the markers peculiar to differentiated cells, such as antigens, enzymes, and hormone receptors. A precise knowledge of these markers is essential for understanding the biochemical lesion peculiar to an individual tumor and for a rational approach to devising a specific therapy.

Quantitative and qualitative changes in hormone receptors have been frequently observed in cancer cells and may reflect the transition to earlier developmental stages of the tissue (Cikes, 1978).

The existence at the membrane or cytoplasmaic level of macromolecules with a specific affinity for hormones opens the way to a selective influence on genomic activity by drugs able to compete with natural agonists. An alternative approach could consist of the use of drugs able to interfere specifically with the synthesis of receptors critical for survival of the cancer cells. A control role in the synthesis of estrogen receptors in normal target tissue, as well as in neoplastic growth [such as the (DMBA)-induced mammary tumors in rats], is exerted by the polypeptidic hormone prolactin (Horrobin, 1975). In developing mammary gland this hormone induces the synthesis of a cAMP-dependent PK most likely involved in the differentiation pathway. In fact, in organ cultures of this tissue, in the presence of cortisol and insulin, a substantial increase occurs in the marker enzyme glucose-6-phosphate dehydrogenase. This effect may be mimicked by exogenous spermidine, in the absence of prolactin, and abolished by indomethacin in the presence of prolactin (Horrobin, 1974, 1975). On the other hand, in the same target tissue prolactin has a stimulating effect on RNA synthesis, which is mimicked by cGMP and prostaglandin F and inhibited by cAMP, phosphodiesterase inhibitors, and prostaglandin E. The dual effect may be understood assuming that the primary effect of the hormone after interaction with the receptor is on the synthesis of prostaglandin E or F, depending on the predominant cell receptors (Russell and Byus, 1976) or the hormone concentration (Fig. 8).

An interaction between cAMP and estrogenic hormones at the nuclear level is suggested by the observation (Cho-Chung *et al.*, 1978) that cAMP-binding proteins accumulate in the nuclei of a regressing tumor after ovariectomy in parallel with the reduced amount of estrogen receptors in the cytosol and nuclei. Translocation of cytoplasmic cAMP binding and PK activity was found in regressing tumors after ovariectomy (Cho-Chung and Redler, 1977; Cho-Chung *et al.*, 1978) or following dibutyryl cAMP treatment. It was suggested that the phosphorylation of nuclear proteins may be involved in the action of cAMP-binding protein.

Our working hypothesis is that cAMP-dependent PK is induced by the hormone prolactin and plays an essential role in modulating gene expression in the normal mammary gland. One interesting possibility is that binding to cAMP achieves conversion of the enzyme to a phosphorylated form which interferes with the transcription of genes essential to cell replication.

The loss of dependence on cAMP of the PK, resulting from the carcinogenic effect at the level of the regulatory subunit, could impair the modulating activity of PK, which could explain the enhancing effect of hormone administration, after the carcinogen, on the development and growth of the tumor. This is in contrast to the antagonistic effect on mammary tumors in rats previously given the carcinogen (Davidson and Britten, 1971; Pearson *et al.*, 1969).

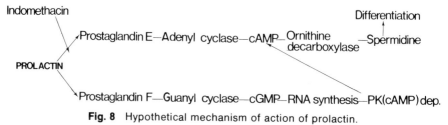

Fig. 8 Hypothetical mechanism of action of prolactin.

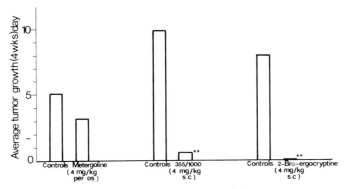

Fig. 9 Activity of DMBA-induced tumors.

The dependence on prolactin of almost half of DMBA-induced tumors in the rat is demonstrated by the regression of these tumors after treatment of intact animals with prolactin secretion inhibitors, such as 2-bromo-α-ergocryptine and the recently synthesized 6-methyl-β-idrossi-acetyl-10 α-ergolynebenzoato (Figs. 9 and 10) (Table II). (Beacco *et al.*, 1978; Formelli *et al.*, personal communication).

This effect could be ascribed to a reduced synthesis of estrophillines or to a more general interference with gene expression in tumor cells bound to the conversion and nuclear translocation of cAMP-binding protein.

The next point to consider is: Can an unreversible change in this control mechanism be responsible for the autonomous growth of nonregressing tumors?

The existence of more primitive mechanisms of control, such as that operating during embryonic development, should be explored. Hormones or other unknown factors produced at definite stages of embryonic de-

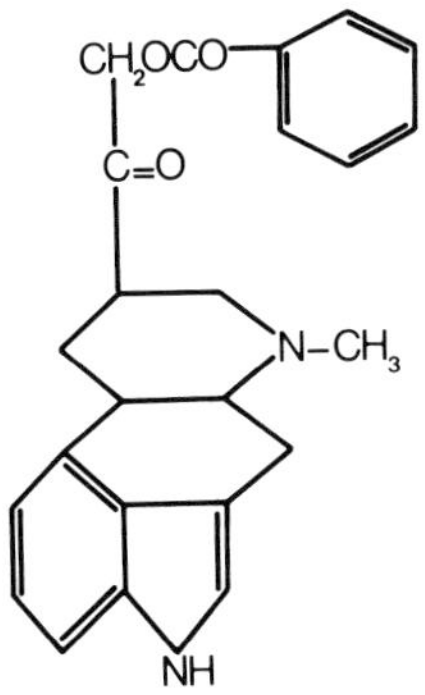

Fig. 10 6-Methyl-β-idrossiacetyl-10-α-ergolynebenzoato.

TABLE II

Activity of DMBA-Induced Tumors

Treatment	Start of treatment (days)	Number of initial tumors per rat	Effect at the end of a 4-week treatment					Toxicity	Death at 5 months
			CR$_1$	PR$_2$	NC$_3$	P$_4$	New tumors		
Control	73–80	1.6	1	1	11	18	13	—	6/11
355/1000	73–80	1.5	9	2	4	5	3	0/11	0/11
Metergolina	80	1.4	1	0	12	9	9	2/9	3/9
CB$_{154}$	94	1.4	4	5	2	0	0	0/8	0/8
355/1000	108	1.7	4	0	4	4	0	0/7	0/7
Late control	123	1.5	0	1	3	6	4	—	0/4

[a] CR$_1$, Complete remission, no tumor palpable; PR$_2$, partial remission, reduction in tumor size to >50% of initial tumor size; NC$_3$, no change, tumor size 51–150%; P$_4$, progression, tumor size >151%.

velopment may bring about coordinated gene expression that leads to the specific regression of tissues and organs no longer required in the adult state. It is well known that the regression of structures (such as the tail in tadpoles) is preprogrammed in the embryo and that the hormone, in this case thyroxine or triiodothyronine, triggers the synthesis of new RNA and protein synthesis preceding the burst of hydrolytic enzyme activity (Tata, 1969). From fetal testes Donahoe has recently isolated a substance that causes the regression of Mullerian ductal carcinomas in animal embryos and the selective inhibition of ovary carcinoma cells in culture (Donahoe, 1978). Similar mechanisms may still be present in the adult; the autolytic reaction triggered in thymocytes by the interaction and subsequent transport to the nucleus of cortisol with its receptors is well known (Rosenau *et al.*, 1972).

III. Conclusion

To conclude it appears that substantial improvement in cancer therapy may be achieved by an increased knowledge of the regulatory mechanisms of gene expression in normal and malignant cells and by the use of the still poorly known agents that affect these processes.

References

Attallah, A. M., and Honck, J. C. (1976). *In* "Chalones" (J. C. Honck, ed.), pp. 355–383. North-Holland Publ./Am. Elsevier, New York.

Beacco, E., Bernardi, L., diSalle, E., Falconi, G., and Patelli, I. (1978). Belg. Pat. No. 861, 480.

Britten, R. J., and Davidson, E. H. (1969). *Science* **165**, 349.

Butcher, F. R., Scott, D. F., Potter, R. V., and Morris, H. P. (1972). *Cancer Res.* **32**, 2135.

Cho-Chung, Y. S., and Redler, B. H. (1977). *Science* **197**, 272.

Cho-Chung, Y. S., Bodwin, J. S., and Clair, T. (1978). *J. Natl. Cancer Inst.* **60**, 1175.

Cikes, M. (1978). *Eur. J. Cancer* **14**, 211.

Coffey, R. G., Hadden, E. M., and Hadden, J. W. (1977). *J. Immunol.* **119**, 1387.

Costa, E., Chuang, D. M., Guidotti, A., and Uzunon, P. (1975). *In* "Chemical Tools in Catecholamine Research" (O. Almgren, A. Carlsson, and I. Engel, eds.), Vol. 2, pp. 283–292. North Holland Publ., Amsterdam.

Costa, E., Kurosawa, A., and Guidotti, A. (1976). *Proc. Natl. Acad. Sci. U.S.A.* **73**, 1058.

Costa, E., Fuller, D. J. M., Russell, D. H., and Gerner, E. W. (1977). *Biochim. Biophys. Acta* **479**, 416.

Davidson, E. H., and Britten, R. J. (1971). *J. Theor. Biol.* **32**, 123.

Di Marco, A. (1967). *In* "Antibiotics" (D. Gottlieb and P. D. Shaw, eds.), Vol. 1, pp. 190–210. Springer-Verlag, Berlin and New York.

Di Marco, A. (1978). *Antibiot. Chemother.* **23**, 216.

Di Marco, A., Arcamone, F., and Zunino, F. (1975). *In* "Antibiotics" (D. Gottlieb and P. D. Shaw, eds.), Vol. 3, pp. 101–128. Springer-Verlag, Berlin and New York.

Donahoe. *Gordon Res. Conf.*

Fildes, F. (1940). *Lancet* **1**, 955.

Gelfant, S., and Candelas, G. (1972). *J. Invest. Dermatol.* **59**, 7.

Gilman, A., and Philips, F. S. (1946). *Science* **103**, 409.

Goldberg, N. D., Haddox, M. K., Nicol, S. E., Acott, T. S., Glass, D. B., and Zeilij, C. E. (1976). *In* "Control Mechanisms in Cancer" (W. E. Criss, T. Ono, and J. R. Sabine, eds.). Raven, New York.

Goodman, L. S., Wintrobe, M. M., Damershek, W., Goodman, M. J., Gilman, A., and McLennan, M. (1946). *J. Am. Med. Assoc.* **132**, 126.

Gursky, G. V., Tumanyan, V. G., Zasedatelev, A. S., Zhuze, A. L., Grokhovsky, S. L., and Gottikn, B. P. (1976). *Mol. Biol. Rep.* **2**, 413.

Hadden, J. W., Hadden, E. M., Haddox, M. K., and Goldberg, N. D. (1972). *Proc. Natl. Acad. Sci. U.S.A.* **69**, 3024.

Hadden, J. W., Hadden, E. M., Johnson, L. D., and Johnson, E. M. (1975). *In* "Lymphocytes and Their Interactions: Recent Observations" (R. C. Williams, Jr., ed.), Kroc Foundation Symposia Series, Vol. 4, pp. 27–45. Raven, New York.

Hadden, J. W., Johnson, E. M., Hadden, E. M., Coffey, R. G., and Johnson, L. D. (1976). *In* "Immune Recognition" (A. Rosenthal, ed.), p. 359. Academic Press, New York.

Honck, J. C., ed. (1976). "Chalones." North-Holland Publ./Am. Elsevier, New York.

Horrobin, D. F. (1974). *Prolactin, Annu. Res. Rev.*

Horrobin, D. F. (1975). *Prolactin, Annu. Res. Rev.*

Insel, P. A., Bourne, H. R., Coffino, P., and Tomkins, G. M. (1975). *Science* **190**, 896.

Johnson, E. M., Hadden, J. W., Karn, J., and Allfrey, V. G. (1974a). *Fed. Proc., Fed. Am. Soc. Exp. Biol.* **33**, 508.

Johnson, E. M., Karn, J., and Allfrey, V. G. (1974b). *J. Biol. Chem.* **249**, 4990.

Johnson, L. D., and Hadden, J. W. (1975). *Biochem. Biophys. Res. Commun.* **66**, 1498.

Jungmann, R. A., and Kranias, E. G. (1977). *Int. J. Biochem.* **8**, 819.

Kostraba, N. C., and Wang, T. Y. (1972). *Cancer Res.* **32**, 2348.

Kuo, J. F., and Greengard, P. (1969). *Proc. Natl. Acad. Sci. U.S.A.* **64**, 1349.

Kupchan, S. M. (1976). *Cancer Treat. Rep.* **60**(8), 1115.

Lewin, B. (1976). "Gene Expression," Vol. 2. Wiley, New York.

Lovie, A. J., Candido, E. P. M., and Dixon, G. H. (1974). *Cold Spring Harbor Symp. Quant. Biol.* **38**, 803.

Pastan, I., and Johnson, G. S. (1976). *In* "Control Mechanisms in Cancer" (W. E. Criss, T. Ono, and J. R. Sabine, eds.). Raven, New York.

Paulus, H., and Sarkar, H. (1976). *In* "Molecular Mechanisms in the Control of Gene Expression" (D. P. Nierlich, W. J. Rutter, C. F. Fox, eds.), pp. 177–194. Academic Press, New York.

Pearson, O. H., Lierena, O., Lierena, L., Molina, A., and Butler, T. (1969). *Trans. Assoc. Am. Physicians* **82**, 225.

Perdue, J. F., and Raizada, M. K. (1976). *In* "Membranes and Neoplasia" (V. T. Marchesi, ed.), Progress in Clinical and Biological Research, Vol. 9, pp. 49–64. Alan R. Liss, New York.

Phillips, D. R., Di Marco, A., and Zunino, F. (1978). *Eur. J. Biochem.* **85**, 487.

Pigram, W. J., Fuller, W., and Hamilton, L. D. (1972). *Nature (London), New Biol.* **235**, 17.

Rion, J. P. (1978). *J. Biol. Chem.* **253**, 656.

Rosenau, W., Baxter, J. D., Rousseau, G. G., and Tomkins, G. M. (1972). *Nature (London), New Biol.* **237**, 20.

Rudland, P. S., Gospodarowicz, D., and Seifert, A. E. (1974). *Nature (London)* **250**, 741.

Russell, D. H., and Byus, C. V. (1976). *Life Sci.* **19**, 1306.

Stein, G. S., Stein, J. L., and Thomson, J. A. (1978). *Cancer Res.* **38**, 1181.

Supino, R., and Di Marco, A. (1978). Personal communication.

Supino, R., Casazza, A. M., and Di Marco, A. (1977a). *Tumori* **63**, 31.

Supino, R., Necco, A., Dasdia, T., Casazza, A. M., and Di Marco, A. (1977b). *Cancer Res.* **37**, 4523.

Tata, J. R. (1969). *Sci. Basis Med.* p. 112.

Tomkins, G. M., Levinson, B. B., Baxter, J. D., and Dethlefsen, L. (1972). *Nature (London), New Biol.* **239**, 9.

Waksman, S. A., and Woodruff, H. B. (1940). *Proc. Soc. Exp. Biol. Med.* **45**, 609.

Wood, D. D. (1940). *Br. J. Exp. Pathol.* **21**, 74.

Yoshida, T., Weissenbach, H., and Kate, E. (1966). *Arch. Biochem. Biophys.* **114**, 252.

Zunino, F., Di Marco, A., Zaccara, A., and Luoni, G. (1974). *Chem.-Biol. Interact.* **9**, 25.

Zunino, F., Zaccara, A., and Di Marco, A. (1978). Personal communication.

22

Isoproterenol-Stimulated Induction of Lactate Dehydrogenase and Modulation of Nuclear Protein Kinase Activity in C_6 Rat Glioma Cells

RICHARD A. JUNGMANN, MARY L. CHRISTENSEN, and DENNIS F. DERDA

Despite present advances in molecular biology, the mechanism of regulation of eukaryotic gene transcription is still poorly understood, in large part because of the genetic and structural complexities of eukaryotic chromosomes. We do know that transcriptional control in eukaryotes requires structural and functional alterations of chromosomal proteins associated with the DNA. These nuclear proteins influence the structure of the genetic material, strengthen or weaken the interaction of the RNA polymerase with the chromatin template, modulate the activity of RNA polymerase, and serve to transmit physiological control signals for gene activation or repression in response to stimuli such as hormones and cyclic nucleotides.

Activation of membrane-bound adenyl cyclase and increased formation of intracellular cyclic AMP (cAMP) is thought to be the mechanism by which a number of effector agents, including a variety of peptide and protein hormones, catecholamines, and many drugs, produce their gene regulatory effects (Jungmann and Kranias, 1977). In addition to the direct acute effect of cAMP and cAMP-dependent protein kinase on metabolic processes not involving transcriptional activity, cAMP and its protein kinase have been implicated in the induction of nuclear RNA and protein synthesis (Jungmann and Russell, 1977). From the presently available evidence it is thought that cAMP-mediated phosphorylation of nonhistone chromosomal proteins plays a major regulatory role in the control of gene expression (Jungmann and Kranias, 1977).

The enhancing effect of catecholamines on C_6 glioma cell lactate dehydrogenase (LDH) activity was initially observed by DeVellis and Brooker (1973) in their experiments with the C_6 subclone of a chemically induced rat glial cell carcinoma. Subsequently, they were able to mimic the effect of isoproterenol with exogenous dibutyryl cAMP and/or theophylline, a phosphodiesterase inhibitor. The suggested involvement of cAMP was further substantiated by the fact that isoproterenol within fractions of a minute after its application to glioma cells raised intracellular cAMP levels for periods of up to 30 minutes. Since actinomycin D and cycloheximide prevented the rise in LDH activity, DeVellis and Brooker (1973) postulated that cAMP-mediated *de novo* LDH synthesis rather than activation of preexisting LDH protein was involved.

I. Effect of Isoproterenol on LDH Activity and Synthesis

Figure 1 illustrates the dose-dependent effect of isoproterenol on the activation of glioma cell LDH and on the level of intracellular cAMP. The inference that *de novo* synthesis rather than activation of preexisting LDH molecules occurred after isoproterenol stimulation of glioma cells was borne out by our direct immunochemical measurement of the rate of LDH synthesis. Figure 2 illustrates the time-dependent changes in LDH enzymic activation as well as in LDH synthesis after isoproterenol stimulation. Synthesis of LDH isozyme was significantly increased as early as 90 minutes after isoproterenol stimulation. No concomitant increase in LDH activity was observed, rather there was a lag period until the LDH

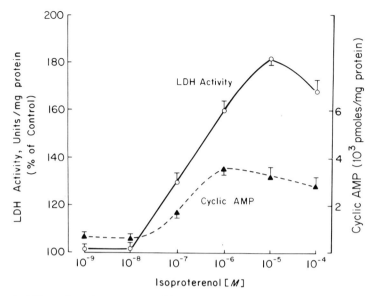

Fig. 1 Effect of varying amounts of isoproterenol on LDH activity and cAMP levels in rat C$_6$ glioma cells. Isoproterenol was added to the culture medium at the indicated concentrations. Intracellular cAMP levels were assayed 15 minutes after isoproterenol addition as described by DeAngelo et al.,(1975). LDH activity in 105,000 g supernatant fractions was assayed by measuring the conversion of pyruvate to lactic acid (Kaplan and Ciotti, 1961). Cultures were 11 days old and in stationary phase for the last 3 days. Each point is the average value obtained from four cultures. Brackets indicate ± SD.

activity was markedly increased. A decline in the rate of LDH synthesis set in 12 hours after isoproterenol stimulation, at which time LDH activity was still increasing. A similar alteration in LDH synthesis and activity could also be achieved after the stimulation of glioma cells with 5×10^{-4}–$10^{-3} M$ dibutyryl cAMP. Evidence that isoproterenol causes an early dose-dependent increase in glioma cell cAMP levels and that the cAMP analogue dibutyryl cAMP mimics the effect of isoproterenol on LDH synthesis strongly indicates the cAMP-dependent nature of the LDH induction. It suggests that cAMP, in an as yet unknown fashion, stimulates the selective synthesis of LDH via a transcriptional or translational mechanism.

The assumption that cAMP acts via a transcriptional mechanism and causes the synthesis or activation of mRNA for LDH has been tested in our laboratory. We recently measured the level of active LDH mRNA in a cell-free wheat germ translational system during isoproterenol-stimulated LDH induction (Miles and Jungmann, unpublished data). The glioma cells were stimulated with $10^{-5} M$ isoproterenol. Under these conditions the

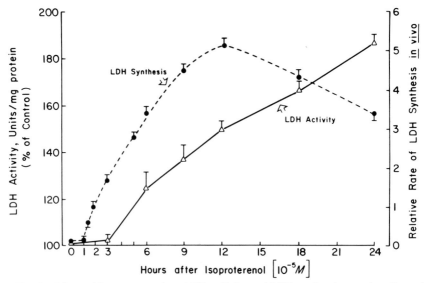

Fig. 2 Effect of isoproterenol on LDH activity and LDH synthesis as a function of time. Isoproterenol at 10^{-5} M was added to stationary 11-day-old cultures. LDH activity was assayed in glioma cell 105,000 g supernatant fractions as described in the legend for Fig. 1. LDH synthesis was determined after pulse-labeling of cultures with [³H]leucine for 1 hour before harvesting cells. Tritium-labeled LDH was collected by immunoprecipitation. The immunoprecipitate was dissociated in 10 mM Tris, pH 7.0, 1 mM EDTA, 0.5% sodium dodecyl sulfate (SDS), and subjected to polyacrylamide gel electrophoresis in the presence of 0.1% SDS. LDH synthesis is represented as the ratio of [³H]leucine incorporated into LDH protein to [³H]leucine incorporated into total protein. Data are means ± SD for three cultures.

levels of active LDH mRNA were significantly increased within 90 minutes after isoproterenol treatment, suggesting that, at least in part, synthesis or activation of LDH mRNA played a functional role in LDH induction.

II. cAMP-Mediated Changes in Protein Kinase Activity during LDH Induction

Whereas the regulation of glioma cell LDH synthesis by cAMP most probably involves changes in the cell content of LDH mRNA, there is as yet no direct experimental evidence of the underlying molecular mechanism by which cAMP triggers the induction of LDH synthesis. Although the proposed mechanisms of cAMP-mediated gene induction in eukaryotes are still largely hypothetical (Jungmann and Russell, 1977; Jung-

mann and Kranias, 1977), our laboratory has been instrumental in elucidating the potential role of cAMP and cAMP-dependent nuclear protein
kinase in controlling gene expression and DNA transcription (Jungmann
and Kranias, 1977). Our working hypothesis is that cAMP, through activation of cAMP-dependent protein kinase and nuclear protein phosphorylation, may selectively control genetic information and determine its repression or derepression.

In view of the markedly isoproterenol-stimulated elevation of glioma
cell cAMP levels (see Figs. 1 and 4), we determined the degree of cAMP-
mediated dissociation of the cAMP-dependent protein kinase holoenzyme
in intact glioma cells. Glioma cell cytosol contains both type I and type II
protein kinase isozymes (Fig. 3). Determination of the DEAE-cellulose
elution profiles of glioma cell protein kinase isozymes at various times
after isoproterenol stimulation revealed a marked reduction in the type I
protein kinase elution area after isoproterenol stimulation, whereas type
II protein kinase elution areas remained essentially unchanged (Fig. 3). A

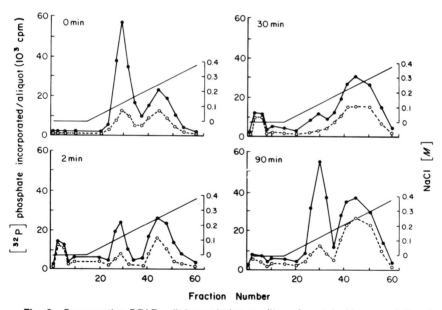

Fig. 3 Comparative DEAE-cellulose elution profiles of protein kinase activity of
glioma cell 10,000 g supernatant fractions obtained before (0 minutes) and at the indicated times after isoproterenol (10^{-5} M) stimulation. The 10,000 g supernatant fractions
(equivalent to 4 mg of protein) from glioma cells were applied on DEAE-cellulose and
elution was carried out with a linear gradient of 0.01–0.4 M NaCl. Aliquots of each fraction were assayed with protamine as substrate (see Hunzicker-Dunn and Jungmann,
1978) in the absence (○) and presence (●) of 10^{-6} M cAMP. —, NaCl.

comparison of the relative elution peak areas of type I and type II isozymes shows a marked reduction in type I isozyme coinciding with the elevation of intracellular cAMP levels. The reduction in type I isozyme occurred as rapidly as 2 minutes after isoproterenol stimulation. The type I isozyme levels remained relatively low but returned to prestimulation levels 2 hours after the initial isoproterenol stimulus (Fig. 4). We interpret the data of Figs. 3 and 4 to indicate that the type I holoenzyme, but not the type II, became significantly and selectively activated (dissociated) by cAMP for a period of about 90 minutes after isoproterenol stimulation of the glial cells.

The marked isoproterenol-stimulated dissociation of type I cAMP-dependent protein kinase suggested the phosphorylation of interacellular substrates, particularly of nonhistone chromosomal proteins which may assume key roles in the mechanism of cAMP-mediated LDH induction. Since we consistently observed a small but significant decrease in the specific and total activity of glioma cell cytosol after isoproterenol stimula-

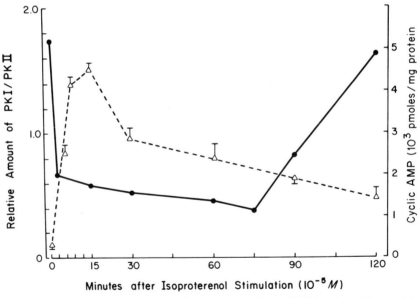

Fig. 4 Effect of isoproterenol ($10^{-5}M$) on intracellular cAMP levels and the protein kinase I(PK I)/protein kinase II (PKII) ratio as a function of time after isoproterenol stimulation of glioma cells. Intracellular cAMP was assayed at the indicated times as described (DeAngelo et al., 1975). The PK I/PK II ratio was obtained from the protein kinase DEAE-cellulose elution areas. The elution areas were determined by weighing the peak paper areas of each DEAE-cellulose elution profile (see Fig. 3) obtained from 10,000 g supernatant fractions of glioma cells at the indicated times after isoproterenol stimulation.

tion, we proceeded to determine the intracellular redistribution of the protein kinase catalytic subunit in subcellular fractions of glioma cells before and after isoproterenol stimulation. Figure 5 reveals that the specific activity of protein kinase in the nuclear and microsomal fractions was significantly increased after isoproterenol stimulation. Additionally, use of the heat-stable protein kinase inhibitor from rabbit skeletal muscle, which selectively inhibits the activity of the catalytic protein kinase subunit (Walsh *et al.* 1971; Ashby and Walsh, 1972), allowed us to show that the increase in protein kinase activity in the nuclear and microsomal fractions was primarily due to increased levels of the catalytic protein kinase subunit in these particulate fractions.

The alterations in nuclear and cytosol protein kinase activity were studied in more detail at various times after isoproterenol stimulation and are illustrated in Fig. 6. Nuclear glioma cell protein kinase activity increased markedly at 5 minutes, reached peak values 10–30 minutes after stimulation, and declined thereafter but remained significantly elevated 2 hours after isoproterenol application. During this time period (0–2 hours after

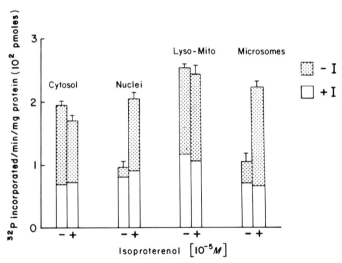

Fig. 5 Effect of heat-stable protein kinase inhibitor on glioma cell subcellular protein kinase activity before and after isoproterenol treatment. Subcellular fractions from 11-day-old unstimulated ($-$I) and isoproterenol-stimulated ($+$I) (15 minutes, 10^{-5} M) stationary cultures were prepared as described by us (Hunzicker-Dunn and Jungmann, 1978). Protein kinase activity was determined with protamine as substrate and with 10^{-6} M cAMP in the absence and presence of saturating amounts of heat-stable inhibitor. The inhibitor was prepared according to Walsh *et al.* (1971). The total bars represent total protein kinase activity measured without inhibitor; open bars represent remaining cAMP-independent protein kinase activity measured in the presence of inhibitor. Data are means $\pm$ SD from four cultures. Lyso-Mito indicates the lysosomal-mitochondrial pellet fraction.

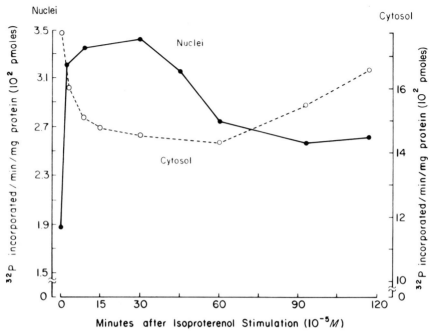

Fig. 6 Effect of isoproterenol on total nuclear and cytosol protein kinase activity as a function of time after isoproterenol stimulation. Eleven-day-old stationary cultures were stimulated with 10^{-5} M isoproterenol. At various times nuclei and 105,000 g cytosol were prepared (Hunzicker-Dunn and Jungmann, 1978), and total protein kinase activity was measured with protamine in the presence of 10^{-6} M cAMP. Data are means from three cultures.

isoproterenol) cytosol protein kinase activity decreased markedly during the first 60 minutes and then recovered to near control levels 2 hours after the stimulus.

The isoproterenol-mediated increase in total nuclear protein kinase activity, occurring concomitantly with a loss of cytosol protein kinase, suggested the possibility of a transfer of cytoplasmic cAMP-dependent protein kinase to the nucleus as a consequence of cAMP action. This possibility is supported by the fact that the acquired nuclear kinase activity was inhibited by the heat-stable protein kinase inhibitor (see Fig. 5). To establish whether the isoproterenol-mediated increase in nuclear protein kinase activity was due to a translocation of cytoplasmic cAMP-dependent protein kinase to nuclear sites, nuclei were analyzed for cAMP-dependent protein kinase activity before and at various times after isoproterenol stimulation. Nonhistone nuclear protein fractions prepared by 0.5 M NaCl extraction of glioma cell nuclei were subjected to Sephadex G-200 gel filtration. The elution patterns are illustrated in Fig. 7. The elution profile of nonhistone proteins isolated from unstimulated glioma cells (0-minute profile) exhibited one main peak of protein kinase activity in fractions 70–79 (PK-I). Stimulation of glioma cells with 10^{-6} M isoproterenol resulted in the appearance in the elution profile of two additional protein

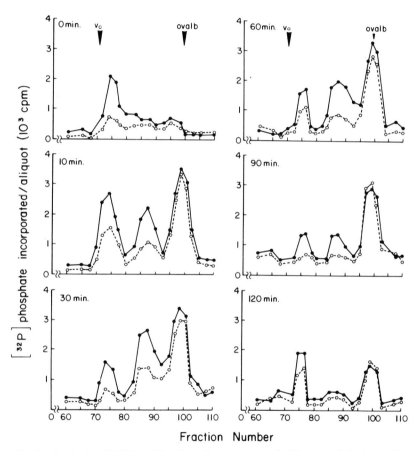

Fig. 7 Sephadex G-200 gel filtration of nuclear protein kinase activity from glioma cells before and after isoproterenol stimulation. Eleven-day-old stationary glioma cell cultures were stimulated with 10^{-5} M isoproterenol for the indicated time periods. After the elapsed stimulation period, nuclei were isolated and 0.5 M NaCl extracts were prepared as described by us (Spielvogel *et al.*, 1977). The extracts were dialyzed overnight against 10 mM NaCl, 10 mM MgCl$_2$, 5% glycerol, 3 mM dithiothreitol, 20 mM Tris, pH 7.4. The dialyzed fractions were subjected to Sephadex G-200 gel filtration. The eluted fractions were assayed for protein kinase activity without cAMP (○) and with 10^{-6} M cAMP (●). The void volume of the column as determined by the elution of blue dextran 2000 is indicated by V_0, and the ovalbumin elution position is indicated by ovalb.

kinase peaks, namely, protein kinase PK-II in fractions 82–92, and protein kinase PK III in fractions 95–104. The elution areas of PK-II and PK-III reached maximal values 10–30 minutes after isoproterenol stimulation and declined but still remained elevated over control values 60–120 minutes after isoproterenol stimulation. Both PK-II and PK-III were inhibited 90–95% by saturating concentrations of heat-stable protein kinase inhibitor, but only PK-II exhibited significant cAMP-binding activity. Determination of the elution positions relative to protein standards of known molecular weight indicate a molecular weight of 150,000 for PK-II and of 44,-000 for PK-III. These characteristics suggest the identity of PK-II with the holoenzyme and of PK-III with the dissociated catalytic subunit of cAMP-dependent protein kinase. This notion was confirmed by conversion of the catalytic subunit PK-III into the holoenzyme PK-II, which occurred after dialysis of the nuclear 0.5 M NaCl extract overnight in the presence of 3 mM Mg^{2+}–ATP.

Evidence for the identity of the nuclear protein kinase PK-II with the cytosol type I cAMP-dependent protein kinase was obtained in several ways. Nuclear protein kinase PK-II and cytosol type I cAMP-dependent protein kinase exhibited identical elution characteristics on DEAE-cellulose and on Sephadex G-200, indicating that both kinases were of similar molecular size and possessed similar ionic charge. Both kinases exhibited an identical K_m for ATP of 7.6 μM and showed similar substrate specificity and identical phosphorylation profiles of nuclear nonhistone proteins. Last, the antigenic properties of the two kinases and their reactivity with antiserum prepared against cAMP-dependent protein kinase were similar. From these data we conclude that the nuclear protein kinase PK-II is related to or identical with the glioma cell cytoplasmic type I cAMP-dependent protein kinase isozyme.

III. Mechanism of Translocation

Based on the above findings isoproterenol-stimulated nuclear translocation of cytoplasmic protein kinase is initiated through a cAMP-mediated dissociation of cytoplasmic type I holoenzyme and subsequent binding of the protein kinase subunits to nuclear acceptor sites. An alternate possibility is the cAMP-mediated transfer of a protein kinase holoenzyme–cAMP complex (R·C–cAMP) to the nuclear site, followed by dissociation of the complex through the action of cAMP or nuclear protein kinase substrates. However, the lack of affinity of the undissociated holoenzyme for chromatin (Jungmann et al., 1974) or for free DNA (Johnson et al., 1975), and the generation of cAMP at the cell membrane followed by dissociation of the cytoplasmic holoenzyme, are incompatible with this alternative.

Previous investigations have allowed us to define the following conditions that have to be met for protein kinase translocation to occur (Jungmann *et al.*, 1974, 1975).

1. Association of the C and R subunits with chromatin requires the presence of cAMP.

2. The intracellular transfer of protein-bound cAMP and of protein kinase from the cytosol toi the nucleus is temperature-dependent.

3. The association of C and R subunits requires "intact" chromatin. Native DNA or reconstituted DNA–histone complexes lack the ability to bind the protein kinase subunits, and the presence of the nonhistone chromosomal protein fraction in the reconstituted chromatin is required for full binding activity.

4. Translocation of cytoplasmic cAMP-dependent protein kinase to chromatin causes the selective phosphorylation of nuclear nonhistone proteins but not of histones.

On the basis of these findings it appears that nuclear translocation of cytoplasmic cAMP-dependent protein kinase provides a precisely regulated, viable mechanism by which biological signals from the cell membrane and cytoplasm are transferred to the nucleus. Details concerning the mechanism of transfer of cytoplasmic protein kinase to the nucleus remain to be established. It is tempting to assume that intracellular structures such as microfilaments, microtubules, and so on, aid and are part of the transfer mechanism. Although our initial experiments testing the participation of microfilaments in the nuclear transfer of protein kinase have yielded inconclusive results because of the lack of effect of cytochalasin B on translocation, studies using inhibitors of microtubule formation have been more successful. Figure 8 illustrates that Colcemid, in a dose-dependent fashion, prevented the isoproterenol-stimulated increase in glioma cell nuclear protein kinase activity. Considering the established inhibitory effect of Colcemid on microtubule formation, one might conclude that microtubules aid in the transfer of protein kinase to the nucleus. However, the effects of Colcemid are too complex to rule out other mechanisms which might prevent an increase in nuclear protein kinase activity, and further studies are required to establish clearly the participation of microtubules in the translocation process.

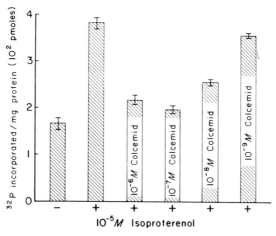

Fig. 8 Effect of varying amounts of Colcemid on isoproterenol stimulation of glioma cell nuclear protein kinase activity. Eleven-day-old stationary glioma cell cultures were stimulated for 15 minutes with 10^{-5} M isoproterenol in the absence and presence of the indicated concentrations of Colcemid. Nuclei were isolated, and total nuclear protein kinase activity was measured with protamine in the presence of 10^{-6} M cAMP. Data are means ± SD from two cultures.

IV. Conclusions

This chapter highlights a number of functional characteristics of the glioma cell cAMP–protein kinase system that are compatible with the concept that catecholamines, via cAMP and cAMP-dependent protein kinase, achieve regulation of glioma cell nuclear protein phosphorylation and of LDH induction via a transcriptional mechanism. The emerging picture strongly suggests that the cAMP-mediated *de novo* synthesis of LDH involves transcriptional activation of LDH mRNA which becomes available for translation about 90 minutes after isoproterenol stimulation of glioma cells. The cAMP-mediated events leading to the initiation of LDH mRNA synthesis are not firmly established. The available evidence allows a correlation of the early initiating molecular steps with LDH mRNA porduction and translation. These early steps consist of (1) interaction of isoproterenol with glioma cell adenyl cyclase and generation of distinctly increased intracellular levels of cAMP; (2) selective cAMP-mediated dissociation and activation of type I protein kinase isozyme for a period of at least 90 minutes but not over 120 minutes after isoproterenol stimulation; (3) an increase in nuclear protein kinase activity for a period of at least 120 minutes caused by the translocation of cytoplasmic type I isozyme to the nucleus, which occurs concomitantly with the decrease in cytosol protein kinase activity; (4) nuclear acquisition of type I isozyme leading to the phosphorylation of specific nonhistone chromosomal proteins. Based on studies with Colcemid it is conceivable that protein kinase translocation requires an intact mechanism of microtubule formation. The possibility that the cAMP-mediated translocation of type I protein kinase isozyme and subsequent phosphorylation of nonhistone proteins act as major regulatory factors in the control of LDH induction must be given serious consideration in the future.

Acknowledgment

The studies described in this chapter were supported by grant GM 23895 from the National Institutes of Health.

References

Ashby, C. D., and Wlash, D. A. (1972). *J. Biol. Chem.* **247,** 6637–6642.

DeAngelo, A. B., Schweppe, J. S., Jungmann, R. A., Huber, P., and Eppenberger, U. (1975). *Endocrinology* **97,** 1509–1520.

DeVellis, J., and Brooker, G. (1973). *In* "Tissue Culture of the Nervous System" (G. Sato, ed.), pp. 231–246. Plenum, New York.

Hunzicker-Dunn, M., and Jungmann, R. A. (1978). *Endocrinology* **103,** 420–430.

Johnson, E. M., Hadden, J. W., Inoue, A., and Allfrey, V. G. (1975). *Biochemistry* **14,** 3873–3884.

Jungmann, R. A., and Kranias, E. G. (1977). *Int. J. Biochem.* **8,** 819–830.

Jungmann, R. A., and Russell, D. H. (1977). *Life Sci.* **20,** 1787–1798.

Jungmann, R. A., Hiestand, P. C., and Schweppe, J. S. (1974). *Endocrinology* **94,** 168–183.

Jungmann, R. A., Lee, S. G., and DeAngelo, A. B. (1975). *Adv. Cyclic Nucleotide Res.* **5,** 281–306.

Kaplan, N. O., and Ciotti, M. M. (1961). *Biochim. Biophys. Acta* **49,** 425–431.

Spielvogel, A. M., Mednieks, M. I., Eppenberger, U., and Jungmann, R. A. (1977). *Eur. J. Biochem.* **73,** 199–212.

Walsh, D. A., Ashby, C. D., Gonzales, C., Calkins, D., Fischer, E. H., and Krebs, E. G. (1971). *J. Biol. Chem.* **246,** 1977–1985.

23

Action of Nitrous Oxide and Griseofulvin on Microtubules and Chromosome Movement in Dividing Cells

S. M. COX, P. N. RAO, AND B. R. BRINKLEY

I. Introduction

It is now well documented that two microtubule systems exist in proliferating cells: the cytoplasmic microtubule complex (CMTC) of interphase cells and the microtubules of the mitotic apparatus (MA) of dividing cells (Brinkley *et al.*, 1975, 1976). Cytoplasmic microtubules appear to play a variety of roles within the cell, including maintenance of cell shape (Porter, 1966), motility (Allison, 1973), mobilization and release of lysosomes (Malawista, 1975), and anchorage of cell surface receptors (Edelman *et al.*, 1973; Edelman, 1976). As cells progress into mitosis, the CMTC disappears during changes in cell shape from flattened anisotropic forms to more rounded structures. During this transition, the CMTC dissociates and is replaced with spindle microtubules which form in association with centriole pairs at each pole of the spindle and with kinetochores of prometaphase chromosomes (Brinkley *et al.*, 1976; Fuller and Brinkley, 1976). The cellular mechanism that regulates the assembly and disassembly of cytoplasmic and spindle microtubules during the cell cycle is poorly understood. Although microtubules in the two systems are morphologically and biochemically similar, we propose that they display dissimilar affinities for various drugs that interfere with microtubule assembly, organization, and function.

Microtubules are composed largely of the protein tubulin, which consists of two similar dimeric polypeptide subunits arranged as heterodimers into 13 protofilaments composing the walls of a hollow tubule (for reviews, see Snyder and McIntosh, 1976; Stephens and Edds, 1976). In addition several classes of microtubule-associated proteins (MAPs) are associated with microtubules (Borisy *et al.*, 1975; Sloboda *et al.*, 1975, 1976). Several drugs such as colchicine, podophyllotoxin, and the *Vinca* alkaloids are known to bind specifically to tubulin and inhibit polymerization of both cytoplasmic and spindle microtubules (Wilson and Bryan, 1974; Wilson, 1975). Another agent, N_2O, has been shown to inhibit mitosis in a variety of cells and tissues (Ferguson *et al.*, 1950; Green and Eastwood, 1963; Kieler, 1957; Ostergren, 1944; Rao, 1968). In an early study, Ostergren (1944) reported that N_2O arrested cells in mitosis in a manner somewhat like that produced by colchicine (C-mitosis). Other investigators using light microscopy have also observed C-mitotic configurations in cells treated with N_2O as well as the noble gases xenon, argon, and krypton (Ferguson *et al.*, 1950). Rao (1968) was able to synchronize HeLa cells by arresting them reversibly in mitosis by the application of N_2O. Ultrastructural and kinetic studies by Brinkley and Rao (1973) showed that N_2O at 80 psi blocked mitosis in HeLa cells but, unlike colchicine and other related agents, had little effect on the assembly of spindle microtubules.

In the present study, a more detailed analysis of the effect of N_2O on spindle microtubules and the elements of the cytoplasmic microtubule complex was carried out using antitubulin immunofluorescence and electron microscopy. The effects of N_2O are discussed in relationship to the action of another C-mitotic drug, griseofulvin, which has also been reported to inhibit mitosis without appreciably altering microtubule polymerization.

II. Methods

A. Cell Culture

1. N_2O Treatment

Human fibroblasts (strain PA_2) obtained from Uta Francke, University of California at San Diego, were routinely grown in Dulbecco's modified Eagle's medium supplemented with 20% fetal calf serum. Cells were seeded into 60-mm tissues culture dishes or on sterile coverslips (11×22 mm) and maintained at 37°C in a humidified atmosphere of 90% air and 10% CO_2. Twenty-four hours after subculture the attached cells were transferred to a pressure bomb and exposed to N_2O or nitrogen under 80 psi (the nitrogen-treated group served as a control). One group of the cells was pretreated for 2.5 hours with 10^{-6} M Colcemid, rinsed, and immediately transferred to the N_2O bomb. After 16 hours, all cells were removed from the pressure bomb and samples obtained for indirect immunofluorescence, electron microscopy, and cell kinetics analysis. Subsequently, some of the cells were transferred to a 37°C incubator and allowed to recover under atmospheric pressure. At 30-minute intervals samples were taken and processed as above.

B. Griseofulvin Treatment

Swiss mouse 3T3 cells from the American Type Culture Collection were grown in a manner identical to that described for PA2 cells. Twenty-four hours after subculture the coverslips with cells attached were treated with increasing concentrations of griseofulvin [1:100 dilution of drug dissolved in spectral grade dimethyl sulfoxide (DMSO)] for 4 hours prior to fixation for fluorescence or electron microscopy. Cells treated with 10^{-4} M griseofulvin were also allowed to reverse in fresh media for 0.5, 1.0, or 2.0 hours before processing for indirect immunofluorescence. As with the N_2O experiments, one group was treated with 10^{-4} M griseofulvin plus 10^{-6} M Colcemid for 2.5 hours and then allowed to recover for 4 hours in medium containing only griseofulvin (10^{-4} M).

Cell survival was determined in asynchronously growing Chinese hamster ovary CHO K1 cells treated with increasing concentrations of griseofulvin. Replicate plates received increasing drug concentrations, while one plate containing only medium served as a control. After incubation in a 5% CO_2 atmosphere at 37°C for either 4 or 18 hours, the medium was decanted, the plates rinsed with Puck's solution A, and the cells removed by trypsinization. Known numbers of cells were seeded into tissue culture plates containing 5 ml medium and fetal calf serum and incubated at 37°C for 7 days. At this time, cells were fixed in methanol, stained with crystal violet, and counted. Survival was based on the ability of a single cell to grow into a colony of 50 or more cells.

C. Immunofluorescence

Indirect immunofluorescence localization of tubulin in the cells was accomplished using rabbit antibodies against purified bovine brain tubulin (Fuller *et al.*, 1975). Coverslips (with cells attached) were rinsed in phosphate-buffered saline (PBS), fixed for 20 minutes in 3% formaldehyde in PBS, and then treated with absolute acetone at −10°C for 7 minutes. The coverslips were briefly rinsed in PBS and incubated with the antibody (0.1 mg/ml in PBS) for 45 minutes at 37°C. The coverslips were again washed in PBS and then incubated for 30 minutes at 37°C in a 1:10 dilution of fluorescein-conjugated goat antiserum against rabbit IgG. After a final wash in PBS, the coverslips were rinsed in distilled water and individually mounted on a glass slide in a drop of glycerol–PBS (9:1, pH 8.5).

Observations were made with a Leitz microscope equipped with a Polemak 2.1 illumination system. A 100-W high-pressure mercury arc lamp was the illumination source and was used with a Leitz KCl heat-absorbing filter and a BG38 red suppression filter. Leitz 40×, 50×, 54×, and 63× objectives were used, and the images recorded on Kodak Plus-X panchromatic film.

D. Electron Microscopy

Cells for transmission electron microscopy were fixed *in situ* with 3% glutaraldehyde in 0.1 *M* PIPES buffer and postfixed in 1% osmium tetroxide in PIPES buffer. After dehydration through an ethanol series, the cells were flat-embedded in Epon according to the method of Brinkley *et al.* (1967b). Following polymerization for 24 hours at 60°C, the culture dish was separated from the Epon wafer. Cells in the Epon wafer were examined with a phase microscope, and selected cells were marked, bored out of the disk, and glued to the tip of a blank Epon peg. Thin sections of the selected cells were cut on a Porter-Blum MT2B ultramicrotome using a diamond knife. Sections were picked up on collodion-coated, slotted grids and stained with alcoholic uranyl acetate followed by lead citrate. The sections were then examined and photographed in a Siemen's 102 electron microscope.

E. *In Vitro* Tubulin Assembly

Microtubule protein was isolated from brains by a modification of the temperature-dependent assembly–disassembly scheme described by Borisy *et al.* (1975). Microtubule protein recycled four times at 2.5 mg/ml was polymerized at 37°C in the assay buffer (50 mM PIPES, 1 mM GTP, 50 mM KCl, 0.1 mM MgSO$_4$, pH 6.94 at room temperature) or in the presence of varying concentrations of griseofulvin (the final concentration assayed contained 1% DMSO). Turbidity was monitored at 350 nm with a Gilford Model 240 spectrophotometer (Gilford Instrument Laboratories, Oberlin, Ohio) equipped with a water-jacketed cuvet chamber, and the temperature maintained at 37°C with a Lauda Model K2 constant-temperature H$_2$O circulator (Sargent-Welch Scientific Company, Skokie, Illinois). The change in OD$_{350}$ with time was recorded on a Varian Aerograph Model 20 strip-chart recorder (Varian Aerograph, Walnut Creek, California).

III. Results

A. Cytoplasmic and Spindle Microtubules

A composite micrograph of control 3T3 cells as observed by antitubulin immunofluorescence is shown in Fig. 1. The elaborate pattern of fluorescent filaments seen throughout the cytoplasm (Fig. 1A) has been described in several studies (Brinkley *et al.*, 1975, 1976; Weber *et al.*, 1975). Figure 1B–F is arranged according to the well-known phases of mitosis, and only a brief summary is given. As prophase begins, the CMTC diminishes and two bright fluorescent spots, presumably centriole pairs, appear near the nuclear membrane (Fig. 1B). Prometaphase is characterized by breakdown of the nuclear membrane and association of the chromosomes with the mitotic spindle (Fig. 1C). The metaphase cell shows the nonfluorescent chromosomes to be arranged on the equatorial plate with bundles of fluorescent filaments extending from the chromosomes to the poles (Fig. 1D). Anaphase is characterized by elongation of the spindle with the fluorescent chromosome-to-pole fibers shorter than in metaphase, and the appearance of interzonal fibers extending from pole to pole. During telophase, cytokinesis begins, and bundles of fluorescent interpolar fibers can be seen (Fig. 1E). Upon completion of cytokinesis, the daughter cells

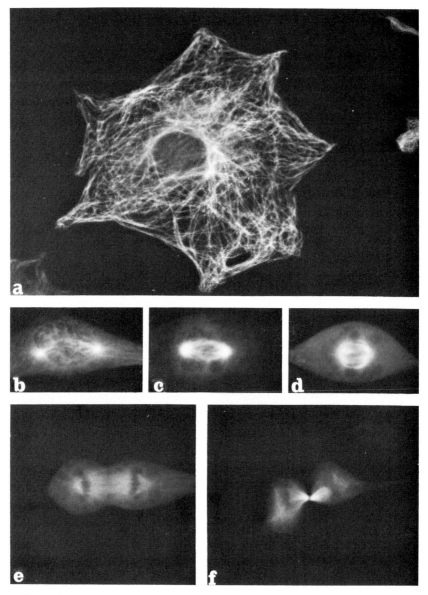

Fig. 1 Tubulin immunofluorescence in 3T3 cells. (a) Interphase cell showing a CMTC. (b) Prophase. (c) Prometaphase. (d) Metaphase. (e) Telophase. (f) Telophase showing midbody.

formed are held together by a narrow, brightly fluorescent cytoplasmic bridge, the midbody (Fig. 1F). Later in telophase or early G_1, the bridge narrows and elongates, and cytoplasmic microtubules reappear in the daughter cells.

B. Colcemid

The inhibitory effect of Colcemid on cytoplasmic and spindle microtubules is well known (Brinkley et al., 1975; Fuller and Brinkley, 1976). The normal CMTC and metaphase spindle of 3T3 cells are shown in Figs. 2 and 4. After treatment of the cells with $10^{-6} M$ Colcemid for 2 hours the CMTC is completely disassembled (Fig. 3). Cells arrested in metaphase, however, display chromosomes grouped around one or two bright fluorescent centers (Fig. 5) which can be shown by electron microscopy to contain centrioles and short kinetochore-associated microtubules (Brinkley et al., 1967a). Such treatments are completely reversible, as described elsewhere (Brinkley et al., 1975; Fuller and Brinkley, 1976; Osborn and Weber, 1976).

C. Nitrous Oxide

Exposure of cultured cells to N_2O treatment for 4 hours resulted in the accumulation of approximately 30% of the cells in metaphase, a level of inhibition comparable to that produced by $10^{-6} M$ Colcemid (Fig. 6). Removal of the cells from the N_2O environment resulted in the rapid and synchronous progression of cells through mitosis into G_1 phase within 60–90 minutes (Rao, 1968). Cells arrested in mitosis displayed two patterns of fluorescence when stained with tubulin antibody. In one the spindle poles were slightly separated with microtubules radiating out in all directions (Fig. 11). In the other, the chromosomes were grouped near the cell center with a single bright fluorescent spot near the center of the chromosome mass (Figs. 9 and 10).

In order to further substantiate the immunofluorescent observations, N_2O-treated cells were examined by transmission electron microscopy. Untreated cells had a well-aligned spindle with the chromosomes arranged on the metaphase plate equidistant between the poles (Fig. 12). Numerous pole-to-pole and chromosome-to-pole microtubules were present and, in general, cell organelles were absent from the area of the mitotic spindle. In contrast, in cells arrested by N_2O, the spindle was irregularly aligned and the chromosomes were distributed randomly, with little apparent positioning between the poles (Fig. 13). Microtubules were seen

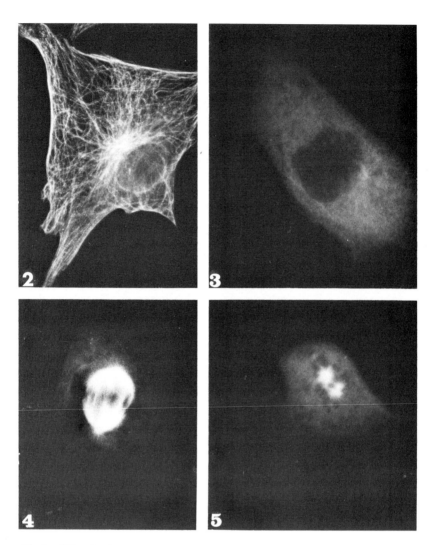

Fig. 2 3T3 cell with a full CMTC.

Fig. 3 3T3 cell treated with 10^{-6} *M* Colcemid for 2 hours. Note the absence of a CMTC.

Fig. 4 Metaphase.

Fig. 5 C-Metaphase after treatment with 10^{-6} *M* Colcemid for 2 hours.

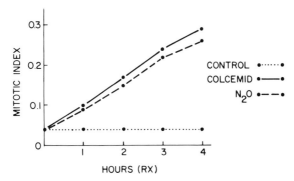

Fig. 6 Arrest and recovery of cells in mitosis after N_2O treatment. N_2O at 80 psi arrests cells in mitosis at approximately the same rate as Colcemid.

associated with both kinetochores and centrioles, but most were not aligned with the spindle axis.

After the cell cultures were removed from the N_2O environment and placed in a CO_2 incubator, a normal spindle formed and the cells progressed through mitosis. Several stages of reversal are shown in Fig. 14A–D. Within 30 minutes a majority of the cells had recovered and progressed to a normal metaphase configuration (Fig. 14A and B). After 60 minutes most of the cells had divided into two daughter cells held together by the midbody (Fig. 14d).

Exposure of cells to the N_2O environment had little or no apparent effect on the organization of the CMTC. As shown in Figs. 7 and 8, cytoplasmic microtubules are extensive in cells exposed to N_2O for up to 16 hours. This is in sharp contrast to the effect of microtubule inhibitors such as Colcemid (Figs. 15a and d) which dissociate microtubules in both the CMTC and MA. In order to evaluate the effect of N_2O on the assembly of the CMTC and spindle microtubules, an experiment was designed in which exponentially growing cells were exposed to Colcemid for 2.5 hours to dissociate both spindle and cytoplasmic microtubules. The cells were then removed from Colcemid and placed in either fresh medium for 60 minutes or fresh medium plus N_2O at 80 psi for periods up to 4 hours. As shown in Fig. 15B and E the CMTC and MA were completely reformed when the Colcemid-arrested cells were placed in fresh medium alone. Likewise, when Colcemid-treated cells were transferred to fresh medium and exposed to the N_2O environment, the CMTC reformed in a manner similar to that observed in control cells (Fig. 15C). Under the same experimental conditions, however, the spindle failed to reform completely, and chromosome movement remained blocked (Fig. 15F). This

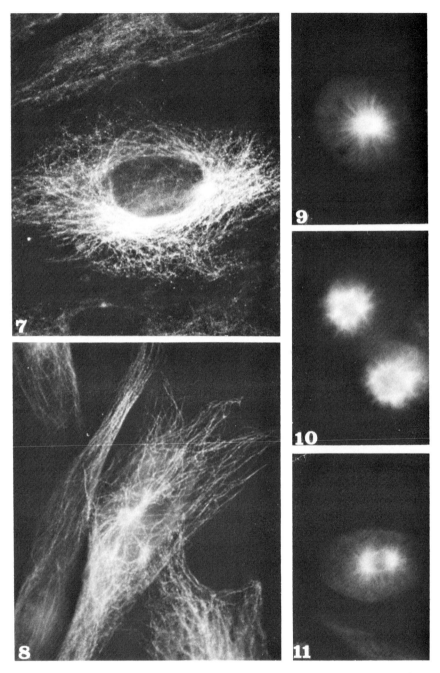

Fig. 7–8 Human PA2 cells showing an extensive CMTC after exposure to a N₂O environment for 8 hours.

Figs. 9–11 PA2 cells arrested in mitosis after exposure to N₂O.

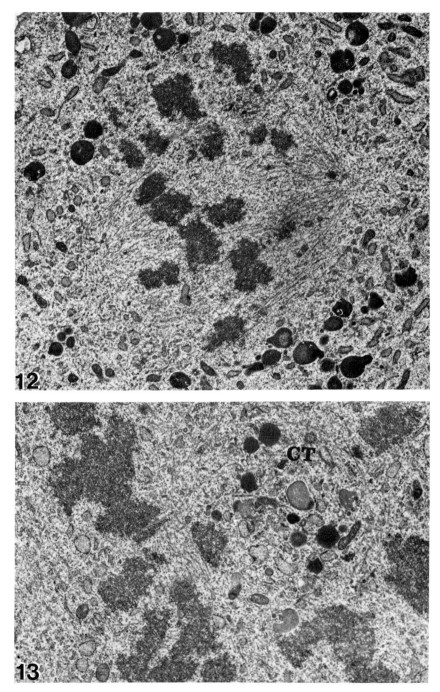

Fig. 12 Electron micrograph of control 3T3 cells in metaphase after treatment with nitrogen at 80 psi. × 7500.

Fig. 13 Electron micrograph of 3T3 cell arrested in metaphase with N_2O. Centrioles (CT) are present along with numerous spindle microtubules. × 16,000.

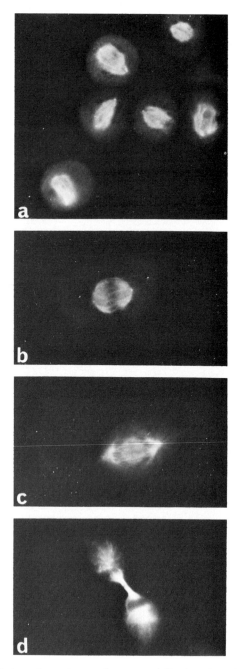

Fig. 14 3T3 cells in various stages of recovery following the release of N_2O arrest. (a) Early stage of recovery. (b) Metaphase with chromosomes at the equatorial plate. (c) Anaphase. (d) Telophase.

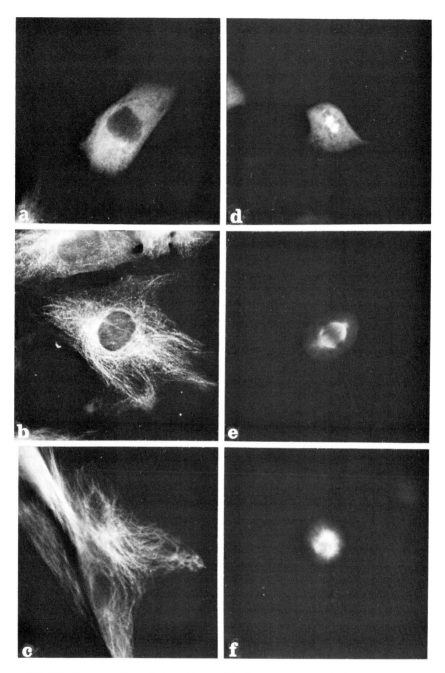

Fig. 15 Recovery from Colcemid arrest in the presence and absence of N₂O. (a) Interphase 3T3 cell after 2 hours of Colcemid. (b) Interphase 3T3 cell exposed to Colcemid for 2 hours and then returned to fresh medium for 60 minutes. Note the extensive CMTC. (c) Interphase 3T3 cell released from Colcemid arrest in a N₂O environment. Note the extensive CMTC. (d) C-metaphase cell after a 2-hour Colcemid treatment. (e) Normal metaphase cell after a 60-minute recovery from Colcemid arrest. (f) Cell arrested in mitosis after a 60-minute recovery from Colcemid but placed in a N₂O atmosphere.

experiment demonstrates conclusively that N_2O has a preferential action on spindle microtubules but little effect on the CMTC.

D. Griseofulvin

Griseofulvin is a mold metabolite obtained from *Penicillium griseoful-vin*, which inhibits mitosis in mammalian cells *in vitro*. Our interest in the drug for present study was due to the finding of Grisham *et al.* (1973) who reported that griseofulvin inhibited mitosis without disrupting spindle microtubules. Thus the drug appeared to affect cells in a manner similar to N_2O.

The action of griseofulvin on 3T3 cells is shown in Fig. 16. A dose of

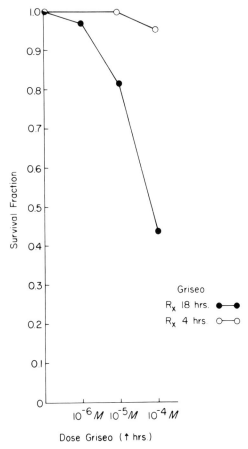

Fig. 16 Survival of CHO cells after exposure to various doses of griseofulvin (griseo).

$1 \times 10^{-4} M$ given for 4 hours caused little alteration in cell survival. The same dose applied for 18 hours, however, resulted in substantial toxicity. Using [^{3}H]griseofulvin to measure uptake of the drug we observed an exponential increase in drug concentration in the cells at 1 to 4 hours. At this time the uptake leveled off, and at 18 hours the concentration was the same as after the 4-hour treatment. This indicates that, with increasing drug exposure, nonrepairable damage is accumulated within the cell. For this reason we chose not to exceed a dose of $1 \times 10^{-4} M$ griseofulvin for more than 4 hours.

Griseofulvin inhibited mitosis in exponentially growing cells in a dose-dependent manner as shown in Fig. 17. At a dose of $10^{-4} M$, griseofulvin arrested cells in mitosis at a level comparable to $10^{-6} M$ Colcemid applied under the same conditions. Examination of griseofulvin-arrested mitotic cells by tubulin immunofluorescence or electron microscopy indicated that the cells were blocked in two general configurations. Some cells were apparently monopolar, with the chromosomes grouped around a single bright fluorescent spot (Fig. 18). Other spindles were more oval in appearance, with the chromosomes arranged on a more typical bipolar spindle (Fig. 19). An electron micrograph of a similar bipolar spindle is shown in Fig. 20. Centrioles are present at each pole, and both kinetochore and interpolar microtubules are present in the spindle. However, the spindle

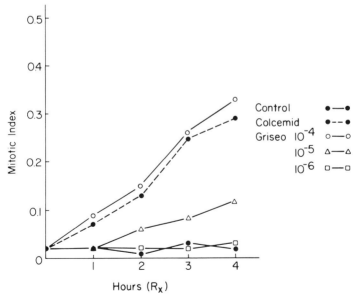

Fig. 17 Mitotic index after the exposure of CHO cells to griseofulvin (griseo) and Colcemid.

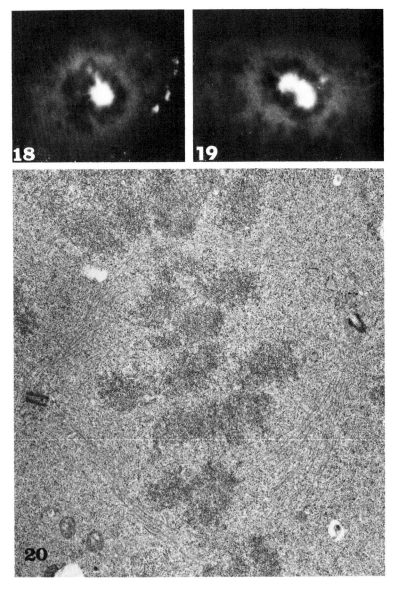

Fig. 18 Antitubulin immunofluorescence of 3T3 cell in mitosis showing a monopolar configuration.

Fig. 19 Same as in Fig. 18 except spindle is more ovoid, a configuration defined as bipolar.

Fig. 20 Electron micrograph of bipolar spindle from griseofulvin-arrested 3T3 cells. Note centrioles at each pole and numerous spindle microtubules. × 18,000.

was considerably shorter than normal. In the monopolar spindle, the centrioles remain near the cell center as shown in Fig. 21A. Microtubules extend from the kinetochores toward the centrioles, and in many instances both sister kinetochores are associated with polymerized microtubules (Fig. 21B). This is in striking contrast to Colcemid-arrested cells which generally display only one of the two sister kinetochores with polymerized microtubules (Brinkley et al., 1967b). Initially both types of metaphase configurations were found in approximately equal numbers in the griseofulvin-treated culture. After more prolonged exposure to the drug, however, mostly monopolar spindles were observed (Table I). Apparently the bipolar spindles become more disorganized and the centrioles become displaced after longer exposure to the drug.

Griseofulvin, unlike N_2O, produced a striking alteration in the structure of the cytoplasmic microtubule system (Fig. 22–25). Although relatively little effect was noted with 10^{-6} and 10^{-5} M treatments, 10^{-4} M griseofulvin for 4 hours resulted in a loss of cell shape and considerable diminution of the CMTC (Fig. 25). However, many cytoplasmic microtubules were still present in most cells (Fig. 26). This effect was completely reversible when cells were removed from the drug and placed in fresh medium (Fig. 27–30).

In an experiment similar to the one described previously for N_2O, the effects of griseofulvin on the assembly of cytoplasmic microtubules were studied in cells pretreated with Colcemid. As shown in Fig. 32, the CMTC was partially reassembled in cells that had been first treated with Colcemid plus griseofulvin for 2.5 hours (Fig. 31) and then transferred to medium containing only 10^{-4} M griseofulvin. It should be pointed out, however, that, although there was partial reformation of the CMTC in the presence of griseofulvin, the cells were still abnormal in shape and contained mostly short, randomly oriented microtubules. Moreover, the assembly of microtubules in the presence of griseofulvin was not asso-

TABLE I
Griseofulvin (10^{-4} M)-Blocked 3T3 Cells

Time (hours)	Monopolar (%)	Bipolar (%)	Total mitotic index
0	—	100	0.04
2	47	53	0.075
4	70	30	0.10
6	84.6	15.4	0.13
8	87.8	12.2	0.165
12	95.5	4.5	0.22
18	92.6	7.4	0.27

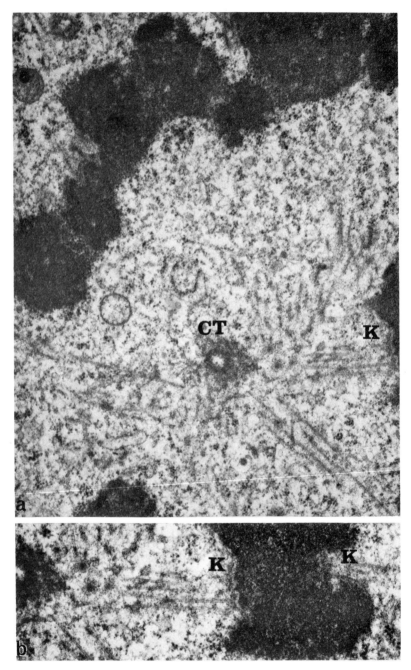

Fig. 21 Electron micrograph of a monopolar spindle. (a) Note centriole with surrounding microtubules. × 13,000. (b) Microtubules are associated with both daughter kinetochores of this metaphase chromosome. × 16,000.

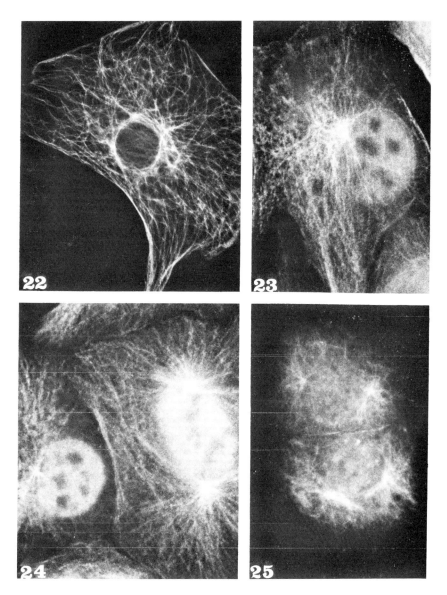

Fig. 22   Control 3T3 cell showing a full CMTC.
Fig. 23   Treated with 10^{-6} M griseofulvin.
Fig. 24   Treated with 10^{-5} M griseofulvin.
Fig. 25   Treated with 10^{-4} M griseofulvin. Note rounded shape and apparent reduction of the CMTC.

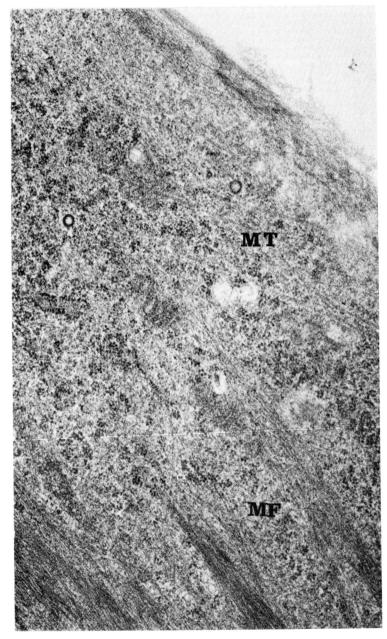

Fig. 26 Electron micrograph of 3T3 cell after exposure to griseofulvin for 4 hours Note numerous microtubules (MT) and microfilament bundles (Mf). × 40,000.

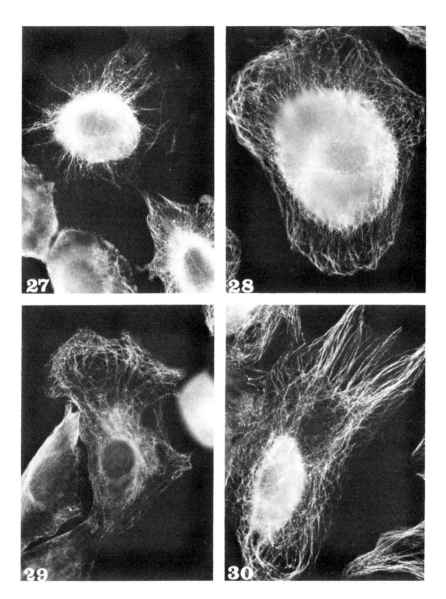

Fig. 27 3T3 cell after a 4-hour treatment with 10^{-4} M Colcemid.

Fig. 28 Thirty-minute recovery after a 4-hour griseofulvin treatment. The CMTC is partially reformed.

Fig. 29 Sixty-minute recovery from griseofulvin.

Fig. 30 One-hundred-twenty-minute recovery from griseofulvin. The CMTC is fully reformed.

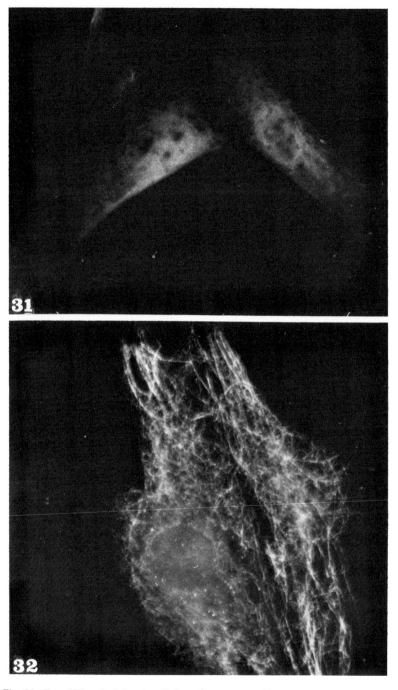

Fig. 31 Two 3T3 cells following Colcemid treatment. Nuclei are apparent, but cytoplasmic microtubules are disrupted.

Fig. 32 Two 3T3 cells after a 60-minute recovery from Colcemid treatment in the presence of 10^{-4} *M* griseofulvin. The CMTC is partially reformed.

ciated with a specific cytoplasmic "organizer" region normally observed in cells recovering from Colcemid (Fuller and Brinkley, 1976; Osborn and Weber, 1976).

The partial reformation of the CMTC in the presence of griseofulvin was in sharp contrast to the situation in metaphase-arrested cells which mostly remained blocked when removed from Colcemid and transferred to medium containing 10^{-4} M griseofulvin (Fig. 33). These results can be taken to indicate that the cytoplasmic microtubules are more resistant to griseofulvin.

In order to evaluate more directly the interaction of griseofulvin with microtubule protein, tubulin was purified by the temperature cycle assembly–disassembly procedure of Borisy *et al.* (1975). Four times recycled microtubule protein was polymerized at 37°C in the presence of varying

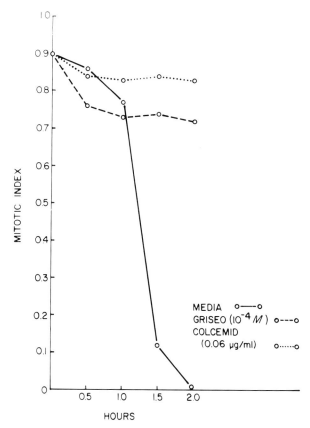

Fig. 33 Recovery from Colcemid arrest in fresh medium (O—O), in 10^{-4} M griseofulvin (O---O), and in Colcemid (O·····O).

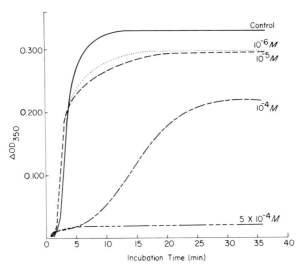

Fig. 34 *In vitro* assembly of bovine brain tubulin in the presence of griseofulvin. Lower concentrations of griseofulvin (10^{-5}–10^{-6} *M*) had little effect on tubulin polymerization. High concentrations of the drug altered the rate and extent of polymerization.

concentrations of griseofulvin. As shown in Fig. 34, lower concentrations (10^{-5}–10^{-6} *M*) had little effect on microtubule polymerization. At 10^{-4} *M*, however, both the rate and extent of assembly were noticeably altered. Increasing the concentration to 5×10^{-4} *M*, a dose toxic to cells in culture, resulted in complete inhibition of polymerization. From these results, it is apparent that griseofulvin can interact directly with some component in the microtubule reassembly system to inhibit *in vitro* polymerization of microtubules.

IV. Discussion

The combined microtubule and microfilament system of eukaryotic cells appears to constitute a dynamic cytoskeleton required for a wide variety of functions including the maintenance of cell shape and motility, mitosis and intracytoplasmic movement, secretion, exocytosis, endocytosis, and cell surface regulation. For the most part, two classes of drugs inhibit the function of the cytoskeleton: colchicine-like drugs including the *Vinca* alkaloids, podophyllotoxin, rotenone, and maytansine, which bind to tubulin and inhibit microtubule assembly, and microfilament inhibitors such as cytochalasin B. Physical agents such as low temperature and increased hydrostatic pressure also inhibit microtubule assembly, whereas D_2O can inhibit several microtubule functions, apparently by stabilizing microtubules and preventing their disassembly.

N_2O and griseofulvin are inhibitors that also appear to interact specifically with microtubules. In the case of N_2O, the nature of this interaction, although unclear, is highly specific, since only spindle microtubules appear to be involved. Moreover, assembly–disassembly of individual microtubules appears not to be affected. Instead, the anesthetic gas disrupts spindle organization such that parallel alignment of microtubules is not achieved. Thus microtubules are assembled at the usual organizing centers, the centrioles and kinetochores, but fail to become organized into a functional spindle.

Due to its specific affect on the mitotic apparatus, the use of N_2O provides additional insight into the role of microtubules in chromosomal movement. Since microtubules can assemble freely in the presence of this gas, but chromosomal movement is inhibited, it can be concluded that movement requires more than just the polymerization of microtubules. Inoue and Sato (1967; Inoue, 1964) have provided considerable evidence that the dynamic assembly and disassembly of spindle microtubules can provide sufficient energy to move chromosomes during mitosis. Their model for chromosomal movement requires that microtubules undergo regulated assembly and disassembly at appropriate stages of mitosis and specifically does not require the involvement of actomyosin-like contractile proteins. Since microtubules are fully assembled in the presence of N_2O, yet chromosome movement is arrested, one can conclude that assembly per se is insufficient for chromosome movement. Thus factors that mediate the interaction of adjacent microtubules also appear to be needed for normal chromosome movement. Several investigators using electron microscopy have described short cross-bridges which connect adjacent microtubules. Although Brinkley and Rao (1973) observed cross-bridges in the N_2O-arrested spindle, they were scarce in comparison with the number of cross-bridges seen in control spindles (McIntosh, 1974). N_2O may therefore interfere with cross-bridge formation, thus preventing the parallel alignment of spindle microtubules needed for chromosomal movement.

The molecular basis of microtubule–microtubule interaction is poorly understood. Dentler *et al.* (1975) observed that fine, whiskerlike filaments associated with reassembled brain microtubules were absent when high-molecular-weight MAPs were chromatographically removed from the tubulin preparations. Similar findings were reported by Murphy and Borisy (1975). Recently, Connolly *et al.* (1977) and Sherline and Schiavone (1978) have shown that antibodies to MAP proteins decorate the spindle when observed by indirect immunofluorescence. Antibodies to another MAP (tau) also decorate the spindle fibers (Connolly *et al.*, 1977). Thus the cross-bridges seen by electron microscopy may be the MAPs, and these may be the target for N_2O inhibition of spindle function.

Another candidate could be a dyneinlike protein recently described as a component of the mitotic spindle (Salmon and Jenkins, 1977; Sakai *et al.*, 1976; Cande, 1978). Dynein is a high-molecular-weight protein which appears as short arms on the A subtubule of the nine outer doublets of the axoneme of cilia and flagella. This protein contains ATPase activity and is necessary for the sliding-tubule mechanism of ciliary motion. The presence of dyneinlike protein in the spindle could account for microtubule-mediated chromosomal movement by a sliding-tubule mechanism. McIntosh and co-workers (1969) have proposed a sliding-tubule model for chromosomal movement in the eukaryotic mitotic spindle. Thus N_2O, by interfering with a dyneinlike protein, may alter the microtubule interaction needed for chromosomal movement. Unfortunately, the molecular interaction of N_2O with microtubule proteins is difficult to ascertain.

One surprising finding of this study was that N_2O had little or no effect on the interphase cytoskeleton. Thus the CMTC, which consists of microtubules essentially identical to those of the spindle, was apparently unaltered by N_2O treatment. When the CMTC was dissociated by Colcemid treatment, the entire apparatus was capable of undergoing normal reassembly upon removal of Colcemid, yet in the presence of N_2O at 80 psi.

Griseofulvin was tested in this study because earlier reports suggested that it might interact with microtubules in a manner somewhat similar to N_2O. Grisham *et al.* (1973) reported that griseofulvin inhibited mitosis in mammalian cells without disrupting microtubule assembly. Our investigations generally support the studies of these investigators. Griseofulvin inhibits mitosis in a dose-dependent manner, and both immunofluorescent and electron microscope studies suggest that many microtubules undergo assembly in the presence of the drug. The spindle, however, fails to form completely and with time becomes highly disorganized.

In this regard, the action of griseofulvin is very similar to that of N_2O. Both agents interrupt mitosis without completely disrupting microtubule assembly and spindle formation. Moreover, neither agent completely disassembles the CMTC under conditions that inhibit the MA. Thus it appears that some process other than microtubule assembly is being altered by such agents. In contrast to our interpretation, Weber and co-workers (1976) investigated the interaction of griseofulvin on microtubules *in vivo* and *in vitro* and concluded that the drug interfered with polymerization in a dose-dependent manner. At lower concentrations ($10^{-5} M$) griseofulvin arrested exponentially growing 3T3 cells in C-metaphase with well-preserved mitotic spindles. At higher doses ($10^{-4} M$) given for 18 hours mitotic figures were absent in the culture, yet cytoplasmic microtubules were diminished in interphase cells. They concluded that the higher dose given for 18 hours delayed cells in interphase due to destruction of cytoplasmic microtubules. This interpretation is questionable, however, since in our hands 10^{-4} M griseofulvin given for a period of 18 hours results in a serious decrease in cell survival. Thus any effect observed at such time could be due to the cytotoxic action of the drug.

The molecular interaction of griseofulvin with microtubule protein is yet unclear. From our *in vitro* experiments we can conclude that the drug alters the rate and extent of polymerization of tubulin at a dose that inhibits mitosis *in vivo*. Thus it must interact with some component in the tubulin reassembly system. The relatively high concentration of griseofulvin needed to achieve inhibition of assembly, however, suggests that this drug acts by a mechanism different from that of colchicine which inhibits polymerization at substoichiometric doses (Margolis and Wilson, 1977).

Wehland *et al.* (1977) found that 10^{-4} M griseofulvin added to a polymerization system consisting of 6 S porcine brain tubulin and 8 M glycerol completely inhibited assembly of microtubules. Since polymerization proceeds under these conditions without the high-molecular-weight MAP proteins, these investigators concluded that griseofulvin blocked polymerization by interacting directly with 6 S tubulin. Obviously more studies are needed before the findings *in vitro* can be applied to microtubules in cells. From our results, we can conclude that, at a dose sufficient to arrest cells in mitosis, some cytoplasmic microtubules cannot only resist depolymerization but can in fact undergo polymerization in the presence of the drug. Thus, if griseofulvin binds directly to 6 S tubulin, some tubulin molecules must be resistant to the drug under the conditions used in our experiments.

V. Summary and Conclusions

The findings in the present study provide additional evidence for two major microtubule populations in proliferating cells; the CMTC of interphase cells and the MA of dividing cells. Although the microtubules comprising these two populations, and perhaps subpopulations within, are morphologically and antigenetically similar, they show varying sensitivity to drugs and inhibitors generally classed as antimitotic agents. Colcemid and other colchicine derivatives interact with 6 S tubulin to inhibit microtubule polymerization in both the CMTC and MA. N_2O and griseofulvin, under the conditions of our experiments, preferentially alter microtubules of the MA with minimal action on the CMTC. Although further work is necessary in order to elucidate the molecular mechanisms associated with agents such as N_2O and griseofulvin, it seems likely that they interfere with the mitotic process without altering spindle microtubule polymerization.

Acknowledgments

The authors are grateful to Peter Redding for technical assistance and his enthusiasm for this study. Appreciation is also extended to Linda Wible and Jan Means for assistance with the manuscript. We are grateful to Dr. Michael Marcum for assistance and advice concerning *in vitro* tubulin assembly. We are also grateful to Debbie Hodges and Donna Turner for technical assistance with the electron microscope. This work was supported in part by NIH grants CA22610 and CA23022.

References

Allison, A. C. (1973). *Ciba Found. Symp., Locomotion Tissue Cells* p. 109.

Borisy, G. G., Marcum, J. M., Olmsted, J. B., Murphy, D. B., and Johnson, K. A. (1975). *Ann. N.Y. Acad. Sci.* **253**, 107–132.

Brinkley, B. R., and Rao, P. N. (1973). *J. Cell Biol.* **58**, 96–106.

Brinkley, B. R., Murphy, P., and Richardson, L. C. (1967a). *J. Cell Biol.* **35**, 279–283.

Brinkley, B. R., Stubblefield, E., and Hsu, T. C. (1967b). *J. Ultrastruct. Res.* **19**, 1–18.

Brinkley, B. R., Fuller, G. M., and Highfield, D. P. (1975). *Proc. Natl. Acad. Sci. U.S.A.* **72**, 4981–4985.

Brinkley, B. R., Fuller, G. M., and Highfield, D. P. (1976). In "Cell Motility" (R. Goldman, T. Pollard, and J. Rosenbaum, eds.), pp. 435–456. Cold Spring Harbor Lab., Cold Spring Harbor, New York.

Cande, Z. W. (1978). *J. Supramol. Struct., Suppl.* **2**, 331.

Connolly, J. A., Kalnins, V. I., Cleveland, D. M., and Kirschner, M. W. (1977). *Proc. Natl. Acad. Sci. U.S.A.* **74**, 2437–2440.

Dentler, W. L., Granett, S., Whitman, G. B., and Rosenbaum, J. L. (1975). *J. Cell Biol.* **65**, 237–241.

Edelman, G. M. (1976). *Science* **192**, 218–226.

Edelman, G. M., Yahara, I., and Wang, J. L. (1973). *Proc. Natl. Acad. Sci. U.S.A.* **70**, 1442–1446.

Ferguson, J., Hawkins, S. W., and Doxey, D. (1950). *Nature (London)* **165**, 1021–1022.

Fuller, G. M., and Brinkley, B. R. (1976). *J. Supramol. Struct.* **5**, 497(349)–514(366).

Fuller, G. M., Brinkley, B. R., and Boughter, J. M. (1975). *Science* **187**, 948–950.

Green, C. D., and Eastwood, D. W. (1963). Anesthesiology 24:341–345.

Grisham, L. M., Wilson, L., and Bensch, K. G. (1973). *Nature (London)* **224**, 294–296.

Inoue, S. (1964). In "Primitive Motile Systems in Cell Biology" (R. D. Allen and N. Kamilya, eds.), pp. 549–598. Academic Press, New York.

Inoue, S., and Sato, H. (1967). *J. Gen. Physiol.* **50**, 259–288.

Kieler, J. (1957). *Acta Pharmacol. Toxicol.* **13**, 301.

McIntosh, J. R. (1974). *J. Cell Biol.* **61**, 166–187.

McIntosh, J. R., Hepler, P. K., and Van Wie, D. G. (1969). *Nature (London)* **224**, 659–663.

Malawista, S. E. (1975). *Ann. N.Y. Acad. Sci.* **253**, 738–749.

Margolis, R. L., and Wilson, L. (1977). *Proc. Natl. Acad. Sci. U.S.A.* **74**, 3466–3470.

Murphy, D. B., and Borisy, G. G. (1975). *Proc. Natl. Acad. Sci. U.S.A.* **72**, 2696–2700.

Osborn, M., and Weber, K. (1976). *Proc. Natl. Acad. Sci. U.S.A.* **73**, 867–871.

Ostergren, G. (1944). *Hereditas* **30**, 429.

Porter, K. R. (1966). *Ciba Found. Symp., Principles Biomol. Organ.* pp. 308–315.

Rao, P. N. (1968). *Science* **160**, 774.

Sakai, H., Mabuchi, I., Shimoda, S., Kuriyama, R., Ogawa, K., and Mohri, H. (1976). *Dev., Growth Differ.* **18**, 211–219.

Salmon, E. D., and Jenkins, R. (1977). *J. Cell Biol.* **75**, 295a.

Sherline, P., and Schiavone, K. (1978). *J. Cell Biol.* **77**, R9–R11.

Sloboda, R. D., Rudolph, S. A., Rosenbaum, J. L., and Greengard, P. (1975). *Proc. Natl. Acad. Sci. U.S.A.* **72**, 177–181.

Sloboda, R. D., Dentler, W. L., and Rosenbaum, J. L. (1976). *Biochemistry* **15**, 4497–4505.

Snyder, J. A., and McIntosh, J. R. (1976). *Annu. Rev. Biochem.* **45**, 699–702.

Stephens, R. E., and Edds, K. T. (1976). *Physiol. Rev.* **56**, 723–724.

Weber, K., Pollack, R., and Bibring, T. (1975). *Proc. Natl. Acad. Sci. U.S.A.* **72**, 459–463.

Weber, K., Wehland, J., and Herzog, W. (1976). *J. Mol. Biol.* **102**, 817–829.

Wehland, J., Herzog, W., and Weber, K. (1977). *J. Mol. Biol.* **111**, 329–342.

Wilson, L. (1975). *Ann. N.Y. Acad. Sci.* **253**, 213–231.

Wilson, L., and Bryan, J. (1974). *Adv. Cell Mol. Biol.* **3**, 21–72.

Wilson, L., Bamburg, J. R., Migel, S. B., Grisham, L. M., and Cuswell, K. M. (1974). *Fed. Proc., Fed. Am. Soc. Exp. Biol.* **33**, 158–166.

Index

8